Traditional and Natural Medicine

Traditional and Natural Medicine

Editor: Violet Edwardson

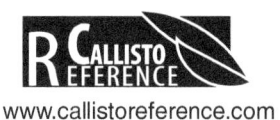

www.callistoreference.com

Callisto Reference,
118-35 Queens Blvd., Suite 400,
Forest Hills, NY 11375, USA

Visit us on the World Wide Web at:
www.callistoreference.com

ISBN: 978-1-64116-078-0 (Hardback)

Cataloging-in-Publication Data

Traditional and natural medicine / edited by Violet Edwardson.
    p. cm.
Includes bibliographical references and index.
ISBN 978-1-64116-078-0
1. Traditional medicine. 2. Naturopathy. 3. Alternative medicine. I. Edwardson, Violet.
R733 .T73 2019
615.5--dc23

Table of Contents

Preface

Traditional medicine is a form of alternative medicine which has been developed on the theories and experiences of varied cultures over centuries. Some of the prevalent practices of this field are acupuncture, Ayurveda, traditional Chinese medicine, etc. Studies of traditional medicine are done through the sciences of herbalism, ethnomedicine, ethnobotany and medical anthropology. This book is a compilation of chapters that discuss the most vital concepts and emerging trends in the study of traditional and natural medicine. Different approaches, evaluations, methodologies and advanced studies have been included in this book. Scientists and researchers will find it a valuable source of information and knowledge.

The researches compiled throughout the book are authentic and of high quality, combining several disciplines and from very diverse regions from around the world. Drawing on the contributions of many researchers from diverse countries, the book's objective is to provide the readers with the latest achievements in the area of research. This book will surely be a source of knowledge to all interested and researching the field.

In the end, I would like to express my deep sense of gratitude to all the authors for meeting the set deadlines in completing and submitting their research chapters. I would also like to thank the publisher for the support offered to us throughout the course of the book. Finally, I extend my sincere thanks to my family for being a constant source of inspiration and encouragement.

Editor

Antiulcer Activity of Patol Churna against Experimental Gastro-duodenal Ulcers in Rats

Varsha J Galani[1]*, Sunita S Goswami[2] and Mamta B Shah[2]

[1]Department of Pharmacology, A.R. College of Pharmacy, Vallabh Vidyanagar-388120, Gujarat, India
[2]Department of Pharmacology, L.M. College of Pharmacy, Navrangpura, Ahmedabad-380009, India

Abstract

Patol churna is a well known ayurvedic formulation of *Trichosanthes cucumerina* Linn. (cucurbitaceae) administered in case of number of alimentary and liver disorders. It is widely used in Indian folk medicine for variety of disease conditions. The aim of present study was to evaluate the antiulcer activity of 50% ethanolic extract of patol churna (PCE) using various experimental models of gastric and duodenal ulceration in rats. Oral administration of 50% ethanolic extract of patol churna was evaluated in rats against ethanol, aspirin and pylorus ligated gastric ulcers as well as cysteamine-induced duodenal ulcers. In all the models studied, the antiulcer activity of PCE compared with that of cimetidine (100mg/kg, p.o.), an H_2 receptor antagonist. PCE showed significant antiulcer activity in ethanol-induced and aspirin-induced gastric ulcer models. In 19 hrs pylorus ligated rats, significant reduction in ulcer index, total acidity and pepsin activity was observed with PCE, when compared with the control group. Mucosal defensive factors such as pH, mucin activity and gastric wall mucous content was found to be increased with PCE. PCE was also, afforded remarkable protection in cysteamine-induced duodenal lesions. The antiulcer activity of PCE was comparable with that of cimetidine. Thus, patol churna extract possess significant antiulcer activity against both gastric and duodenal ulcers in rats. The antiulcer activity may be attributed to its cytoprotective action and inhibition of acid secretary parameters.

Keywords: Antiulcer activity; Duodenal ulcer; Gastric ulcer; *Trichosanthes cucumerina* Linn; Patol churna

Introduction

Trichosanthes cucumerina Linn. (cucurbitaceae) is an annual climber and widely distributed throughout India, Ceylon, Malaya and North Australia. In Gujarat, the plant is known as 'Patola' or 'Kadvi Parval'. Patol churna is a well known ayurvedic formulation of *T. cucumerina* administered in case of number of alimentary and liver disorders. Whole plant is reputed for the treatment of hepatic and alimentary canal disorders. Fruits of *Trichosanthes cucumerina* are used as laxative, purgative, antipyretic, alexiteric and antiulcer agent. The leaves are good for bilious disorders [1]. Antidiabetic [2], hepatoprotective [3], anti-inflammatory [4], antifertility [5], antioxidant [6], antibacterial [7], antifungal [8] and antiviral [9] activities of the plant were reported. The fruits contain ascorbic acid, lycopene, phenols, flavonoids, alkaloids, tannins and saponins [6,10]. Present study was undertaken to evaluate the effect of 50% ethanolic extract of patol churna (PCE) in various experimental ulcer models.

Materials and Methods

Plant material and extraction

Patol churna, a readymade formulation powder was procured from the local market of Ahmedabad, India and authentication was done in the department of Pharmacognosy, L. M. College of Pharmacy, Ahmedabad. It was found to be a mixture of all the aerial parts of *Trichosanthes cucumerina*. The powder was extracted exhaustively with 50% ethanol by maceration at room temperature for 2 days with occasional shaking. The crude extract was dried at 40°C under vacuum (Yield – 11% w/w of dried powder). The pharmacological assays were arried out with aqueous solution of dried extract (PCE). The doses were expressed as mg of dried extract per kg of rat.

Drugs and chemicals

Cimetidine (Cadila, Ahmedabad) was used as reference standard. Aspirin (Cadila, Ahmedabad) and Cysteamine (Merck, Germany) were used for experimental induction of gastric and duodenal ulcers respectively.

Animals

Wister rats (200-250g) of either sex bred in Central Animal House facility of the institute were used. The animals were housed under standard conditions, maintained on a 12 hrs light/dark cycle and had free access to food and water up to the time of experimentation. The animals were acclimatized to the laboratory environment 1 hr before the experiments. Animals were randomly distributed into groups of 10 animals each. All experiments were conducted during the light period (08.00-16.00 hrs). All the protocols were approved by the Institutional Animal Ethical Committee (IAEC) and conducted according to the guidelines of CPCSEA (Committee for the Purpose of Control and Supervision of Experiment on Animals).

Treatment

Freshly prepared aqueous solution of dried extract of patol churna (PCE) in suitable dilution was administered orally in the test animals. For the ethanol induced ulcer model, animals were divided in to five groups, each group consisting of six animals. Group 1 served as control group received distilled water (vehicle) 1 ml/kg, p.o., group 2-4 served as test groups received PCE (300, 500 and 800mg/kg, p.o.) and group

*Corresponding author: Varsha J Galani, Department of Pharmacology, A.R College of Pharmacy, Vallabh Vidyanagar-388120, Gujarat, India
E-mail: vrp173@yahoo.com

5 served as positive. In all other models animals were divided in to 3 groups (n = 6) viz. control, test and reference standard. Test group received PCE at the dose of 500mg/kg, p.o. in aspirin induced, pylorus ligated and cysteamine induced ulcer model. Cimetidine (100mg/kg, p.o.) was used as reference standard in all experimental models.

Ethanol- induced gastric ulcer model: 1ml of 80% ethanol was administered orally to 36 hrs fasted rats [11]. PCE at the dose of 300, 500 and 800mg/kg was administered orally 1 hr before ethanol treatment. After 2 hrs of ethanol administration, animals were sacrificed and ulcer index of glandular mucosa was determined [12].

Aspirin-induced gastric ulcer model: Aspirin was suspended in 1% CMC in water and administered orally at the dose of 500mg/kg to 36 h fasted rats [13]. PCE (500mg/kg) was administered orally, 1hr before aspirin treatment. The rats were sacrificed 6 h after aspirin administration, the stomachs removed and opened along the greater curvature to determine ulcer index of glandular mucosa [12].

Pylorus ligation-induced gastric ulcer model: In 36 hrs fasted rats pylorus ligation were performed under light ether anaesthesia, care being taken not to cause bleeding or to occlude blood vessels. PCE at the dose of 500 mg/kg was administered orally immediately after pylorus ligation. 19 hrs after ligation, the rats were sacrificed. The stomachs were removed and opened along the greater curvature. The glandular portion of stomach was observed for measurement of ulcer index [14]. The contents were drained into tubes, centrifuged and subjected to analysis for various biochemical parameters. The volume and pH of gastric juice were measured. Total acidity [15], Total acid output [16], Pepsin activity [17], total carbohydrate [18] and protein content [19] were estimated. Finally, the total carbohydrate to protein (TC/PR) ratio i.e, mucin activity was derived. Gastric wall mucus content (GWMC) was measured from glandular portion of stomach [20] and was expressed as mg of alcian blue per g of wet glandular tissue [21].

Cysteamine-induced duodenal ulcer model: Cysteamine hydrochloride was administered in two doses of 400 mg/kg in 10% aqueous solution at an interval of 4 hrs to rats [22]. PCE was administered in a single dose (500 mg/kg, p.o.) 1 hr before the first dose of cysteamine. Parameters studied in this model were percentage mortality, total lesion area, score of intensity and ulcer index. Ulcer index was calculated as the sum of arithmetic mean of the intensity in a group and the ratio of the positive/total multiplied by 2.

Statistical analysis

The results were expressed as mean ± SEM. Data were analysed using one way ANOVA followed by Tukey's multiple range test A 'p' value less than 0.05 was considered as statistically significant.

Results

Ethanol-induced gastric ulcer model

The results are summarized in Table 1. PCE showed significant dose dependent reduction in ulcer index at 300, 500 and 800mg/kg, when compared with the control group (p< 0.05). Similarly, cimetidine produced significant reduction in ulcer index as compared with control.

Aspirin-induced gastric ulcer model

As shown in Table 2, PCE treatment showed significant reduction in ulcer index when compared with the control group (p< 0.05).

Positive control, cimetidine treated animals also showed significant reduction in ulcer index as compared to control animals (p< 0.05).

Pylorus ligation-induced gastric ulcer model

As shown in Table 3, PCE and cimetidine showed significant reduction in ulcer index (p < 0.05) as compared to control. None of the treatment groups showed any marked change in volume of gastric acid secretion parameter. There was significant rise in gastric pH by PCE and cimetidine as compared to control group (Table 3). The treatment groups viz. PCE and cimetidine showed significant reduction in total acidity when compared with the control group (Table 3). Total acid output remained unaltered in all the treatment groups. Along with total acidity, pepsin activity was significantly reduced by PCE and cimetidine treatment (Table 3). Significant rise in total carbohydrate content was observed in treatment groups as compared with the control

Treatment	Dose (mg/kg, p.o.)	Ulcer Index	% Protection
Control	-	2.19 ± 0.36	-
PCE	300	0.91 ± 0.14*	58.45
	500	0.59 ± 0.08*	73.06
	800	0.39 ± 0.08*	82.19
Cimetidine	100	1.17 ± 0.08'	46.58

n = 6 Expressed as mean ± SEM. One way Anova followed by Tukey's multiple range test; *p < 0.05 when compared with control group.

Table 1: Effect of PCE against ethanol–induced gastric ulcer model in rats.

Treatment	Dose (mg/kg, p.o.)	Ulcer index	% protection
Control	--	1.23 ± 0.08	-
PCE	500	0.62 ± 0.10*	49.59
Cimetidine	100	0.48 ± 0.04*	60.98

n = 6 Expressed as mean ± SEM. One way Anova followed by Tukey's multiple range test; *p<0.05 when compared with control group.

Table 2: Effect of PCE against aspirin-induced gastric ulcer model in rats.

Parameters	Control	PCE (500 mg/kg) (p.o.)	Cimetidine (100 mg/kg) (p.o.)
Ulcer index	0.66 ± 0.11	0.11 ± 0.03*	0.14 ± 0.05*
Vol. of gastric content (ml/100g)	3.67 ± 0.24	4.00 ± 0.56	4.15 ± 0.13
pH	2.20 ± 0.19	3.62 ± 0.19*	5.20 ± 0.07*
Total acidity (mEq/L)	14.77 ± 0.94	5.03 ± 0.33*	9.83 ± 0.20*
Total acid output (mEq/100 g)	54.04 ± 4.70	46.27 ± 15.3	40.22 ± 0.88
Pepsin activity (µg/ml)	750 ± 41.03	299.83 ± 17.62*	310.0 ± 31.97*

n= 6 Expressed as mean ± SEM. One way Anova followed by Tukey's multiple range test; *p<0.05 when compared with control group.

Table 3: Effect of PCE on ulcer index and acid secretory parameters in pylorus ligated gastric ulcers in rats.

Parameters	Control	PCE (500 mg/kg, p.o.)	Cimetidine (100 mg/kg, p.o.)
Total carbohydrate (µg/ml)	496.67 ± 46.69	1506.33 ± 100.16*	880.5 ± 54.45*
Protein content (µg/ml)	294.7 ± 67.04	129.5 ± 21.78*	46.17 ± 1.14*
TC : PR ratio	2.18 ± 0.41	13.64 ± 2.24*	19.08 ± 1.12*
GWMC	57.63 ± 7.90	59.18 ± 6.12	74.21 ± 7.99

n= 6 Expressed as mean ± SEM. One way Anova followed by Tukey's multiple range test; *p<0.05 when compared with control group.

Table 4: Effect of PCE on mucoprotective parameters in pylorus ligated gastric ulcer in rats.

Treatment	Ulcer incidence No %	Mortality No. %	Ulcer score	Total lesion area (mm²)	Ulcer index	% inhibition
Control	8/8 100	3/8 37.5	2.50 ± 0.28	88.38 ± 3.87	4.5	-
PCE (500 mg/kg, p.o.)	8/8 100	1/8 12.5	1.00 ± 0.12	43.75 ± 1.79*	3.0	33.33
Cimetidine (100mg/kg, p.o.)	8/8 100	0/8 0.0	0.90 ± 0.12*	41.2 ± 3.04*	2.9	35.56

n= 6 Expressed as mean ± SEM. One way Anova followed by Tukey's multiple range test; *$p<0.05$ when compared with control group.

Table 5: Effect of PCE on cysteamine-induced duodenal ulcer in rats.

group (Table 4). At the same time, protein content was significantly reduced in both the treatment groups (Table 4). Based on the results of total carbohydrate and protein content, mucin activity was determined in terms of TC: PR ratio increased significantly as compared to control. Gastric wall mucous content was increased significantly in PCE treated group as compared to control (Table 4).

Cysteamine-induced duodenal ulcer model

In cysteamine-induced duodenal ulcer model, PCE and cimetidine showed significant reduction in the total lesion area when compared with control group (Table 5).

Discussion

50% ethanolic extract of patol churna showed significant antiulcer effect against ethanol and aspirin-induced gastric ulcers. Ethanol administration may evoke gastric secretion through a more direct action on the stomach, involving the release of gastrin, histamine [23] and endogenous endothelin (ET-1) from vascular endothelial cells in the fundic mucosa [24]. Also, certain prostaglandins are capable of protecting rats against gastric mucosal lesions caused by necrotizing agents like ethanol and strong acid [25]. Aspirin has been recorded to cause mucosal damage by several factors such as inhibiting prostaglandin synthesis, enhancing acid secretion, increasing back diffusion of H^+ ions, decreasing mucin secretion and breaking of mucosal barrier [26]. Thus, the antiulcer activity of the patol churna extract in these models can be related to the cytoprotective action.

Gastric hypersecretion plays an important role in production of experimental ulcers by pylorus ligation [27]. Increased biosynthesis of nucleic acids and increased metabolism of carbohydrates and thereby exhaustion of carbohydrates and other compensatory mechanisms could also be responsible for ulceration due to pylorus ligation [28]. It is evident from the biochemical parameters that PCE has antiulcer effect in pylorus ligation model. The mechanism of their antiulcer activity can be related to the acid neutralizing property, reduction in acid-pepsin secretion and increase in mucin activity.

Cysteamine-induced ulcers are considered to be due to continuous hypersecretion of gastric acid [29]. The pathogenesis of cysteamine-induced duodenal ulcers includes enhanced gastric acid secretion [29], increased duodenal motility [30], delayed gastric emptying [31] and decreased duodenal bicarbonate secretion in response to acid [31]. It is suggested from our results that patol churna and cimetidine possess significant antiduodenal ulcer activity. The mechanism of this activity can be related to inhibitory effect of acid and pepsin activity.

Conclusion

The results of the present study indicate that 50% ethanolic extract of patol churna has protective effect against experimental gastro-duodenal ulcers in rats.

References

1. Kirtikar KR, Basu BD, ICS (1981) Indian medicinal plants. (2ndedn) Lalit Mohan Basu, Allahabad, India.

2. Kirana H, Srinivasan B (2008) *Trichosanthes cucurmerina* Linn Improves glucose tolerance and tissue glycogen in non insulin dependent diabetes mellitus induced rats. Indian J Pharmacol 40: 103-106.

3. Kumar SS, Kumar RB, Krishna Mohan G (2009) Hepatoprotective activity of *Trichosanthes cucumerina* Var *cucumerina* L on carbon tetrachloride induced liver damage in rats. J Ethnopharmacol 123: 347-350.

4. Kolte RM, Bisan VV, Jangde CR, Bhalerao AA (1996) Anti-inflammatory activity of root tubers of *Trichosanthes cucumerina* (Linn) in mouse's hind paw oedema induced by carrageenan. Indian J Indigenous Med 18: 117-121.

5. Kage DN, Malashetty VB, Seetharam YN, Suresh P, Patil SB (2009) Effect of ethanol extract of whole plant of *Trichosanthes cucumerina* var. *cucumerina* L. on gonadotropins, ovarian follicular kinetics and estrous cycle for screening of antifertility activity in albino rats. Int J Morphol 27: 173-182.

6. Adebooye OC (2008) Phyto-constituents and antioxidant activity of the pulp of snake tomato *Trichosanthes cucumerina* L. Afr J Tradit Complement Altern Med 5: 173-179.

7. Hariti M, Rathee PS (1995) Antibacterial activity of the unsaponifiable fractions of the fixed oils of (*Trichosanthes*) seeds. Asian J Chem 7: 909-911.

8. Harit M, Rathee PS (1996) Antifungal activity of the unsaponifiable fractions of the fixed oils of (*Trichosanthes*) seeds. Asian J Chem 8: 180-182.

9. McGrath MS, Luk KC, Abrams HD, Gaston I, Santulli S, et al. (1992) Antiviral studies with trichosanthin, a plant derived single chain ribosome inactivating protein: Natural Products as Antiviral Agents. Plenum Press New York.

10. Edeoga HO, Osuagwu GGE, Omosun G, Mbaebie BO, Osuagwu AN (2010) Pharmaceutical and therapeutic potential of some wild cucurbitaceae species from South-east Nigeria. Rec Res Sci Tech 2: 63-68.

11. Robert A, Nezamis JS, Lancaster C, Hanchar AJ (1979) Cytoprotection by prostaglandin in rats prevention of gastric necrosis produced by alcohol, HCl, NaOH, hypertonic, NaCl and thermal injury. Gastroenterology 77: 433-443.

12. Ganguly AK, Bhatnagar OP (1973) Effect of bilateral adrenalectomy on the production of restraint ulcer in the stomach of albino rats. Canad J Physiol Pharmacol 51: 748-750.

13. Hemmati H, Rezvani A, Djahanjuiri B (1973) Prevention of aspirin induced ulceration in rats with α-methyldopa and disulfiram. Pharmacology 9: 374-376.

14. Shay H, Komarov SA, Fcis SE, Meraze D, Gruenstein M, et al. (1973) A simple method for the uniform production of gastric ulceration in the rat. Gastroenterology 5: 43-61.

15. Hawk PB, Oser BC, Summerson WH (1954) Practical Physiological chemistry, (13thedn) Blakiston Company Inc., Toronto, New York.

16. Goel RK, Chakrabarti A, Sanyal AK (1985) The effect of biological variables on the antiulcerogenic effect of vegetable plantain banana. Planta Medica 2: 85-88.

17. Debnath PK, Gode KD, Govinda D, Sanyal AK (1974) Effect of propranolol on gastric secretion in albino rats. Br J Pharmacol 51: 213-216.

18. Nair BR (1974) Investigation on the venom of South Indian scorpion *Heterometrus scaber* (Ph.D Thesis), Trivendrum (Kerala), University of Kerala.

19. Lowry OH, Rosenberg NJ, Farr AL, Randall RJ (1951) Protein measurement with folin phenol reagent. J Biol Chem 193: 265-275.

20. Corne SJ, Motrisser SM (1974) A method for the quantitative estimation of gastric barrier mucus. J Physiol 242: 116-117.

21. Kulkarni SK, Goel RK (1996) Gastric antiulcer activity of UL-409 in rats. Indian J Exp Biol 34: 683-686.

22. Szabo S (1978) Duodenal ulcer disease. Animal model: cysteamine-induced acute and chronic duodenal ulcer in the rat. Am J Pathol 93: 273-276.

23. Glass GBJ, Slomiany BL, Slomiany A (1979) Biochemical and pathological derangements of the gastrointestinal tract following acute and chronic digestion of ethanol: Biochemistry and pharmacology of ethanol. Plenum Press, New York.

24. Ogawa A, Yabana T (1993) Pathogenic role of endothelin-1 on ethanol-induced gastric mucosal lesion of rat. Sapporo Igaku Zasshi 62: 203-211.

25. Robert A (1979) Cytoprotection by prostaglandins. Gastroenterology 77: 761-767.

26. Goel RK, Bhattacharya SK (1991) Gastroduodenal mucosal defence and mucosal protective agents. Indian J Exp Biol 29: 701-714.

27. Kitagawa H, Kurahashi K, Fujiwara M, Kohei H (1978) Antiulcerogenic effect of a pyrido-benzodazepine derivative (L-S519) on experimental ulcers. Arzneim Forsch 28: 2122-2127.

28. Mozsik GY, Kiss B, Javor J, Kraus M, Toth E (1969) Effect of cholinesterase inhibitor treatment on phosphorus and nucleic acid metabolism in the stomach wall. Pharmacology 2: 45-59.

29. Takeuchi K, Nishikawa H, Okabe S (1987) Role of local motility changes in the pathogenesis of duodenal ulcers induced by cysteamine in rats. Dig Dis Sci 32: 295-304.

30. Tanaka H, Takeuchi K, Okabe S (1989) Effects of the duodenal ulcerogens, mepirizole and cysteamine on gastric motility and emptying in rats. Scand J Gastroenterol. 24: 104-107.

31. Briden S, Flemstrom G, Kivilaasko E (1985) Cysteamine and propionitrile inhibit the rise of duodenal mucosal alkaline secretion in response to luminal acid in rats. Gastroenterology 24: 104-107.

The Model of Superfluid Physical Vacuum as a Basis for Explanation of Efficacy of Highly Diluted Homeopathic Remedies

Liudmila B. Boldyreva[1]* and Elena M. Boldyreva[2]*

[1]*The State University of Management, Moscow, Russia*
[2]*Peoples' Friendship University, Moscow, Russia; Weston Learning Center, Ontario, Canada*

Abstract

The results of using homeopathic remedies for treatment of milking cows with mastitis and calves with gastrointestinal disorders are described. An explanation of effects of highly diluted homeopathic remedies, based on a model of superfluid physical vacuum, is provided.

Under assumption that physical vacuum has the properties of superfluid ^{3}He-B, the effects of ultra-low doses can be taken due to spin supercurrents between spin structures produced in the superfluid physical vacuum by the biologically active substance and the target biological object. The properties of the spin supercurrents are similar to those in superfluid ^{3}He-B.

Keywords: Homeopathy; Veterinary; Ultra-low doses; Model of superfluid physical vacuum; Spin structures in physical vacuum; Spin supercurrents

Introduction

The homeopathic remedies used nowadays represent dilutions of D30 and higher. Note that the probability of the event that a D30 dilution of 1 mole of a substance contains at least one molecule will be ~0.001%. This makes explanation of the efficacy of highly diluted homeopathic remedies extremely difficult in the framework of existing physical conceptions.

That is why along with attempts to explain the effects of highly diluted remedies on organisms from the physical standpoint, there are explanations based on the placebo effect. The latter is associated with a therapeutic effect caused by suggestion or autosuggestion inducing a positive response of the immune system.

However, the efficacy of using highly diluted homeopathic remedies for treating animals, including evidence given in this paper, cannot be accounted for by the placebo effect, which applies to humans only.

It is noteworthy that the positive results of homeopathic treatment of animals, i.e. cows, as described in this paper, are often achieved by using the same homeopathic medicines that are used in treating similar diseases in humans. Thus both for humans and for animals there seem to be the same mechanism of "correcting" the organism's functions (No doubt, the placebo effect may take place as concerns humans, however, there should be a different mechanism determining the efficacy of treating an organism with a highly diluted homeopathic remedy).

Looking at the problem from the physical standpoint, it is natural to use the formalism of quantum physics. Firstly, in quantum physics the size of a particle is determined by its de Broglie wavelength. The de Broglie wavelength of a quantum object can exceed the classical size of the quantum object by some orders of magnitude (e.g. the de Broglie wavelength of the electron in a hydrogen atom in the ground state is five orders of magnitude greater than the electron's "classical" radius). As a result of this, the notion of substance concentration ceases to have its conventional meaning in this case. Secondly, there are effects, relating to quantum nonlocality, which suggest that quantum correlations may exist between any quantum objects, including correlations between the remedy and target organism as consisting of quantum objects.

There are a number of works where the explanation of some effects of homeopathic remedies is based on concepts of patient-practitioner-remedy entanglement, [1-3]. But to the authors' knowledge, no physical process in physical vacuum has been proposed so far for explanation of the effects of highly diluted homeopathic remedies.

Note that the effects of highly diluted homeopathic remedies on organisms are similar to those of low-intensity electromagnetic radiation and low-density streams of quantum particles (electron, proton, neutron, etc.) [4,5]. This suggests that there is the same physical mechanism underlying the effects of ultra-low doses on biological systems.

It is shown in this paper that under assumption that physical vacuum has the properties of superfluid ^{3}He-B [6-8] the effects of ultra-low doses (ULD) of biologically active substances (BAS) on biological objects (BO) can be taken to be due to spin supercurrents between spin structures produced in such physical vacuum (hereinafter referred to as the superfluid physical vacuum - SPV) by the BAS and the target BO [8-10]. The properties of these spin supercurrents are similar to those of spin supercurrents in superfluid ^{3}He-B.

Thus the main feature of the approach discussed here is that it is based on accounting for the properties of physical vacuum.

Treatment of Cows Using Homeopathic Remedies

Experiments described below were initiated in Russia in 1999, a period of a considerable fall in agricultural production, caused by economic situation in the country; they had been conducted before the implementation of the government-supported National Project of development of agriculture.

The experiments were carried out on two large farms of the Moscow region. Out of date equipment (e.g. dairy machines), wear-

*Corresponding authors: Liudmila B. Boldyreva, The State University of Management, Moscow, Russia, E-mail: boldyrev-m@yandex.ru

Elena M. Boldyreva, Weston Learning Center, ON Canada
E-mail: elena-boldyreva@hotmail.com

out of ventilation systems, wear-out of the barn premises led to a high incidence of various diseases of the cows and calves. In these "extreme" conditions homeopathic remedies were used in the therapy of the milking cows with mastitis [11].

A great advantage of the use of homeopathic remedies over the administration of antibiotics in the case of mastitis is that after the treatment milk can be used without any restrictions. In the research conducted, conventional and homeopathic methods of treating cows with serous and catarrhal mastitis were studied. Mastitis was caused mainly by improper milking machine functioning and had traumatic etiology. In summer period cows were also fetched to pasture that increased the incidence of traumatic mastitis. There was a loss in milk production; milk had a watery appearance and flakes in it. Udder quarters affected were reddened, edematous, painful and hot to the touch. California Mastitis Test was conducted additionally to estimate somatic cell count that proved to be elevated.

Two experiments were conducted at an interval of six months, that is, with different weather conditions. In the 1st experiment 44 lactating cows with mastitis were equally allocated to the control and the experimental groups; in the second experiment 32 cows with mastitis were divided into two equal groups, the control and the experimental ones. At the beginning of both experiments the cows of both the control and experimental groups had the same symptoms of mastitis described above.

Table 1 shows the schedule of administering antibacterial medications to the cows of the control group in both experiments, and homeopathic remedies to the cows of experimental group in the 1st experiment, and those of experimental group in the 2nd experiment.

The homeopathic remedies used were as follows. *Traumeel ad us. vet.* and *Echinacea compositum ad us. vet.* are complex homeopathic remedies produced by *Biologische Heilmittel Heel GmbH,* Germany (www.heel.de). *Traumeel ad us. vet.* contains fifteen plant, mineral and metallic ingredients in homeopathic dilutions from D3 to D11 [12]. Its "symptom picture" includes pain, inflammation, swelling and fever; this remedy is widely used in veterinary and human medicine in trauma-related conditions. It explains the choice of this remedy for the treatment of cows with mastitis, taking into account such dominant predisposing factor as trauma.

Echinacea compositum ad us.vet. contains eight ingredients of plant and animal origin, minerals and metals in homeopathic dilutions from D3 to D10 [13]. Its "symptom picture" is associated with inflammation, fever, swelling, reddening; this remedy is prescribed for stimulation of defense mechanisms of the organism.

A cow was considered to be cured clinically if the symptoms resolved completely (udder not swollen or painful, not hot), milk had normal organoleptic properties (normal color and consistency), and California Mastitis Test did not reveal high level of somatic cells.

The percentage of animals cured in the 1st experiment in various

time intervals in days (the day number is counted off from the beginning of the experiment) is shown in Figure 1. A similar characteristic for the 2nd experiment is shown in Figure 2. An average duration of mastitis in the experimental groups of the 1st and the 2nd experiment was 2.4 and 1.9 days less than that in the control ones correspondingly. In the control groups of the 1st and 2nd experiments 27.3% and 25% of cows recovered only after the 10th day (up to 3 weeks) respectively, while in both experimental groups all the animals were cured by the 10th day. A peculiarity of *Echinacea compositum ad us.vet.* is that in many cases at the beginning of its use a temporary exacerbation of the symptoms is noticed (1-2 days), but after that a quick recovery takes place. This is likely to be able to explain the lower percentage of recovered animals of the experimental group in the 2nd experiment in the first three days of treatment in comparison with that in the 1st experiment. The different percentages may also be associated with that the experiments were conducted in different seasons.

Note: At the same period of time, a series of experiments on homeopathic treatment of calves with gastrointestinal disorders (diarrhea) was conducted [14]. In the experiments, treatment of 94 calves at the age of 0-21 days was conducted. The calves were allocated to two equal groups: control and experimental. At the beginning of the experiment the calves of the control and the experimental groups had the same symptoms of diarrhea: very loose feces, severe dehydration of the organism, loss of appetite, depression, loss of skin elasticity, coat dullness, anemic mucous membranes, sinking of the eye within the orbit. Antibacterial medications, namely, *Trimerazin* per os and *Bicillinum* intramuscular were used in the control group. In the experimental group, complex homeopathic remedies, namely, *Mucosa compositum ad us. vet.* and *Berberis-Homaccord ad us. vet.* produced by *Biologische Heilmittel Heel GmbH,* Germany (www.heel.de), were administered subcutaneously every day.

Mucosa compositum ad us. vet. is a unique remedy that is composed of extracts of mucous membranes derived from different organs of pig. All the extracts have dilution of D8. It also contains plant, mineral and metallic ingredients in dilutions from D4 to D28. This remedy is used in human and veterinary medicine for those patients who suffer from the inflammation of mucous membrane of various organs, including intestine [15]. *Berberis-Homaccord ad us. vet.* is a combination of three plant ingredients having 4 dilutions each, from D4 to D200 [16].

As a result, in the experimental group the recovery from diarrhea took 2.8 days, without use of antibiotics; in the control group the recovery from diarrhea took 5.0 days. The calves were considered to be cured clinically if the symptoms of diarrhea resolved completely.

The Model of Superfluid Physical Vacuum: A Brief Description

According to the model, physical vacuum has the properties of a superfluid and consists of pairs of oppositely charged particles possessing spins. In the unperturbed state the total spin of a pair equals

	Control group	Experimental group 1	Experimental group 2
1 day of treatment	Mastijet Forte, intramammary infusions.	*Traumeel ad us. vet.* Injected subcutaneously.	*Traumeel ad us. vet.* and *Echinacea compositum ad us. vet.* Injected subcutaneously.
2 day of treatment	Mastijet Forte, intramammary infusions.	*Traumeel ad us. vet.* Injected subcutaneously.	*Traumeel ad us. vet.* and Echinacea compositum ad us. vet. Injected subcutaneously.
3 day of treatment	Streptomycin injected intramuscular.	*Traumeel ad us. vet.* Injected subcutaneously and then every other day.	*Traumeel ad us. vet.* and *Echinacea compositum ad us. vet.* Injected subcutaneously and then every other day.
4 day of treatment and other days	Streptomycin injected intramuscular and then every day.	*Streptomycin* injected intramuscular and then every day.	*Streptomycin* injected intramuscular and then every day.

Table 1: The schedule of administering antibacterial medications (Control groups of the 1st and 2nd experiments) and homeopathic remedies (Experimental groups).

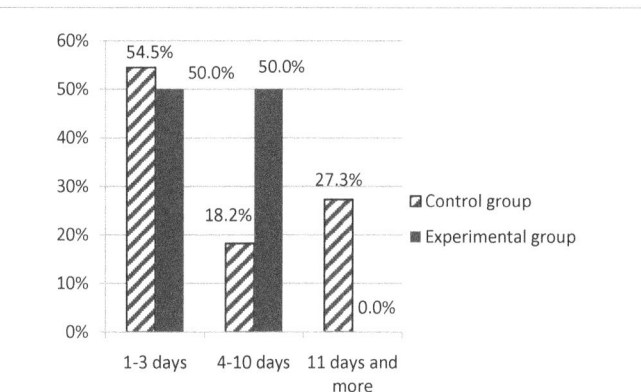

Figure 1: Percentage of animals cured in the 1st experiment in various time intervals, in days. The day number is counted off from the beginning of the experiment.

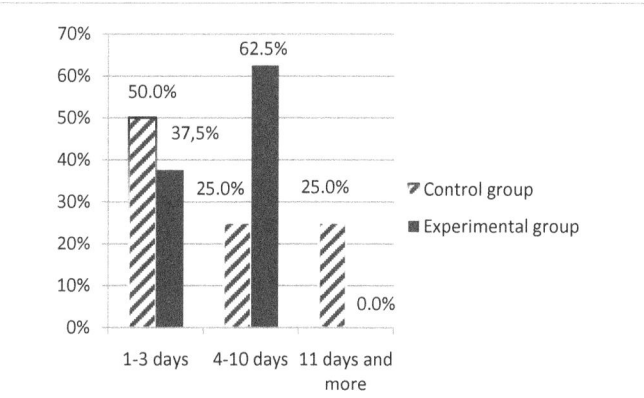

Figure 2: Percentage of animals cured in the 2nd experiment in various time intervals, in days. The day number is counted off from the beginning of the experiment.

zero. The model is based on the properties of superfluid ³He-B, whose atoms have non-zero spin as well and form pairs whose total angular momentum (the sum of the orbital and spin angular momenta) is zero in the pure state. One of the properties of superfluid ³He–B is that areas with coherently precessing spins of ³He atoms, the so-called homogeneously precessing domains (HPDs) [17-21], may exist there.

A HPD is characterized by spin S, precession angle (or precession phase) α, nutation angle β, and precession frequency ω (Figure 3). In a homogeneously precessing domain, energy U is related to the frequency ω of precession as

$$U = S\omega. \qquad (1)$$

According to the model, a quantum object is a HPD in the SPV [8].

The precession and nutation angles are angles of orientation of the order parameter, and there are processes that tend to make respectively equal both the values of precession angles and the values of nutation angles throughout the liquid volume. Such processes in superfluid ³He-B are spin supercurrents. For example, the value of spin supercurrent in the direction of axis **z**, J_z, is determined as follows:

$$J_z = -b_1 \frac{\partial \alpha}{\partial z} - b_2 \frac{\partial \beta}{\partial z}, \qquad (2)$$

where, b_1 and b_2 are proportionality factors depending on β and the properties of the medium.

There exists such a phenomenon in ³He–B as phase slippage. At a

certain difference in precession angles, $\Delta\alpha_c$, for two HPDs there takes place a precession phase slippage, or phase drop, by $2\pi n$ (n = 1, 2…). The critical spin supercurrent J_c corresponds to $\Delta\alpha_c$ [21]. Figure 4a and 4b show examples of the character of dependence of normalized spin supercurrent J/J_c between two HPDs with respective precession frequencies ω_1 and ω_2 ($\omega_1 \uparrow\uparrow \omega_2$) on the hypothetical difference in the precession angles, $\Delta\varphi$, which is defined as $\Delta\varphi = (\omega_1 - \omega_2)t$, t being time. Up to the value of $\Delta\varphi$ equal to $\Delta\alpha_c$, the hypothetical difference is equal to the precession angles difference determining the spin supercurrent, $\Delta\alpha$, that is, $\Delta\varphi = \Delta\alpha$. On the curves, the line 1–1 corresponds to the change in the supercurrent in the process of phase slippage, the 2π phase slip taking place. In Figure 4a, we have $\Delta\alpha_c = \pi$ [17]. In Figure 4b, $\Delta\alpha_c \approx 3\pi$ [20].

Generally, the determination of time dependency of the magnitude of the spin supercurrent between two regions with precessing spins (for example, homogeneously precessing domains – HPDs, see Figure 3) is a difficult problem, because the speed of transmission of information of the existence of a gradient of the order parameter is, in theory, infinite, and the speed of the spin supercurrent is finite [21]. Besides, a possibility of phase slippage should be taken into account. The respective precession and nutation angles of interacting HPDs will become equal, provided the distance X between them and the difference between their precession frequencies, $\Delta\omega$, satisfy the following conditions:

$$\Delta\omega \to 0 \qquad (3)$$

$$X \to 0 \cdot \qquad (4)$$

The Mechanism of Action of Biologically Active Substances in Ultra-Low Doses on Biological Objects

According to the SPV model, a quantum object is a homogeneously precessing domain in physical vacuum, i.e. it is a spin structure in physical vacuum. The biologically active substance and the target biological object consist of quantum entities: electrons, protons, etc. Therefore, the biologically active substance and the biological object produce spin structures in physical vacuum.

We shall assume that the spin structure produced in the SPV by a BO is characterized by a single value of the precession frequency and single values of the angles of precession and nutation, that is, the structure is a homogeneously precessing domain in the SPV.

In the model discussed here, it is convenient to express ULDs of BAS in terms of so-called quanta. A "quantum" is such a dose of substance which produces in the SPV a spin structure that is characterized by single values of the precession frequency, the angle of precession and angle of nutation, and thus the structure can be thought of as being, like that of the BO, a HPD in the SPV.

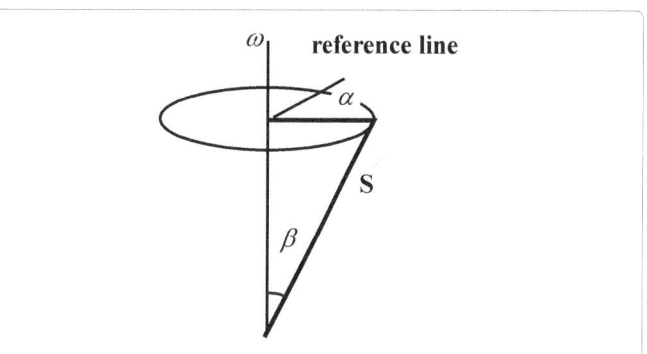

Figure 3: Precession of spin S with frequency ω; α is the precession angle relative to a reference line, β is the nutation angle.

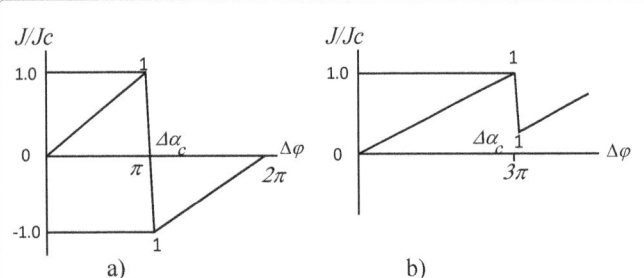

Figure 4: Dependences of the normalized spin supercurrent J / J_c on the hypothetical difference in the phases of precession, $\Delta\varphi$. Up to point $\Delta\varphi = \Delta\alpha_c$, $\Delta\varphi = \Delta\alpha$. The phase slippage is shown by line 1-1. The 2π phase slippage is taking place.
a) $\Delta\alpha_c = \pi$.
b) $\Delta\alpha_c \approx 3\pi$.

To describe the spin structures produced in the SPV by a "quantum" of ULD of BAS and by that of a BO, we shall introduce a number of notions relating to time t: ω_{1t} will be the frequency of precession in the spin structure produced by the ULD of BAS, ω_{2t} the frequency of precession in the spin structure produced by the BO, and $\Delta\alpha_t$ the difference in the precession angles of the structures. Let us assume that the interaction of the ULD of BAS and the biological object starts at time $t = \tau_1$. The difference in the precession angles, $\Delta\alpha_{\tau_1}$, at time τ_1 is determined as

$$\Delta\alpha_{\tau_1} = \left(\omega_{1\tau_1} - \omega_{2\tau_1}\right)\tau_1 + \Delta\alpha_0, \tag{5}$$

where $\Delta\alpha_0$ is the difference in the angles of precession of spin structures at time $t = 0$. In the special case of $\Delta\alpha_0 = 0$ the equation (5) takes the form:

$$\Delta\alpha_{\tau_1} = \left(\omega_{1\tau_1} - \omega_{2\tau_1}\right)\tau_1. \tag{6}$$

Note. There is lack of experimental data available on the character of dependence of spin supercurrents on the difference in the nutation angles of spin structures. Therefore, the nutation angles are not considered in the analysis of interaction between an ULD of BAS and a BO.

If the difference $\Delta\omega = \omega_{1\tau_1} - \omega_{2\tau_1}$ meets the condition (3) (condition (4) is taken to be always met), then according to the properties of spin supercurrents there will be equalization of the precession angles. As follows from equations (5) and (6), the precession angles equalization results in a decrease in the difference in the precession frequencies in the spin structures produced by the ULD of BAS and the BO in the SPV, that is, for time $\tau_2 > \tau_1$ (provided that ω_{1t} does not change within the time τ_2-τ_1, and equals $\omega_{1\tau_1}$) we can write:

$$\Delta\alpha_{\tau_2} \approx 0,$$
$$\left|\omega_{1\tau_1} - \omega_{2\tau_2}\right| < \left|\omega_{1\tau_1} - \omega_{2\tau_1}\right|, \tag{7}$$

where variables $\Delta\alpha_{\tau_2}$, $\omega_{2\tau_2}$ correspond to respective $\Delta\alpha_{\tau_1}$, $\omega_{2\tau_1}$, but their values are taken at $t = \tau_2$.

Thus the action of the ULD on the BO within the time τ_2-τ_1, provided the conditions (3) and (4) are satisfied, will result in that the characteristics of the spin structure produced by the BO will tend to become the same as those of the spin structure produced by the ULD. (From this viewpoint, one can speak of sensitivity of the BO to the action of ULD.)

The SPV model discussed makes it possible to explain the features

of the effects of biologically active substances in ultra-low doses on biological objects, as observed in a lot of studies [4,5,22]:

1. The kinetic paradox: the effect of an ULD of a BAS on a cell or an organism is the strongest when the latter contain the same substance but in doses that are some orders of magnitude greater than the ULD used.

2. A change in sensitivity (generally, an increase) of the BO with respect to a subsequent exposure to a BAS in an ultra-low dose.

3. Dependence of the "sign" of the effect (inhibition or stimulation) on the initial state of the BO being treated.

4. A non-monotonic, polymodal ("oscillatory") dose-response (or dose-effect) dependence. In most cases the activity maxima are observed within definite ranges of doses, which are separated by so-called dead zones. In some cases, the same effects are produced by doses of biologically active substances differing in 5 to 8 orders of magnitude. There are also cases where a change in the "sign" of the effect is observed in the dose dependence.

5. Disappearance of side effects with a decreased dose of BAS (but with persisting activity of the BAS in ULD).

Let us show that the above features of effects of BAS in ULD on BO can be explained by the properties of spin supercurrents emerging between the spin structures in the SPV.

1. The kinetic paradox

Note that condition (3) is always valid for the BAS which has been already contained in the BO but in a dose some orders of magnitude higher than the ultra-low dose used. The high concentration of such a substance in the BO results in that the spin structure produced by the BO in the SPV will have the characteristics determined by the properties of the substance, in particular, resulting in the minimum difference between the frequencies $\omega_{2\tau_1}$ and $\omega_{1\tau_1}$.

2. A change in sensitivity (generally, an increase) of the BO with respect to a subsequent exposure to a BAS in ULD.

According to (7), the action of a BAS in ULD on a BO results in that the frequency of precession in the spin structure produced by the BO changes. The change may result in that in the action of a second ULD on the same BO the BO sensitivity with respect to the second ULD will depend on the properties of the first ULD. Indeed the condition (3) may become invalid for the second ULD while it was valid before the action of the first ULD. Or, on the contrary, condition (3) may become valid for the second ULD although it was not valid before the action of the first ULD.

Let us consider the case where the frequency of precession in the spin structure produced by the first ULD (which was designated above as $\omega_{1\tau_1}$) is equal to the precession frequency in the spin structure produced by the second ULD. As follows from (7), after the action of the first ULD on the BO over the time τ_2-τ_1 the quantity $\Delta\omega = \omega_{1\tau_1} - \omega_{2\tau_2}$ (used in condition (3)) becomes of a smaller order of magnitude than it was before the action of the first ULD when it was equal to $\omega_{1\tau_1} - \omega_{2\tau_1}$. This increases the sensitivity of the BO to subsequent actions of an ULD of BAS whose spin structure has the same precession frequency $\omega_{1\tau_1}$ as that of the first ULD.

3. The dependence of the "sign" of the effect on the initial state of BO.

In point 1 above, the action of an ULD of BAS on a BO over the time τ_2-τ_1 results in that, under (7), the frequency of precession associated with the BO changes by the quantity $\omega_{2\tau_2} - \omega_{2\tau_1}$. Consequently, taking into account (1), the energy of the spin structure produced by the BO in the SPV (and, as may be supposed, the energy of the object itself) will change by ΔU as follows:

$$\Delta U = S(\omega_{2\tau_2} - \omega_{2\tau_1}), \tag{8}$$

where S is the total spin of the spin structure produced by BO in the SPV.

Thus depending on the sign of $\omega_{2\tau_2} - \omega_{2\tau_1}$ biologically active substances can be classified into two categories: "cooling" and "heating" with respect to the specific BO. If at time τ_1 the difference between the precession angles $\Delta\alpha_{\tau_1}$ is determined by (6), then, according to (7) and (8), at $\omega_{2\tau_1} < \omega_{1\tau_1}$ the energy flow occurs towards the BO, and at $\omega_{2\tau_1} > \omega_{1\tau_1}$ the direction of energy flow is opposite. According to (2), (6) and (7), the direction of energy flow is the same as that of the spin supercurrent.

In the general case, as follows from (5) and (2), the sign of spin supercurrent $(J)_{\tau_1}$ determining its direction at time τ_1 depends not only on the difference $\omega_{2\tau_1} - \omega_{1\tau_1}$, but on the magnitude and the sign of $\Delta\alpha_0$. It can be assumed that the sign of spin supercurrent determines the "sign" of the effect of ULD of BAS on the BO.

4. A non-monotonic, polymodal dose-effect curve; in some cases a change in the "sign" of the effect.

Let us examine the action of a BAS in ULD on a BO provided the ULD consists not of a single "quantum", as in the above cases, but of Z "quanta". Let j_i be the spin supercurrent between the spin structures produced by the i-th "quantum" of the ULD and the BO. Then the total spin supercurrent, J_{sum} caused by all "quanta" will be determined by the expression $J_{sum} = \sum_{i=1}^{Z} j_i$. Assuming that for every i the spin supercurrents j_i are equal to each other in both magnitude and sign, namely, $j_i = j$, then:

$$J_{sum} = Z \cdot j. \tag{9}$$

According to the properties of the spin supercurrents, there will be slippage of the angle (phase) of precession by the value of $2\pi n$ ($n = 1, 2\ldots$) at a certain $\Delta\alpha_c$ and respective J_c. Taking into account (9), we shall introduce the critical value of the number of "quanta", Z_c, at which the quantity J_{sum} takes the value of J_c whereby a slippage takes place:

$$Z_c = J_c / j. \tag{10}$$

As follows from the experiments whose results are shown in Figures 4a and 4b the dependence of spin supercurrent j on $\Delta\alpha$ is non-monotonic and polymodal. The phase slippage may lead to a change in the sign of the spin supercurrent (Figure 4a) and thus to a decrease of the latter (Figure 4b). This makes both the value of Z_c and the sign of the effect variable for the same pair "ULD–BO". Therefore, the phase slippage phenomenon makes the dependence of the total spin supercurrent between the spin structures produced by BAS in ULD and the BO on the number of "quanta" non-monotonic and polymodal.

5. The disappearance of side effects with a decreased dose of BAS (but with persisting activity of the BAS).

According to the definition of "quantum" introduced in this work, a quantum is such a dose of substance which produces in the SPV a spin structure with a single precession frequency of spins of microparticles that constitute the SPV, that is, under the notation introduced earlier,

the frequency ω_{1t}. If the dose consists of several quanta, this means that the spin structure produced in the SPV by the BAS used is characterized by several values of ω_{1t} and, accordingly, may affect simultaneously several biological objects for which conditions (3) and (4) are satisfied. That is, the less the dose, the less the number of biological objects that interact with the BAS in ULD.

Discussion

I. The interaction of quantum objects through spin supercurrents is performed on a level different from the molecular one, namely, in the superfluid physical vacuum. Therefore, spin supercurrents cannot be shielded by molecular substances. This property of spin supercurrents agrees with the evidence given in the book by P. Bellavite and A. Signorine "The Emerging Science of Homeopathy" [23]: "There is some preliminary evidence demonstrating a homeopathic effect not only of solutions but also of closed ampoules containing solutions and placed in contact with the system to be regulated (human or animal)."

It follows from the above that an organism can "infect" another organism, although the "disease" is absolutely non-contagious from the standpoint of medical science. This contagious effect may take place due to an interaction between a sick organ of one organism and a healthy organ of another organism provided the organs produce spin structures in the SPV having closely spaced frequencies of precession. However, a sanative effect can take place as well if the interaction gives rise to the appropriate change in the characteristics of the spin structures produced by the sick organ. It is well known that up to the 19th century it was a common belief that one could get rid of a disease by "transferring" it to an animal. For example, according to J. G. Frazer, the famous ethnologist, the "ancients held that if a person suffering from jaundice looked sharply at a stone-curlew, and the bird looked steadily at him, he was cured of the disease" [24].

II. Since there is a spin structure for any quantum object in physical vacuum, low-density streams of quantum particles (electrons, neutrons, protons, etc.) can act on a biological object as a BAS in ULD. The study of effects of such streams on a biological object is an efficient way of determining the precession frequency of spins in the spin structure produced by the biological object in physical vacuum (the BO spin structure precession frequency has been denoted as ω_{2t}). This is due to the simplicity of determining the precession frequency of spins in the spin structure produced by a quantum particle in physical vacuum. Under the SPV model, this frequency is equal to $E/\hbar$, where E is the particle energy. Under equation (3), the effect of a quantum particle is maximum if $\omega_{2t} \approx E/\hbar$.

III. Electromagnetic radiation consists of quantum entities, photons, and consequently, according to the SPV model, produces in physical vacuum spin structures that may interact with the spin structures of biological objects. It was empirically established that the effects characteristic of the action of ULDs of biologically active substances on biological objects take place as well at the action of low-intensity EM radiation [4]. (Electromagnetic radiation is referred to as a low-intensity radiation if its flux density is less than 1 μW/cm².) Since spin supercurrents cannot be shielded by molecular substances, including the substances of which electromagnetic screens are made, a somewhat paradoxical, from the standpoint of mainstream physics, situation may arise: electromagnetic radiation, as producing spin supercurrents, can affect biological objects through electromagnetic screens.

A low-intensity EM radiation will produce an effect (in particular, a therapeutic one) on a BO provided the difference between the radiation frequency and the precession frequency of spins in the spin structure produced by the BO in the SPV meets the condition (3). A change in the above spin precession frequency means a change in the frequency of low-intensity EM radiation on which the radiation may produce an effect on the BO. (It is noteworthy that in the spin structure produced in the SPV by EM radiation there is a spin precession frequency equal to the frequency of the EM radiation.) Thus the study of effects of low-intensity electromagnetic radiation on a biological object, as well as the above mentioned study of effects of low-density streams of quantum particles, is an efficient way of determining the precession frequencies of spins in the spin structure produced by the biological object in physical vacuum.

IV. According to the SPV model, spin supercurrents may arise between spin structures produced by any quantum objects in the SPV. This makes it possible for a BAS to effect a BO indirectly, through an intermediary which has acquired the properties of the BAS as a result of the preceding interaction with the latter.

That is, if there is an object or medium and the precession frequency of its spin structure becomes equal to that of the spin structure of the BAS as a result of interaction between the spin structures (the frequency has been denoted as ω_{1t}), then the object or medium acquires a capacity to produce the same effect on the BO as the BAS. There are a number of experiments where the properties of water were affected by low-intensity electromagnetic radiation, weak magnetic fields, cosmophysical and geophysical factors of the environment [4,25], thus water can be considered to be such an intermediary.

V. According to the SPV model, the precession frequency of spins in the spin structure produced by a quantum object is determined by the energy of the object. But the energy of a quantum object determines as well the spectrum of its natural frequencies. Therefore, the spin precession frequency in the spin structure produced by a biological object (it has been denoted as ω_{2t}) may coincide with one of the frequencies of the electromagnetic radiation of the object (ω'). Since according to the SPV model the frequency of a photon is equal to the frequency of precession of spins in the spin structure produced by it in physical vacuum, the effect of a flux of photons having frequency ω' on such a BO will be the greatest because equation (3) will be met. This can elucidate the long-lived principle of treatment of various diseases: "Like cures like." Here are some well-known recommendations based on that principle: erysipelatous inflammation having red color is treated by application of red cloth; choledochitis by yellow cloth. In fact, this principle is a manifestation of the "kinetic paradox" described.

Conclusions

The effect of a biologically active substance (BAS) in ultra-low dose (ULD) on a biological object (BO) can be performed through spin supercurrents arising between spin structures produced by the BAS and the BO in physical vacuum having properties of superfluid ^{3}He-B.

From the standpoint of the model of superfluid physical vacuum, the study of characteristics of spin structures (specifically, the spin precession frequencies) produced by a biological object in physical vacuum is best to perform as a study of effects of low-intensity electromagnetic radiation or low-density streams of quantum entities (neutrons, electrons, etc.) on the biological object.

References

1. Walach H (2003) Entanglement model of homeopathy as an example of generalized entanglement predicted by weak quantum theory. Forsch Komplementarmed Klass Naturheilkd 10: 192-200.

2. Milgrom LR (2006) Towards a new model of the homeopathic process based on quantum field theory. Forsch Komplementmed 13: 174-183.

3. Hankey A (2009) Macroscopic quantum coherence in patient-practitioner-remedy entanglement: the quantized fluctuation field perspective. Evid Based Complement Alternat Med 6: 449-451.

4. Burlakova EB, Konradov AA, Maltseva EL (2008) The effects of ultra-low doses of biologically active substances and low-intensity physical factors. Proceedings of the IV International Symposium on Action Mechanisms of Ultra-low Doses. The Russian Academy of Sciences, Moscow: 123-149 (in Russian).

5. Burlakova EB, Kondradov AA, Khudiakov IV (1990) [The action of chemical agents at ultralow doses on biological objects]. Izv Akad Nauk SSSR Biol 22: 184-193.

6. Sinha KP, Sivaram C, Sudarshan ECG (1976) The Superfluid Vacuum State. Time-Varying Cosmological Constant and Nonsingular Cosmological Models. Foundations of Physics 6: 717-726.

7. Boldyreva LB, Sotina NB (1992) Superfliud Vacuum with Intrinsic Degrees of Freedom. Physics Essays 5: 510-513.

8. Boldyreva LB (2012) What does this give to physics: attributing the properties of 3He-B to physical vacuum? URSS, Moscow.

9. Boldyreva LB (2009) A quantum-mechanical model of action of ultra low doses of biologically active substances and low intensity electromagnetic radiation on biological objects. Abstracts and Articles of International Seminar in Tallinn. "Radiating fields of Earth, related architectural geometry of forms and their influence on organisms", Estonian geopathic society and other organizations: 106-114.

10. Boldyreva LB (2011) An analogy between effects of ultra-low doses of biologically active substances on biological objects and properties of spin supercurrents in superfluid 3He-B. Homeopathy 100: 187-193.

11. Boldyreva EM (2003) Mastitis of cows and the use of homeopathic preparations for the treatment. Book of abstracts of the 54th Annual Meeting of the European Association for Animal Production. Italy. Rome 9: 278.

12. http://www.heel.de/upload/Heel_de_Traumeel_adusvet_Inj_V_017864_03_BPZ_7_2975.pdf

13. http://www.heel.de/upload/Heel_de_Echinacea_compositum_adusvet_Inj_V_016146_04_BPZ_2961.pdf

14. Boldyreva EM (2001) The use of homeopathic preparations for the treatment of intestinal disorders. Dairy and beef cattle farming 8: 30-32 (in Russian).

15. http://www.heel.de/upload/Heel_de_Mucosa_compositum_adusvet_Inj_V_016484_BPZ_2969.pdf

16. http://www.heel.de/upload/Heel_de_Berberis_Homaccord_adusvet_Inj_V_015688_02_BPZ_2953.pdf

17. Bunkov YM (2009) Spin superfluidity and coherent spin precession. J Phys Condens Matter 21: 164201.

18. Dmitriev VV, Fomin IA (2009) Homogeneously precessing domain in 3He-B: formation and properties. J Phys Condens Matter 21: 164202.

19. Borovic-Romanov AS, Bunkov YM, Dmitriev VV, Mukharskii YM, Sergatskov DA (1989) Investigation of Spin Supercurrents in 3He-B. Physical Review Letters 62: 1631-1634.

20. Dmitriev VV (2005) Spin Superfluidity in 3He. Physics Uspekhi 48: 77-83.

21. Fomin IA (1987) Critical superfluid spin current in 3He-B. JETP Letters 45: 135-138.

22. Bonamin LV, Endler PC (2010) Animal models for studying homeopathy and high dilutions: conceptual critical review. Homeopathy 99: 37-50.

23. Bellavite P, Signorine A (2002) Emerging science of homeopathy. North Atlantic Books, Berkeley, California: 6-9.

24. Frazer GG (1923) The Golden Bough. London.

25. Tsetlin VV (2010) Studies into water reactions to variations of cosmophysical and geophysical factors of the environment. Aviakosmicheckaya i ekologicheskaya meditsina 44: 26-30 (in Russian).

Ayurvedic Concepts in Thirukkural

Thirunavukkarasu MS* and Kapoorchand H

Government Ayurveda Medical College and Hospital, Kottar, Nagercoil, Tamilnadu, India

Abstract

Ayurveda, the ancient Indian medicine is applauded all over the world for its application in overcoming the maladies of human race. Many medical and non-medical treatises elaborate on various aspects of Ayurveda, though several texts have caught our attention still there are many, which are yet to be explored. Thirukkural is one such ancient scripture in Tamil literature that has gained so much importance and has seen many translations and commentaries into almost all major languages of the world. This paper is an attempt to discuss various references in couplets of Thirukkural with regard to Medicine i.e., Ayurveda and its similarity between concepts like Causes of the disease, Nutritional disciplines, treatment principles and importance of four pillars in the treatment.

Keywords: Ayurveda; Thirukkural; Medicine; Couplets

Introduction

Ancient Indian medicine is applauded all over the world for its application in overcoming the maladies of human race. Many medical and non-medical treatises elaborate on various aspects of Ayurveda, though several texts have caught our attention still there are many which are yet to come into limelight. One such poetic masterpiece is 2,200 year old south Indian Dravidian classic "Thirukkural" [1]. Researchers are now slowly gaining foot focusing on the unpublished and unexplored manuscripts, which deals with the basic principles of this science. CCRAS and other such institutions are imparting stress on such research activities. Apart from the classical Ayurvedic texts, principles of Ayurveda are found in numerous manuscripts written during post Vedic era. A Critical appraisal of one such work "Thirukkural" is being detailed in this article. Thirukkural is one of the ancient scripture in Tamil literature and it is universally accepted and was written by Thiruvalluvar in 2nd century A.D [2]. It is the only Tamil literary work which has gained so much importance and has seen many translations and commentaries into almost all major languages of the world [3]. As Dr. Albert Schweiteitzer had rightly said "There hardly exists in the literature of the world a collection of maxims in which we find such lofty wisdom" [4]. Thirukkural consists of 133 chapters each containing 10 couplets, collectively to 1330 couplets and were grouped into 3 sections namely Virtue, Wealth and Love. The first part deals with the moral value of human life and has 38 chapters. The second part is on socio economic values of men in a civilized society and has 70 chapters and the third part is on psychological values of life and has 25 chapters. In the second part, the last chapter is dedicated to Medicine (Chapter 95) [5]. The word Ayurveda means Knowledge of Life or Science of Life. Ayurveda is a traditional system of medicine native to India and is in the process of evolving into Integrative medicine. The science originated from Lord Brahma and received by Dhanvantari more than 3000 years ago and is an *upaveda* (auxiliary knowledge) of Atharvaveda. Golden period of Ayurveda ranges from 800 B.C. to 1000 A.D. The three most important treatises in Ayurveda appeared during this period, they are Charaka Samhita, Sushruta Samhita and Ashtanga Samgraha. Thirukkural came into existence subsequently i.e., after Ayurveda, as the author had explored certain ideas like Life skills, Education, Politics, Medicine, sexual life, etc., in his work. This paper is an attempt to discuss those various instances referred in couplets with regard to Medicine. To explore the medical related information cited in the manuscript "Thirukkural".

Materials and Methods

1. Thirukkural.

2. Available Ayurvedic texts.

The materials are compared and summarized on the basis of similar existing theories.

Results are based on a qualitative aspect rather than quantitative.

Observation and Discussion

The chapter of Medicine in Thirukkural consists of 10 couplets. Among them the first couplet explains about the causes of diseases. The next consecutive six couplets explain about the maintenance of Health by adopting the right kind of food regimen. Eighth and ninth couplet explains about the method of treatment and the last one explains the importance of four limbs (Chatuspadas) in the treatment of a patient.

Causes of Disease

In the foremost couplet of kural, Thiruvalluvar says that the excess or deficiency of the three life forces viz   *Vata, Pitta* and *Kapha* leads to diseases.

மிகினும் குறையினும் நோய்செய்யும் நூலோர்
வளிமுதலா எண்ணிய மூன்று. (941)

Similarly Ayurveda categorizes three basic types of functional principles (Doshas) namely *Vata, Pitta* and *Kapha*. These principles are essential for basic function of human body. *Vata* is essential for movement, *Pitta* for digestion and *Kapha* for Stability. Imbalance of these principles causes disease. The references pertaining to the causes for increase and decrease of these three functional principles are also available [6].

Nutritional Discipline

Valluvar has explained and given more importance to dietetic regimen for maintaining health in six couplets. Second couplet says

*Corresponding author: Thirunavukkarasu MS, Lecturer, Govt. Ayurveda Medical College and Hospital, Kottar, Nagercoil, Tamilnadu, India, E-mail: thiru.dr@gmail.com

that the one who takes the food after digestion of previous food will never suffer illness. Third couplet mentions that one who wishes long life should take diet in moderate quantity after being assured of digestion of the previous meal. In the next couplet, the person should take compatible diet only when he is hungry. Fifth couplet says that one who is interested in healthy life should take suitable diet in proper quantity. Sixth couplet explains that the disease will occur if food is taken in excess quantity [4,5]. Seventh couplet says that one who takes large quantity of food beyond the capacity of digestive fire suffers from various diseases.

மருந்தென வேண்டாவாம் யாக்கைக்கு அருந்தியது
அற்றது போற்றி உணின் (942)

அற்றல் அளவறிந்து உண்க அஃதுடம்பு
பெற்றான் நெடிதுய்க்கு மாறு (943)

அற்றது அறிந்து கடைப்பிடித்து மாறல்ல
துய்க்க துவரப் பசித்து (944)

மாறுபாடு இல்லாத உண்டி மறுத்துண்ணின்
ஊறுபாடு இல்லை உயிர்க்கு (945)

இழிவறிந்து உண்பான்கண் இன்பம்போல் நிற்கும்
கழிபே ரிரையான்கண் நோய் (946)

தீயள வன்றித் தெரியான் பெரிதுண்ணின்
நோயள வின்றிப் படும் (947)

In Ayurveda, *Ahara* (Diet/Food) is one among the three pillars/supports of life i.e., *trayopasthambha*. The three supports of life are intake of food, sleep and observance of *brahmacarya*; supported by these three well regulated factors of life, the body is endowed with strength, complexion and growth [7]. Ayurveda aims to maintain health. Health as well as disease is dependent on various factors, among which Diet is the most important one. Hence, Ayurveda emphasizes on the diet and dietetic regimen, as diet is the cause of health as well as diseases. And also Acharya's have explained clinical features of a disease and its management based upon the properties and actions of diet and its regimen which was prevalent during that period [8]. Diet may be healthy or unhealthy. A healthy diet depends upon the variation in quantity, time of consumption, method of preparation, habitat and constitution of body, disease and the age of an individual. Even though a person is taking healthy diet, the amount of diet should not disturb the equilibrium of *Doshas* and *Dhatus* of the body, gets digested as well as metabolized in proper time is to be regarded as the proper quantity of food. Acharyas have also explained the signs and symptoms of the intake of food in proper quantity, i.e. the diet should not create pressure in the stomach and flanks, no obstruction to the function of heart, no heaviness in the abdomen, there should be proper nourishment of the senses, relief in hunger and thirst, feeling of comfort in regular work like standing, sitting, sleeping, walking, exhaling, inhaling, laughing and talking [9]. Acharyas have explained the concept of *Jirna–Ajirna*. So, one should take diet after the digestion of previous diet is considered as proper time for diet, which is most important factor for the health. By following the proper diet in proper time, it promotes longevity by motivating the Agni and it opens the channels of circulations, produces Pure belching, enthusiasm, elimination of *malas* (Urine and Stool) at the proper time, lightness of the body, appearance of hunger and thirst are the symptoms of good digestion [10]. Symptom of proper digestion is specifically mentioned under the dietetics because intake of food before the previous food

is digested may aggravate all the three *Doshas* leading to serious consequences. Healthy individuals as well as the patients should observe the following, even while using food articles which are more wholesome by nature; one should eat food in proper quantity which is hot, unctuous and not contradictory in potency and that too, after the digestion of the previous meal. Food should be taken in proper place equipped with all the accessories, without talking or laughing, with concentration of mind and paying due regard to oneself.

Paying due consideration to the quality and time, a self-controlled men should regularly take such useful food and drinks as are conductive to the internal power of digestion, including metabolism like an Ahiitagni (a men who perform *Yajna*), who takes diet conductive over of digestion being aware of wholesomeness of food and drinks, who resort to meditation of "Brahma" and charity, enjoys bless without any disease during the present as well as future lives [11].

Treatment of Disease

In the eighth couplet, the physician who needs success in treatment should understand the stage of disease, cause of disease and then treat the disease. The next couplet says the physician who treats by understanding the patient's strength, nature of the disease and season will succeed in his carrier.

நோய்நாடி நோய்முதல் நாடி அதுதணிக்கும்
வாய்நாடி வாய்ப்பச் செயல் (948)

உற்றான் அளவும் பிணியளவும் காலமும்
கற்றான் கருதிச் செயல் (949)

Hetu (aetiology), *Linga* (sign and symptoms), *Ousadha* (drug and therapy) are the three principles of Ayurveda [12]. Without the knowledge of *Hetu* (cause of a disease) and *Linga* (sign and symptoms), the implication of *Ousadha* (drug and therapy) is not possible. In the classics, the Acharyas said that "*rogamadou pareekshet tathonantaram aoushadam*" it is very essential that before planning any treatment one should have complete knowledge of *Desha, kala, Rogibala, Rogabala* and *Agni*. To understand the nature of disease, one should adopt three fold (*Trividha pariksha*), six fold (*Shadvidha pariksha*), eight fold (*Asta sthana pariksha*) and tenfold (*Dashavidha pariksha*) examinations. To understand the cause and pathogenesis of the diseases, *Nidana Panchakas* are explained. Examination of patient is conducted for the knowledge of lifespan, degree of strength and intensity of morbidity. Detailed examination of the patient is the initial step for planning suitable/appropriate therapy.

Fourfold of Treatment

The last couplet says that four pillars namely Physician, Medicine, medical attendant and patient for responsible for prognosis of a disease.

உற்றவன் தீர்ப்பான் மருந்துஉழைச் செல்வானென்று
அப்பால்நாற் கூற்றே மருந்து (950)

Ayurveda also explains the importance of these four pillars for successful execution of a treatment. They are physician, medicaments, nursing personnel and the patient. The physician is considered as the foremost among them and should possess technical skill, scientific knowledge, purity and dexterity human understanding. Next, comes the drugs and they should possess of high quality, wide application, with high potency and should be available adequately. Attendant or nursing personnel is the third component of treatment and should have good knowledge of nursing, skilled in their art and be affectionate, clean and resourceful. The fourth component is the patient himself, who should be cooperative, obedient, fearless and able to communicate or describe his ailment. These sixteen qualities are needed for successful treatment [13]. Here within the scope of an article we could discuss only a few things related to the topic, while Valluvar has encapsulated these details in just two lines giving prime importance to treatment; detailed descriptions are available in the classics regarding Cause of the disease, Nutritional discipline, treatment principles and importance of four pillars of treatment. The similarity between Ayurveda and Thirukkural is not only in the concept of medicine, but also with regard to the code and conduct of life, sexual and seasonal regimen etc.

Conclusion

This presentation is a sincere and honest effort to put forth the various references pertaining Ayurveda principles mentioned in one of the well-known Tamil literary classic. We further suggest that this would form a wonderful and invaluable work, if carried out as a research topic which would bring to lime light various aspects, unknown to our present and future generation.

Acknowledgement

I would like to thank my brother Dr. Sundara BR Kasinath, who motivated this topic and also I would like to thank my friend Dr. Sathish. HS; and my student Dr. P Jeeva, who have helped me with valuable suggestions and guidance in this work.

References

1. https://www.himalayanacademy.com/media/books/tirukural/tirukural.pdf

2. Somasundaram O (1986) Sexuality in Thirukural, The great Tamil book of ethics. Indian J Psychiatry 28: 83-85.

3. Norman C (1992) Interpreting Thirukkural: the role of commentary in the creation of a text. J Am Orient Soc 112: 549-566.

4. https://www.researchgate.net/publication/281281689_Life_Skills_in_Classical_Tamil_Literature_Thirukural

5. http://www.indicabooks.com/Books.asp?category_id=49

6. Dr. Anna Moreshwar Kunte (2005),Vagbhata, Ashtanaga Hridaya, Sarvangasundara of Arunadatta and Ayurveda Rasayana of Hemadri commentary, Chaukambha orientalia, Varanasi, 956: 14.

7. Yadavji Trikamji Acharya (2001), Agnivesha, Charaka Samhita, Chaukhamba Surbharati Prakashan, Varanasi, 5th edition, 738; 74.

8. Yadavji Trikamji Acharya (2001), Agnivesha, Charaka Samhita, Chaukhamba Surbharati Prakashan, Varanasi, 5th edition, 738; 152.

9. Yadavji Trikamji Acharya (2001), Agnivesha, Charaka Samhita, Chaukhamba Surbharati Prakashan, Varanasi, 5th edition, 738; 238.

10. Shivprasad Sharma, Vrddha vagbhata, Astanga Samgraha, Chaukambha Sanskrit Series, Varanasi, ISBN – 81-7080-186-9; 965; 116.

11. Yadavji Trikamji Acharya (2001), Agnivesha, Charaka Samhita, Chaukhamba Surbharati Prakashan, Varanasi, 5th edition, 738; 174.

12. Yadavji Trikamji Acharya (2001), Agnivesha, Charaka Samhita, Chaukhamba Surbharati Prakashan, Varanasi, 5th edition, 738; 7.

13. Yadavji Trikamji Acharya (2001), Agnivesha, Charaka Samhita, Chaukhamba Surbharati Prakashan, Varanasi, 5th edition, 738; 63.

Characterization of Human Aortic Endothelial Cells, Endothelial Progenitor Cells, and Cardiomyocytes

Ching-Hung Chen[1] and Chan-Yen Kuo[2]*

[1]Department of Anesthesiology, Show Chwan Memorial Hospital, Changhua, Taiwan
[2]Graduate Institute of Systems Biology and Bioinformatics, National Central University, Chung-li, Taiwan

Abstract

Despite advances in therapy, heart failure remains a significant disease burden, with poor outcomes, worldwide. Reactive Oxygen Species (ROS) damage cardiomyocytes. Endothelial progenitor cells promote the repair of the endothelium of arteries damaged by ROS. However, gene expression profiles of Human Aortic Endothelial Cells (HAECs), Endothelial Progenitor Cells (HEPCs), and Cardiomyocytes (HCMs) are unclear. In the present study, we determined the expression profiles of different genes in HAECs, HEPCs, and HCMs by performing quantitative PCR. Results showed that p53 and Cx37 were up-regulated, but VEGF, Cx43, and eNOS were down-regulated in HEPCs. Cx40 and eNOS were up-regulated in HAECs. Moreover, we determined the effect of hydrogen peroxide-derived ROS on HCMs. Results showed that Cx40, Cx45, VCAM-1, ICAM-1, p53, and p21 were up-regulated, but E-cadherin was down-regulated after high concentration of hydrogen peroxide treatment.

Keywords: Human aortic endothelial cells (HAECs); Endothelial progenitor cells (HEPCs); Cardiomyocytes (HCMs); Reactive oxygen species (ROS)

Introduction

Coronary artery disease is a large disease burden in several countries. Endothelial dysfunction caused by oxidative stress and inflammation is an essential process underlying the progression of heart failure [1-3]. Tissues engineering aims to apply the principles of engineering and life science in developing biological substitutes that maintain, restore, or improve tissues. In clinical, new drugs and vascular bypass have improved the quality of life of patients with Cardiovascular Disease (CVD) but have not decreased morbidity or mortality [4]. Tateishi-Yuyama et al. reported that autologous transplantation of bone marrow-derived progenitor cells is a potential therapy of angiogenesis for patients with limb ischemia [5]. Autologous cell therapies involving bone marrow or circulating blood-derived progenitor cells are safe and exert beneficial therapeutic effects by inducing angiogenesis/vasculogenesis in patients with ischemic diseases [6,7]. In addition, human embryonic stem cell (hESC)-derived endothelial cells could be beneficial for potential applications such as engineering of new blood vessels, endothelial cell transplantation into the heart for myocardial regeneration, and induction of angiogenesis for treating regional ischemia [8]. However, because of ethical issues associated with ESCs, peripheral blood-derived epithelial progenitor cells (EPCs) are used for cell therapy [9]. EPCs are a potential inexhaustible source of functional vascular cells that have important features of mature ECs for regenerative medicine. However, it is difficult to define EPCs generated from different sources because they lack a unifying phenotype [10]. Glaser et al. suggested that different types of EPCs include colony-forming unit Hill cells, circulating cells, and endothelial colony-forming cells [11]. Therefore, it is very important to functionally characterize EPCs.

Gap junctions form conduits between adjacent cells that are composed of connexin subunits; these conduits allow direct intercellular communication [12]. Gap junctions also promote intercellular communication in the cardiovascular system and are essential for normal vascular function [13,14]. Connexins expressed in the vascular wall include Cx37, Cx40, Cx43, and Cx45 and those expressed by endothelial cells include Cx37 and Cx40 [12,14]. However, the role of these connexins in Human Aortic Endothelial Cells (HAECs), Human Endothelial Progenitor Cells (HEPCs), and Human Cardiomyocytes (HCMs) is unclear. Nitric Oxide (NO) is very important for regulating endothelial function. Increasing in NO production is either increased by Endothelial Nitric Oxide Synthase (eNOS) enzymes [15-17] or reduced by Reactive Oxygen Species (ROS) [18]. Ischemic preconditioning causes ROS overproduction in the mitochondria under hypoxia [19,20]. However, the effect of hypoxia on Cx37, Cx40, Cx43, and Cx45 is unclear. In this study, we characterized HAECs, HEPCs, and HCMs. In addition, we examined the effect of hypoxia on the expression of the abovementioned connexins in each cell model.

Materials and Methods

Cell lines and cell culture

HAECs (PromoCell GmbH, Heidelberg, Germany) were cultured in T-25 flasks (Corning Glassworks, Corning, NY, USA) containing endothelial cell growth medium MV (PromoCell GmbH) supplemented with 0.05 ml/ml fetal calf serum, 0.004 ml/ml endothelial cell growth supplement, 10 ng/ml epidermal growth factor, 90 µg/ml heparin, and 1 µg/ml hydrocortisone at 37°C and in an atmosphere of 5% CO_2/95% air.

HEPCs (Amsbio, UK) were cultured in T-25 flasks containing EPC growth medium (Cat#Z7030073; Bio Chain Institute Inc., CA, USA) at 37°C and in an atmosphere of 5% CO_2/95% air.

HCMs (PromoCell GmbH) were cultured in T-25 flasks containing myocyte growth medium (PromoCell GmbH) supplemented with 0.05 ml/ml fetal calf serum, 0.5 ng/ml epidermal growth factor, 2 ng/ml basic fibroblast growth factor, and 5 µg/ml insulin at 37°C and in an atmosphere of 5% CO_2/95% air.

***Corresponding author:** Chan-Yen Kuo, Graduate Institute of Systems Biology and Bioinformatics, National Central University, Chung-li, Taiwan
E-mail: cykuo@thu.edu.tw

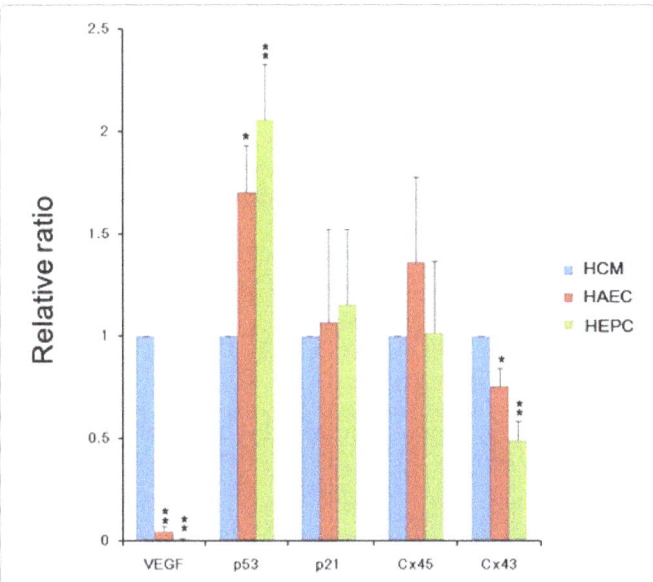

Figure 1: Relative mRNA levels of genes encoding different connexins, vascular endothelial growth factor (VEGF), p21, and p53 in human aortic endothelial cells (HAECs), human endothelial progenitor cells (HEPCs), and human cardiomyocytes (HCMs). All data are presented as mean ± SEM (n=3); $p<0.05$ and $p<0.01$ compared with control.

Culture medium was replaced every 2 days. After reaching 70–80% confluency, the cells were trypsinized and were seeded in six-well plastic dishes for performing subsequent experiments. Passages 3–6 HAECs, 3–10 HEPCs, and 3–9 HCMs were used in subsequent experiments.

RNA isolation and quantitative PCR

Total RNA was isolated from the cells by using TRIzol reagent (Invitrogen, Thermo Fisher Scientific, CA, and USA). Primer sequences and procedure used for quantitative PCR (qPCR) analysis of genes encoding vascular endothelial growth factor (VEGF), p53, p21, Cx37, Cx40, Cx43, Cx45, eNOS, VE-cadherin, vascular cell adhesion molecule-1 (VCAM-1), intercellular adhesion molecule-1 (ICAM-1), and β-actin. cDNAs of genes encoding VEGF, p53, p21, Cx37, Cx40, Cx43, Cx45, eNOS, VE-cadherin, VCAM-1, ICAM-1, and β-actin were synthesized using the following primer sets: 5′-TGC AGA TTA TGC GGA TCA AAC C-3′ and 5′-TGC ATT CAC ATT TGT TGT GCT GTA G-3′ for the gene encoding VEGF, 5′-GCC CAA CAA CAC CAG CTCC T-3′ and 5′-CCT GGG CAT CCT TGA GTT CC-3′ for the gene encoding p53, 5′-GAG GCC GGG ATG AGT TGG GAG GAG-3′ and 5′-CAG CCG GCG TTT GGA GTG GTA GAA-3′ for the gene encoding p21, 5′-GTT GCT GGA CCA GGT CCA GG-3′ and 5′-GGA TGC GCA GGC CAC CAT CT-3′ for the gene encoding Cx37, 5′-GTA CAC AAG CAC TCG ACC GT -3′ and 5′-GCA GGG TGG TCA GGA AGA TT-3′ for the gene encoding Cx40, 5′-CAA TCA CTT GGC GTG ACT TC-3′ and 5′-GTT TGG GCA ACC TTG AGT TC-3′ for the gene encoding Cx43, 5′-GGA GCT TTC TGA CTC GCC TG-3′ and 5′-CGG CCA TCA TGC TTA GGT TT-3′ for the gene encoding Cx45, 5′-CGG CAT CAC CAG GAA GAA GA-3′ and 5′-CAT GAG CGA GGC GGA GAT-3′ for the gene encoding eNOS, 5′-CAT GAG CCT CTG CAT CTT CC-3′ and 5′-ACA GAG CTC CAC TCA CGC TC-3′ for the gene encoding VE-cadherin, 5′-GAT ACA ACC GTC TTG GTC AGC CC-3′ and 5′-CAG TTG AAG GAT GCG GGA GTA TAT G-3′ for the gene encoding VCAM-1, 5′-CGA TGA CCA TCT ACA GCT TTC

CGG-3′ and 5′-GCT GCT ACC ACA GTG ATG ATG ACA A-3′ for the gene encoding ICAM-1, and 5′-TCC ACC TTC CAG CAG ATG TG-3′ and 5′-GCATTTGCGGTGGACGAT-3′ for the gene encoding β-actin. qPCR was performed using Platinum SYBR Green qPCR kit (Invitrogen, Thermo Fisher Scientific) in iCycler (Bio-Rad).

Statistical analysis

Data are shown as mean ± SEM. Treatment groups were compared using a two-tailed t-test by using a SAS software.

Results and Discussion

Gene profiles of HAECs, HEPCs, and HCMs

We validated the expression of genes encoding Cx37, 40, 43, 45, eNOS, VEGF, p21, and p53 by performing qPCR (Figures 1 and 2). EPCs play a critical role in neovascularization and re-endothelialization after ischemia and endothelial injury, respectively [21,22]. Interestingly, we observed that the expression of VEGF was decreased in HAECs and HEPCs (Figure 1). Previous studies have reported that VEGF is expressed in cardiac myofibroblasts, non-endothelial cells with the morphological features of fibroblasts in rat myofibroblasts isolated from heart infarcts [23,24]. However, limited anti-VEGF antibody-based therapeutic approaches are available for preventing cellular senescence in patients with CVD because these approaches exert different therapeutic effects in animal experiments and clinical trials [25]. Therefore, it is important to determine the gene expression profiles of HAECs, HEPCs, and HCMs.

Effect of hypoxia on HCMs

Mitochondria play a crucial role in regulating intrinsic pathways of apoptosis or programmed cell death [26]. Mitochondria are the major source of endogenous ROS in cells because they contain the electron transport chain required for oxidative phosphorylation [27,28]. However, the effect of hypoxia on HCMs is limited. We used hydrogen peroxide (H_2O_2) to mimic hypoxic condition [29] and determined the gene expression profiles of HAECs, HEPCs, and HCMs under hypoxia. Our results showed that the expression of genes encoding Cx40, Cx45, VCAM-1, ICAM-1, p21, and p53 was upregulated and that of the gene encoding E-cadherin was downregulated in cells treated with high concentration of H_2O_2 (200 µM) (Figure 3).

ROS upregulate VCAM-1 expression in endothelial cells [30]; however, this was not observed in HCMs. H_2O_2 increases the secretion of ICAM-1 in canine myocytes [31], which is consistent with the results of the present study. Long et al. reported that the expression of p21/WAF-1/CIP-1, a well-characterized target of p53 transactivation, also increases under hypoxia. Furthermore, hypoxia-induced rat cardiac myocytes to apoptosis via p53 activation [32]. Thus, our results suggest that H_2O_2-derived ROS trigger the apoptosis of HCMs. However, further studies should be performed to confirm this hypothesis.

Interestingly, ST2 (suppression of tumor formation) is a receptor for the interleukin-33 and critical to coronary artery disease. Marzullo et al. suggested that ST2/IL-33 pathway may play a central role in the novel mechanism of plaque development and eventually rupture [33].

Acknowledgement

This study was supported by grant RD105056 from Show Chwan Memorial Hospital, Changhua, Taiwan.

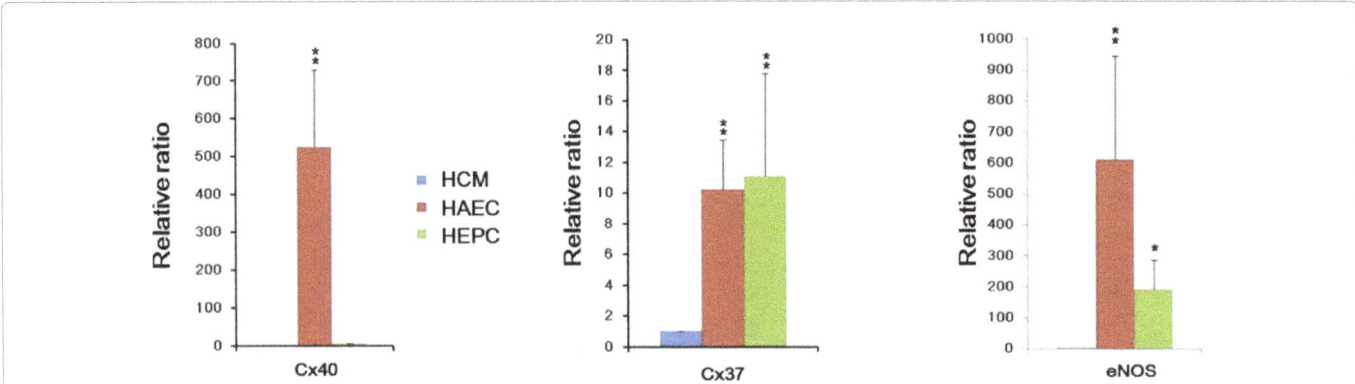

Figure 2: Relative mRNA levels of genes encoding various connexins and endothelial nitric oxide synthase (eNOS) in human aortic endothelial cells (HAECs), human endothelial progenitor cells (HEPCs), and human cardiomyocytes (HCMs). All data are presented as mean ± SEM (n=3); $p<0.05$ and $p<0.01$ compared with control.

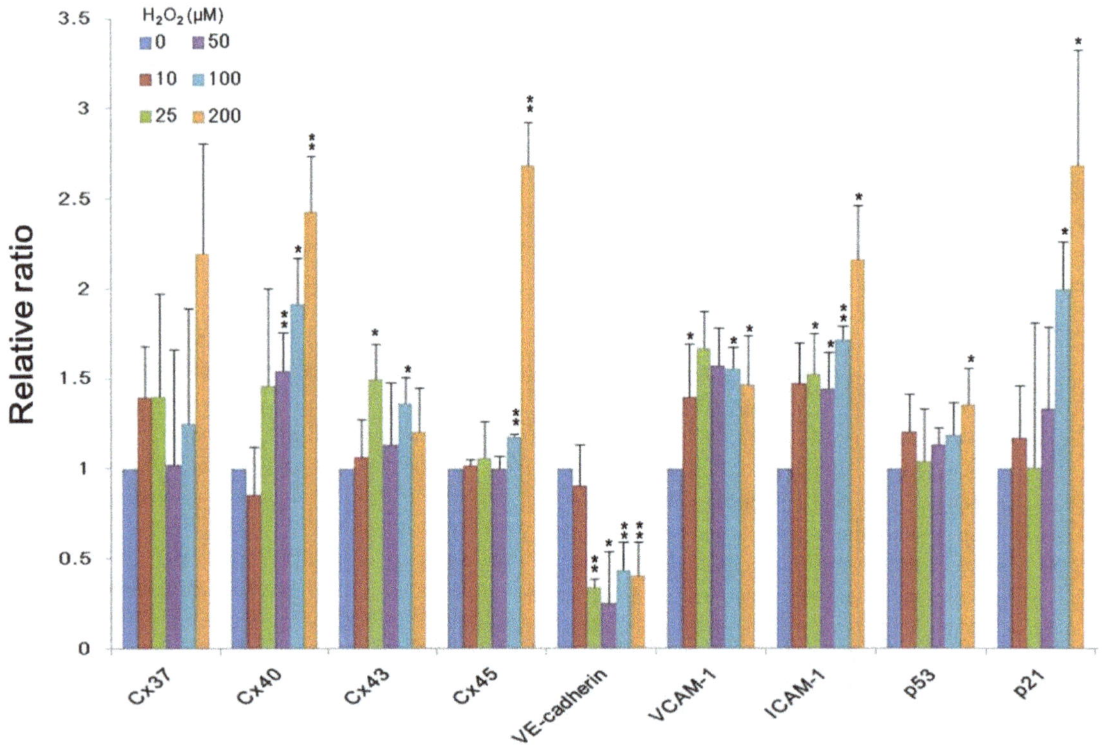

Figure 3: Effect of hydrogen peroxide (H_2O_2) on human cardiomyocytes (HCMs).

References

1. Scott J (2004) Pathophysiology and biochemistry of cardiovascular disease. Curr Opin Genet Dev 14: 271-279.

2. Sun HJ, Hou B, Wang X, Zhu XX, Li KX, et al. (2016) Endothelial dysfunction and cardiometabolic diseases: Role of long non-coding RNAs. Life Sci.

3. Jensen HA, Mehta JL (2016) Endothelial cell dysfunction as a novel therapeutic target in atherosclerosis. Expert Rev Cardiovas Ther 14: 1021-1033.

4. Nugent HM, Edelman ER (2003) Tissue engineering therapy for cardiovascular disease. Circul Res 92: 1068-1078.

5. Tateishi-Yuyama E, Matsubara H, Murohara T, Ikeda U, Shintani S, et al. (2002) Therapeutic angiogenesis for patients with limb ischaemia by autologous transplantation of bone-marrow cells: a pilot study and a randomised controlled trial. The Lancet 360: 427-435.

6. Li Z, Han Z, Wu JC (2009) Transplantation of human embryonic stem cell-derived endothelial cells for vascular diseases. J Cell Biochem 106: 194-199.

7. Huang PP, Li SZ, Han MZ, Xiao ZJ, Yang RC, et al. (2004) Autologous transplantation of peripheral blood stem cells as an effective therapeutic approach for severe arteriosclerosis obliterans of lower extremities. Thromb Haemost 91: 606-609.

8. Levenberg S, Golub JS, Amit M, Itskovitz-Eldor J, Langer R (2002) Endothelial cells derived from human embryonic stem cells. Proc Natl Acad Sci 99: 4391-4396.

9. Asahara T, Murohara T, Sullivan A, Silver M, van der Zee R, et al. (1997) Isolation of putative progenitor endothelial cells for angiogenesis. Science 275: 964-966.

10. Hirschi KK, Ingram DA, Yoder MC (2008) Assessing identity, phenotype, and fate of endothelial progenitor cells. Arterioscler Thromb Vasc Biol 28: 1584-1595.

11. Glaser DE, Gower RM, Lauer NE, Tam K, Blancas AA, et al. (2011) Functional characterization of embryonic stem cell-derived endothelial cells. J Vasc Res 48: 415-428.

12. Sohl G, Willecke K (2004) Gap junctions and the connexin protein family. Cardiovasc Res 62: 228-232.

13. Michela P, Velia V, Aldo P, Ada P (2015) Role of connexin 43 in cardiovascular diseases. Eur J Pharmacol 768: 71-76.

14. Morel S (2014) Multiple roles of connexins in atherosclerosis- and restenosis-induced vascular remodelling. J Vasc Res 51: 149-61.

15. Alderton WK, Cooper CE, Knowles RG (2001) Nitric oxide synthases: structure, function and inhibition. Biochem J 357: 593-615.

16. Dudzinski DM, Igarashi J, Greif D, Michel T (2006) The regulation and pharmacology of endothelial nitric oxide synthase. Annu Rev Pharmacol Toxicol 46: 235-276.

17. Hambrecht R, Adams V, Erbs S, Linke A, Krankel N, et al. (2003) Regular physical activity improves endothelial function in patients with coronary artery disease by increasing phosphorylation of endothelial nitric oxide synthase. Circulation 107: 3152-3158.

18. Adams V, Linke A, Krankel N, Erbs S, Gielen S, et al. (2005) Impact of regular physical activity on the NAD(P)H oxidase and angiotensin receptor system in patients with coronary artery disease. Circulation 111: 555-562.

19. Duranteau J, Chandel NS, Kulisz A, Shao Z, Schumacker PT (1998) Intracellular signaling by reactive oxygen species during hypoxia in cardiomyocytes. J Biol Chem 273: 11619-11624.

20. Bagheri F, Khori V, Alizadeh AM, Khalighfard S, Khodayari S, et al. (2016) Reactive oxygen species-mediated cardiac-reperfusion injury: Mechanisms and therapies. Life Sci 165: 43-55.

21. Urbich C, Dimmeler S (2004) Endothelial progenitor cells: characterization and role in vascular biology. Circ Res 95: 343-53.

22. Hur J, Yoon CH, Kim HS, Choi JH, Kang HJ, et al. (2004) Characterization of two types of endothelial progenitor cells and their different contributions to neovasculogenesis. Arterioscler Thromb Vasc Biol 24: 288-293.

23. Chintalgattu V, Nair DM, Katwa LC (2003) Cardiac myofibroblasts: a novel source of vascular endothelial growth factor (VEGF) and its receptors Flt-1 and KDR. J Mol Cell Cardiol 35: 277-286.

24. Harmey JH, Bouchier-Hayes D (2002) Vascular endothelial growth factor (VEGF), a survival factor for tumour cells: implications for anti-angiogenic therapy. Bioessays 24: 280-283.

25. Sanada S, Taniyama Y, Azuma J, Yuka, II, Iwabayashi M, et al. (2014) Endothelial progenitor cells in clinical settings. J Stem Cells 9: 117-125.

26. Green DR, Reed JC (1998) Mitochondria and apoptosis. Science 281: 1309-1312.

27. Murphy MP (2009) How mitochondria produce reactive oxygen species. Biochem J 417: 1-13.

28. Stowe DF, Camara AK (2009) Mitochondrial reactive oxygen species production in excitable cells: modulators of mitochondrial and cell function. Antioxid Redox Signal 11: 1373-1414.

29. Hool LC, Arthur PG (2002) Decreasing cellular hydrogen peroxide with catalase mimics the effects of hypoxia on the sensitivity of the L-type Ca^{2+} channel to beta-adrenergic receptor stimulation in cardiac myocytes. Circ Res 91: 601-609.

30. Cook-Mills JM, Marchese ME, Abdala-Valencia H (2011 Vascular cell adhesion molecule-1 expression and signaling during disease: regulation by reactive oxygen species and antioxidants. Antioxid Redox Signal 15: 1607-1638.

31. Lu H, Youker K, Ballantyne C, Entman M, Smith CW (2000) Hydrogen peroxide induces LFA-1-dependent neutrophil adherence to cardiac myocytes. Am J Physiol Heart Circ Physiol 278: H835-H842.

32. Long X, Boluyt MO, Hipolito ML, Lundberg MS, Zheng JS, et al. (1997) p53 and the hypoxia-induced apoptosis of cultured neonatal rat cardiac myocytes. J Clin Invest 99: 2635-2643.

33. Marzullo A, Ambrosi F, Inchingolo M, Manca F, Devito F, et al. (2016) ST2L Transmembrane Receptor Expression: An Immunochemical Study on Endarterectomy Samples. PLoS ONE 11: e0156315.

5

Homeopathic Medicines Protect Environment, Health and Development by Controlling Mulberry Diseases

Subhas Chandra Datta[1]* and Rupa Datta[2]

[1]Eco-club Research Unit, Kanchannagar D.N.Das High School, Kanchannagar, Burdwan-713102, West Bengal, India
[2]Life Science Unit, Burdwan Model School, Dewandighi, Burdwan-713101, West Bengal, India

Abstract

Plant diseases, caused by pathogens, significantly reduce food production particularly in the developing world where farmers have little knowledge of these pests. In sericulture, mulberry is an economical plant because silk production depends on the nutritive quality of the leaves which is hampered by various pathogen attacks like nematodes, fungus, virus, bacteria and insects etc. Recently, synthetic- and chemical- pesticides are the most effective means of control, but they are both expensive and environmentally unfriendly. The "evils" of synthetic- and chemical- pesticides has been a major concern to environmentalists. The use of chemical pesticides may achieve a measure of control of those mulberry diseases but there remains the problem of residual toxicity in the treated plants and this toxicity results in reduced palatability of the leaves to the feeding silkworm larvae, reduction in growth of the larvae and also in silk production. These are serious issues which directly cause crises of financial losses, food productions, and climatic changes, but in combination, their impact could be catastrophic for the global economy. To move forward will require new and more efficient solutions, technologies and products. Climate change and resource productive economies are now universally recognized as a significant global environmental challenge. To meet the challenge of the problems, a number of plant bio-nematicides though effective and easily biodegradable are not easily available in large quantities from natural sources and isolation of only a small quantity of an effective metabolites requires huge quantities of plant materials. This would result in rapid depletion of natural resources, particularly in tropical regions. Indiscriminate use of plant resources have already created problem of biodiversity conservation in the world. Bio-nematicides from animal origin (like nematode extract) reduce nematodes infestation in different plants and root callous by using their defense-response against nematode infection. But it remains as a problem.

To conquer this situation, the only 'Homeopathy' can solve all the above mentioned problems. Here, Homeopathic medicines; Cina, prepared from the flowering meristems of *Artemisia nilagirica* (Clarke) pamp and Aakashmoni, prepared from the funicles of *Acacia auriculiformis* A. Cunn, mixed with distilled water @ 7.2 mg/ml, were applied by foliar spray once daily for 15 days @ 10ml/plant on mulberry (Morus alba L., cv. S1) are highly effective in ameliorating mulberry diseases: root-knot [Meloidogyne incognita (Kofoid and White) Chitwood], leaf spot [Cercosporam moricola (Cooke)], powdery mildew [Phyllactinia corylea (Pers.) Karst], mosaic disease (mosaic virus) and tukra disease [*Maconellicoccus hirsutus* (Green)]. Both the drugs also improve the plant growth effectively which directly increase photosynthesis rate and significantly reduce CO_2 in the environment. Both the drugs also improve the growth of silkworms, shell weight, sex ratio percentage [SR%] and egg laying capacity of mother moth and also increase silk production and effective rate of silkworms rearing [ERR] commercially which directly enriches sericulture industry as well as agriculture sector. These cost-effective homeopathic medicines are easily available, biodegradable, non-phytotoxic and non-pollutant as well as conserve our biodiversity which will contribute towards "Sustainable Environment, Health and Development".

Keywords: Homeopathic medicines; Cina; Aakashmoni; Control; Mulberry disease; Sericulture; Environment

Introduction

Mulberry (*Morus alba* L.) is an important economical crop plant in sericulture and it grows under a wide range of ecological condition. It holds a special place as a major foreign exchange earner for many tropical and temperate countries. India secures the second position for the production of raw silk in the world, which is short about 30% to fulfill the home requirements [1]. The reasons for this deficiency as well as low quality of raw silk are, however, generally attributed to build up of the diseases of mulberry and silkworms, inadequate employment of improved culture and rearing practices [1,2-11]. Right from sprouting and throughout growing seasons, it is largely affected by a number of pathogens like plant parasitic nematodes, fungus, bacteria, virus and insects causing various diseases forming disease-complex and break the host resistance [1,2-12]. These pathogens are the main obstacles causing considerable loss in yield and nutritive value of mulberry foliage. Feeding of the diseased leaves affect the health of the silkworms adversely and the cocoon yield in terms of quality and quantity [2-11,13,14]. Root-knot disease, caused by *Meloidogyne incognita* (Kofoid and White) Chitwood, reduces 10-12% leaf yield in addition to affecting the leaf quality for silkworms feeding [3-14]. Leaf spots disease caused by *Cercosporam moricola* (Cooke) fungus, losses 10-35% leaf yield reducing moisture, proteins adversely and ultimately the quality and quantity of cocoons. *Phyllactinia corylea* (Pers.) Karst fungus, causing powdery mildew disease, is the most common and wide spread economically important disease reducing 10-30% leaf yield and reducing the crude protein content by as much as 33%. The mosaic disease caused by mosaic virus results in inward curling of leaves, particularly leaf margins and tip with chlorotic lesions on the leaf surface, stunted growth and suppressed leaf size [1-14]. Tukra

*Corresponding author: Subhas Chandra Datta, Masterpara (New Traffic Colony), P.O. & P.S.- Andal, Burdwan, Pin-713321, West Bengal, India
E-mail: dattasubhas@rediffmail.com

disease, caused by *Maconellicoccus hirsutus* (Green) (*Pseudococcidae*), tremendously reduces the leaves, depleting the nutritive value and plant growth, leaf yield and leaf protein content significantly [1-14].

Recently, synthetic and chemical pesticides are the most effective means of control, but they are both expensive and environmentally unfriendly. For sustainability of agriculture therefore, farmers should divorce the synthetic and chemical pesticides strategy and marry the phytochemicals option which is non-toxic to man and the environment, biodegradable and affordable to the peasant farmer in the developing world. The "evils" of synthetic and chemical pesticides has been a major concern to environmentalists. Recently efforts have therefore been shifted towards the use of plant extracts against pathogens as alternative to synthetic compounds. But it is not cost effective and it affects our biodiversity conservation directly [1-15].

To overcome this situation, it has been already observed that the extract prepared from the funicles of *Acacia auriculiformis* A. Cunn. and it's pure compounds acaciasides (A&B), are effective in reducing mulberry diseases leaving no residual toxicity in the leaves to affect the growing silkworm larvae [2,3,16-18] And recently it has also been observed that the use of Cina, prepared from the flowering meristems of *Artemisia nilagirica* (Clarke) pamp and Aakashmoni prepared from the funicles of *Acacia auriculiformis* A. Cunn. on mulberry reduced root-knot disease and enriched sericulture industry [10].

Aims and objectives

The purpose of the present investigation is to see the efficacy of the homeopathic medicines; Cina 200C, prepared from the flowering meristems of *Artemisia nilagirica* (Clarke) pamp and Aakashmoni 200C, prepared from the funicles of *A. auriculiformis*, in ameliorating root-knot disease of mulberry (*M. alba*, cv. S$_1$) caused by *M. incognita* root-knot nematodes pathogens and also to find out if the Aakashmoni 200C can reduce the four foliar diseases, caused by pathogens, under field condition. The foliar diseases were: leaf spot disease caused by *Cercosporam moricola* (Cooke) fungus pathogens, powdery mildew disease caused by *Phyllactinia corylea* (Pers.) Karst fungus pathogens, mosaic disease caused by mosaic virus pathogens and tukra disease caused by *Maconellicoccus hirsutus* (Green) mealy bug pathogens. The effects of the leaves of the Cina 200C- and Aakashmoni 200C- treated plants on the leaf consumption, growth of silkworm's larvae, silk gland weight and effective rate of rearing (ERR) were also observed.

In course of our experiments with anti-nematode agents, Aakashmoni 200C, it was observed that the mulberry plants besides being infected with root-knot nematodes were also naturally infected with above mentioned four foliar diseases (leaf spot, powdery mildew, mosaic viral and tukra disease). Thus both the root-knot and foliar diseases, caused by various plant pathogens, were taken in to consideration during the evaluation of the effects of Aakashmoni 200C. The result would be more realistic in terms of the potentiality of the Aakashmoni 200C, use as potential bio-agents, in controlling various plant pathogens.

Materials and Methods

Site of the experimental plots

The field experiment was carried out at the Sriniketan Sericultural Composite Unit, Government of West Bengal, India where temperature was 28 ± 5°C and relative humidity was 75 ± 5%. Soil and root samples [19-22] were taken at random from a sericulture field spreading over an area of 5.6 acre of land with a view to determining the extent and intensity of *Meloidogyne incognita* (Kofoid & White) Chitwood nematode pathogen infestation. Later, three areas (in the same locality and climatic condition) each measuring 0.02 has one naturally root-knot disease infected- untreated field and other two naturally root-knot disease infected Cina 200C and Aakashmoni 200C- treated field, were demarcated in the mulberry field where there were no soil differences as well as environmental factor.

The first area nematode infected (2863 ± 55 J$_2$/1 kg of soil) sandy soil was mixed with yard manure (2: 1 vol/vol). Every day, at least 40 random sampling of moist rhizospheric soil (200g of soil i.e., each sample collected by making a hole of 1.8 cm wide and 6 cm deep) were done in the nematode infected area for 30 days and were assessed the *M. incognita* population [19,20] and this naturally infected soil-filled area, demarking untreated field, was replicated thrice.

The other two areas of naturally *M. incognita* infected sandy soil field was also prepared by mixing yard manure (2:1 vol/vol), removing weeds, irrigating water and interchanging among the soil for uniform distribution of manure and nematodes in the naturally infected field which was estimated by regular soil sampling like a same process of previous one. These naturally infected soil-filled areas, demarking treated fields, were also replicated thrice.

Mature three years old mulberry cutting, *Morus alba* L., cv. S$_1$ (average 25cm length and 20g fresh weight) collected from same sericulture field, were planted with a gap of 45cm throughout the experimental fields where there were no soil difference and climatic conditions. The planted mulberry cuttings were allowed to grow for a period of three months. Regular rhizospheric soil and root sampling (at random) were done for estimation of nematode population during this three month growth period of mulberry in all fields [19,20,23]. At least 80 random rhizospheric soil samples (200g in each sample) were collected from rhizospheric root-soil area of root (10-15cm X 10-15cm) and at least 40 random root samples (2g fresh root in each sample) were collected from newly formed roots (or gall roots) for determining the intensity or presence of nematodes in all the experimental fields [2,3,9].

After three months growth of mulberry, *M. incognita* populations were estimated in the rhizospheric soil as well as roots [19-22] (at least 40 at random sampling in each area) of mulberry plants in each areas of mulberry field. The *M. incognita* infected mulberry plants achieved growth of 50-60 cm in height. All the infected mulberry plants were divided into batches. The batches were; untreated- batches, Cina 200C- and Aakashmoni 200C- treated batches and each batch had 8-plots (20 plants/plot).

At first all the plants were pruned, manured with NPK and irrigated every 7 days. Rhizospheric soil was interchanged among the plants to keep the nematode infestation as uniform as possible in the naturally infected field. After pruning, the plants were allowed to grow for a period of 135 days when their root-knot, leaf spot, powdery mildew, viral and tukra diseases were assessed [1-3,24-26]. The field trial was replicated three times.

Plant pathogens caused mulberry diseases

Root-knot disease: Rhizospheric soil and root sample were taken at random from all the infected plots. *Meloidogyne incognita* populations (10 samples/plot in each plant group) were estimated in the rhizospheric soil as well as roots [2-9,19,20] of infected mulberry plants. Total number and surface area of leaves of all plant groups were counted [2,3,10]. Total number of root-galls/plant were counted in the infected roots of mulberry plants [2,23,27,28]. The total protein content of the leaf and root samples (10 at random sampling/plot) from plots was determined [27-29]. All the data from experiments were counted for statistical analysis by student's t- test. In this field trial, sacrifices of mulberry plants were not done due to well reported pathological characters from our previous experiments [2,3].

Foliar diseases: The main foliar diseases, observed in the sericulture field, were: leaf spot disease caused by *Cercosporam moricola* (Cooke) fungus pathogens, powdery mildew disease caused by *Phyllactinia corylea* (Pers.) Karst fungus pathogens, mosaic disease caused by mosaic virus pathogens and tukra disease caused by *Maconellicoccus hirsutus* (Green) mealy bug pathogens. All the disease identified according to their characteristic symptoms by the experts concerned [1-4,12,24]. Diseased leaves of each type were counted in each plot [30]. The percentage of disease infection was based on diseased leaf surface area [30-32].

Preparation of homeopathic mother tincture (MT)

Air-dried and powdered flowering meristems of *Artemisia nilagirica* (Clarke) Pamp- and funicles of *Acacia auriculiformis* A. Cunn, were extracted with 90% ethanol at room temperature (25 ± 2°C) for 15 days and were filtered for collecting extract. Later, the ethanol from the extracts was removed by evaporation at room temperature (25 ± 2°C). The residues were dried in a desecrator over anhydrous calcium chloride. The crude residues were dissolved in 90% ethanol at 1mg/ml concentration and were formed homeopathic mother tincture of *A. nilagirica* called Cina MT and *A. auriculiformis,* named Aakashmoni MT (Original solution or crude extract) respectively [7,10,11,14].

Preparation of potentized Liquid medicine

The homeopathic mother tinctures of Cina MT and Aakashmoni MT were diluted respectively with 90% ethanol (1:100) proportionate in a round vial. The vial were filled up to two-third of its space, tightly corked. And then were given 10 powerful down ward strokes of the arm. This process of mechanical agitation is called succession. This was the 1st centesimal potency named Cina 1C and Aakashmoni 1C. All the subsequent potencies were prepared by further diluting each potencies with 90% ethanol in the same proportion (1:100) and the mixture were given 10 powerful down ward strokes. In this way potencies up to Cina 200C and Aakashmoni 200C were prepared respectively [10].

Preparation of medicated globules

Both the homeopathic potencies in liquid form can be kept in globules. A vial were filled up to two-third of its empty space with sucrose globules of a particular size. Few drops of a liquid potency of Aakashmoni 200C were poured in to the vial to just moisten all the globules. The vial were corked and then shaken so that all globules were uniformly moistened. The cork was loosened and the vial was turned upside down to allow excess liquid drain out. After keeping the vial in the inverted position for nine to ten hours, the vial were turned upright, well corked and kept in a cool dry place away from light. The dry globules were then kept in a vial and medicated globules were known to retain their properties for many years. In this process the drug soaked globules Cina 200C and Aakashmoni 200C was prepared [10,11].

Preparation of control globules

A vial were filled up to two-third of its empty space with sucrose globules of a particular size. Few drops of 90% ethanol were poured in to the vial to just moisten all the globules. The vial were corked and then shaken so that all globules were uniformly moistened. The corks were loosened and the vial is turned upside down to allow excess liquid to drain out. After keeping the vial in the inverted position for nine to ten hours, the vial were turned upright, well corked and kept in a cool dry place away from light. The dry globules were then kept in a vial to retain their properties for many years. In this process the 90% ethanol soaked control sucrose globules were prepared. The control globules were prepared in the same way for comparison to the preparation of medicated Cina 200C- and Aakashmoni 200C- globules which were prepared with the 90% ethanol media [10,11].

Preparation of test- and control- solutions

The drug soaked globules of Cina 200C- and Aakashmoni 200C- were then be mixed with sterile distilled water in the proportion of 7.2 mg globules/ml of water [10,11]. The 90% ethanol soaked globules were then mixed with sterile distilled water in the proportion of 7.2 mg globules/ml of water and the Cina 200C- and Aakashmoni 200C- control solutions were prepared for comparison to the preparation of test solutions [10,11].

Mortality test

Three sets of cavity block with 1ml distilled water containing 50 larvae (J_2) of *M. incognita* were taken; one set was treated as control and other two were treated as treatment sets of Cina 200C and Aakashmoni 200C. To assess the direct effect of Cina 200C- and Aakashmoni 200C- test solutions, the water was removed by pipette from all the treatment sets, and immediately replaced by 1ml of test solutions - Cina 200C and Aakashmoni 200C (7.2 mg globules/ml concentration) were added respectively. To assess the direct effect of control solution, the control set was received 1 ml of control solution and observed with every 30 minutes interval for a period of 12 hours exposure period at room temperature (25 ± 2°C). This mortality test [33] was replicated five times. It was noted that both the control (without drugs) and treatment (with drugs) sets were received sucrose globules [10]. This mortality tests were replicated five times.

Treatment

Seventy six days after pruning, of mulberry plants, all the treatment were done by foliar spray @ 10ml/plant (7.2mg/ml concentration) once daily for 15 days with Cina 200C- and Aakashmoni 200C - test solutions and control solutions respectively. Treatments were given in such a way that all the leaves of the plants were completely sprayed with solutions. During spraying, the soil surface underneath each plant was covered with polyethylene sheet [2-4,10]. All Cina 200C- and Aakashmoni 200C- treated groups were received 10ml/plant test solutions (7.2 mg Cina 200C- and Aakashmoni- globules/ml concentration) respectively. The infected untreated with Cina- and Aakashmoni- (control) groups were similarly received 10 ml/plant control solutions (7.2mg- 90% ethanol soaked globules/ml concentration) [2-4,10]. It is noted that the infected untreated with Cina- and Aakashmoni (controls), were not untreated, but treated with the solution made from sugar pills soaked in the alcohol medium. The infected untreated (controls) were only treated with the solutions made from sugar globules in the alcohol medium (i.e. without medicine Cina - and Aakashmoni). At fifteen days after the second treatment all the parameters of diseases were assessed again for each group [2-4,10]. All the data were used for statistical analysis by student's t-test.

Analysis of residue

A thin layer chromatography plate (TLC) was made with silica gel [34]. Mulberry leaves, collected one day after last treatment were homogenized in a blender and extracted with ethanol. The residue was applied at one end of the plate as a small circular spot. The initial spot should be compact for reproducible R_f values and zones should always be placed at the same distance from the surface of developer [34]. Here, the residues run in thin layer chromatography plate (TLC) with the standard from the Cina 200C- and Aakashmoni 200C- test substances [10, 34].

Rearing of silkworms

The eggs of a mother moth of the multivoltine 'Nistari' race (*Bombyx mori* L.) supplied by Regional Sericultural Research and Training Institute, Berhampore-742101, India, after hatching (93% hatching rate) and brushing 1st stage silk worm larvae in the rearing tray, the larvae were divided into three batches (180 silkworm larvae/batch) and reared [2-4,7-9,35]. The larvae of infected untreated batch (control) were fed with the leaves of pathogen infected diseased leaves of mulberry plants from infected untreated (control) plots and the larvae of infected treated two-batches were fed with the leaves of Cina 200C- and Aakashmoni 200C -treated leaves of mulberry plants from infected treated respectively. Fresh leaves were given to the larvae 4-times daily. Mulberry leaves were used for feeding fifteen days after the last treatment with both the drugs. The larvae were kept inside the rearing chamber at 27±2°C and 70 ± 15% RH. The fresh weight of the larvae and that of the leaves served were recorded daily for each batch until the larvae started spinning. The consumption of fresh leaves [(Fresh leaves served – Dry leaves residues - Fresh leaves initially consumed) X Moisture loss], number of feeding and number of feeding day to cocoon formation, number of escaping feeding during moulting, moulting span days and mortality rate were recorded. The fresh silk gland weight of mature 5th instar larvae (before start spinning), starting time to spinning, span of spinning, fresh cocoon weight, fresh shell weight, silk layer ratio (SR% = Shell weight/Cocoon weight×100), effective rate of rearing (ERR % = Number of cocoon harvested/

Number of silk worm hatched ×100), sex ratio percentage (Number of male adult emerged/Number of female adult emerged×100) and egg laying capacity of mother moth were determined [2-4,7-9,35]. For statistical analysis by student's t- test, ten mature 5th instar silkworm larvae for fresh silk gland weight and ten cocoons for fresh shell weight were dissected out in each batches including replica of all batches [2-4,7-10,35]. All the data from rearing trial were used for statistical analysis by student's t- test.

Results

Estimation of the nematode population from field trial

The initial nematode populations [Meloidogyne incognita (Kofoid & White) Chitwood], stretching over an area of 5.6acre of mulberry plantation, were 1779 ± 43 J_2 per 200g of soil and 830 45 J_2 per 2g of root. The nematode populations in the demarcated 0.16 acre, were 1950 ± 11 J_2 per 200g of soil and 615 ± 15 J_2 per 2g of root [before treatment (Day-0)].

Mortality test

It was observed that Cina 200C- and Aakashmoni 200C- had no toxic effects on nematodes mortality within the exposure period of 12 hours at room temperature (25 ± 2°C). For this reason, no data were presented in the results section.

Analysis of residue

There had left no toxic residues of Cina 200C- and Aakashmoni 200C- in all the infected -treated plants by thin layer chromatography plate (TLC). For this reason, no data were presented in the results section.

Root-knot disease

Table 1 shows the effects of Cina 200C- and Aakashmoni 200C- on *Meloidogyne incognita* pathogens infected mulberry plants in a field trial replicated thrice (P<0.01 by 't'- test). All naturally infected plants (treated plant group) treated with Cina 200C- and Aakashmoni 200C- showed increase number and surface area of leaves, and higher protein content in leaves and root than infected untreated (control) plants (untreated plant group). In all infected Cina 200C- and Aakashmoni 200C- treated plants, the population of root-knot nematodes decreased

Treatment batches (20plants / plots & 8 plots/ batches)*	Average No. of leaves/plant*		Average Surface area of leaves (sq.cm)*		Average Protein content (%)+				Average Nematode population +				Average No. of rootgalls/plant +	
					Leaf		Root		Soil (200g)		Root (2g)			
	Day-0	Day-30	Day-0	Day-30	Day-0	Day-30	Day-0	Day-30	Day-0	Day-30	Day-0	Day-30	Day-0	Day-30
Infected Untreated (Control)	380ax ±12.67	430by ±13.43	7885ax ±157.70	24516by ±408.60	2.98ax ±0.13	6.75by ±0.25	4.38ax ±0.16	7.82by ±0.30	1937ax ±74.50	78by ±3.39	639ax ±24.57	107by ±5.09	1197ax ±46.03	221by ±8.50
Infected Cina 200C -treated	382ax ±12.83	434by ±10.12	7883ax ±143.30	25217dy ±387.91	2.99ax ±0.12	6.78by ±0.24	4.38ax ±0.15	7.88cy ±0.26	1935ax ±74.30	66cy ±2.35	639ax ±22.03	55dy ±2.39	1207ax ±46.42	187cy ±6.67
Infected Aakashmoni 200C -treated	380ax ±12.83	436by 12.12±	7882ax ±143.30	25215dy ±327.02	2.99ax ±0.8	6.78by ±0.12	4.38ax ±0.15	7.89cy ±0.22	1933ax ±74.34	62cy ±2.32	639ax ±22.03	54dy ±2.32	1208ax ±40.42	184cy ±6.64

''- Means average values of 40 plants in triplicate.
'+'- Means average values of 20 samples in triplicate.
'Day-0'- Means before treatment.
'Day-30'- Means after treatment.
'a,b'- Significant difference by t-test (P<0.01) in the same column.
'x,y'- Significant difference by t-test (P<0.01) in the same row between day-0 and day-30 of each character.
Table 1: Effects of Cina 200C- and Aakashmoni 200C- on *Meloidogyne incognita* infected mulberry plants in a field trial.

significantly in rhizospheric soil and as well as in roots than infected untreated (control) plants. The number of root galls also decreased significantly after Cina 200C- and Aakashmoni 200C- treatment.

Foliar diseases

Table 2 shows only the effects of Aakashmoni200C on leaf spot, powdery mildew, mosaic viral and tukra diseases of mulberry plants in a field trial replicated thrice assessed initially (Day- 0) and after a period of 30 days (Day- 30) by 't'- test (P<0.01). Aakashmoni 200C significantly reduced the number of leaves infected with leaf spot, powdery mildew, mosaic viral and tukra as compared to the pre-treatment condition (Day- 0). The percentage of control achieved were 62.08 for leaf spot, 77.89 for powdery mildew, 64.91 for mosaic virus and 38.42 for tukra infection as compared to the pre-treatment level (Day- 0). In case of infected untreated plots leaf spot, powdery mildew, mosaic viral and tukra diseases showed naturally 27.80%, 17.76%, 29.37% and 21.20% reduction respectively, in 30 days (Day -30).

Effects on feeding silkworms

Table 3 shows the effects of Cina 200C- and Aakashmoni 200C- on diseased infected mulberry plants in a silkworm rearing and field trial replicated thrice on the feeding, growth and mortality of silkworms (P<0.01 by 't'-test). The average consumption of leaves by the 5th instars, average number of feeding to cocoon formation, average number of feeding day to cocoon formation, average number of escaping– feeding during moulting and average moulting span days were less for Cina

200C- and Aakashmoni 200C- treated plants than for infected untreated (control) ones. The average mortality rate (%) was nil with Cina 200C- and Aakashmoni 200C- treated plants groups and 56% with infected untreated (control) one. However, the average fresh weight of the 5th instars larvae were higher with Cina 200C-and Aakashmoni 200C-treated plants than with infected untreated (control) one.

Effects on silk production and rearing practices

Table 4 shows the effects of feeding Cina 200C- and Aakashmoni 200C- treated mulberry leaves on silk production, spinning characters and rearing practices in a silkworm rearing and field trial replicated thrice (P<0.01 by 't'-test). The average fresh silk gland weight, average fresh cocoon weight, average fresh shell weight and average shell ratio (SR%) were higher with Cina 200C- and Aakashmoni200C - treated plants than with infected untreated (control) one. It is notable that average starting time to spinning day and average span of spinning day (i.e. duration of span) were fewer with the Cina 200C- and Aakashmoni 200C - treated plants than with infected untreated (control) ones. Average effective rate of rearing (ERR %), average sex ratio percentage and average egg laying capacity were significantly higher with all Cina 200C- and Aakashmoni 200C- treated groups.

Discussion

The homeopathic drugs; Cina 200C- and Aakashmoni 200C- ones again confirm that the cost effective drugs not only reduced root-knot, leaf spot, powdery mildew, viral and tukra diseases but also improved

Treatment groups (20plants/ Plot & 8 plots/ group)	Average number of disease-infected leaves / plant (%)							
	Leaf spot		Powdery mildew		Mosaic		Tukra	
	Day-0	Day-30	Day-0	Day-30	Day-0	Day-30	Day-0	Day-30
Infected Untreated (Control)	70.58ax ± 2.28	98.38ay ± 3.93 (<27.80%)	80.75ax ±3.23	98.51ay ±3.94 (<17.76%)	68.68ax ±2.74	98.05ay ±4.10 (<29.37%)	57.15ax ±2.38	78.35ay ±3.26 (<21.20%)
Infected Aakashmoni 200C -treated	70.53ax ±2.71	8.45by ±2.71 (>62.08%)	80.86ax ±3.11	2.97by ±0.01 (>77.89%)	68.32ax ±2.62	3.41by ±0.13 (>64.91%)	57.11ax ±2.37	18.69by ±0.81 (>38.42%)

Day-0 Means before treatment. Day-30 means after treatment.
a, b - Significant difference by 't'-test (P<0.01) in the same column.
x, y - Significant difference by 't'- test (P<0.01) in the same row between day-0 and day-30 of each character.
( ) - Figures in the parentheses show percentage of reduction on day-30 as compared to the initial level on day-0 in the same row.
Table 2: Effects of Aakashmoni 200C- on leaf spot, powdery mildew, mosaic and tukra diseases of mulberry plants in a field replicated thrice assessed initially (Day-0) and after a period of 30 days (Day-30).

Treatment batches (180 larvae/ batch)*	Average number of						
	Consumption of leaves(g) (5th instar)*	Feeding to cocoon formation*	Feeding- day to cocoon formation*	Escaping feeding during moulting*	Moulting span day (1st to 5th instar)*	Larval fresh weight (g) (5thinstar)*+	Mortality rate (%)*
Infected Untreated (Control)	4.03a ±0.15	76.00a ±2.37	19.00a ±0.50	51.00a ±1.75	13.00a ± 0.39	1.48a ±0.03	56.00 ±2.43
Infected Cina 200C -treated	2.46b ± 0.09	62.00b ± 1.93	15.00b ± 0.44	20.00b ± 0.68	5.00b ± 0.15	2.63b ± 0.06	Nil
Infected Aakashmoni 200C -treated	2.42b ± 0.04	60.00b ± 1.92	15.00b ± 0.40	20.00b ± 0.62	5.00b ± 0.13	2.61b ± 0.05	Nil

a,b - Different small letters in a column show significant difference by 't'- test (P<0.01).
* - Average values of 180 silk worm larvae in triplicate.
+ - Average values of 10 silk worm larvae were dissected in triplicate.

Table 3: Effects of disease-infected and Cina 200C- and Aakashmoni 200C - treated mulberry plants in a field on the feeding and growth of silkworms in the silkworms rearing trials (replicated thrice).

Treatment batches (180 larvae/ batch)*	Average								
	Silk gland fresh weight(g) (5th instar)+	Starting time to spinning (at day-)*	Span of spinning day*	Cocoon fresh weight (g)*	Shell fresh weight (g)+	Shell ratio (SR %)+	Effective rate of rearing (ERR %)*	Sex ratio (Male / Female %)	Egg laying capacity
Infected Untreated (Control)	0.98a ± 0.03	34.00a ± 1.30	10.00a ± 0.45	0.85a ± 0.03	0.11a ± 0.01	12.94a ± 0.49	21.37a ± 0.63	76.00a ± 1.94	320.00a ± 13.91
Infected Cina 200C -treated	1.98b ± 0.07	20.00b ± 0.51	3.00b ± 0.09	1.09b ± 0.04	0.24b ± 0.02	22.01b ± 0.67	97.43b ± 2.16	68.00b ± 1.74	540.00b ± 11.73
Infected Aakashmoni 200C -treated	1.98b ± 0.04	20.00b ± 0.42	3.00b ± 0.06	1.09b ± 0.02	0.24b ± 0.01	22.01b ± 0.42	97.48b ± 2.16	68.00b ± 1.72	540.00b ± 11.71

a,b - Different small letters in a column show significant difference by 't'- test (P<0.01).

* - Average values of 180 silk worm larvae in triplicate.

+ - Average values of 10 silk worm larvae and cocoon were dissected in triplicate.

Table 4: Effects of disease-infected and Cina 200C- and Aakashmoni 200C - treated mulberry plants in a field on the growth of silk gland, spinning time, cocoon, shell, rearing, sex ratio and egg laying capacity in the silkworms rearing trials (Replicated thrice).

the nutritive value of the treated leaves of infected plants [10].

- From this field trial, we confirm that Cina 200C and Aakashmoni 200C also improves the nutritive value of the treated leaves [2,6-10] which directly influences on the consumption of leaves, number of feeding and number of feeding day to cocoon formation, and indirectly affects on moulting stage in all the Cina 200C- and Aakashmoni 200C- treated groups from these trials.

- And due to ill development of infected untreated (control) batches larvae took more time to moult which is proved from the number of escaping feeding during moulting [2,6-10].

- Higher nutritive value of treated plants contribute to higher growth of silkworm larvae, silk gland weight, cocoon weight and shell weight which increase silk production significantly [2,6-10] for commercial purpose [10].

- The improved health of the larvae, cocoon weight, silk gland and shell weight from the Cina 200C- and Aakashmoni 200C- treated groups of the infected plants might have resulted in the fewer starting time to spinning and span of spinning day and the total elimination of the mortality rate [2,6-10]. However, Cina 200C- and Aakashmoni 200C is too dilute to contain drug molecules [2,6-10,36]. Naturally, the drug might not have affected the nematode directly [2,6-10] and for this reason, no mortality occurs.

- The effective rate of rearing (ERR %) is very high in all Cina 200C- and Aakashmoni 200C- treated treatment batches which enriches the sericulture industry in many ways, specially for commercial purpose [2,6-10].

- The mulberry leaves did not contain any toxic residues of the Cina 200C- and Aakashmoni 200C- test substances by the thin layer chromatography (TLC). It is reported that Cina- and Aakashmoni- at ultra high dilution has physical basis in the form of charge transfer interaction and altered rate of tumbling in the specific part of the molecules of the diluents medium [2,6-10,36].

- Rather, the drug Cina 200C- and Aakashmoni 200C- might have induced natural defense response in the test plants against nematode parasites and has conferred defense response on growing larvae [2,6-10,36].

- In fact, it is surprising that all infected Cina 200C- and Aakashmoni 200C- treated plants not only are less affected by nematodes but also have a better growth than the infected untreated with Cina 200C- and Aakashmoni 200C (control) plants [2,6-10,36].

- And the positive effects of growth may be responsible for defense resistance against pathogens [2,6-10,36,37]. Both the drugs also improve the plant growth effectively which directly increase photosynthesis rate and significantly reduce CO_2 in the environment. So we can say that Cina 200C- and Aakashmoni200C might have induced synthesis of many new proteins which have stimulated increased photosynthesis rate, stomatal activity and water retention capacity of Cina 200C- and Aakashmoni 200C- treated plants [2,6-10,36,37,38].

- The positive effects of growth on infected Cina 200C- and Aakashmoni 200C- treated plants may not only be responsible for defense resistance to nematodes pathogen but also improves growth of silkworm larvae and silk gland weight, cocoon weight, shell weight and effective rate of rearing (ERR %) [2,6-10,36,37,38] which increase silk production for commercial purpose. It is proved from the result that silk production is higher in the Cina 200C- and Aakashmoni200C- treated groups than infected untreated with Cina 200C- and Aakashmoni 200C- (control) groups.

Conclusion

These results once again suggest that plant diseases (like nematodes, fungus, virus, bacteria and insects etc) might be effectively controlled by the potentized cost effective homeopathic medicines Cina 200C- and Aakashmoni 200C- at an extremely low dose and also increases silk production and effective rate of rearing commercially which directly enriches sericulture industry as well as agriculture sector. Both the potentized-biopesticide-homeopathy-drugs also improve the plant growth effectively which directly increase photosynthesis rate and significantly reduce CO_2 in the environment. These cost-effective homeopathic medicines are easily available, biodegradable, non-phytotoxic and non-pollutant as well as conserve our biodiversity which will contribute towards "Sustainable Environment, Health and Development".

Acknowledgements

The work described here has been supported by Rtd. Prof. N.C.Sukul, Dept.

of Zoology, Visva-Bharati and Joint Director, Sriniketan Sericultural Composite Unit, Sriniketan, Govt. of West Bengal and Mr. Achintya Mondal, Secretary, BIMS, BMS & BIMLS,West Bengal,India. Lastly, for help in statistical analysis we are immensely indebted to Dr. Tapan Mondal, Asst. teacher of Secondary School. Sri Basudev Mondal, Assistant English-Teacher of Kanchannagar, D.N.Das High School, Kanchannagar, Burdwan, who has revised the English of the manuscripts.

References

1. Teotia RS, Sen SK (1994) Mulberry disease in India and their control. Sericologia 34: 1-18.

2. Datta SC, Sinhababu SP, Sukul NC (1997) Improved growth of silkworms from effective treatment of mulberry diseases by *Acacia auriculiformis* extract. Sericologia 37: 707-715.

3. Datta SC (1999) Bio-nematicides in the control of root-knot nematode. Ph.D thesis, Department of Zoology, Visva-Bharati, Santiniketan-731235, West Bengal, India (unpublished).

4. Datta SC (2006) Effects of *Cina* on root-knot disease of mulberry. Homeopathy 95: 98-102.

5. Datta SC (2006) Possible use of amaranth as catch crop for root-knot nematodes intercropped with okra. Phytomorphology 56: 113-116.

6. Datta SC, Datta R (2006) Liquid homeopathic medicine *Cina* enriches sericulture industry. Journal of Environmental & Sociobiology 3: 55-60.

7. Datta SC, Datta R (2007) Increased silk production by effective treatment of naturally infected root-knot and black leaf spot diseases of mulberry with acaciasides. Journal of Environmental & Sociobiology 4: 209-214.

8. Datta SC, Datta R (2008) Potentized *Artemisia nilagirica* extract Cina increases silk production and effective rate of rearing in a field trial. Hpathy Ezine.

9. Datta SC (2010) The Role of Cina in the Field of Enriched Sericulture. Hpathy Ezine.

10. Datta SC, Datta R (2011) Control root-knot disease of mulberry by homeopathic medicines: Aakashmoni [MT, 30C, 200C & 1000C] prepared from the funicles of *Acacia auriculiformis*. Hpathy Ezine.

11. Sukul NC, Sinhababu SP, Datta SC, Nandi B, Sukul A (2001) Nematotoxic effect of *Acacia auriculiformis* and *Artemisia nilagirica* against root-knot nematodes. Allelopathy Journal 8: 65-72.

12. Powell NT (1971) Interaction between nematodes and fungi in disease complexes. Annual Rev Phytopathology 9: 253-274.

13. Govindaiah, Sharma DD (1994) Root-knot nematode, *Meloidogyne incognita* infesting mulberry - a review. Indian Journal of Sericulture 33: 110-113.

14. Datta SC (2007) Mulberry disease: Problem in sericulture. SEBA Newsletter, Environment & Sociobiology 4: 7-10.

15. Datta SC, Datta R, Sinhababu SP, Sukul NC (1998) Acaciasides and root-knot nematode extract suppress *Melodogyne incognita* infection in lady's finger plants. Proceeding of the National Seminar on Environmental Biology 98: 205-209.

16. Datta SC, Datta (Nag) R (2007) Increased silk production by effective treatment of naturally infected root-knot and black leaf spot diseases of mulberry with acaciasides. Journal of Environmental & Sociobiology 4: 209-214.

17. Datta SC, Datta R, Sinhababu SP, Sukul NC (1998) Acaciasides and root-knot nematode extract suppress *Melodogyne incognita* infection in lady's finger plants. Proceeding of the National Seminar on Environmental Biology 98: 205-209.

18. Mahato SB, Pal BC, Nandi AK (1992) Structure elucidation of two acylated triterpenoid bioglycosides from *Acacia auriculiformis* Cunn. Tetrahedron 48: 6717-6728.

19. Christie JR, Perry VG (1951) Removing nematodes from soil. Proceeding of Helminthological Society. Washington 18: 106-108.

20. Sukul NC (1987) Soil and plant nematodes. West Bengal State Book Board Publisher 1-271.

21. Sukul NC (1992) Plants antagonistic to plant parasitic nematodes. Indian

Review of Life Science 12: 23-52.

22. Sukul NC (1994) Control of plant parasitic nematodes by plant substances. Allelopathy in Agriculture and Forestry, (Edited by S.S. Narwal and P. Tauro), Scientific Publisher, Jodhpur, India, 183-211.

23. Chatterjee A, Sukul NC (1981) Total protein of galled roots as an index of root-knot nematode infestation of lady's finger plants, Phytopathology 71: 372-274.

24. Gunasekhar V, Govindaiah, Datta RK (1994) Occurrence of *Altemaria* Leaf blight of mulberry and a key for disease assessment. Int J Tropical Plant Dis 12: 53-57.

25. Datta SC (2005) Plant Parasitic nematodes – an agricultural problem and its solutions. Visva-Bharati Quarterly 11: 89-100.

26. Datta SC (2005) Possible use of amaranth as catch crop for root-knot nematodes intercropped with mulberry. Journal of Environ & Sociobiol 2: 61-65.

27. Das S, Sukul NC (1986) Biochemical changes of some crop plants due to root-knot nematode infection. Proceeding of National Symposium of New Dimension in Parasitology, Allahabad, India 86: 122-125.

28. Das S, Sukul NC, Mitra D, Sarkar H (1989) Distribution of lectin in nematode infested and uninfested roots of Hibiscus esculentus. Nematologica Mediterranea 17: 123-125.

29. Lowry OH, Rossebrough NJ, Farr AR, Randall RJ (1951) Protein measurement with the Folin-phenol reagent. Journal of Biological Chemistry 193: 265-275.

30. James WC (1971) An illustrated series of assessment keys for plant diseases, their preparation and usage. Can Plant Disease Surv 51: 39-65.

31. Allen SJ, Brown JF, Kochman JK (1983) Production of inoculums and field assessment of Atemaria helianthi on sunflower. Plant Disease 67: 665-668.

32. Sengupta K, Govindaiah, Pradip K, Murthuza B (1990) Hand book on pest and disease control of mulberry and silkworm- Disease of mulberry and their control. United Nations Economic and Social Commission for Asia and Pacific, Bangkok, Thailand 1-14.

33. Fenner LM (1962) Determination of nematode mortality. Plant Disease Reporter 46: 383.

34. Consden R, Gordon AH, Martin AJP (1944) Qualitative analysis of proteins: a partition chromatographic method using paper. J Biol Chem 38:224.

35. Krishnaswamy S, Narasimhanna MN, Suryanarayana SK,Kumararaj S (1972) Manual on sericulture, Silkworm rearing, Agric Services Bul 15, FAO, Rome.

36. Anonymous (1920) The American Homeopathic Pharmacopoeia. 9th edn, Philadelphia, USA: Boericke and Tafel.

37. Field B, Jordan F, Osbourn A (2006) First encounters – development of defense – related natural products by plants. New Phytologist 172: 193-207.

38. Zarter CR, Demmig-Adams B, Ebbert V, Adamska I, Adams WW III (2006) Photosynthetic capacity and light harvesting efficiency during the winter-to-spring transition in subalpine conifers. New Phytologist 172: 283-292.

6

Erythrocyte and Plasma Antioxidants in Bronchial Asthma Before and After Homeopathic Treatment

Shiefa Pinto[1], Ashalatha V Rao[2] and Anjali Rao[3]*

[1]Department of Biochemistry, Fr. Muller Medical College, Mangalore, Karnataka, India
[2]Department of Biochemistry, K. S. Hegde Medical Academy, Deralakatte Mangalore, Karnataka, India
[3]Department of Biochemistry, Kasturba Medical College, Manipal, India

Abstract

Objective: Oxidative stress is involved in the pathophysiology of bronchial asthma. The present study was done to assess the effectiveness of practicing homeopathy in modulating free radical toxicity in bronchial asthma by measuring some parameters of oxidant stress and antioxidant defenses in blood, before and after homeopathy treatment.

Methods: In the present study, erythrocyte lipid peroxidation (LP), erythrocyte antioxidants viz., glutathione (GSH), glutathione reductase (GR), superoxide dismutase (SOD), catalase (CT) and plasma antioxidants viz., ceruloplasmin, glutathione-S-transferase (GST), vitamin C, total antioxidant activity (AOA) have been determined in 41 patients with bronchial asthma and 53 control subjects. Twenty three patients who were treated with homeopathic remedies were considered for the follow-up studies.

Results: Erythrocyte LP (0 hour, $p<0.001$; 2 hours, $p<0.001$; and susceptibility to LP, $p<0.01$) and SOD ($p<0.05$) were significantly higher, whereas plasma vitamin C ($p<0.001$) and AOA ($p<0.001$) were significantly lower in bronchial asthma patients when compared to controls. In follow-up patients the erythrocyte LP (0 hour, $p<0.01$; 2 hours, $p<0.001$; and susceptibility to LP, $p<0.001$) and SOD ($p<0.01$) were significantly lower when compared to their pretreatment values. Plasma vitamin C attained a normal range. The AOA activity after treatment was not significantly different from that observed before treatment.

Conclusion: The present study showed an imbalance between antioxidants and oxidants in bronchial asthma. Oxidative stress had increased as indicated by increased LP, increased SOD, decreased vitamin C and decreased AOA. On homeopathic treatment the LP had decreased in the erythrocytes which shows that homeopathic treatment has some effect in reducing oxidative stress. This is further evidenced by returning of plasma vitamin C and erythrocyte SOD to the normal levels, but oxidant stress has not been completely overcome within the period of study as plasma AOA has still not returned to normal control levels. Thus, a prooxidant mileu exists in asthma patients which tends to normalize after homeopathic treatment.

Keywords: Free radicals; Homeopathy; Bronchial asthma

Introduction

Homeopathy, is a system of alternative medicine that strives to treat "like with like" [1,2]. It is used extensively throughout the world [3] being particularly popular in Europe and India [4,5]. The WHO definition of asthma is that it is a disease characterized by recurrent attacks of breathlessness and wheezing, which vary in severity and frequency from person to person. In an individual, they may occur from hour to hour and day to dayIn common with conventional medicine, homeopathy regards diseases as morbid derangements of the organism [1,2]. However, it differs in preferring to view each case of sickness as a strictly individual phenomenon. Homeopathy rests on the premise of treating sick persons with extremely diluted agents that in undiluted doses are deemed to produce similar symptoms in a healthy individual. Belief in the effectiveness of homeopathy in general is wide-spread and growing among the physicians and public [5-7]. Homeopathic treatment has also been found to be effective in treatment of respiratory tract disorders [4].

Asthma is a lower airways disease characterized by enhanced responsiveness to a variety of stimuli and manifested by airways obstruction that changes spontaneously or therapeutically [8]. Airways are unique in both their exposure to high levels of environmental oxidants and their unusually high concentration of extracellular antioxidants. Oxidative stress may play an important role in the pathophysiology of asthma [9-12] and may be a final common

pathway leading to tissue damage. Variety of different substances such as allergens, gaseous pollutants, chemicals, drugs, bacteria and viruses [13] leads to the recruitment and activation of inflammatory cells which have an exceptional capacity for producing oxidants in asthmatic airways. Activated eosinophils, neutrophils, monocytes, macrophages and also resident cells such as bronchial epithelial cells, generate oxidants [10,14-19]. Allergen-specific reactions involving the acquired immune system are characterized by the production of interleukin (IL-5) and the subsequent recruitment and activation of eosinophils. In contrast, stimuli that act *via* the innate immune system lead to the production of IL-8 and the subsequent recruitment and activation of neutrophils. However, both of these pathways lead to the production of ROS, primarily due to the respiratory burst of activated inflammatory cells [20].

***Corresponding author:** Anjali Rao, Professor of Biochemistry, Kasturba Medical College, Manipal – 576104, Karnataka, India
E-mail: dranjalirao@hotmail.com

Oxidative stress can have many detrimental effects on airway function including airway smooth muscle contraction [21], induction of airway hyper responsiveness [22,23], mucus hypersecretion [24,25], epithelial shedding [26] and vascular exudation [27,28]. Furthermore, ROS can induce cytokine and chemokine production through induction of the oxidative stress-sensitive transcription of nuclear factor-κB in bronchial epithelial cells [29].

In the present work, a study has been carried out on the levels of few oxidant and antioxidant parameters in plasma and RBC in order to find out whether they correlate with reported findings in respiratory airways and epithelium and also to find out whether homeopathic treatment has any influence on them.

Material and Methods

Study design

The study plan was approved by the Ethics Committee of the Medical Faculty, and all subjects volunteered for the trial.

Exclusion/inclusion criteria

Patients coming for the first time for homeopathic treatment were considered. They were advised not to take any other medications. Exclusion criteria included pregnancy, human immunodeficiency virus infection, and history of respiratory infection in the previous 6 weeks.

Blood samples were obtained from 41 bronchial asthma patients (males 17, females 24), aged 20-70 (mean age 36.71$\pm$ 0.624) years. They were on homeopathic services at Fr. Muller Homeopathic Hospital during the period July 2004 to July 2006. These patients suffered from one or more of the following symptoms-wheezing, breathlessness, sneezing and cough. Classical homeopathy was followed where a comprehensive homeopathic history was taken, followed by prescription of a single individualized remedy in response to changing symptoms. For follow-up studies only 23 patients were available. From these patients, another blood sample was collected after 3 months of treatment. Different oxidant and antioxidant parameters were estimated in blood samples obtained before and after treatment. Following treatment with homeopathic drugs 75% of the patients who had come for followup studies felt a relief in their symptoms. The results were compared with those obtained in age and sex matched healthy non hospitalized individuals who were considered as normal controls. The control group consisted of 53 individuals (36 males, 17 females), aged 24 to 64 (mean age 45.42 $\pm$ 1.36) years. They had no history of bronchial asthma. They did not suffer from any one or more of the following symptoms-wheezing, breathlessness, sneezing and cough. A consent form was taken from them before blood samples were taken from them. Subjects who had come to the OPD for normal routine health checkups and had all parameters normal were taken for the study.

Methodology

Random blood samples were collected in heparinised bottles from normal subjects and bronchial asthma patients. Plasma and RBC's were separated. 50% erythrocyte suspensions were prepared according to the method of Kartha and Krishnamurthy [30]. These suspensions were used for some of the assays performed. The assays performed in the erythrocytes were lipid peroxidation (LP), glutathione (GSH), glutathione reductase (GR), catalase (CT), and in plasma were glutathione-S-transferase (GST), vitamin C, ceruloplasmin, antioxidant activity (AOA).

The hemoglobin content of the erythrocytes was determined by the cyanmethemoglobin method. Erythrocyte LP was determined by incubating RBC suspension in saline phosphate buffer containing 0.44M H_2O_2 at 0 hour and 2 hours. Aliquots were drawn from the above mixture at 0 hour and 2 hours. Lipid peroxidation in RBC was determined by estimating malondialdehyde (MDA) produced using thiobarbituric acid [31]. Erythrocyte GR activity was determined by recording the decrease in absorbance due to depletion of NADPH for a period of 5 minutes at 340nm [32]. SOD was determined according to the method of Beauchamp and Fridovich [33] based on inhibition of nitrozolium reduction. CT activity in the hemolysate was determined by adopting the method of Brannan et al. [34]. The assay is based on the disappearance of H_2O_2 in the presence of the enzyme source at 26°C. The GSH content of erythrocytes was determined as described by Beutler et al. [35].

Plasma ceruloplasmin was determined by p-phenylene diamine

Names of homeopathic Medications	Number of lines	Total homeopathic medications	
		%	Total (%)
Arsenicum alb	24	19.67	19.67
Pulsatilla	12	9.83	29.50
Antimonium tartaricum	10	8.20	37.7
Natrum sulphuricum	8	6.56	44.26
Kali carbonicum	8	6.56	50.82
Ferrum Phosphoricum	6	4.91	55.73
Ammonium carbonicum	6	4.91	60.64
Phosporus	5	4.1	64.74
Sepia officinalis	5	4.1	68.84
Lycopodium clavatum	4	3.28	72.12
Natrum muriaticum	4	3.28	75.40
Magnesia Phosphorica	4	3.28	78.68
Nihilina	4	3.28	81.96
Calcarea flourica	3	2.46	84.42
Rhus toxicodendron	3	2.46	86.88
Nux Vomica	3	2.46	89.34
Sulphur	3	2.46	91.80
Others	10	8.20	100.00
Total medications	122	100.00	....

Table 1: The 17 most prescribed homeopathic medications in 41 patients.

Names of homeopathic Medications	Number of lines	Total homeopathic medications	
		%	Total (%)
Arsenicum alb	16	21.62	21.62
Pulsatilla	8	10.81	32.43
Antimonium tartaricum	6	8.11	40.54
Natrum sulphuricum	6	8.11	48.65
Ferrum Phosphoricum	7	9.46	58.11
Kali carbonicum	4	5.40	63.51
Sabedella	4	5.40	68.91
Magnesia Phosphorica	4	5.40	74.31
Ammonium carbonicum	3	4.06	78.37
Lycopodium clavatum	3	4.06	82.43
Nihilina	3	4.06	86.49
Others	10	13.51	100.00
Total medications	74	100.00	-------------

Table 2: The 11 most prescribed homeopathic medications for the 23 patients whose follow up blood sample were taken.

oxidase activity [36]. Plasma vitamin C was determined chemically using dinitrophenyl hydrazine as a colour compound [37]. Plasma GST was determined by incubating CDNB (1 chloro 2, 4 dinitro benzene) with reduced GSH in the presence of serum containing glutathione-S-transferase. 2, 4-dinitrophenylglutathione (adduct) formed was read at 340nm [38]. AOA activity was measured as given by Koracevic et al. [39].

The package used for statistical analysis was SPSS/PC+ (version 11.0).

Homeopathetic Treatment of Bronchial asthma patients

A total of 122 prescription lines were prescribed for 41 patients i.e. 2.9 medications per patient, on an average. One prescription line corresponds to one medication prescribed to one patient at the inclusion visit. Medications were given simultaneously or sequentially depending on the condition of the patient. Homeopathic treatment was prescribed for all the patients.

Table 1 shows the 17 homeopathic medications most prescribed in the study group (i.e, 41 patients) during this study, the main ones are: *Arsenicum alb, Pulsatilla, Antimonium tartaricum, Natrum sulphuricum, Kali carbonicum, Ferrum Phosphoricum* and *Ammonium carbonicum.*

Arsenicum alb, Pulsatilla, Antimonium tartaricum, Natrum sulphuricum, Kali carbonicum and *Ammonium carbonicum* were most often prescribed at a dilution of 30°c, whereas *Ferrum Phosphoricum* at 6x. 54% of the 41 patients received *Arsenicum alb* and 29% received *Pulsatilla. Antimonium tartaricum, Natrum sulphuricum, Kali carbonicum, Ferrum Phosphoricum* and *Ammonium carbonicum* were prescribed for 24%, 17%, 19%, 14% and 13% of the patients respectively.

Group	TBARS as nmol MDA/ g Hb (Mean ± SEM)		
	0 Hour	2 Hours	Susceptibility to LP
Normal Controls(NC) n=53	77.8 ± 4.46 (20.8 – 181.6)	384.5 ± 18.54 (102.8 – 898.7)	306.0± 16.65 (72.0-735.6)
Bronchial asthma n=41	101.9 ± 8.01 *** (20.3 – 299.1)	514.4 ± 31.32 *** (118.9 – 936.3)	412.5±30.00 ** (98.9-833.5)
% change	30.97%>NC	33.78% >NC	34.80%>NC

Statistical significance of results vs. NC:　** p< 0.01, *** p< 0.001.
Ranges of TBARS levels observed are given in parentheses
n= number of cases
(Mann-Whitney Test)

Table 3: Lipid peroxidation in bronchial asthma.

Clinical status	TBARS as nmol MDA/ g Hb Mean ± SEM		
	0 Hours	2 Hours	Susceptibility to LP
Before treatment n=23	118.2±12.10 (20.3-299.1)	552.7±47.20 (118.9-936.3)	434.5±45.87 (98.6-833.5)
After treatment n=23	77.0 ± 7.52 ** (20.9 – 169.9)	354.7 ± 23.90 *** (140.8 – 605.2)	277.8±22.10*** (86.1-465.7)
% change	34.80%< before Treatment	35.82%< before treatment	36.07 %< before treatment

Statistical significance of values obtained after treatment vs. values before treatment: ** p< 0.01, *** p< 0.001.
Ranges of TBARS levels observed are given in parentheses
n= number of cases
(Paired T-Test)

Table 4: Lipid peroxidation in bronchial asthma before and after treatment.

Diagnosis	GSH (µmol/g Hb)	SOD (units/g Hb)	Catalase (units/g Hb)	GR (units/g Hb)
Normal Controls(NC)	4.71 ± 0.209 (2.36 – 10.25) N=53	9214 ± 492.5 (4046 – 21990) n=53	245996 ± 10410.2 (27920 – 413385) n=53	1.77 ± 0.153 (0.10 – 4.09) n=51
Bronchial asthma	5.39 ± 0.382 (1.46 – 10.38) n=41 NS	11787 ± 986.4 * (2396 – 36053) n=41	283870 ± 23404.0 (77978 – 881356) n=41 NS	1.88 ± 0.199 (0.22 – 5.79) n=39 NS
% change	12.52%>NC	27.92%>NC	15.39% > NC	6.21%>NC

Statistical significance of results vs.NC:　p< 0.05, NS = Not significant.
The figures in the parentheses indicate the ranges of antioxidant levels observed
n= number of cases.
(Mann-Whitney Test).

Table 5: Erythrocyte antioxidant levels in bronchial asthma (Mean ± SEM).

Table 2 shows the 11 homeopathic medications most prescribed for 23 patients whose follow up blood sample was taken. *Arsenicum alb, Pulsatilla, Antimonium tartaricum, Natrum sulphuricum* and *Ferrum phosphoricum* were the main homeopathic treatments prescribed for the patients.

Results

Erythrocyte LP and susceptibility towards LP in bronchial asthma patients was significantly high compared to normal controls (Table 3). After treatment a significant decrease was observed in LP. Susceptibility was also decreased significantly (Table 4). SOD activity in the erythrocytes was found to be significantly increased in pre-treated asthmatic patients, compared with normal control subjects (Table 5). The enzyme activity decreased significantly in post-treated patients when compared to corresponding pretreated subjects (Table 6). A comparison of erythrocyte GSH, CT and GR in bronchial asthma

patients with those in normal controls showed no significant change (Tables 5, 6).

Plasma vitamin C level and AOA were significantly decreased in asthmatic patients, when compared with that of normal control subjects (Table 7). A comparison of vitamin C levels before and after treatment showed a significant increase in the latter (Table 8). After treatment, AOA remained significantly low when compared to normal subjects. There was no significant difference in the ceruloplasmin levels and GST in asthmatic patients when compared to normal controls before and after homeopathic treatment (Table 7, Table 8).

Discussion

Asthma prevalence has increased dramatically in the recent years [40]. Epidemiological evidence suggests that changes in diet, in particular reduced antioxidant intake, have contributed to increases in asthma prevalence and severity and raises the

Clinical Status	GSH (μmol/g Hb)	SOD (units/g Hb)	Catalase (Units/g Hb)	GR (Units/g Hb)
Pre-treatment	6.02+0.470 (1.46-10.38)	13276+1527.8 (3274 – 36053)	283221+35677 (77978 -881356)	2.02+0.0300 (0.28- 5.79)
Post-treatment	4.73 ± 0.278 (2.82 – 8.70) n=23 NS	9991 ± 999.9 ** (2340 – 23545.2) n=23	260732 ± 17343 (117935– 390472) n=23 NS	1.34 ± 0.259 (0.00 – 5.10) n=22 NS
% change	21.42%< before treatment Treatment	32.87%<before Treatment	7.94%< before treatment	33.66%<before treatment

Statistical significance of values obtained after treatment vs. values before treatment: NS = Not significant, ** p< 0.01.
The figures in the parentheses indicate the ranges of antioxidants levels observed
n= number of cases.
(Wilcoxon Signed Ranks Test).

Table 6: Follow up studies of various erythrocyte antioxidants in bronchial asthma patients.

Diagnosis	Vitamin C (μmol/L)	Ceruloplasmin (g/L)	GST (IU/L)	AOA (mmol/L)
Normal Controls(NC)	22.5 ± 1.23 (3.5 – 49.5) n=53	0.479 ± 0.0268 (0.225 – 1.400) n=53	4.31 ± 0.450 (0.41 – 15.41) n=53	1.03 ± 0.060 (0.32 – 2.20) n=53
Bronchial asthma	12.4 ± 1.40*** $ (0.7 – 42.3) n=41	0.580 ± 0.055 (0.046 – 2.140) n=41 NS	4.27 ± 0.583 (0.00 – 20.80) n=41 NS	0.54 ± 0.035 *** # (0.22 – 1.05) n=36 NS
% change	44.88%<NC	21.08>NC	0.92%<NC	47.57%<NC

Statistical significance of results vs. NC: ** p< 0.01, *** p< 0.001, NS = Not Significant.
The figures in the parentheses indicate the ranges of antioxidant levels observed
n= number of cases.
($=Anova, # =Mann-Whitney Test)

Table 7: Plasma antioxidant levels in bronchial asthma patients (Mean± SEM).

Clinical Status	Vitamin C (μmol/L)	Ceruloplasmin (g/L)	GST (IU/L)	AOA (mmol/L)
Pre-treatment	13.1 ± 2.12 (3.1- 42.3)	0.597 ± 0.8300 (0.150 – 2.140)	3.84 ± 0.485 (0.50 -10.41)	0.47 ± 0.043 (0.22-1.02)
Post-treatment	26.0 ± 2.55 ** (4.2 – 46.6) n=23	0.519 ± 0.0875 (0.75 – 2.300) n=23 NS	4.62 ± 0.612 (0.31 – 11.45) n=23 NS	0.53 ± 0.045 (0.22 – 1.04) n=21 NS
% change	98.47%>before treatment	13.06%<before treatment	20.31%>before treatment	12.76%>before treatment

Statistical significance of values obtained after treatment vs. values before treatment: NS = Not significant.
The figures in the parentheses indicate the ranges of antioxidant levels observed
n= number of cases.
(Wilcoxon Signed Rank test)

Table 8: Follow up studies of plasma antioxidants in bronchial asthma patients (Mean± SEM).

possibility that dietary interventions may improve asthma [41]. Lipid peroxidation is of particular significance inasthma. Recent studies have demonstrated [42] elevated plasma lipid peroxidation in asthma, as measured by 8-iso-PGF$_{2\alpha}$ Elevated MDA levels have been observed in both plasma [43-46] and breathe condensate in asthmatics [47]. Studies done by Nadeem et al. [48] showed increased plasma levels of lipid peroxidation products, measured as TBARS in asthmatic patients. The results of present work are also in agreement with these findings as judged by increased RBC lipid peroxidation. In vitro lipid peroxidation of RBC has significantly increased at 0 hour in asthmatic patients when compared to normal controls. The TBARS concentration at 2 hours is also significantly increased in asthmatic patients when compared to control subjects. Even the susceptibility towards lipid peroxidation has increased significantly.

Important antioxidants in the respiratory tract lining fluid include reduced GSH, mucin, uric acid, vitamin C and albumin [49]. GSH is a key antioxidant in the lining fluid of the respiratory tract. It is 100-fold more concentrated in the airway epithelial lining fluid compared with plasma. The glutathione system is a central mechanism for reducing H$_2$O$_2$. It complements catalase as a reducing system for H$_2$O$_2$ but exceeds catalase in its capacity to eliminate additional varieties of toxic peroxides [50]. Disturbed GSH status is reported in asthma, with total [51] and oxidized [52] GSH being elevated in bronchoalveolar larvage (BAL) fluid and reduced GSH being elevated in erythrocytes [53]. Studies done by Nadeem et al. [48] showed similar results suggesting that GSH synthesis and/or transport has increased in response to the presence of excess oxidants and has subsequently been oxidized as it performs its antioxidant role. However, in the present study no increase was observed in the GSH levels in asthmatic patients.

Reports on SOD enzymatic antioxidant status in asthma are inconsistent. Studies done by Kurosawa et al. [54] in platelets of bronchial asthmatic patients showed significantly higher levels of SOD activity than those of normal healthy subjects. Nadeem et al [55] have shown an increase in SOD activity in the erythrocytes. In the present work also an increase in SOD activity in the erythrocytes was observed and this is in agreement with the above findings. This increase in SOD in the RBC cells might be a compensatory mechanism for increased oxidative stress. However, Powell et al [55] did not find increased activity of erythrocyte SOD in their study. Smith [56] reported unchanged levels of SOD in BAL. Tekin et al. [57] and Fenech [58] have reported decreased SOD activity in erythrocytes of asthmatics compared with controls. De Raeve et al [59] have reported decreased SOD activity in bronchial epithelial cells. Zn, a cofactor of SOD, has also been reported to be decreased [60] or unchanged [61].

Catalase is most effective in the presence of high H$_2$O$_2$ concentrations. In the present study, the red blood cell catalase activity was not found to be changed. Similar studies done by Nadeem et al. [48] and Tekin et al. [57] in the erythrocytes of asthmatics showed no change in catalase activity when compared to control subjects. This might be because the hydrogen peroxide formed after dismutation of superoxide anion by SOD can be actively scavenged by normal levels of catalase.

A study by Yang et al. [62] have emphasized on the critical role of the copper containing enzyme, ceruloplasmin in defence against oxidative damage and infection in the lungs. However in the present study, no significant alteration in plasma ceruloplasmin levels was observed when compared to control subjects.

Olusi et al. [63] have reported a decrease in plasma vitamin C level in asthmatic patients when compared to control subjects. Similar results were obtained in the present work. There was a marked decrease in plasma vitamin C level in asthmatic patients when compared to control subjects. Olusi et al [63] have also reported decrease vitamin C levels in leucocytes of asthmatics. Recent studies found that supplementation with vitamin C reduced ozone related decrement in lung function in asthmatic subjects, particularly in those with genetically determined increased susceptibility to oxidative stress [64].

In the present study, the plasma total antioxidant capacity in asthmatic patients was significantly lower than that in control subjects. Rahman et al. [65] also reported a decreased total antioxidant capacity of plasma in asthmatic patients. The decrease in the total plasma antioxidant level may partly be because of decrease in plasma vitamin C which is an important antioxidant. Following treatment with homeopathic drugs 75% of the patients who had come for followup studies felt a relief in their symptoms. The concentration of lipid peroxides in these patients decreased significantly both at 0 hour and 2 hours. This indicates that the homeopathic drugs had the effect of reducing lipid peroxidation in asthmatics. However, they had no significant antioxidant activity invitro.

The erythrocyte antioxidant enzyme SOD significantly decreased after treatment compared to pre-treatment values almost reaching normal levels. The antioxidant vitamin of plasma i.e. vitamin C increased to normal range. But total antioxidant activity remained significantly low. This seems to indicate that other antioxidants which contribute to total antioxidant activity are not affected by the treatment. Glutathione reductase activity was increased after treatment. Probably this is a reflection of increase in antioxidant capacity of erythrocytes to counter the oxidant change.

While it is difficult to compare the data due to differences in the disease severity it is clear that, overall status of the antioxidant enzymes and their cofactors is often altered in asthma, indicating a disturbed oxidant/antioxidant balance. Following homeopathic treatment the oxidative stress is decreased at least partially. This is evidenced by significant decrease in lipid peroxidation, increase in vitamin C and decrease in SOD.

Limitation of this study

Although this study is the first of its kind in homeopathy it has certain limitations. Biomarkers like eosiophil count (Eosinophilia), NF-KB, neutrophils, monocytes, macrophages, macrophage degranulation assay, B-cell, IgE estimation, allergen-specific reactions (interleukin) IL-5, IL-8 IL-4, CD^4, CD^8 cell or secondary messenger assays etc. could have been performed to make the study more complete. However, these assays could add on to the future scope of this study.

References

1. Andrew L, Nicola G (1995) In: The complete guide to homeopathy, edited by Blanche S. Dorling Kindersley London, NewYork 11-19.

2. Andrew L, Stephanic F, Dorling Kindersley (2000) In: Encyclopedia of Homeopathy. London, NewYork 200: 12-25.

3. Ernst E (2005) Is homeopathy a clinically valuable approach?. Trends in Pharmacological Sciences 26: 547-548.

4. Medhurst R (2004) The use of homeopathy around the world. J Australian Traditional Medicine Society 10: 153.

5. Samir M, Bhatia GS, Pandhi P (2001) Patterns of use of unconventional therapies in the medical outpatient department of a tertiary care hospital in India. J Etnopharmacology 75: 71-75.

6. Knipschild P, Kleijnen J, Riet TG (1990) Belief in the efficacy of alternative medicine among general practitioners in the Netherlands. Soc Sci Med 31: 625-626.

7. Ernst E, Resch KL, White AR (1995) Complementary medicine-what physicians think of it; a meta-analysis. Arch Inter Med 155: 2405-2408.

8. David PS, Philip F (2006) Asthma. In: Atlas of allergies and clinical immunology. Philadelphia, Pennsylvania 81-113.

9. Niki LR, Emiel FM, Yvonne MWJ (2007) Modulation of Glutaredoxin-1 Expression in a mouse model of allergic airway disease. Am J Respir Cell Mol Biol 36: 147-151.

10. Barnes PJ (1990) Reactive oxygen species and airway inflammation. Free Rad Biol Med 109: 235-243.

11. Doelman CJA, Bast A (1990) Oxygen radicals in lung pathology. Free Rad Biol Med 9: 381-400.

12. Mak JCW, Chang-Yeung MW (2006) Reactive oxidant species in asthma. Curr Opinion Pulm Med 12: 7-11.

13. Levine SJ (1995) Bronchial epithelial cell-cytokine interactions in airway inflammation. Invest Med 43: 241-249.

14. Barnes PJ, Chung KF, Page CP (1998) Inflammatory mediators of asthma: an update. Pharmacol Rev 50: 515-596.

15. Andres LE, Irfan R, Victor P, Joan AB, Josep R, et al. (2005) Lack of systemic oxidative stress during PAF challenge in mild asthma. Respiratory medicine 99: 519 -523.

16. Bowler RP, Crapo JD (2002) Oxidative stress in allergic respiratory diseases. J Allergy Clin Immunol 110: 349–356.

17. Dworski R (2000) Oxidant stress in asthma. Thorax 55: 51-53.

18. Henricks PA, Nijkamp FP (2001) Reactive oxygen species as mediators in asthma. Pulm Pharmacol Ther 14: 409-420.

19. Rahman I, MacNee W (2002) Reactive oxygen species. In: Asthma and COPD, edited by Barnes PJ, Drazen J, Rennard S, London, Academic Press 243-254.

20. Aldridge RE, Chan T, Dalen CJ (2002) Eosinophil peroxidase produces hypobromous acid in the airways of stable asthmatics. Free Radic Biol Med 33: 847-856.

21. Rhoden KJ, Barnes PJ (1989) Effect of hydrogen peroxide on guinea-pig tracheal muscle in vitro: role of cyclo-oxygenase and airway epithelium. Br J Pharmacol 98: 325-330.

22. Katsumata U, Miura M, Ichinose M et al. (1990) Oxygen radicals produce airway constriction and hyperresponsiveness in anesthetized cats. Am Rev Respir Dis 141: 1158-1161.

23. Weiss EB, Bellino JR (1986) Leukotriene-associated toxic oxygen metabolites induces airway hyperreactivity. Chest 89: 709-716.

24. Adler KB, Holden-Stauffer WJ, Repine JE (1990) Oxygen metabolites stimulate release of high-molecular weight glycoconjugates by cell and organ cultures of rodent respiratory epithelium via arachidonic acid dependent mechanism. J Clin Invest 85: 75-85.

25. Phipps RJ, Denas SM, Sielczak MV, Wanner A (1990) effects of 0.5ppm ozone on glycoprotein secretion, ion and water fluxes in sheep trachea. J Appl Physiol 60: 918-927.

26. Doelman CJA, Leurs R, Oosterom WC, Bast A (1990) Mineral dust exposure and free radical-mediated lung damage. Exp Lung Res 16: 41-55.

27. Maestro DRF, Bjork J, Arfors K (1981) "Increase in microvascular permeability induced by enzymatically generated free radicals." I. In vivo study. Microvasc Res 22: 239-254.

28. Tate RM, Benthuysen VKM, Shasby DM, McMurtry IF, Repine JE (1992) Oxygen-radical-mediated permeability edema and vasoconstriction in isolated perfused rabbit lungs. Am Rev Respir Dis 126: 802–806.

29. Biagioli MC, Kaul P, Singh I, Turner RB (1999) The role of oxidative stress in rhinovirus Induced elaboration of IL-8 by respiratory epithelial cells. Free Rad Biol Med 26: 454-462.

30. Kartha VN, Krishnamurthy S (1978) Factors affecting in vitro lipid peroxidation of rat brain homogenate. Ind J Physiol Pharmacol 22: 44-52.

31. Stocks J, Dormandy TL (1971) The auto-oxidation of human red cell lipids induced by hydrogen peroxide. B J Haematol 20: 95-111.

32. Horn HD, Burns FH Glutathione reductase. In: Bergmeyer HV editor. Methods of Enzymatic Analysis. Academic Press, NewYork 1978: 875.

33. Beauchamp C, Fridrovich I (1971) Superoxide dismutase: improved assays and an assay applicable to acrylamide gels. Anal Biochem 44: 276-287.

34. Brannan TS, Maker HS, Raes IP (1989) Regional distribution of catalase in the adult rat brain. J Neurochem 36: 307-309.

35. Beutler E, Duron O, Kelly BM (1963) Improved method for the determination of blood glutathione. J Lab Clin Med 61: 882-888.

36. William SF, Shozo N (1970) Measurement of Serum ceruloplasmin by its p phenylenediamine oxidase activity. Clinical Chemistry 16: 903-909.

37. Norbert WT (1986) In: Nobert WT editor. Text book of Clinical Chemistry 960.

38. Adachi Y, Horii K, Takahashi Y, Tanihata M, Ohba Y, et al. (1980) Serum glutathione-S-transferase activity in liver diseases. Clin Chim Acta 106: 243-255.

39. Koracevic D, Koracevic G, Djordjevic V, Andrejevic S, Cosic V (2001) Method for the measurement of antioxidant activity in human fluid. J Clin Pathol 54: 356-361.

40. Downs SH, Marks GB, Sporik R, Belosouva EG, Car NG, et al. (2001) Continued increase in the prevalence of asthma and atopy. Arch Dis Child 84: 20–23.

41. Fogarty A, Britton J (2000) The role of diet in the aetiology of asthma. Clin Exp Allergy 30: 615-627.

42. Wood LG, Fitzgerald DA, Gibson PG, Cooper DM, Garg ML (2000) Lipid peroxidation as determined by plasma isoprostanes is related to disease severity in mild asthma. Lipids 35: 967-974.

43. Rahman I, Morrison D, Donaldson K, MacNee W (1996) Systemic oxidative stress in asthma, COPD and smokers. Am J Respir Crit Care Med 154: 1055-1060.

44. Kalayci O, Besler T, Kilinc K, Sekerel BE, Saraclar Y (2000) Serum levels of antioxidant vitamins (alpha tocopherol, beta carotene, and ascorbic acid) in children with bronchial asthma. Turkish J Pediatr 42: 17–21.

45. Shanmugasundaram KR, Kumar SS, Rajajee S (2001) Excessive free radical generation in the blood of children suffering from asthma. Clinica Chimica Acta 305: 107-114.

46. Ozarus R, Tahan V, Turkmen S, Fahrettin T, Kazim B et al (2000) "Changes in malondialdehyde levels in bronchoalveolar fluid and serum by the treatment of asthma with inhaled steroid and beta2-agonist." Respirology 5: 289–292.

47. Antczak A, Nowak D, Shariati B, Krol M, Piasecka G, et al. (1997) "Increased hydrogen peroxide and thiobarbituric acid-reactive products in expired breath condensate of asthmatic patients." Eur Respir J 10: 1235-1241.

48. Nadeem A, Chhabra SK, Masood A, Raj HG (2003) Increased oxidative stress and altered levels of antioxidants in asthma. J Allergy and Clinical Immunology 111: 72-78.

49. Cross CE, van der Vliet A, O'Neill C, Louie S, Halliwell B (1994) Oxidants, antioxidants, and respiratory tract lining fluids. Environ Health Perspect 102: 185–191.

50. Ross D, Norbeck K, Moldeus P (1985) The generation and subsequent fate of glutathionyl radicals in biological systems. J Biol Chem 260: 15028-15032.

51. Smith LJ, Houston M, Anderson J (1993) Increased levels of glutathione in

bronchoalveolar lavage fluid from patients with asthma. Am Rev Respir Dis 147: 1461-1464.

52. Kelly FJ, Mudway I, Blomberg A, Frew A, Sandstrom T (1999) Altered lung antioxidant status in patients with mild asthma. Lancet 354: 482-483.

53. Vural H, Uzun K (2000) Serum and red blood cell antioxidant status in patients with bronchial asthma. Can Respir J 7: 476-480.

54. Kurosawa M, Kobayashi H, Nakano M (1993) Cu-Zn superoxide dismutase activities in platelets from stable bronchial asthmatic patients. Int Arch Allergy Immunol 101: 61-65.

55. Powell CVE, Nash AA, Powers HJ, Primhak RA (1994) Antioxidant status in asthma. Pediatr Pulmonol 18: 34-38.

56. Smith LJ, Shamsuddin M, Sporn PHS, Denenberg M, Anderson J (1997) Reduced superoxide dismutase in lung cells of patients with asthma. Free Rad Biol Med 22: 1301-1307.

57. Tekin D, Ayse SB, Mungan D, Misirligil Z, Yavuzer S (2000) The antioxidant defense in asthma. J Asthma 37: 59-63.

58. Fenech AG, Ellul-Micallef R (1998) Selenium, glutathione peroxidase and superoxide dismutase in Maltese asthmatic patients: effects of glucocorticoid administration. Pulm Pharmacol Ther 11: 301-308.

59. DeRaeve HR, Thunnissen FBMJ, Kaneko FT, Guo FH, Lewis M, et al. (1997) Decreased Cu,Zn-SOD activity in asthmatic airway epithelium: Correction by inhaled corticosteroid in vivo. Am J Physiol 272: 148-154.

60. Vural H, Uzun K, Uz E, Kocyigit A, Cigli A, et al. (2000) O Concentrations of copper, zinc and various elements in serum of patients with bronchial asthma. J Trace Elements Med Biol 14: 88-91.

61. Goldey DH, Mansmann HC, Rasmussen AI (1984) Zinc status of asthmatic, prednisone-treated asthmatic and non-asthmatic children. J Am Dietetic Assoc 84: 157-163.

62. Yang F, Friedrichs WE, deGraffenried L, Herbert DC, Weaker FJ, et al. (1996) "Cellular expression of ceruloplasmin in baboon and mouse lung during development and inflammation." Am J Respir Cell Mol Biol 14: 161-169.

63. Olusi SO, Ojutiku OO, Jessop WJ, Iboko MI (1997) Plasma and white blood cell ascorbic acid concentrations in patients with bronchial asthma. Clinica Chimica Acta 92: 161-166.

64. Romieu I, Sienra-Monge JJ, Ramirez M, Moreno-Macías H, Reyes-Ruiz NI, et al. (2004) Genetic polymorphism of GSTM1 and antioxidant supplementation influence lung function in relation to ozone exposure in asthmatic children in Mexico City. Thorax 59: 8-10.

65. Katsoulis K, Kontaklotis T, Leonardopoulos I, Kotsovili A, Legakis IN, et al. (2003) Serum total antioxidant status in severe exacerbation of asthma: Correlation with the Severity of the disease. J Asthma 40: 847-854.

7

Management of Urolithiasis (Mutrashmari) by an Ayurvedic Preparation *VarunaMulatwak Kashaya*

Siddaram Arawatti[1]*, Seema Murthy[2], Pandey BB[1] and Shringi MK[1]

[1]Department of Shalya tantra, National Institute of Ayurveda, Jaipur, India
[2]NKJ Ayurvedic Medical College, Bidar, Karnataka, India

Abstract

Introduction: In the present study an effort was made to evaluate the efficacy of *Varunamulatwak kashaya* (decoction of *Crataeva nurvala* rootbark and *Moringa oleifera* bark). The main aim of this particular study was inclined towards the disintegration, dissolution, dislodgement and expulsion of renal stones. These drugs are easily available, economical and are easy to administer, which are having anti-inflammatory, diuretic and Antilithic properties. Total 30 patients were selected randomly and were divided into two groups i.e. Group-I and Group-II each group contains 15 patients. Group-I: This group was treated with *Varunamulatwak kwatha* in a dose of 45 ml, twice daily, after food for a period of 45 days. Group-II: This group was treated with Flush out therapy (hydro therapy). After completion of the study with *Varunamulatwak Kashaya* for 45 days, the results were encouraging. The efficacy of *Varunamulatwak kashaya* in relief of Pain (76%), Haematuria (83%), Dysuria (76%), Size of calculi (74%) and Number of calculi (68.7%) was highly significant. Hence it was concluded that traditional ayurvedic management is effective and have no adverse effects on the patients of Urolithiasis.

Keywords: Mutrashmari; Urolithiasis; *Varunamulatwak kashaya*; *Crataeva nurvala*

Introduction

Urinary stone constitute one of the commonest diseases in our country and pain due to kidney stones is known as worse than that of labour pain. Among all the pain, abdominal pain always drags not only patient's attention but also the curiosity of the surgeon. The information regarding *Ashmari* [1,2] is available in almost all *samhita* (Ancient treatise) of Ayurveda. In India, approximately 5-7 million patients suffer from stone disease [3,4] and at least 1/1000 of Indian population needs hospitalization due to kidney stone disease. Thus, the disease is as widespread as it is old, particularly in countries with dry, hot climate [5]. These are "stone belt regions". The incidence of calculi varies as per geographical distribution, sex and age group. The recurrence rate is 50 to 80%. Males are more frequently affected than the female and their ratio is 4:3 [6]. The incidence is still higher in the age group between 30-45 years and incidence declines after age of 50.

In *Ayurveda* numbers of drugs are mentioned to treat *mutrashmari* [5]. Among them the '*Varunamulatwak kwatha*', which is mentioned in *Chakradatta* text 34/25 [7], was selected for the study. This compound drug is advised in decoction form. This drug can be given on O.P.D basis and is administered without requiring hospitalization. These drugs are easily available, economical and are easy to administer. These are also using since ancient period traditionally. These are having anti-inflammatory [8], diuretic and Antilithic [9] properties. Hence the clinical study has been undertaken to evaluate the efficacy of '*Varunamulatwak kwatha*' in the management of Urolithiasis.

Aims and objectives of the study were:

- To evaluate therapeutic effect of *Varunamulatwak kwatha* in *Mutrashmari*.

- To know the efficacy of the conservative medical treatment.

Materials and Methods

The present clinical study was a single blind clinical study where 30 patients were selected by random sampling procedure, attending the OPD (Out Patient Department) of NKJ Ayurvedic Medical College and Hospital, Bidar, Karnataka. The selection of cases was done on the bases of clinical presentation and the diagnosis was established accordingly. The selected patients were divided into two groups, 15 in each.

Group-A (Trail group): This group was treated with *Varunamulatwak kwatha* in a dose of 45 ml, twice daily, after food for a period of 45 days.

Group-B (Control group): This group was treated with oral fluid intake if patient unable to take orally then flush out therapy (hydro therapy).

Patients of both the groups were advised for a follow up on every Fifteen days (2 weeks) for 3 times, during treatment. The patient was advised to drink 3-4 litres of water per day and to consume suitable diet with proper sleep and excretion of natural urges. Patients were advised to avoid milk, tomato, cauliflower, spinach, fish and meat (incompatible diets and regimen) during the period of treatment [10].

Inclusion criteria

Patients were selected between 20 to 50 yrs age group, irrespective of sex, having calculi size less than 8 mm anywhere on KUB. Patient's those who were ready to give written consent.

Exclusion criteria

Patients with size of calculi greater than 8 mm, patients with systemic pathology and any acute urinary obstructive condition.

Diagnostic phase

The patients complaining of pain abdomen and other related

---

*Corresponding author: Dr. Siddaram Arawatti, M.S.(Ay), Ph.D. Scholar, Shalya Tantra Department, National Institute of Ayurveda, Zoravar singh Gate, Amer Road, Jaipur -302002, India, E-mail: drsidd1273@gmail.com

symptoms like Dysuria, Haematuria and burning micturition were selected and all these patients were subjected to through general and systemic examination i.e. microscopic examination of urine, X-ray KUB and USG. After the diagnosis was confirmed the patients were registered for the clinical study.

Varunamulatwak kwatha

This is the drug used in the study. The ingredients of this yoga are *Varunamula twak* [11] + *Shigru mula* [11] + Water.

Preparation of *Varunamulatwak kwatha*

Varunamulatwak + Shigru mula ↓

Added 32 parts of water ↓

Boild in *Mandagni*(low flame) ↓

Reduced for ¼ part ↓

Kwatha(decoction) is preparid ↓

(**Varunamula twak kwatha**)

Dosage: 45 ml of kwatha both the times is advice after meals for 45 days [12].

Flush out therapy

The procedure in which intravenous fluids are administered to the patient (in an attempt to flush them out). Intravenous fluid administration is a standard therapy for stones.

Materials: IV stand, IV set, scalp vein needle, spirit swab, adhesive plaster strips and IV Fluid bottle-NS 0.9%.

Procedure: The distal limb was compressed with hand in pumping motion to press the blood into the vein then the vein was palpated and cleaned with spirit swab. Then the vein was punctured with the scalp vein needle and the compressing hand was released and IV was connected, set to the Scalp vein needle. The regulating clamp was opened and the flow was adjusted to 20 drops/minute. The scalp vein needle was fixed securely with 3 to 4 adhesive strips.

Dosage: 2 L 0.9% saline over 4 hours.

Assessment phase

The patients were assessed on the basis of subjective and objective parameters before and after treatment.

A. **Subjective criteria**

• Pain abdomen

• Haematuria

• Dysuria

B. **Objective criteria**

• Size of stone

• Site of stone

• Number of the stone

Assessment criteria

Subjective criteria: Pain abdomen [13]**:** Pain was assessed by VAS (Visual Analogue Scale): In terms of sufferer it is Grade 0: Absence of pain/No pain; Grade I: 1 to 3 mark on scale (mild pain); Grade II: 4 to 6 mark on scale (moderate pain cannot be ignored, interferes with function, and needs treatment from time to time); Grade III: 7 to 10 mark on scale (severe-requires constant attention) [6].

Haematuria: was assessed by routine urine examination and presence and absence of RBC. Grade 0: Absence of RBC's in urine; Grade I: Presence of RBC's in urine; Grade II: More than 3-5 RBCs in urine; Grade III: More than 3-5 RBC.

Dysuria: was assessed by history of pain and radiation during micturition. Grade 0-Absence of pain during micturation; Grade 1-Mild pain during micturition; Grade 2-Moderate pain during micturition; Grade 3-Severe pain during micturition.

Objective criteria: Size of stone: was assessed by USG every week in mm. Grade 0 (good): More than 50% of decrease in size; Grade 1 (fair): In between 25% to 50% of decrease size; Grade 2 (poor): Less than 25% of decrease in size; Grade 3 (no response): No change in size.

Site of stone: was assessed under USG guidance and graded as follows. Grade 0: Expelled; Grade 1: Stone in bladder; Grade 2: Stone in ureter; Grade 3: Stone in renal pelvis.

PH of urine: was assessed by biochemical examination of urine.

Blood urea: was assessed by routine urine examination.

Serum creatinine: was assessed by routine urine examination.

X-ray KUB: was assessed before treatment and after treatment and was presented with Present (1) and Absent (0).

USG: was assessed before treatment and after treatment and was presented with Present (1) and Absent (0).

Assessment of result: For the purpose of the assessment of result we have used some grade points considering the severity of different sign and symptoms and clinical assessment of result of result was done as:- cure: 100% free from cardinal sign and symptoms (pain abdomen, haematuria, dysuria, site of stone and dislodgement). Maximum improvement: 75% to 99% improvement of the above mentioned cardinal sign and symptom. Moderate improvement: 50% to 75% improvement of the above mentioned cardinal sign and symptom. Mild improvement: 25% to 50% improvement of the above mentioned cardinal sign and symptom. No improvement: less them 25% improvement of the above mentioned cardinal sign and symptom.

Observations and Results

All the patients were advised to take similar dietary regimen. The duration of treatment was 45 days in maximum. The clinical assessment was done in every 15th day's interval. The initial finding through clinical, pathological and radiological statements were compared with the result of progressive 15th day, 30th day and 45th day and so on of investigations. Grading and grouping according to the assessment criteria concerned to each item categorically differentiated the findings among the patients in the clinical study. And finally the assessment as a whole was presented in percent value. In order to present the study in a scientific manner the statistical assessment of the result were assessed of result mean ± S.D of each sign and symptom before treatment was compared with mean ± S.D value of after treatment, *t*-test was used for the purpose of the test of significance the effectiveness *Varunamulatwak kwatha* and was assessed through p-value (Tables 1- 4) (Figure 1).

Discussion

From the present study it becomes evident that the urological

Observations	Predominance	Percentage
Age	30-39 and 40-49	33.33%
Sex	Male	73.33%
Religion	Hindu individuals	76.66%
Habitat	Urban area	66.66%
Marital status	Married	73.33%
Educational status	Higher secondary	43.33%
Socio-economic status	Lower Middle class	56.66%
Occupation	Service	43.33%
Dietary habits	Mixed	73.33%
Site of the Stone	Ureteric	50%

Table 1: Demographic observations of total registered patients.

Sign / symptom	Mean ± S.D			Df	p-value	t-value	Effective ness %	Remark
Pain	2.14 ± 0.77	BT AT1	1.42 ± 0.51		<0.01	4.28	33%	HS
		AT2	0.85 ± 0.36		<0.01	5.1	60%	HS
		AT3	0.5 ± 0.51		<0.01	9.2	76%	HS
Haematuria	0.85 ± 0.36	BT AT1	0.35 ± 0.49		>0.01	2.8	58%	NS
		AT2	0.28 ± 0.46		>0.01	3.2	66%	S
		AT3	0.14 ± 0.36		<0.05	5.54	83%	HS
Dysuria	1.5 ± 0.65	BT AT1	0.78 ± 0.80		<0.01	5.5	47.6%	HS
		AT2	0.71 ± 0.72		<0.01	4.9	52.3%	HS
		AT3	0.35 ± 0.49		<0.01	6.2	76.1%	HS
Size of stone	4.42 ± 0.58	BT AT1	2.7 ± 1.8		<0.01	3.5	37%	HS
		AT2	1.78 ± 1.62		<0.01	5.6	59%	HS
		AT3	0.5 ± 0.6		<0.01	19.7	88%	HS
Site of stone	22.2 ± 0.8	BT AT1	1.5 ± 0.8	14	<0.05	2.2	29%	S
		AT2	1.07 ± 0.7		<0.05	3.6	51%	S
		AT3	0.5 ± 0.7		<0.01	5.5	74%	HS
Number	1.14 ± 0.36	BT AT1	0.71 ± 0.46		>0.01	2.45	37.5%	NS
		AT2	0.71 ± 0.46		>0.01	2.45	47.5%	NS
		AT3	0.35 ± 0.4		<0.01	4.9	68.7%	HS
X-ray	1±0	BT AT1	0.64 ± 0.49		<0.01	2.66	35.7%	HS
		AT2	0.42 ± 0.51		<0.01	4	57.1%	HS
		AT3	0.28 ± 0.46		<0.01	5.5	71.4%	HS
USG	1 ± 0	BT AT1	0.85 ± 0.36		<0.01	1.4	14.2%	HS
		AT2	0.5 ± 0.51		<0.01	3.5	50%	HS
		AT3	0.28 ± 0.46		<0.01	5.5	71.4%	HS

S.D–Standard deviation, B.T–Before treatment, A.T–After treatment, df– Degree of freedom, t–Test of significant, p–Probability, H.S- Highly significant N.S.- Non significant

Table 2: Showing effectiveness of drug in group-A.

problems form an important part of medical deliberations. Perhaps, this can be the reason for detailed description of the urinary system related disease i.e. *Mutrashmari* (Urolithiasis) in our Ayurvedic texts. Old literature gives a clear idea of the disease that it has come into existence from the very beginning. In *Ayurveda madhura* (sweets) and *guru* (heavy for digestion) diets and hot climate are the main cause for the formation of *Ashmari* (stones) [5]. As this can be understood hypothetically with the present contemporary science that these types of food may reduce the solubility crystals in the urine, this may lead into precipitations and formation of the stone. Where as in Modern Science they have considered many causative factors for the stone formation, but stone has been seen even in those patients also, where these factors are absent. So in total, the etiology of the disease is still unknown.

Discussion upon the Observation

All cases were analyzed for the incidence of *Mutrashmari* in relation to age, sex, socio-economic status etc.

In the present series of observation it was found that 33.33% of patients were in the age group 30-39 yrs, and 33.33% in the age group 40-49 yrs. This indicates that the incidence is higher in 3rd and 4th decade of life. Excessive work and by the excessive sweating leads to decrease in urine output in turn helps for the formation of stone. The incidence of *Mootrashmari* was relatively more in males (73.33%) than in females (26.66%) in the present study and the ratio was almost 2:1. The incidence of calculogenesis will be same in female compared to men after menopausal age, as citrates are not secreted during menstrual cycle and after menopause.

On observing the distribution of incidence among Hindu, Muslim and Christian, the prevalence was seen more in Hindu, (76.66%), then in Muslim (20%) and then Christian (3.33%). This does not indicate the incidence as higher in Hindus. This percentage is synchronous with their general percentage in the population. People of any community appear to be equally susceptible to the disease. Incidence of socio-economic status shows predominance of Lower middle class (56.66%). It will indicate that there is no any particular socio-economic status for stone formation.

Discussion on mode of action of drug

The major component isolated from this plant is lupeol, which is used to treat hypercrystalluria, hyperoxaluria and hypercalciuria. The

Sign /symptom	Mean ± S.D			Df	p-value	t-value	Effective ness %	Remark
Pain	2.13 ± 0.83	BT AT1	1.46 ± 0.51		<0.01	5.29	31.20%	HS
		AT2	1.2 ± 0.56		<0.01	5.13	43.75%	HS
		AT3	0.8 ± 0.67		<0.01	4.93	62.50%	HS
Haematuria	0.73 ± 0.45	BT AT1	0.6 ± 0.5		<0.05	1	18.10%	HS
		AT2	0.4 ± 0.5		<0.05	2	45.40%	HS
		AT3	0.2 ± 0.41		<0.01	4	72.20%	HS
Dysuria	1.93 ± 0.79	BT AT1	1.06 ± 0.88		<0.05	6.5	44.80%	S
		AT2	0.46 ± 0.51		<0.01	8.87	75.80%	HS
		AT3	0.33 ± 0.48		<0.01	6.8	82%	HS
Size of stone	4.2 ± 0.7	BT AT1	3.7 ± 0.9		<0.05	3.7	11	S
		AT2	2.4 ± 1.9		<0.01	4.4	43.30%	HS
		AT3	1.2 ± 1.7	14	<0.01	7.5	70%	HS
Site of stone	2.06 ± 0.70	BT AT1	1.7 ± 0.5		<0.05	2.6	16.10%	S
		AT2	1.06 ± 1.7		<0.01	3.8	48.30%	HS
		AT3	0.7 ± 0.45		<0.01	5.7	64.50%	HS
Number	1.2 ± 0.41	BT AT1	0.9 ± 0.25		<0.05	2.25	22.20%	S
		AT2	0.53 ± 0.51		<0.01	5.29	55.50%	HS
		AT3	0.33 ± 0.48		<0.01	9.53	72.20%	HS
X-ray	1 ± 0	BT AT1	0.53 ± 0.51		<0.01	3.5	46.60%	HS
		AT2	0.4 ± 0.50		<0.01	4.58	60%	HS
		AT3	0.2 ± 0.4		<0.01	7.4	80%	HS
USG	1 ± 0	BT AT1	0.53 ± 0.51		<0.01	3.5	46.6%	HS
		AT2	0.4 ± 0.50		<0.01	4.58	60%	HS
		AT3	0.13 ± 0.35		<0.01	9.5	86.60%	HS

Table 3: Showing effectiveness of drug in group-B.

RESULT	GROUP – A			GROUP – B		
	15 days	30 days	45 days	15 days	30 days	45 days
Cured	0	0	2	0	0	0
Maximum Improve	0	2	6	0	6	9
Moderate Improve	2	5	4	5	3	5
Mild Improve	5	7	2	7	5	1
No Improve	8	1	1	3	1	0

Table 4: Overall clinical assessment of result.

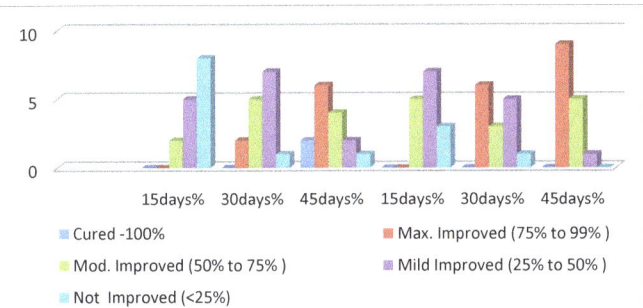

Figure 1: Overall clinical assessment of result. Group –A: Overall Clinical assessment on 45th day showed that 1 patient had no improvement, 6 patients had maximum improvement, 4 patients had moderate improvement; whereas 2 patients had mild improvement and 2 patients had completely cured. Group –B: Overall Clinical assessment on 45th day showed that 9 patients had maximum improvement, whereas 5 patients had moderate improvement, and 1 patient had mild improvement.

compound is also widely used to treat urinary disorders like urolithiasis, and it decreases elevated concentration of oxalate, phosphorous and magnesium in renal tissue. Lupeol also possesses antipyretic, analgesic, anti-inflammatory activity.

Discussion on result's of subjective criteria

The effectiveness of the treatment adopted in both the groups in respect to each parameter is tabulated on the basis of the difference between the scores before treatment and after treatment.

Pain: The effectiveness of *Varunamulatwak kwatha* is 76% with *t*-value 9.21 and the level of significance of p-value is <0.01, which is highly significant. The effectiveness of group-B is 62.5%with *t*-value 4.93 and the level of significance of p-value is <0.01. It shows that *Varunamula twak kwatha* having the analgesic and anti-inflammatory [8,9] properties.

Haematuria: The effectiveness of group-A is 83.33% with *t*-value 5.54 and the level of significance of p-value is <0.01, which is highly significant. The effectiveness of group-B is 72.7% with *t*-value 4 and the level of significance of p-value is <0.01. The effectiveness of *Varunamulatwak kwatha* over the group-A patients are showing good response to the treatment, because of the effectiveness of the intended drugs over the *mutrashmari* showing anti-inflammatory properties.

Dysuria: The effectiveness of group-A is 76.1% with *t*-value 6.23 and the level of significance of p-value is <0.01. The effectiveness of group-B is 82.7% with *t*-value 6.80 and the level of significance of p-value is <0.01, which is highly significant. Administration of fluids causes the increase urine output by this dysuria is subsided so flush out therapy is highly significant then *varunamulatwak kwatha*.

Objective criteria

Size of stone: The effectiveness of group-A is 88% with *t*-value 23.4 and the level of significance of p-value is <0.01, which is highly significant. The effectiveness of group-B is 71.42% with *t*-value 6.99 and the level of significance of p-value is <0.01, which is highly significant. It indicates that *Varunamulatwak kwatha* having the *Ashmaribhedana* (Anti-lithic) [5] property.

Site of stone: The effectiveness of group-A is 74.1%with *t*-value 5.52 and the level of significance of p-value is <0.01, which is highly significant. The effectiveness of group-B is 64.5% with *t*-value 5.7 and the level of significance of p-value is <0.01, which is highly significant.

It is due to stagnation of the urine in the specific area causes the precipitation of crystals by which stone is formed.

Number of stones: The effectiveness of group-A is 68.7% with *t*-value 4.95 and the level of significance of p-value is <0.01, which is highly significant. The effectiveness of group-B is 72.2% with *t*-value 9.53 and the level of significance of p-value is <0.01, which is highly significant.

Overall clinical assessment of result

Finally the clinical assessment was carried out on overall results of the effect of *Varunamula twak kwatha* on each individual sign and symptoms and collectively presented in the form of cured, maximum improvement, moderate improvement, mild improvement and no improvement. However it was evident that in group-A after 45 days 2 (100%) patients were cured, 6 (75%-99%) had maximum improvement, 4 (50%-75%) had moderate improvement, 2(25%-50%) had mild improvement and 1 (<25%) patient with no improvement. In group-B, 9 (75%-99%) had maximum improvement, 5 (50%-75%) had moderate improvement, 1 (25%-50%) had mild improvement. *Varunamula twakkwatha* has a significant role in the management of *Mutrashmari* as majority of patients showed highly significant response.

Conclusion

Following conclusion were drawn after analysis of review (Ayurvedic, Modern and Drug), clinical observation and interpretations on the parameters.

- In the observation it was found that, the lithotryptic [9] action of the *Varunamula twak kwatha* was showing significant effect.

- *Varunamulatwak kwatha* was capable of reducing Pain intensity (76%) than flush out therapy (62.5%).

- *Varunamulatwak kwatha* was capable of reducing Haematuria (84%) than flush out therapy (70%).

- *Varunamulatwak kwatha* was capable of reducing Dysuria (76.1%) and flush out therapy (82.7%).

- *Varunamulatwak kwatha* was capable of reducing Size of stone (88%) than flush out therapy (71.42%).

- *Varunamulatwak kwatha* was capable of reducing Site of stone (65.5%) than flush out therapy (61.6%).

- *Varunamulatwak kwatha* was capable of reducing number of stone (68.7%) and flush out therapy (72.2%).

References

1. Kashinath Shastri (2006) Charaka Samhita of Agnivesha with Vidyotini Hindi commentary, Chikisa sthan 26/59-60. (reprint edition), Chaukhambha Sanskrit sansthan, Varanasi.

2. Kaviraj Ambikadutt Shastri (2001) Sushrut Samhita with Ayurved tatva Sandipika Hindi commentary, Nidaansthan 3/7. (12thedn), Choukhambha Sanskrit Sansthan, Varanasi.

3. Norman S Williams (2010) Bulstrode. Bailly & Love's short practice of Surgery. Chapter 71. (25thedn), Hodder Arnold publishers, London.

4. Townsend CM, Beauchamp D, Mattox KL (2010) Sabiston Textbook of Surgery. In editor. Sabiston Textbook of Surgery. Elsevier publications, Newdelhi.

5. Kaviraj Ambikadutt Shastri (2001) Sushrut Samhita with Ayurved tatva Sandipika Hindi commentary, Nidaansthan ¾. (Reprint edition), Choukhambha Sanskrit Sansthan, Varanasi.

6. Amitkumar singh (2009) Comparativeclinical Study in the Management of Mootrashmari with Kulattha Churna and Swetaparpati, MD Thesis. RGUHS, Bangalore.

7. Chakrapani dutta, Chakra Dutta (2010) Reprint edition, Choukhambha Sanskrit Bhavan; Varanasi.

8. Bhattacharjee SK (2008) Handbook of Medicinal Plants. (1stedn), Pointer Publication, Jaipur.

9. Ashok Sheth (2005) The Herbs of Ayurveda. (1stedn), Hiscan Pvt Ltd, Bhavnagar.

10. Sharma PV, Dravyaguna Vignyan (2009) part II, Reprint edition, Choukhambha Bharati Academy, Varanasi.

11. Brahmashankar Mishra Shastri (1997) Bhava Prakash with Vidyotini hindi commentary, Uttaradha, Ashmari Rogadhikar. (6thedn), Choukhambha Sanskrit Sansthan, Varanasi.

12. Adhomalla, Sarangadhara Samhita with Gudhartha Deepika commentary, edited by Parashuram Shastri (2006) Madhyam Khanda. (Reprint edition),Choukhambha Surabharati, Varanasi.

13. Tripathy RN, Otta SP, Siddaram A (2011) A traditional approach in wound healing. IJTK 10.

8

Comparative Phytochemical Analysis of Fermented and Unfermented Seeds of *Dialium giuneense*

Utubaku AB[1], Yakubu OE[2]* and Okwara DU[2]

[1]Department of Medical Biochemistry, Cross River University of Technology, Calabar, Nigeria
[2]Department of Biochemistry, Federal University Wukari, Nigeria

Abstract

The present study was designed to study the fermentation process and to scientifically evaluate its phytochemical components. Fermentation was carried out using traditional method. Exactly 160 g of the seeds were soaked in water, washed, and cooked for 2 h, after which they were washed, sieved and parboiled for 20 min, the seeds sieved, cotyledon poured into fermenting pot covered tightly to prevent heat escape, fermented for 72 h while still hot, and the final product was gotten and sundried. The phytochemical analysis of *Dialium guineense* was carried out, and the results of the analysis shows the presence of the following phytochemicals in varied proportion across the different samples; saponin, flavonoids and phenolic compounds. Findings from this study suggest that *D. guineense* contains agents (secondary metabolites) capable of ameliorating certain disease conditions, therefore, its use as condiment for food preparation is encourage.

Keywords: *Dialium guineense;* Phytochemical; Fermentation; Antioxidants; Nutrition

Introduction

Dialium guineense also known as Black Velvet Tamarind (BVT) is an indigenous tropical forest fruit tree of the family Leguminosae. BVT is an important non-timber multipurpose agroforestry crop with a high potential [1]. The potentials of BVT as food supplement, in herbal medicine and as source of energy are well documented [2-4]. According to Agbani [5], BVT is a lesser known tropical forest fruit with high consumption but given a less priority in terms of research, production, improvement, storage and hence not domesticated. *D. guineense* is also one of food and medicinal plants of Lama Forest reserve [5]. Black velvet tamarind *(D. guineense),* a forest tree, is well known in many localities especially in West Africa. Small black velvet fruits are characteristic of the genus. The tree grows to about 20 m in height, 0.8 m in diameter, low-branching, rarely straight, bearing a compact densely leafy crown but is often shrubby [6].

Phytochemicals are a large group of plant-derived compounds hypothesized to be responsible for much of the disease protection conferred from diets high in fruits, vegetables, beans, cereals, and plant-based beverages such as tea and wine [7]. Based on their chemical structure, phytochemicals can be broken into the following groups; Flavonoids which are the most diverse group of phytochemicals, Phenolic Acids, Stilbenes/Lignans, Alkaloids, Saponinn, Tannin, Steroids, Phenols etc. [8]. Fermentation is a metabolic process that converts sugars to acids, gases and/or alcohol. It occurs in yeast and bacteria but also in oxygen-starved muscle cell as in the case of lactic acid fermentation. The science of fermentation is known as zymology. Fermentation takes place in lack of oxygen (when the electron transport chain is unusable) and becomes the cell's primary means of ATP (energy) production, it turns NADH and pyruvate produced in the glycolysis steps into NAD^+ and various small molecules depending on the type of fermentation. In the presence of O_2 NADH and pyruvate are used to generate ATP in respiration. This is called oxidative phosphorylation and it generates much more ATP than glycolysis alone.

Materials and Methods

Preparation of the sample (*Dialium guineense*)

The African Velvet Tamarind *Dialium guineense* needed for this research was purchased in a local market at Bedia village in Obudu Local Government Area of Cross River State, Nigeria, and transported to Medical Biochemistry laboratory of Cross River University of Technology, Okuku campus for processing.

Processing of *Dialium guineense*

Traditional method of processing *D. guineense* was used with the help of two local scientists specialized in the fermentation of *D. guineense*. The seeds were soaked in water, washed (160 g) of seed sample cooked for 2 h, after which it was washed and sieved, parboiled for 20 min, the seeds sieved, cotyledon poured into native fermenting pot covered tightly to prevent heat escape, fermented for 72 h while still hot, and the final product gotten and sundried.

Phytochemical screening of *Dialium guineense* seeds

The methods and procedures for the phytochemical analysis of *D. guineense* were from Wadood et al. [9].

Determination Flavonoid

1 g of pulverized *Dialium guineense* was put into a test tube and 10 ml of distilled water added and mixed rigorously with whirl mixer and filtered with a filter paper and funnel and the filtrate was divided into 2 test tubes, drops of lead acetate and NaOH was added each yellow and colour precipitate indicates the presence of flavonoids.

Tests for saponin

1 g of pulverized *D. guineense* was measured into a test tube, 10 ml of distilled water was added, and the solution was mixed with whirl mixer then heated to boil on hot plate, it was left to cool and was filtered into a clean test tube and then 1 ml of the filtrate was measured into 2

*Corresponding author: Yakubu OE, Department of Biochemistry, Federal University Wukari, Nigeria, E-mail: oj4real_2007@yahoo.co.uk

test tubes each. In one, filtrate in the test tube ferric chloride solution was added with few drops and into the other, drops of benedict solution and ferric chloride.

Tests for tannin

1 g of pulverized *D. guineense* was measured into test tube and 20 ml of distilled water was added and heated with the help of a hot plate and was allowed to cooled and filtered into a clean test tube. 1 ml of the sample was measured into a test tube and few drops of bromine solution was added showing the presence of tannin by coloured precipitate.

Tests for alkaloids

1 g of pulverized *D. guineense* was measured and 10 ml (10%) HCL was added and mixed rigorously by whirl mixer for about 10 min and it was then filtered, the filtrate was divided into 2 test tubes. Mayer's test and Dragendorff test was carried out in each of the sample respectively.

Tests for steroids

Into a test tube was 1 g of pulverized *D. guineense*) seeds. 10 ml of chloroform was added and then 2 drops of salkowki's reagent was also added.

Tests for phenols

The sample *D. guineense* was weight, 1 g of the pulverized seed was placed into test tube, 10 ml of distilled water was added and mixed, then was filtered into test tubes with filter paper and funnel and 1 ml of the filtrate was measured into test tube and phenol was added, a precipitate indicate the presence of phenolic acid.

Results

This study has revealed the presence of phytochemicals considered as active medicinal chemical constituents. Important medicinal phytochemicals such as flavonoids, saponin, and phenolic compounds were present in the samples. The result of the phytochemical analysis shows the plant is rich in at least one of flavonoids, saponin and phenolic compounds.

Discussion

From the research, it was seen that biologic compounds (phytochemicals) such as flavonoids, saponin and phenolic compounds were present in the three samples in varied proportion whereas alkaloid and tannin were absent. Saponins are extremely poisonous, as they cause hemolysis of blood and are known to cause cattle poisoning [10,11]. They possess a bitter and acrid taste, besides causing irritation to mucous membranes. They are mostly amorphous in nature, soluble in alcohol and water, but insoluble in non-polar organic solvents like benzene and n-hexane. Saponins are also important therapeutically as they are shown to have hypolipidemic and anticancer activity. Saponins are also necessary for activity of cardiac glycosides. The two major types of steroidal sapogenin are diosgenin and hecogenin. Steroidal saponins are used in the commercial production of sex hormones for clinical use. For example, progesterone is derived from diosgenin. From the result obtained, there was a high concentration of saponin in the crude seed (+++) as compared to the fermented seed (+), therefore fermentation reduces the concentration of saponin. Hence fermentation of *Dialium guineense* seed before consumption is advice sable. Concentrations of flavonoids in the fermented seed (++) is higher than that of the crude seed (+). Numerous reports

Family of Compounds	Aqeous Extract of Fermented Seed	Aqeous Extract of Unfermented Seed	Aqeous Extract of Uncooked Shell
Flavonoids	++	+	+
Saponin	+	+	+++
Tannin	–	–	–
Phenolics	+	–	+
Alkaloids	–	–	–

(-): Negative test
(+): Weakly positive
(+ +): Moderately positive
(+ + +): Strongly positive

Table 1: Phytochemical test of fermented seed, crude seed and uncooked shell of *Dialium guineense.*

support their use as antioxidants or free radical scavengers [12]. Phenolic compounds are very important to plants and have multiple functions. The most important role may be in plant defense against pathogens and herbivore predators, and thus are applied in the control of human pathogenic infections. Phenolics essentially represent a host of natural antioxidants, used as nutraceuticals, and has been found to have enormous ability to combat cancer and are also thought to prevent heart ailments to an appreciable degree and sometimes are anti-inflammatory agents. These phytochemicals plays unique roles in the biologic system, hence fermented products of *D. guineense* seed should be recommended to our daily dietary intake (Table 1).

Conclusion

The phytochemical analysis of *Dialium guineense* seed shows the presence of various biological secondary metabolites which plays an important role in the normal functioning of the body. Beside their nutritional and protective function, they also serve as medicinal plant. Hence, Nutritionist and pharmacologist should support research on this seed as further research will bring out the potentials in this plant for being processed for drug development and nutritional satiety.

References

1. Nwaoguala CNC, Osaigbovo AU, Orhue ER (2007) Seed treatment for development of seedlings of Black Velvet Tamarind (*Dialium guineense*). Afr J Gen Agr 3: 49-51.

2. Ogbe OF, Egharevba RKA (1992) Indigenous food plant. Field survey of indigenous and useful plants, their preparation for food and home garden, Edo/Delta States of Nigeria. University programme on National Research in Africa 1: 132-134.

3. Aghatise OV, Egharevba RK (1994) Response of *Dialium guineense* to pre-germination treatments. Nitrogen Fixing Tree Report 12: 54-55.

4. Aoguala CNC, Osaigbovo AU (2009) Enhancing seedling production of Black Velvet Tamarind (*Dialium guineense*). J Appl Nat Sci 1: 36-40.

5. Agbani P (2002) Phytosociological studies of forest clusters longitudinal parbands at large scales: Case of the central nucleus of the semi-deciduous semi-deciduous forest of the Lama in Benin.Mémoire de DEA, Faculté des Lettres, Arts et Sciences Humaines, Université d'Abomey Calavi (Bénin).

6. Okegbile EO, Taiwo EA (1990) Nutritional potentials of velvet tamarind (*Dialium guineense* Wild). Niger Food J 8: 115-121.

7. Arts IC, Hollman PC (2005) Polyphenols and disease risk in epidemiologic studies. Am J Clin Nutr 81: 317-325.

8. Martinko MMT, John M, Parker J (1996) Brock biology of microorganisms (8th edn.). Prentice Hall, USA.

9. Wadood A, Ghufran M, Jamal SB, Naeem M, Khan A, et al. (2013) Phytochemical analysis of medicinal plants occuring in local area of Mardan. Biochem Anal Biochem 2: 144.

10. Sarker SD, Nahar L (2007) Chemistry for pharmacy students general, organic and natural product chemistry. England: John Wiley and Sons.

11. Kar A (2007) Pharmaocgnosy and pharmaco-biotechnology (Revised-Expanded Second Edition). New Age International Limited Publishers, New Delhi, India pp: 332-600.

12. Puupponen-Pimiä R, Nohynek L, Ammann S, Oksman-Caldentey KM, Buchert J (2008) Enzyme assisted processing increases antimicrobial and antioxidant activity of bilberry. J Agr Food Chem 56: 681-688.

9

Effect of Preparation Method on Antioxidant Activity of Ayurvedic Formulation Kumaryasava

Rahul Manmode[1]*, Jagdish Manwar[2], Mustafa Vohra[3], Satish Padgilwar[2] and Nitin Bhajipale[2]

[1]Department of Chemistry, University of Massachusetts, Lowell-01854, USA
[2]Department of Quality Assurance, Institute of Pharmacy, Akola-444 004, India
[3]Department of Alcohol Technology, Vasantdada Sugar Institute, Pune-412 307, India

Abstract

Kumaryasava is an alcoholic Ayurvedic formulation prepared by the fermentation of *Aloe vera*. Flowers of *Woodfordia fruticosa* are added as inoculums for fermentation process. The aim of the present investigation to find the effect of its preparation method on antioxidant activity of *Kumaryasava*. Three different formulations of *Kumaryasava* were prepared by fermentation using three different inoculums viz. *Woodfordia fruticosa* flowers, *Madhuca indica* flowers and yeast *Saccharomyces cerevisiae SC1011*. During fermentation process, relationship between alcohol generation and sugar utilization in each formulation was studied. *In vitro* antioxidant activity of all formulations was evaluated by 1,1-diphenyl-2-picryl hydrazyl (DPPH) scavenging, hydrogen peroxide scavenging and total reducing power. The results were compared to standard antioxidant ascorbic acid. All the tested formulations showed marked *in vitro* antioxidant activity in which *WFKA* (*W. fruticosa* flowers based *Kumaryasava*) showed prominent activity. Obtained IC_{50} values of *WFKA* in DPPH scavenging assay, hydrogen peroxide scavenging assay and total reducing power assay were 481.78, 50.13 and 49.60, respectively. From the results it is concluded that formulation (*WFKA*) prepared by traditional method showed higher *in vitro* antioxidant activity relative to others.

Keywords: Aloe Vera; *Woodfordia fruticosa*; *Madhuca indica*; Alcohol; Antioxidant activity

Introduction

The use of Ayurvedic formulations has led to the sudden increase in the number of Ayurvedic drug manufactures due to the toxicity and side effects of allopathic medicines. *Kumaryasava* is an Ayurvedic formulation containing *Aloe Vera* (leaves) is the major crude drug along with 17 other minor ingredients [1]. *A. vera* (Synonym: *Aloe barbadensis*, family *Liliaceae*), also known as *Kumaari*, is a shrubby plant with succulent and elongated leaves. The plant is widely cultivated throughout India, especially in the coastal region of Maharashtra, Gujarat and South India [2]. Leaves of the plant were reported to exhibit various effects like wound healing, anti-inflammatory and immunomodulatory activity [3-6]. Topical polyherbal formulation containing pulp of *A. vera* leaves as a main ingredient is used for the treatment of acne [7]. Ayurvedic Pharmacopoeia of India recommends *Kumaryasava* for the treatment of abdominal lump, epilepsy, digestive impairment and menopause [1].

Traditionally, *Kumaryasava* is prepared by the fermentation of leaves of *A. vera*. During the preparation, flowers of *Woodfordia fruticosa* (Family-*Lythraceae*) are added as inoculums for alcoholic fermentation. This fermentation process uses the natural yeasts present on the flowers of *W. fruticosa* [8,9]. The yeast present on the flowers may vary depending on the source location and hence about one month period is recommended to complete the fermentation process. Alcohol generated during the fermentation process causes the extraction of water insoluble active principle components from the crude drugs. According to Ayurvedic Pharmacopoeia of India, *Kumaryasava* should contain not less than 5% v/v and not more than 10% v/v self-generated alcohol (40-80 g/l). *W. fruticosa* flowers, based formulations are useful in various conditions like leucorrhoea, dysfunctional uterine bleeding, burning sensation in stomach, weakness and rheumatoid diseases [10-12].

Madhuca indica (synonym: *Madhuca latifolia*) belonging to family *Sapotaceae* is a large forest tree found largely in the central and north Indian plains and forests [13]. Flowers of the tree contain 28.1-36.3%

w/w of fermentable sugars [14]. Presence of yeast *Saccharomyces cerevisiae*, well known for alcohol production, was documented in the literature [15]. Therefore, these flowers are used to produce fermented alcoholic drink *mahuwa* (country liquor). Tribals of Bastar in Chattisgarh, Orissa and Jharkhand consider the *mahuwa* drink as part of their cultural heritage. The flowers are also used in making of some Ayurvedic formulations like *Abhayarista, Kutajarista, Partadyarista* etc. [1].

Inspite of availability of numerous sources of inoculums like flowers of *M. indica* or yeast strain *S. cerevisiae*, even today *Kumaryasava* is being prepared by traditional method using *W. fruticosa* flowers [16,17]. This process takes upto 1-month period to complete the fermentation process. Therefore, there is urgent need to reduce this long time to fewer days by trying the other inoculums those contain fermentation yeast. Literature survey indicated that no report on kinetics of alcohol generation and sugar utilization during making of *Kumaryasava* by traditional method. We are the first to report the kinetics of fermentation process in traditional method of preparation of same formulation. This data will be helpful to decide when to stop fermentation process.

Antioxidant molecules are able to reduce oxidative stress the by preventing the oxidation of other molecules. This stress is caused by free radicals which initiate chain reaction and seek stability through electron pairing with biomolecules like lipids, proteins, DNA in the cells and causes lipid peroxidation along with protein and DNA damage

*Corresponding author: Dr. Rahul Manmode, Department of Chemistry, 1st University Avenue, University of Massachusetts Lowell, Lowell, USA
E-mail: rahulmanmode@gmail.com

[18]. Antioxidant activity of extract of *A. vera* leaves is well documented [19-21]. During the making of *Kumaryasava,* minor ingredients like *Nordostachys jatamansi, Piper cubeba, Syzygium aromaticum* etc., also contribute to the antioxidant activity. Therefore, all minor ingredients were omitted to avoid their interference in antioxidant activities [22-24]. *In vitro* antioxidant activity of formulations was evaluated by 1,1-diphenyl-2-picryl hydrazyl (DPPH) scavenging, hydrogen peroxide scavenging and total reducing power. The data of antioxidant study will explain at least in part how preparation method affects the biological activity. Jaggery was used as source of sugar to produce alcohol.

Materials and Methods

Plant material and chemicals

Leaves of *A. vera* were collected from nearest farm (Figure 1). Flowers of *W. fruticosa* were collected from the Solapur district and flowers of *M. indica* were collected from Washim district of Maharashtra, India. All the samples were then immediately transferred into the sterilized plastic bag. The plant materials were authenticated from Agharkar Research Institute, Pune, India. Commercial grade of jaggery was purchased from local market. The chemicals and solvents used in this experimental work were of the highest quality available.

Collection of *S. cerevisiae SC1011*

Standard culture of yeast *S. cerevisiae SC1011* was collected from Vasantdada Sugar Institute, Pune, India. The strain was maintained on MGYP agar slants (3 g malt extract, 10 g glucose, 3 g yeast extract, 5 g peptone and 20 g agar per liter of water, pH 4.5) and preserved at 4°C for routine use.

Preparation of Jaggery Media (12°brix)

About 6-7 g of jaggery was dissolved in 350 ml of distilled water. This media was then transfered to measuring cylinder (250 ml capacity). Brix hydrometer of range 10-20 was dipped into the media and brix value was observed. The brix value was adjusted to 12 by addition of water or jaggery and pH was adjusted to 4.5. To the media, 0.01% w/v of diamonophosphate and 0.01% w/v of urea was added as a source of nitrogen, autoclaved at 15 lbs at 121°C for 15 min, cooled and used in further experimental work.

Preparation of inoculums of *S. cerevisiae SC1011*

The inoculums of *S. cerevisiae SC1011* was prepared by transferring one loopful of yeast culture into 100 ml of sterile 12°brix jaggery medium and incubated at 32.5°C for 24 h in shaker incubator at 180 rpm. After incubation, cell count of yeasts were measured using neubauer counting chamber (methylene blue indicator was used to stain viable cells).

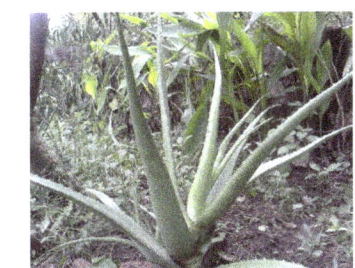

Figure 1: Plant of Aloe Vera plant.

Preparation of formulations

Leaves of *A. vera* were cut into bits and the skin was removed to obtain a pulp. In three separate 1 L conical flasks, 250 g jaggery was dissolved in 300 ml of distilled water by boiling. The flasks were cooled and final volumes of media were made up to 500 ml. To each flask, 100 g of pulp was added and they were autoclaved at 121°C for 20 min. After sterilization, flasks were cooled and flasks were inoculated with *W. fruticosa flowers* (16 g), *M. indica* flowers (10 g) and inoculums of *S. cerevisiae SC1011* (10 ml, cell count- 3×10^7 cells/ml), separately. Formulation inoculated with *W. fruticosa* flowers, *M. indica* flowers and yeast *S. cerevisiae SC1011* were named as *WFKA, MIKA* and *SCKA,* respectively. All the flasks were incubated in BOD incubator at 32.5°C for 30 days. At the intervals of 3 days, 15 ml of fermentation broth was withdrawn from each formulation aseptically, centrifuged at 6000 rpm, and supernatant layers were used for the analysis of alcohol generated (g/l) and residual sugar (% w/v).

Analysis of broth

Kinetics of fermentation was studied by determining the relationship between alcohol generation and sugar utilization. Amount of alcohol generated was determined by dichromate oxidation method and that of residual sugar was determined by titration method [25,26].

Evaluation of *in-vitro* antioxidant activity

After completion of fermentation process, all the formulations were filtered through three layers of muslin cloth over other. Filtered formulations were centrifuged at 3000 rpm for 20 min and were used for evaluation of *in vitro* antioxidant activity by various assay methods. Ascorbic acid (100 μg/ml) was used as standard antioxidant for comparing results of sample solution.

DPPH scavenging assay

Ability of formulation to scavenge DPPH free radical was carried out by slightly modifying the procedure given in the literature [27]. Solution of DPPH was prepared by dissolving 33 mg of compound in 1 L of analytical grade methanol and was then store in dark amber colored bottle. 1 ml of various concentration (100, 200, 400, 800 and 1000 μl/ml) of formulation in water were taken in different test tubes. To each tube, 5 ml of DPPH solution was added, shaken and tubes were immediately kept in dark at 27°C for 20 min. After incubation, the tubes were centrifuged at 3000 rpm for 5 min and absorbance of supernatant layer was measured at 517 nm using UV-Vis Spectrophotometer (Shimadzu, model 160). Control solution was also prepared and zero was set using solvent methanol. Percentage DPPH scavenging effect was calculated from the following formula:

$$\%DPPH\ Scavenging\ effect = \frac{Ac - As}{Ac} X100$$

Where, Ac is the absorbance of control solution, and As is the absorbance of sample solution.

Hydrogen peroxide scavenging assay

Ability of formulation to scavenge hydrogen peroxide (H_2O_2) was carried out by method reported in literature [28]. H_2O_2 solution (100 mM) was prepared in phosphate buffer (pH 7.4). About 0.5 ml of solution of each formulation of various concentration (10, 20, 40, 60 and 100 μl/ml) of formulations in water was added to test tube separately containing 4.5 ml of H_2O_2 solution. Tubes were incubated at room temperature for 10 min and absorbance of solution was measured at 230 nm against a solution in phosphate buffer without

H_2O_2. Percentage of H_2O_2 scavenging activity was calculated from the following formula:

$$\% \, Hydrogen \, peroxide \, scavenging \, activity = \frac{Ac - As}{Ac} X100$$

Where, Ac is the absorbance of control solution, and As is the absorbance of sample solution.

Reducing power assay

Reducing ability of formulations was measured according to procedure given in literature [29]. The different concentrations of formulation (10, 20, 40, 60 and 100 μl/ml) were mixed with phosphate buffer (2.5 ml, 0.2 M, pH 6.6) and potassium ferricyanide (2.5 ml, 1%). To this, about 2.5 ml of trichloroacetic acid (10%v/v) was added, and mixture was incubated at 50°C for 20 min. After incubation, mixture was centrifuged at 3000 rpm for 20 min. 2.5 ml of supernatant layer was mixed with 2.5 ml of water and 0.5 ml of $FeCl_3$ (0.1%), and absorbance was measured at 700 nm wavelength.

Statistical analysis

The data of antioxidant testing are expressed as mean ± standard error of mean (SEM). Statistical analysis was performed using a one-way analysis of variance (ANOVA) and differences were considered to be significant at $p < 0.05$.

Results

Alcohol generation in formulation SCKA, MIKA and WFKA was stopped after 6 days, 15 days and 21 days, respectively. In SCKA, fermention process was stopped after 6 days with the alcohol generation of 85.21 g/l. this amount of alcohol was remained constant till 30 days. Initial amount of residual sugar was 29.27 g/100 ml. Within a period of first 6 days, 86.91% of initial sugar was utilized for this alcohol production and then no further utilization was observed. In finished SCKA formulation, amount of alcohol and residual sugar was 84.70 g/l and 3.26 g/100 ml, respectively. In MIKA, flowers of M. indica have produce 71.53 g/l of alcohol after 15 days using 56.05% of initial amount of sugar. Initial amount of residual sugar was 30.81 g/100 ml. Over the period of next 15 days, negligible (0.167% w/v) reduction in amount of alcohol was noted. Nevertheless, amount was sugar was constant in this period. In finished formulation, amount of alcohol and residual sugar was 69.86 g/l and 13.54 g/100 ml, respectively. In WFKA, which was prepared traditionally using flowers of W. fruticosa, fermentation process was completed after 24 days. Initial amount of residual sugar was 34.3 g/100 ml. In this period, amount of alcohol produced was 70.65 g/l at a rate of production was 2.94 g/l per day. Over the remaining period, amount of alcohol and sugar was nearly constant. Till last day, 62.36% of initial amount sugar was utilized for production of 69.21 g/l of alcohol. In finished formulation, 12.91 g/100 ml of sugar was present (Figure 2).

Evaluation of in vitro antioxidant activity of all formulations was carried out using three model systems viz. DPPH scavenging assay, reducing power assay and hydrogen peroxide scavenging assay. All the formulations and ascorbic acid solution were found to decreases the concentration of DPPH significantly ($p < 0.05$) with the concentration of 100 μl/ml to 1000 μl/ml. The order of DPPH scavenging activity was WFKA>MIKA>SCKA >ascorbic acid. IC_{50} values WFKA, SCKA, MIKA and ascorbic acid were 481.78, 607.16, 642.64 and 723.77, respectively (Figure 3). Hydrogen peroxide scavenging capacity of formulations was carried out using different concentration. SCKA indicated lesser activity than those of WFKA and MIKA. The order of activity shown by formulations was WFKA> MIKA >SCKA>ascorbic acid. IC_{50} values of WFKA, MIKA, SCKA and ascorbic acid were 50.13, 71.41, 86.18 and 92.91, respectively (Figure 4). In reducing power assay, the order of reducing power shown by formulations was WFKA>MIKA >SCKA>ascorbic acid. IC_{50} values of WFKA, MIKA, SCKA and ascorbic acid were 49.6, 53.4, 59.4 and 64, respectively (Figure 5).

Discussion

Three different formulations of Kumaryasava i.e. WFKA, MIKA and SCKA were prepared by fermentation using various sources of inoculums like W. fruticosa flowers, M. indica flowers and yeast S. cerevisiae SC1011, respectively. To avoid any interference with activity, all minor ingredients were omitted during preparation. For all, jaggery media (50% w/v) was as source of sugar for alcohol [30]. Both non-traditional inoculums (M. indica flowers, S. cerevisiae SC1011) have produced recommended amount of alcohol i.e. 40 to 80 g/l within a shorter period relative to traditional method. In SCKA, rate of alcohol generation and rate of sugar utilization was faster than other formulation. In this case, fermentation process was stopped after 6 days. Flowers of M. indica were found to intermediate type of inoculums. It minimizes the duration of fermentation time of 30 days to just 15 days. In WFKA, it takes about 24 days to complete the fermentation process. In this case, rate of alcohol generation and sugar utilization was much less than others. Slow alcohol generation

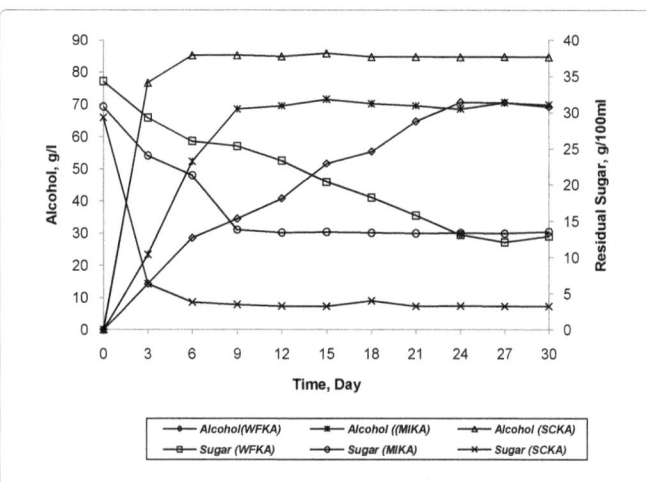

Figure 2: Kinetic relationship between alcohol generation and sugar utilization.

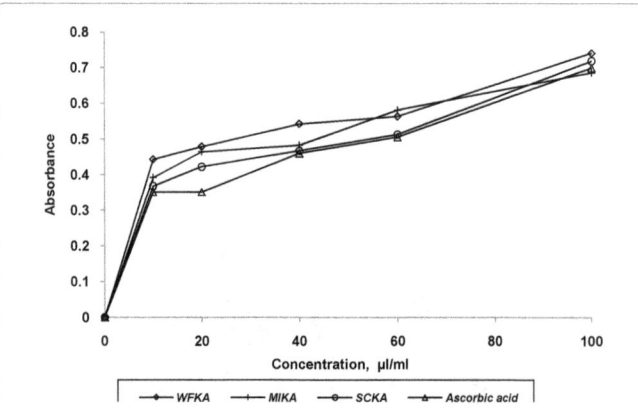

Figure 3: DPPH scavenging activity of different formulations. The values are expressed as mean ± SEM (n=3). WFKA = Kumaryasava prepared using W. fruticosa flowers; MIKA = Kumaryasava prepared using M. indica flowers; SCKA = Kumaryasava prepared using yeast S. cerevisiae

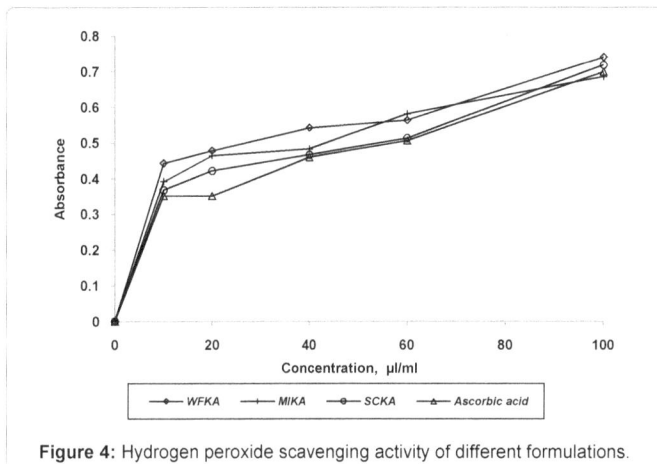

Figure 4: Hydrogen peroxide scavenging activity of different formulations.

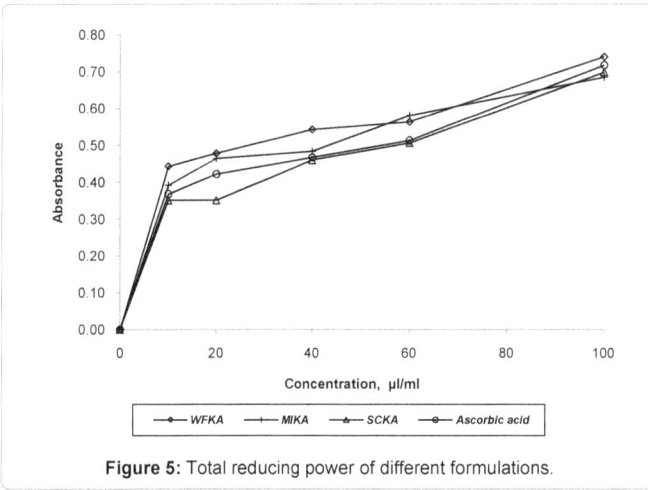

Figure 5: Total reducing power of different formulations.

may cause incomplete extraction of water insoluble active principles of crude drugs, and perhaps Ayurvedic Pharmacopoeia of India might have recommended enough time (one month) for complete extraction. In all formulations, good co-relationship was observed between the alcohol generation and sugar utilization. These data of fermentation may be used as a new method to classify the inoculums with respect to their maximum for alcohol generation capacity.

Medicinal plants contain phenolic compounds, which are responsible for different kinds of biological effects including antioxidant activity [31,32]. The free radical scavenging activities of all formulations were evaluated using metabolic solution of DPPH. DPPH is a stable nitrogen-centered free radical. DPPH has advantages of being unaffected by such a metal ion due certain side reactions, such as metal ion chelation and enzyme inhibition brought about by various additives. Antioxidant molecule quench DPPH radicals (by providing hydrogen atom or by electron transfer, conceivably via a free radical attack on the DPPH molecule) and convert them to a colorless/yellow product (2,2-diphenyl-1-hydrazine or a substituted analogs of hydrazine) resulting in a decreasing absorbance at a 517 nm [33]. Substances to perform this above reaction can be considered as antioxidants [34]. Lower absorbance of the reaction mixture indicated higher DPPH scavenging activity. In biochemical systems, superoxide radicals are converted to hydrogen peroxide (H_2O_2) by superoxide dismutase. H_2O_2 has ability of penetrating biological membranes. It is very reactive but in presence of certain transition metal ions such

as iron and copper, it can subsequently produce extremely reactive hydroxyl radicals [35]. Results show all formulations possess significant H_2O_2 scavenging activity. It has reported that the reducing power of plant is related to the antioxidant potential of active principles present [36]. Color change from yellow to different shades of green and blue depends upon the reducing power of each formulation. The presence of antioxidants in the Ayurvedic formulation causes the reduction of Fe^{3+} (Ferric cyanide complex) to Fe^{2+} (ferrous form). This Fe^{++} complex can be monitored by measuring the formation of Perl's Prussian blue at 700 nm [37]. In this assay, absorbance of sample solution was increased with increase in concentration of formulations. Hence, the increase in absorbance indicates increasing trend of reducing power. Higher absorbance of the reaction mixture indicated greater reducing power. The reducing power of formulations was increased with increasing concentration.

Though the alcohol is earlier in formulation using non-traditional *inoculums (M. indica* flowers, *S. cerevisiae SC1011),* but they did not showed activity equal to formulation *WFKA* prepared by traditional method. All the formulations were found to exhibit higher antioxidant activity than that of ascorbic acid. This increase in activity may be due to presence of potent antioxidant principles in the leaves of *A. vera* and or may be due to the presence of jaggery in higher concentration. Jaggery also reported as good antioxidant agent [38]. Beside its use as a sugar, it may act as good antioxidant agent in the formulation. Among all, *W. fruticosa* flowers based *Kumaryasava WFKA* showed highest antioxidant activity by all models. This increased of in activity might be due to the presence of phenolic compounds in the flowers of *W. fruticosa* that possesses potent antioxidant activity [39,40].

Conclusion

Even though the fermentation process is much slower using inoculums of *W. fruticosa* flowers relative to other inoculums, experimentally it is proved that their presence in the *Kumaryasava* highly contributes to the antioxidant activity. The phenolic compounds of the flowers might be responsible for this activity. Therefore, it has been concluded that the formulation prepared by traditional method reported in Ayurvedic Pharmacopoeia is the best formulation in respect of antioxidant activity.

References

1. The Ayurvedic Pharmacopoeia of India (2009). (1stedn), New Delhi, India.

2. Mohammed Ali (2007) Textbook of Pharmacognosy. (2ndedn), CBS Publishers and Distributors, New Delhi, India.

3. Chithra P, Sajithlal GB, Chandrakasan G (1998) Influence of aloe vera on the healing of dermal wounds in diabetic rats. J Ethnopharmacol 59: 195-201.

4. Vazquez B, Avila G, Segura D, Escalante B (1996) Antiinflammatory activity of extracts form Aloe vera gel. J Ethnopharmacol 55: 69-75.

5. Langmead L, Makins RJ, Rampton DS (2004) Anti-inflammatory effects of Aloe vera gel in human colorectal mucosa in vitro. Aliment Pharmacol Ther 19: 521-527.

6. Iamnishi K (1993) Aloctin A, An Active Substance of Aloe Arborescens Miller As An Immunomodulator. Phytother Res 7: S20-S22.

7. Baskar G, Arshia S, Priyadarshini SRB (2009) Formulation and evaluation of topical polyherbal antiacne gels containing Garcinia mangostana and Aloe vera. Phcog Mag 5: 93-99.

8. Atal CK, Bhatia AK, Singh RP (1982) Role of Woodfordia fruticosa Kurtz (Dhataki) in the preparation of Asavas and Aristhas. J Res Ayurved Sidd 3: 193-199.

9. Maheshwari DK, Lal R (1999) Role of microflora associated with Dhataki flowers (Woodfordia fruticosa Kurtz) in the production of Ayurvedic tonic Amritarishta. J Ind Bot Soc 78: 91-94.

10. Kirtikar KR, Basu BD (1935) Indian Medicinal Plants. Lalit Mohan Basu Publishers and Distributer: Allahabad, India.

11. Kroes BH, Van den Berg AJ, Abeysekera AM, de Silva KT, Labadie RP (1993) Fermentation in traditional medicine: the impact of Woodfordia fruticosa flowers on the immunomodulatory activity, and the alcohol and sugar contents of Nimba Aristha. J Ethnopharmacol 40: 117-125.

12. Tewiri PV, Neelam, Kulkiro MK (2001) A study of lukol in leucorrhoea, pelvic inflammatory diseases and dysfunctional uterine bleeding. Anc Sci Life 21: 139-149.

13. Khare CP (2007) Indian Medicinal Plants: An illustrated Dictionary. Springer.

14. Swain MR, Kar S, Sahoo AK, Ray RC (2007) Ethanol fermentation of mahula (Madhuca latifolia L.) flowers using free and immobilized yeast Saccharomyces cerevisiae. Microbiol Res 162: 93-98.

15. Dandu MM, Dhabe AS (2011) Saccharomyces cerevisiae strains from nectar for wine production. Bioinfolet 8: 314.

16. Dombek KM, Ingram LO (1987) Ethanol production during batch fermentation with Saccharomyces cerevisiae: changes in glycolytic enzymes and internal pH. Appl Environ Microbiol 53: 1286-1291.

17. Van Maris AJ, Abbott DA, Bellissimi E, Van den Brink J, Kuyper M, et al. (2006) Alcoholic fermentation of carbon sources in biomass hydrolysates by Saccharomyces cerevisiae: current status. Antonie Van Leeuwenhoek 90: 391-418.

18. Ali KM, Chatterjee K, De D, Maiti S, Pathak TK, et al. (2011) Evaluation of antioxidant activity of seed of Holarrhena antidysenterica: An approach through different in vitro models. J Nat Pharm 2: 115-118.

19. Hu Y, Xu J, Hu Q (2003) Evaluation of antioxidant potential of Aloe vera (Aloe barbadensis Miller) extracts. J Agric Food Chem 51: 7788-7791.

20. Zhang ZT, Du YJ, Liu QG, Liu Y (2001) Determination of the antioxidative effect of Aloe vera. Nat Prod Res Develop 13: 45-46.

21. Hu Q, Hu Y, Xu J (2005) Free radical-scavenging activity of Aloe vera (Aloe barbadensis Miller) extracts by supercritical carbon dioxide extraction. Food Chem 91:85-90.

22. Sharma SK, Singh AP (2012) In vitro antioxidant and free radical scavenging activity of Nardostachys jatamansi DC. J Acupunct Meridian Stud 5: 112-118.

23. Nahak G, Sahu RK (2011) Phytochemical evaluation and antioxidant activity of Piper cubeba and Piper nigrum. J Appl Pharm Sci 01: 153-157.

24. Kumar P, Jaiswal P, Singh VK, Singh DK (2011) Medicinal, therapeutic and pharmacological effects of Syzygium aromaticum (Laung). Pharmacologyonline 1: 1044-1055.

25. Crowell EA, Ough CS (1979) A modified procedure for alcohol determination by dichromate oxidation. Am J Enol Vitic 30: 61-63.

26. Lane JH, Eynon L (1923) Determination of reducing sugars by means of Fehling's solution with methylene blue as internal indicator. J Soc Chem Ind Trans: 32-36.

27. Chidambara Murthy KN, Singh RP, Jayaprakasha GK (2002) Antioxidant activities of grape (Vitis vinifera) pomace extracts. J Agric Food Chem 50: 5909-5914.

28. Ruch RJ, Cheng SJ, Klaunig JE (1989) Prevention of cytotoxicity and inhibition of intercellular communication by antioxidant catechins isolated from Chinese green tea. Carcinogenesis 10: 1003-1008.

29. Oyaizu M (1986) Studies on products of the browning reaction. Antioxidative activities of browning reaction products prepared from glucosamine. Jpn J Nutr 44: 307-315.

30. Mary Anupama P, Guru MD, Ayyanna C (2010) Optimization of fermentation medium for the production of ethanol from jaggery using box-behnken design. Int J Appl Biol Pharm Tech 1: 34-45.

31. Ricardo da Silva JM, Darmon N, Fernandez Y, Mitjavila S (1991) Oxygen free radical scavenger capacity in aqueous models of different procyanidins from grape seeds. J Agric Food Chem 39: 1549-1552.

32. Sato M, Ramarathnam N, Suzuki Y, Ohkubo T, Takeuchi M, et al. (1996) Varietal differences in the phenolic content and superoxide radical scavenging potential of wines from different sources. J Agric Food Chem 44: 37-41.

33. Brand-Williams W, Cuvelier ME, Berset C (1995) Use of a free radical method to evaluate antioxidant activity. LWT - Food Science and Technology 28: 25-30.

34. Rekka E, Kourounakis PN (1991) Effect of hydroxyethyl rutosides and related compounds on lipid peroxidation and free radical scavenging activity. Some structural aspects. J Pharm Pharmacol 43: 486-491.

35. Halliwell B, Gutteridge JM (1981) Formation of a thiobarbituric-acid-reactive substance from deoxyribose in the presence of iron salts: the role of superoxide and hydroxyl radicals. FEBS Lett 128: 347-352.

36. Duh PD, Tu YY, Yen GC (1999) Antioxidant activity of water extract of Harng Jyur (Chrysanthemum morifolium Ramat). LWT - Food Science and Technology 32: 269-277.

37. Duh PD, Yen GC (1997) Antioxidant activity of three herbal water extracts. Food Chemistry 60: 639-645.

38. Harish Nayaka MA, Sathisha UV, Manohar MP, Chandrashekar KB, Dharmesh SM (2009) Cytoprotective and antioxidant activity studies of jaggery sugar. Food Chem 115: 113-118.

39. Finose A, Devaki K (2011) Phytochemical and Chromatographic studies in the flowers of Woodfordia fruticosa (L) Kurz. Asian J of Plant Sci Res 1: 81-85.

40. Chandan BK, Saxena AK, Shukla S, Sharma N, Gupta DK, et al. (2008) Hepatoprotective activity of Woodfordia fruticosa Kurz flowers against carbon tetrachloride induced hepatotoxicity. J Ethnopharmacol 119: 218-224.

10

Attitudes among Elderly towards Complementary and Alternative Medicine use as a Suicide Prevention Program in Korea: A Preliminary Study

Bethsaida Yanain Rojas[1], Eric Richardson[2], Dong-Hyun Ahn[3]

[1]College of Medicine, Hanyang University, Seoul, South Korea.
[2]Graduate School of Biomedical Science & Engineering, College of Medicine, Hanyang University, Seoul, South Korea.
[3]Department of Neuropsychiatry, Institute of Mental Health, Hanyang Center for Behavioral Development, Hanyang University, Seongdong-gu, Seoul, South Korea.

Abstract

Introduction: Suicide among Korean elderly persons continues to be a major issue, with most suicides being in the over 65 years old demographic population. It has the highest suicide rate of all Organization for Economic Cooperation and Development (OECD) member countries and ranking 31st out of 38 member nations in terms of overall life satisfaction. It is well known that depression is the psychiatric diagnosis most strongly associated with suicide; therefore, the aim of this research was to explore how to address depression using Complementary and Alternative Medicine (CAM) among senior citizens.

Methods: A cross-sectional study was conducted among 326 subjects aged 65 years and over, attending senior citizen halls located in Seoul, Korea. The survey instrument was designed to explore whether CAM is a good adjuvant in suicide prevention programs within senior citizen halls. Data entry was done by using Excel and exported to SPSS version 21.0 software package for analysis.

Results: Among 326 participants, 93.3% reported using one or more CAM modalities for depression-related outcomes. Prayer, traditional Korean medicine, sports, diet, medicinal herbs and fungi were the leading complementary and alternative therapies used to improve mood disorders. Almost half of respondents, 49.7% used some complementary health therapy while receiving conventional depressive treatment.

Conclusion: The findings support the urgent need to resolve the social problem of suicide among elderly population, especially isolated elders. CAM appears to be widely accepted and used by a high percentage of Korean elderly people to improve mood disorders. Most herbs were self-prescribed and undisclosed to health care providers. This result highlights the need of in-depth study into Complementary Health approaches and their potential effects as adjunctive treatment for elders at risk of suicide.

Keywords: Depression; Suicide; Prevention; Elderly; South Korea; Complementary and Alternative Medicine (CAM)

Introduction

Despite South Korea's economic success over the past several decades, the generation of elderly responsible for its economic miracle has been poorly rewarded. South Korea has received the nickname as "suicide capital of the world" partly because so many of its elders end their own lives and due to the rise of suicides rates, to date the problem persists [1]. Despite policies to reduce this number, it has the highest suicide rate of all Organization for Economic Cooperation and Development (OECD) member countries (28.1 per 100,000 in 2012, while the average rate for all of the OCED countries was 12.1), topping all other nations for more than a decade [2].

Rising poverty among the elderly correlates with an increase in their suicide rate from 34 per 100 thousand persons in 2000 to 72 in 2010, far above the OECD average of 22 deaths per 100,000 populations. One-half of Korea's population aged 65 and over lives in relative poverty, nearly four times higher than the OECD average of 13% [3]. The high elderly poverty rate reflects the decline in family support before other private and public sources of old-age income have matured. Korea ranks last in supporting its elderly population and is the least prepared to care for its rapidly aging population among the OECD countries. Many elderly assumed that their children would care for them, thus making it unnecessary to prepare financially. The increase in the number of elderly living alone–from 0.54 million in 2000 to 1.25 million (a quarter of the elderly) in 2010–also indicates declining family support. South Korea has the fastest aging population among the advanced economies and the factors shown to lead elderly to commit suicide are economic hardship, unemployment, psychological despair, physical pain and family problems. In the near future, when 30-year-old Koreans become 65, the country's employment rate for the elderly is expected to top 40%, with more than 7.3 million elders aged 65 years and older participating in economic activities. The rise in the elderly employment rate comes as life expectancy increases, as most retirees are unprepared for a longer life after retirement. Korea's life expectancy was around 77 years in 2002, but it is expected to rise to 82.5 years in 2020 [3,4].

The issue of "suicide and depression" has had an economic impact on the nation. The costs derived from suicides and depression increased 42% between 2007 and 2011 to 10.4 trillion won (10.2 billion dollars). About two-thirds of that comes from lost potential income and nearly a third from the consequent fall in productivity [5]. By the

*Corresponding author: Dong-Hyun Ahn, Director, Department of Neuropsychiatry, Institute of Mental Health, Hanyang Inclusive Clinic for Development Disorders, Hanyang Center for Behavioral Development, College of Medicine, Hanyang University, 222-1, Wangsimni-ro, Seongdong-gu, Seoul, 04763, South Korea
E-mail: adndh@hanyang.ac.kr

year 2020, depression is projected to show the second greatest increase in morbidity after cardiovascular disease, inducing a significant socioeconomic burden [6]. Depression in the elderly increases the risk for medical illness and is often missed and untreated, resulting in fatal consequences [7]. Some studies report a low degree of willingness to express suicidal thoughts by the elderly, while others suggest that the absence of treatment in those elderly with depression is associated with the occurrence of suicide attempts [8]. It is well known that depression is a leading factor linked to self-destruction; therefore, addressing clinical depression and improving psychological well-being of the elderly may be beneficial in preventing suicidal ideation and reduce suicide risk by implementing community-based prevention [9].

To date, research related to suicide prevention and intervention strategies using Complementary and Alternative Medicine (CAM) has been limited to programs conducted for veterans, military personnel and prisoners. However, no research has been undertaken to assess the attitudes and perceptions toward use of CAM as a strategy to prevent suicides among elderly people. This paper describes the quantitative evaluation of the perceptions and attitudes among the elderly population regarding the use of CAM, whether its use could be implemented as a strategy within senior citizen halls to prevent suicides and for increasing their quality of life. The study aims were to evaluate the current knowledge, prevalence and preference of CAM use in a sample of Korean elderly aged 65 years and over that use the senior citizen halls, the application of CAM as an adjuvant in suicide prevention programs within senior citizen halls, and its relationship with social demographic characteristics.

Methods

Research design

This research was a cross-sectional and descriptive study collecting quantitative survey data. The questionnaire consisted of Closed-Ended and Open-Ended Questions written in Korean.

Research area

This study was carried out in Seoul, South Korea from January to August 2016 among 326 elders, attending Senior Citizen Halls (SCH), in Korean "경로당". Seoul city has 25 districts, with a total of 3338 facilities at the time of the study. Although there are existing Suicide Prevention Programs running for the last several years at Elderly Welfare Centers, many elderly that attend the neighborhood Senior Citizen Halls do not attend Elderly Welfare Centers due to many factors including distance, convenience, economic factors and attraction to the environment of the facility. From the available Senior Citizen Halls, four were selected from the official data of the [Korean CDC], three from among the districts with the highest suicide rates, and one from amongst the districts with the lowest suicide rates.

Study population

The study population was apparently healthy elderly aged 65 years and over, being free from any terminal illness, willing to participate in the survey and living in the selected districts. Sample size was calculated using the single population proportion formula as follows: $n=z^2 \cdot p \cdot q/e^2$ [10].

Sampling method

The survey was divided into two stages, the first one was cluster sampling, a total of forty-eight senior citizen halls were selected. Second, the number of participants per Senior Citizen Halls was proportionally determined based on the total number of SCHs and total members per hall in each selected district.

Data collection

Elders who met the criteria received the information in verbal form about the research and those persons willing to participate in the survey gave consent and filled out the questionnaires. Participants were interviewed by the principal investigator, three Korean teachers and eight Korean interviewers with previous experience in interviewing elders, who were trained to administer the questionnaire and taught on CAM as defined in the questionnaire. Participants were offered two options for completing the survey: either independently completing the survey, or being interviewed and asked each question by the interviewer.

Quality control

The questionnaire was pre-tested among twenty elders over 65 years old, workers from Hanyang, Korea, Seoul and Hanguk Universities to check ambiguity, incomprehensible and leading questions. Following the pilot-test's feedback, the survey instrument was rewritten and restructured six times; the translation was made and reviewed by two Korean students of English language and a Korean English teacher.

Data analysis

The closed-ended questions from the questionnaires were initially coded using Microsoft Office Excel and transferred to the Statistical Package for the Social Science (SPSS) v.21 for analysis. Chi square test for single variance, P-values, and logistic regression's tests for comparison of variables were used to compare categorical groups. Quantitative data was summarized and analyzed with descriptive statistics and results was expressed as percentage, organized and presented using frequency tables.

Ethical considerations

Ethical approval was obtained from the Institutional Review Board on Human Subjects Research and Ethics Committees, Hanyang University and the additional permissions were requested to each Senior Citizen Hall selected. The survey was conducted under privacy, confidentiality and the questionnaires were anonymous. To ensure voluntary participation from each participant, an informed consent form signed was obtained from them.

Results

Socio-demographic characteristics

The population included in the analysis for this study was 326 subjects between 65-96 years old from Senior Citizen Halls (SCH). No participant was discarded because the survey was not self-administered; the research was conducted one by one (interviewer-respondent) (Table 1).

Prevalence

Overall, 93.3% (n=304) of the participants that reported depressive feelings or those diagnosed with depression have used one or more complementary therapies as a personal treatment.

Preference

The most commonly used alternative or complementary therapies by elders were prayer 22% (n=67), traditional Korean medicine 16.4% (n=50) sports 12.9% (n=39), diet 8.9% (n=27) and medicinal herbs and fungi 8.3% (n=25). Although the findings indicate a broad selection

Variable	Classification	Senior Citizen Hall	
		Frequency (N=326)	Percentage (100%)
Gender	Female	265	81.20%
	Male	61	18.80%
Age	The "Young Old" 65-74	69	21.10%
	The "Old" 75-84	161	49.40%
	The "Oldest-Old" 85+	96	29.50%
Religion	Roman Catholic	33	10.10%
	Christian	86	26.30%
	Protestant	9	2.80%
	Buddhist	105	32.20%
	Muslim	0	0%
	No religion	93	28.60%
	Others	0	0%
Marital Status	Married	153	47%
	Separated	14	4.20%
	Divorced	28	8.60%
	Widowed	131	40.10%
	Single/Never Married	0	0%
Accompanier of residence	Alone	94	28.90%
	With Spouse	108	33.10%
	With Spouse and Family	89	27.30%
	Relatives	35	10.70%
Level of Education	Illiterate	107	32.90%
	Elementary School	97	29.70%
	Middle School	49	15.00%
	High School	50	15.30%
	College	4	1.20%
	Bachelor's Degree	15	4.60%
	Master's Degree	0	0%
	Doctorate's Degree	1	0.30%
	Other	3	1.00%
Occupation	Employed	3	0.90%
	Self-Employed	6	1.90%
	Housewife	95	29.10%
	Retired	48	14.80%
	Out of work and looking for work	10	3.00%
	Out of work but not currently looking for work	10	3.00%
	Unable to work	152	46.70%
	Others	2	0.60%
Average monthly Income	Less than 1 million won	74	22.70%
	1 million-2.5 million won	52	16.00%
	2.5 million-5 million won	12	3.60%
	More than 5 million won	1	0.30%
	No Income	187	57.40%
Health insurance	National Health Insurance	166	51.00%
	National Health Insurance+Individual Health Insurance	79	24.20%
	Medical Care	9	2.80%
	None	72	22%

Table 1: Social demographic characteristics.

of CAM practices, for the majority of the participants the perceived efficacy of their preferred CAM modality was positive (Table 2).

Distance between participant home and welfare facility

The majority of users 98.5% (n=321) responded that the most convenient facility in terms of distance from home and comfort was the Senior Citizen Hall. The results showed that 43% (n=140) of participants have used the services of SCH for a period of five to ten years, 31.9% (n=104) one to five years, followed by periods of less than 1 year 15% (n=49) and more than ten years 10.1% (n=33) respectively. Elders most

commonly use the SCH facility daily 34% (n=111), followed by 3 weeks in the month 32% (n=104), and 2 weeks per month 23% (n=75), and averaged spending from 4 to 10 h per day there 60% (n=198). The rest of the population was spread out between less than 4 h per day or more than 10 h per day.

Decision to use the Senior Citizen Hall (SCH)

Elders reported the following reasons for using the SCH, in descending percentages: loneliness (51.5%), meeting new friends (13.8%), boredom (11.7%), engage in activity for enjoyment (10.7%), others (8%) and for learning (4.3%) respectively. They report feeling the following benefits from visiting the SCH: "I am not alone and I have friends" (95.4%), followed by "I forget my problems when I stay in SCH" (89.9%), "I can trust and express my feelings and thoughts" (54%).

Attitudes

In the surveyed population, nearly half (49.8%) report that they believe programs and activities that teach and promote CAM at the SCH would be helpful to improve the quality of life and help learn how to deal with problems that lead to depression. Only (14.3%) of the respondents disagree with this statement (Table 3).

Discussion

This research provides a first estimate of the prevalence of use and knowledge toward use of CAM treating depression among Korean elderly, as well as, the attitudes for developing suicide prevention programs using CAM in Senior Citizen Halls.

The World Health Organization (WHO) recognizes "suicide" as a public health priority accounting for more than half of the world's 1.5 million violent deaths annually [11]. In 2013, the 66th World Health Assembly, with 194 Member States, adopted the WHO's Comprehensive Mental Health Action Plan 2013–2020, the first in its history. The plan sets a central role for provision of community based care and emphasis on human rights, and in addition, promotes moving away from a purely medical model to address various social factors including income, education, housing, and other social service, that impact on mental health as a more comprehensive [12]. South Korea has implemented Strategies to Prevent Suicide (STOPS), a program of "initiatives aimed at increasing public awareness, improving media reporting of suicide, restricting access to means, screening and improving treatment for persons at high risk of suicide." This program includes national guidelines for media coverage to focus more on warning signs and possibilities of treatment, rather than factors that lead to suicide [13]. Various CAM modalities can provide social and non-traditional interventions in relation to these programs.

The use of alternative medicine modalities as an isolated therapy is uncommon because most people use non-mainstream approaches along with conventional medicine, which is more accurately defined as complementary medicine. Alternative medicine would be defined as treatments that replace conventional medical care *in toto* [14]. Evidence-based data that suggest CAM therapies are effective adjuvants for treating mental health disorders. Evidence-based integrative complementary medicine treatment models, such as ALPS (Antidepressant-Lifestyle-Psychological-Social) [15] have been previously used to treat clinical depression (characterized by psychophysiological changes in energy, sleep, appetite, low mood, feelings of worthlessness or guilt, loss of pleasure and/or suicidal thoughts) [16]. Other studies show physical therapies such as Tai Chi and physical exercises have a positive effect on maintaining elders' mobility and thus are beneficial to maintaining mental health [17-19]. Research of Korean senior citizen halls found that community programs for better quality of life and improved physical and mental health are satisfactory and successful if the population served participates in their selection and planning [20-23].

Globally, the use of CAM therapy for various kinds of diseases is continuing to increase across many cultures, social backgrounds, and across all ages for multiple and diverse reasons, so it is important to know the prevalence of use and current knowledge on CAM to address

Division	Senior Citizen Hall	
	Frequency (N=304)	Percentage (100%)
Harmful	0	0%
Not at all effective	10	3.30%
Neutral	61	20.10%
Effective	212	69.70%
very effective	21	6.90%

Table 2: CAM use satisfaction.

Do you think that CAM could help to treat mental illness and prevent suicides?		
Division	Senior Citizen Hall	
	Frequency (N=326)	Percentage (100%)
Yes	211	64.80%
No	115	35.20%
If you know someone desiring to die would you recommend the use of CAM?		
Yes	210	64.40%
No	116	35.60%

Table 3: Attitudes regarding to use of CAM to treat mental illness and preventing suicide.

the epidemic of depression and suicide among the elderly. It is especially important to document the use of CAM that is occurring alongside allopathic medicine, to know the efficacy of the various therapies and prevent negative effects that could come from the unreported combining of therapies.

The results of our research show a high prevalence of CAM use (93.3%), alongside a surprisingly low level of knowledge (36.9%) concerning their use by healthcare providers. In addition (49.7%) of CAM users were taking concurrent prescription medication, a high percentage compared to another study showing that 13% of participants were taking herbs along with allopathic medicine, obtaining as a presumed result higher depression and anxiety scores than other herb users [24]. This imbalance between use and knowledge will seriously affect the health of those elderly who use CAM to treat their symptoms of depression caused by problems other than mental illness. Ventegodt and Merrick have suggested that even for patients with serious mental and physical disorders, nondrug CAM therapies appear to be safe [25]. The use of CAM is likely not the problem, instead it is the low level of knowledge towards what they are using, especially the use of phyto-therapeutics that is not communicated to their doctors; it is a dangerous combination. This finding is in agreement with a previous study, suggesting that the prevention of negative herbal-medicinal interactions requires training healthcare personnel to obtain more detailed patient information regarding CAM usage, especially oral and other physical therapies [26].

Mind/Body Interventions Therapies (44.1%) to treat symptoms of depression were the preferred CAM treatment among elderly people in our study; these include prayer (22%), sports (12.9%), humor therapy (4.3%), and dance and music therapy (3.6%). Other studies support the findings in this research, indicating that mind and body practices relieve the symptoms of depression and provide benefits in mood alterations [27-31]. The second most used group of CAM modalities were Biologically Based Therapies (28.4%), which includes diet (8.9%), medicinal herbs and fungi (8.3%), dietary supplements (6.9%), and megavitamin therapy (3.3%); these therapies, including dietary changes, belong to the natural product therapies. These results are in agreement with a previous study, showing that 34% of patients used herbal medicines to treat mood disorders, that most of these patients self-prescribed the herbal remedies and their use was undisclosed to their healthcare providers [24]. Significantly, Traditional Korean Medicine (16.4%) was the most used alternative medical system, which is within the group of other approaches (16.7%). These results provide compelling evidence for the integration of CAM into Evidence-Based Clinical Practice.

Information about CAM use was commonly obtained from family (21.5%), advertising on TV, streets, buildings, etc. (17.8%), others (traditional market) (14.7%), oriental medicine healthcare workers (13.5%) and friends (11%); similar results have been reported from a National Survey in 2006 in a general population in South Korea [32]. Regarding reasons for CAM use, the main cause was: "dissatisfaction toward allopathic medicine and/or treatments were not available for a specific illness" (39.8%), "traditional background, belief in the alternative system and individual philosophical viewpoint" (16.9%), "others" (in case of hearing good comments on certain alternative therapy or personal experience of positive side effects) (16.3%), and "a hope for fewer side effects" (14.4%). A lower but significant percentage were motivated by economic factors believing that "alternative medicine is cheaper than allopathic medicine" (4.6%), others began complementary therapies out of curiosity (4.6%) or by recommendation from a medical doctor (3.4%). These reports suggest that the use of CAM may be positively influenced by culture, background, family, friends, environment and oriental medicine healthcare workers. These results found are similar to other studies done [33,34].

Our research clearly shows that the elderly perceive CAM as a helpful adjunct to help treat mental illness and prevent suicide (64.8%), and would recommend the use of CAM (64.4%) to someone with suicidal thoughts. The factors statistically associated with perceptions toward use of CAM for suicide prevention were predicted by previous attitudes when treating symptoms of depression using alternative therapies, age, and marital status, accompanier of residence, income and health insurance. Regarding to attitudes: Age, income, health insurance and their perceived effectiveness of complementary and alternative treatments for mental health, were the independent predictors. In this respect, the strongest predictors were an average monthly income between 2.5-5 million won (p-value ≤ 0.001) perceived effectiveness (p-value ≤ 0.001) and previous attitudes (p-value ≤ 0.001) toward using CAM for mental health. Our observations are in agreement with findings of the WHO traditional medicine strategy 2002-2005, where it is mentioned that in most developed countries the use of CAM appears to be related to factors other than cost and tradition, because the traditional medicine use is quite different from country to country and region to region [35].

Despite South Korea's status as a developed country, there are people with "low income, no income nor health insurance" and that population turns to alternative medicine for the most common reasons: necessity, affordability and accessibility. This is also in agreement with the WHO traditional medicine strategy 2014-2023, wherein factors such as low income, inadequate education, poor health and inequality (found in high proportions in developing countries), force the populace to use alternative therapies because they are cheap, available and accessible [36]. This suggests that regardless of whether individuals are lower or higher income and education, with or without health insurance, young or old, in search of "just health" or "a good human life with quality," people are using CAM to achieve that purpose. Therefore, we conclude our hypothesis that perceptions and attitudes among Korean elderly people toward use of CAM as an adjuvant in suicide prevention

programs within senior citizen halls to help to decrease suicide rates was found positive.

Limitations

Three districts studied have the highest elderly' suicide rate in Seoul (2010-2014), and one district among the lowest suicide rate, but not nationally. Therefore, the results do not represent the whole aging society of South Korea.

Conclusion

The study gave a perspective of knowledge, use, attitudes and perceptions towards use of CAM as a preventive strategy in senior citizen halls to help to reduce suicide risk. It may be helpful for the understanding of elders' concerns, expectations and anxieties about the research question. This information may be helpful in assisting to know how to decrease the older people's suicide rate through CAM program research conducted within senior citizen halls. Notwithstanding their limitations, this pilot study may generate new information or ideas as a contribution to the appropriate authorities, focusing on CAM use as a tactic for preventing suicides in senior citizen halls and the outcomes of this study may be helpful as a reference for future related studies.

Funding and sponsorship

This research was supported by Hanyang Institute of Mental Health.

Authors' Contribution

Rojas BY wrote the proposal, participated in data collection, analyzed the data and drafted the paper. Richardon E and Ahn Dong-Hyun approved the proposal, participated in data analysis, revised subsequent drafts of the paper and approved the final manuscript.

Acknowledgments

We are very grateful to Hanyang Institute of Mental Health for financial support and to Institutional Review Board on Human Subjects Research and Ethics Committees, Hanyang University for approval of ethical clearance and technical support of this preliminary study. Then, we would like to thank the Korean senior citizens who participated in this study for their commitment in responding to our interviews. We are also grateful to those Senior Citizen Hall facilities who accepted participate, for their assistance and permission to undertake the research. Finally, our sincere thanks to the Koreans students and teachers for their great effort, especially to Lee Kwang-Il for his unconditional support during the survey.

References

1. Kwon JW, Chun HR, Cho SI (2009) A closer look at the increase in suicide rates in South Korea from 1986–2005. BMC Public Health 9: 72.

2. World Health Organization (WHO) (2012) Suicide rates by country. Global Health Observatory Data Repository.

3. Jones RS, Urasawa S (2014) Reducing the high rate of poverty among the elderly in Korea. OECD Economics Department Working Papers.

4. Jackson R, Howe N, Nakashima K (2010) The global aging preparedness index. Center for Strategic and International Studies.

5. Hyun KR (2015) Analysis of Social-economic Cost on Major Illnesses to Set Priority of Health Security Policies. Health Insurance Policy Research Institute. National Health Insurance Service.

6. World Health Organization (WHO) (2011) World Health Organization. Mental health: Depression.

7. NAMI National Alliance on Mental Illness (NAMI) (2014) Depression in Older Persons Fact Sheet.

8. Kim SM, Ha JH, Yu JH, Park DH, Ryu SH (2014) Path analysis of suicide ideation in older people. International Psychogeriatrics 26: 509-515.

9. McGirr A, Renaud J, Séguin M, Alda M, Turecki G (2008) Course of major depressive disorder and suicide outcome: A psychological autopsy study. J Clin Psychiatry 69: 966-70.

10. Wayne WD, Chad LC (2013) Biostatistics: A foundation for analysis in the health sciences. Tenth edition.

11. http://www.who.int/mediacentre/news/releases/2014/suicide-prevention-report/en/

12. World Health Organization (WHO) (2013) World Health Organization. WHO's mental health action plan 2013–2020.

13. Hendin H, Xiao S, Li X, Huong TT, Wang H, Hegeel U, Philips MR (2015) Suicide Prevention in Asia: Future Directions.

14. https://nccih.nih.gov/

15. Sarris J (2011) Clinical Depression: An Evidence-based Integrative Complementary Medicine Treatment Model. Altern Ther Health Med 17: 26-37.

16. APA American Psychiatric Association (APA) (2013) Diagnostic and statistical manual of mental disorders.

17. Huh MD, Ha CK (2006) Comparative analysis of satisfaction in physical activity of the aged in welfare center and in the hall for the aged. Korea J Sport Sci 15: 633-646.

18. Kim SJ (2007) The effect of Tai Chi exercise on the wellness in the elderly who use senior citizen's club. Journal Korean. Soc Living Environ Sys 14: 229-238.

19. Chu SK, Lee CY, Yoo JH (2012) The effects of an aerobic exercise program on mobility, fall efficacy, balance, and stress in the elderly at senior centers. J Korean Acad Commun Health Nurs 23: 22-30.

20. Rim CS, Kim KH, Kim MS, Lee KH, Lee IS (2006) A study on current status and future aspects of the senior citizen halls in Seoul. Journal of Welfare for the Aged 31: 313-343.

21. Min BG (2006) The activate plan and the present status of hall for the old. Korean Academy of Social Welfare Support 2: 255-270.

22. Lee HW, Song YH, Lee JS, Choi SY (2005) A comparative study on the facilities type of gyungrodang in urban single housing district and present condition of welfare service of the elderly. J Korean Hous Assoc 16: 17-25.

23. Lee JY, Kim EC, Sohn TJ (2005) A study on improving plan and using condition for age hall as leisure facilities in Chung-Ju. Composition of the Academic Conference of the Korean Architecture Society 1: 105-110.

24. Edwards D, Heufelder A, Zimmermann A (2012) Therapeutic effects and safety of Rhodiola rosea extract WS® 1375 in subjects with life-stress symptoms–results of an open-label study. Phytother Res 26: 1220-1225.

25. Ventegodt S, Merrick J (2009) A review of side effects and adverse events of non-drug medicine (nonpharmaceutical complementary and alternative medicine): psychotherapy, mind-body medicine and clinical holistic medicine. J Complement Integr Med 6: 16.

26. McCrea CE, Pritchard ME (2011) Concurrent herb-prescription medication use and health care provider disclosure among university students. Complement Ther Med 19: 32-36.

27. Yeung AS, Ameral VE, Chuzi SE, Fava M, Mischoulon D (2011) A pilot study of acupuncture augmentation therapy in antidepressant partial and non-responders with major depressive disorder. J Affect Disord 130: 285-289.

28. Monti DA, Beitman BD (2010) Integrative Psychiatry. Oxford, UK: Oxford University Press.

29. Muskin PR (2000) Complementary and Alternative Medicine and Psychiatry. Arlington, VA: American Psychiatric Press Inc.

30. Mischoulan D, Rosenbaum JF (2008) Natural Medications for Psychiatric Disorders (2nd edn.). Philadelphia, PA: Lippincott Williams & Wilkins.

31. Koch S, Morlinghaus K, Fuchs T (2007) The joy dance: specific effects of a single dance intervention on psychiatric patients with depression. Arts Psychother 34: 340-349.

32. Ock SM, Choi JY, Cha YS, Lee J, Chun MS, et al. (2009) The use of complementary and alternative medicine in a general population in South Korea: results from a national survey in 2006. J Korean Med Sci 24: 1-6.

33. McFadden KL, Hernández TD, Ito TA (2010) Attitudes Towards Complementary and Alternative Medicine Influence Its Use. Explore (NY) 6: 380-388.

34. Da Silva TL, Ravindran LN, Ravindran AV (2009) Yoga in the treatment of mood and anxiety disorders: A review. Asian J Psychiatr 2: 6-16.

35. World Health Organization (WHO) (2002) World Health Organization. Traditional Medicine Strategy 2002-2005. Geneva.

36. World Health Organization (WHO) (2013) World Health Organization. Traditional Medicine Strategy 2014-2023. Geneva.

11

Current Approaches of Research in Naturopathy: How Far is its Evidence Base?

Rajiv Rastogi*

Central Council for Research in Yoga & Naturopathy (CCRYN) 61-65, Institutional Area, Janakpuri, New Delhi-110058, India

Abstract

Naturopathy is a system of health care comprises a traditional system of healing based on philosophical principles vogue to ancient India. It has its own concepts of health and disease and also principles of treatment. Ancient scriptures like *Vedas* give a comprehensive detail about these practices. This system laid more importance on the preventive health rather than curative one. This is one of the reasons that Naturopathy system is gaining popularity day by day.

Naturopathy is a science of health and healthy living. It teaches us how to live healthy? What to eat? And how our daily routine should be? And help a person in attaining freedom from disease and with the help of their regular use, positive and vigorous health can be acquired. The main objectives of Naturopathy are to change the unhealthy living habits of people and to teach them the healthy and positive lifestyle in accordance to the laws of Nature with the effective help of different Naturopathy modalities.

Naturopathy system is found very effective in the management of various disorders where there is no cure. However, in depth clinical studies are required to be conducted to establish its efficacy in prevention and management of diseases especially in Naturopathy. Some efforts have been made but not adequate.

The present paper states the current approaches of research in Naturopathy highlighting its basic principles. It also throws light on the reasons behind and explores new areas of research indicating the need of evidence base.

Keywords: Naturopathy; Naturopathy research; Evidence base

Introduction

Naturopathy comprises a traditional system of healing based on philosophical principles vogue to ancient India. Many techniques of Naturopathy system like ushapanam and upvas (fasting) were part of routine living practices peculiar to early days. Ancient scriptures like *Vedas* give us a comprehensive detail about these practices [1].

Naturopathy is a system of health care. It is called as science of healthy living. It is a drugless system of healing based on well founded philosophy. Naturopathy has its own concepts of health and disease and also principles of treatment. It lays more importance on the preventive aspect of health care rather than curative one. This is one of the reasons that Naturopathy system is gaining popularity day by day.

Naturopathy is a system of man building in harmony with constructive principles of nature on physical, mental, moral and spiritual planes of living. It has great health promotive, diseases preventive and curative as well as restorative potential [2] (Figure 1).

Naturopathy is also defined as a system of medicine for cure of diseases by encouraging natural curative reactions inherent in every diseased cell through methods and treatments based upon the fundamental laws which govern health.

Naturopathy is basically a preventive system of treatment. It believes that man is a complete health unit and treat the body physically, mentally, socially (morally) and spiritually for all round health [3]. If one follows the laws of nature he may prevent himself from various diseases (Figure 2).

According to Naturopathy as defined by Lindlahr [4], "The primary cause of disease, barring accidental or surgical injury to the human organism and surroundings hostile to human life, is violation of Nature's laws. The effects of violation of Nature's laws on the physical human organism are:

- Lowered Vitality

- Abnormal composition of blood and lymph

- Accumulation of waste matter, morbid materials and poisons"

To prevent the diseases one has to obey the universal laws of nature in life by adopting the natural methods of living and of treatment. These methods which are applicable in the prevention and management of most of the disorders have been described by Lindlahr [4], as under:

- **Return to Nature** by the regulation of eating, drinking breathing, bathing, dressing, working, resting, thinking, the moral life, sexual and social activities, etc. establishing them on a normal and natural basis.

- **Elementary remedies,** such as water, air, light, earth cures, magnetism, electricity, etc.

- **Chemical remedies**, such as scientific food selection and combination, homeopathic medicines, simple herb extracts and the vito chemical remedies.

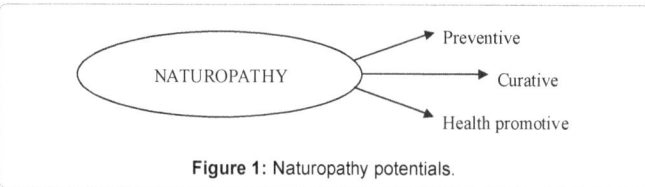

Figure 1: Naturopathy potentials.

*Corresponding author: Rajiv Rastogi, Central Council for Research in Yoga & Naturopathy (CCRYN) 61-65, Institutional Area, Janakpuri, New Delhi-110058, India
E-mail: rrastogi2009@gmail.com

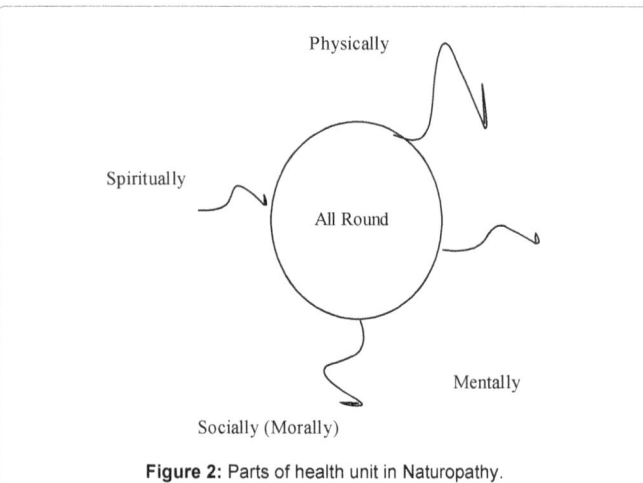

Figure 2: Parts of health unit in Naturopathy.

- **Mechanical remedies,** such as corrective gymnastics, massage, magnetic treatment, structural adjustment and in cases of accident, surgery.

- **Natural and spiritual remedies,** such as scientific relaxation, normal suggestion, constructive thought, the prayer of faith etc.

The difference between Naturopathy and other systems of medicine is that in Naturopathy the methods and treatments used to encourage the inherent curative reaction within each cell are based upon the five fundamental laws which govern health. The cure is obtained, not by reactions to the medicines introduced but because the very vitality and the health of diseased cells improve with the help of the methods and treatments used. According to Naturopathy for sound health tranquility of mind, balanced food, regular exercise and proper rest are essential [3] (Figure 3).

The main principles of Naturopathy are as under [2]:

1. All disease, their cause and their treatment are one.

2. The primary cause of disease is not bacteria. Bacteria develop only after the accumulation of morbid matter when a favorable atmosphere for their growth develops in the body. Hence, the primary cause of disease is morbid matter not the bacteria.

3. Acute diseases are self healing efforts of the body. Hence they are our friends, not the enemy. Chronic diseases are the outcome of wrong treatment and suppression of the acute diseases.

4. Nature is the greatest healer. Body has a capacity to prevent itself from disease and regain health, if unhealthy.

5. Patient is treated not the disease.

6. Treats physical, mental, social (moral) and spiritual all the four aspects together.

7. Treats body as a whole instead of giving treatment to each organ separately.

8. Naturopathy does not use medicines. According to Naturopathy, 'Food is Medicine.'

9. According to Gandhiji "*Ramanama* is the best natural treatment", means doing prayer according to one's spiritual faith is an important part of treatment.

Naturopathy is a science of health and healthy living. It teaches us how to live healthy? What to eat? And how our daily routine should be? The methods of Naturopathy helps a person in attaining freedom from disease and with the help of their regular use, positive and vigorous health can be acquired. Hence, Naturopathy is also called as Natural life. Its main objective is to change the unhealthy living habits of people and to teach them the healthy lifestyle in accordance with the laws of Nature. Different modalities of Naturopathy are very effective in the fulfillment of this pursuit.

It believes that the human body has remarkable recuperative power. It is composed of five great elements i.e. Panchamahabhootas, imbalance of these creates disease. Treatment of the diseases by these elements i.e. Air, Water, Earth, Fire and Ether is known as Naturopathy (Figure 4).

Modalities of Naturopathy

The main modalities of Naturopathy are comprised of:

Diet therapy

It is the main modality under Naturopathy which stresses that the food must be taken in natural or maximum natural form only. Fresh seasonal fruits, fresh green leafy vegetables and sprouts are excellent form of natural foods. These diets are further broadly classified into following three types:

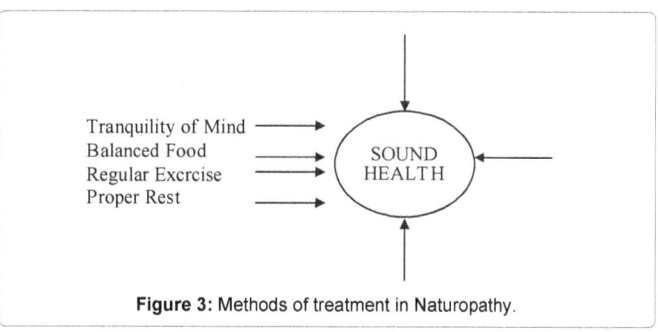

Figure 3: Methods of treatment in Naturopathy.

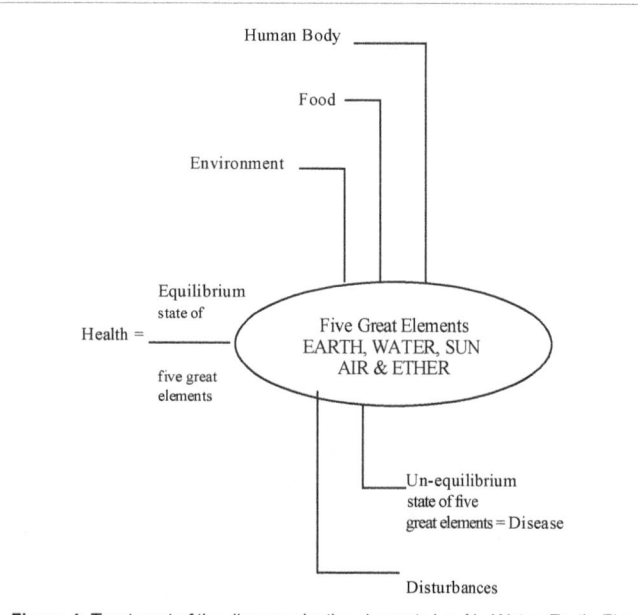

Figure 4: Treatment of the diseases by the elements i.e. Air, Water, Earth, Fire and Ether in Naturopathy.

- **Eliminative Diet:** Liquids- Lemon water, Citric juices, Tender Coconut water, Vegetable soups, Butter milk, Wheat grass juice etc.

- **Soothing Diet:** Fruits, Salads, Boiled or Steamed Vegetables, Sprouts, and Vegetables etc.

- **Constructive Diet:** Wholesome flour, Unpolished rice, little pulses, Sprouts, Curd etc.

These diets are alkaline in nature and purify the body, improve health and render it immune to disease. Naturopathy believes that for preserving health the diet should consist of at least 20% acidic (cooked) and 80% alkaline (uncooked) food. Considering the importance of food in Naturopathy it is regarded as Basic Medicine [5].

Stange R [6] stated that when applied to functional disorders, dietary treatment- the most important measure in natural medicine - has its greatest effect when these disorders affect the gastrointestinal tract, in particular epigastric dyspepsia and irritable bowel syndrome. On the basis of a comprehensive dietary anamnesis, it is often possible to identify foodstuffs and eating behavior capable of aggravating the patient's symptoms. The underlying basic principle of treatment is that the gastrointestinal tract first undergoes a temporary period of rest before being gradually re-accustomed to a biologically high-quality diet. A central approach includes various forms of fasting therapy, in particular in the case of severe conditions, which can usefully be supported by additional relaxation techniques, psychotherapy, hydrotherapy, massage and special manual techniques.

In a study responses to cooked and uncooked food in 32 outpatients with essential hypertension was examined; 28 were also overweight. By varying cooked and uncooked food percentages and salt intake, patients acted as their own control subjects in this unblinded study. After a mean duration of 6.7 months, average intake of uncooked food comprised 62% of calories ingested. Mean weight loss was 3.8 kg and mean diastolic pressure reduction 17.8 mm Hg, both statistically significant (P less than 0.00001). Eighty percent of those who smoked or drank alcohol abstained spontaneously [7].

Fasting therapy

It is an important modality comes under Naturopathy. Mental preparedness is essential to yield effective results in fasting. According to Naturopathy there is only one cause of disease i.e. accumulation of morbid matter and only one cure i.e. elimination of morbid (toxic) matter from the body. Fasting is an effective treatment for removing the disorders of mind and body and is a process of providing rest to digestive system. The vital energy which digests the food is wholly engaged in the process of elimination during fasting.

To determine the effects of short-term fasting on carbohydrate tolerance, 10 obese women with noninsulin-dependent diabetes mellitus (NIDDM) were studied with meal tolerance tests before and after 3 days of fasting. The study revealed that Carbohydrate tolerance improves in obese diabetic (NIDDM) women after 3 days of fasting, in contrast to the impairment of glucose tolerance seen in lean or obese nondiabetic subjects after fasting [8].

Mud therapy

It is one of the important modality, which is very simple but highly effective. The mud used for therapeutic purpose is neat and clean and free from contamination of stone pieces or chemicals, manure etc., and is taken from 5 to 6 ft. depth from the surface of the ground.

Mud therapy gives coolness to the body. It dilutes and absorbs the toxic substances of body and ultimately eliminates them from body. Mud packs and Mud baths are the main forms of treatment. Mud is used effectively in constipation, headache due to tension, high blood pressure and skin diseases etc. Mud pack is applied on forehead also in headache and high blood pressure. Gandhiji also used to take mud packs for getting rid of his constipation.

A study was conducted to evaluate the short-term effects of mud-pack therapy on pain relief and functional improvement in knee osteoarthritis in comparison with intra-articular hyaluronic acid injections.

The study included 23 patients who were diagnosed as having knee osteoarthritis according to the ACR (American College of Rheumatology) criteria, and had complaints lasting for more than three months. All the patients had stage 2 or 3 osteoarthritis radiographically according to the Kellgren-Lawrence criteria. Twelve patients (3 males, 9 females; mean age 54±6 years; range 46 to 67 years) received mud therapy bilaterally. Mud packs were heated to 45ºC and applied on both knees for 30 minutes daily for a total of 12 weekdays. Eleven patients (2 males, 9 females; mean age 53±9 years; range 40 to 66 years) received a total of three bilateral intra-articular hyaluronic acid injections, each interspersed by weekly intervals. The study revealed that Mud-pack therapy is a noninvasive, complication-free, and cost-effective alternative modality for the conservative treatment of knee osteoarthritis [9].

Hydrotherapy

Water is a main component of Naturopathy. It is an ancient method of treatment used mainly for preserving health, relieving the inner congestion [10] and curing different types of diseases. Taking bath in clean and fresh water is very effective as it opens up the pores of skin, imparts lightness and alertness to the body, all systems and muscles of body are activated and the blood circulation improves. It is believed that the old tradition of taking bath in rivers, ponds or water falls on specific occasions in India is virtually a form of Hydrotherapy only. Hip bath, Enema, Hot and Cold fomentation, Hot foot bath, Spinal bath, Steam bath, Immersion bath, Hot and Cold packs on Abdomen, Chest and other parts of the body are the recent developments in Hydrotherapy.

In naturopathy, application of a cold chest pack for 30 min daily over a period of time is believed to improve lung functions in bronchial asthmatics. For scientific evaluation of this treatment, a study was carried out on 15 medication-free bronchial asthma patients (2 males) with ages from 19 to 42 years. The peak expiratory flow rate (PEFR, in l/min) was recorded before, during and after a 30 min application of a cold chest pack. This treatment was carried on for 21 days, during which the patients received other naturopathy treatments such as fasting, diet changes, hydro therapy, massage, magneto therapy, color therapy and application of mud packs, along with yoga therapy. The results suggest that (I) an application of a cold chest pack increase the PEFR as an immediate effect and (ii) this effect is augmented following 21 days of other naturopathy treatments along with yoga [11].

Massage therapy

It plays an important role in Naturopathy treatment procedure. It is a scientific and systemic manipulation of the tissues and organs of the body, aims at improving the blood circulation and also at strengthening muscles and bodily organs. Taking Sun bath after massaging the whole body is a well known health practice in India during winters. It bestows combined benefits of massage and Sun rays therapy. To overcome different disease symptoms, specific techniques of massage are used and necessary therapeutic effects are obtained through it. Mustard oil, sesame oil and coconut oil are generally used in massage for lubrication as well as for creating therapeutic effects.

A randomized controlled trial including 60 participants was conducted in Sweden between 2005 and 2007 to evaluate change in health-related quality of life for people with constipation receiving abdominal massage. The control group continued using laxatives as before and the intervention group received additional abdominal massage. Health-related quality of life was assessed using the EQ-5D and analyzed with linear regression. The study revealed that abdominal massage may be cost-effective in the long-term and it is relevant to consider it when managing constipation [12].

Chromo therapy

The seven colours of spectrum i.e. Violet, Indigo, Blue, Green, Yellow, Orange and Red are used in Naturopathy as therapy which have different therapeutic properties and effects. Chromo therapy is applied by coloured bottles filled with water or oil and exposed to Sun rays for specified hours. This colour charged water is used as an external application for skin disorders and is also ingested as a tonic for digestive disorders. Specific colours are applied on specific parts with the help of lamps with the specific coloured glasses. These devices of Chromo therapy are used effectively in prevention and treatment of different diseases. These colours are also applied in daily life in various ways like coloured light in the room, coloured clothing, colours in dining form, foods charged by specific colours, wall paints, colour of furniture etc.

Air therapy

Fresh air, an important part of Naturopathy is most essential for good health. The advantage of air therapy is achieved by taking air bath daily for at least 20 minutes. Walking in fresh air is a best form of air bath. It is more advantageous when combined with morning cold rub and exercises. Air bath has soothing and tonic effect upon the millions of nerve endings all over the surface of the body and enhances the elimination process. It has shown good results in nervousness, neurasthenia, rheumatism, skin, mental and various other chronic disorders.

As Lindlahr [4] says, 'Walking is a splendid form of exercise, provided it is made vigorous enough to set in motion all the muscles of the body and to produce perspiration. There is no better form of elimination than natural perspiration' [13].

Naturopathy provides a systemic schedule to all its patients consisting of a diet prescription followed by certain Naturopathy treatments and do's and don'ts with a view to change their life style in a positive manner as under.

Daily Routine and Diet Chart

5.00 a.m. 5.30 a.m.

Get up from bed. Drink about half a liter of water (Ushapanam). Attend natural calls and prayer. Brisk walk/Suryanamaskara/Yogasanas/Games/Gardening/Swimming and Pranayama or Breathing exercises followed by Shavasana or Yoga Nidra.

6.15 a.m.

One glass of lemon water (Half/ one lemon + one/two table spoonful of honey or jaggery + 300 ml. of water Or tender coconut

water / triphala water / amla water / Bittergourd juice / Methi water / Diabetic Herbal Juice / Herbal Tea etc.)

6.30 a.m.

Treatments if necessary.

* Enema if constipated during fasting.
* Cold Hip Bath – 10 mts or Cold towel pack on the abdomen for 20 to 30 minutes / Mud packs for 20 minutes. Weekly thrice / daily.
* Cold / Neutral wet spinal pack for 20 to 30 minutes. Weekly thrice / daily.
* Affusion with hot and cold water alternatively 3 minutes / 1 minute daily.
* Cold neutral wet knee pack / chest pack for 30 to 45 minutes daily.

7.15 a.m.

Cold / Neutral water full bath

Breakfast 9.00 a.m.

Seasonally available fruits / Sprouts / Salads / Butter Milk – 1 cup / Soup / Fruit or Vegetable Juice

Lunch 1.00 p.m.

Uncooked diet i.e. raw salads 100-200 gms (Cucumber, carrot, radish, beetroot, tomato, dhania patti / palak /pudina / cabbage etc.). Seasonal fruits i.e. papaya, apple, mosambi, orange, guava, pineapple, mango, grapes, etc. 300 gms. Vegetable chutney 2 to 4 tablespoon, Sprouts-100 gms (Wheat, moong, moth, chana, methi, ragi, alfalfa etc.) Vegetable soup or Buttermilk 200 to 300 ml. Or Cooked / steamed vegetables 300 to 400 gms; Sprouts / cooked whole soaked pulses ½ to 1 cup Whole grams Roti 1 to 2/ Wheat Dalia 1 or 2 cups / unpolished cooked rice 1 to 2 cups; Vegetable soup or Buttermilk 200 to 300 ml.

6.00 p.m.

* Attend natural calls.
* Bath with cold / neutral water and do prayer or meditation. If necessary drink one glass of seasonal fruit juice / tender coconut water / one glass of buttermilk / barley water or drink only water.

Dinner 7.00 p.m.

Salad 100 grams, 300-400 gms Steamed green vegetables, Vegetable soup or Buttermilk, vegetable chutney, Roti-1 or 2.

Avoid

* Coffee, tea, smoking, tobacco chewing, pan masala, jarda, alcohol, soda etc.
* Non vegetarian food, eggs.
* Frozen / processed / fast / preserved / refined / coloured / flavoured / deodorized Food / Bottled aerated drinks.
* White flour (Maida), White sugar etc.
* Saturated fats / hydrogenated oils.
* Overeating / untimely eating.

- Late lunch / dinner, late sleep.
- Oily and fried foods.
- Stress, anger, worry, hurry, depression, anxiety etc.
- Polluted Air, Noise.
- Avoid indulgence in all unnatural physical / psychological habits.
- Water immediately before and after food.

Reduce

- Salt
- Sweets
- Chilies and Spices
- Dal (Pulses)

Follow

- Regular eating of natural diet preferably two times in a day.
- Chew well and eat with a peaceful mind.
- Drink at least three liters of water in a day, (300 ml. at 2 hours gap)
- Practice exercise in any form.
- Fasting one day in a week with only liquids – seasonal fruits and vegetable juices 4 to 6 glasses in a day or with water only.
- Prayer / Yoganidra / meditation or relaxation twice in a day.
- Expose body to sunlight / fresh air as far as possible [14].

Yoga & Naturopathy systems, recently, are found to have a global spurt evidenced by a constant growth of their followers across the world [15].Their low cost structures; simplicity, inclination towards natural modalities and a consideration of psyche besides other causes of an ailment are possibly the best reasons explaining this spurt. For past many years, these non-pharmacological techniques have also shown their potential to prevent and intervene in a variety of systemic and life style disorders [16-20].

Close interconnection between Body-Mind-Soul has become a widely accepted phenomenon now. Subsequently, psyche and soma thus are taken up as two expressions of one integrated body in an undulating manner representing the dominant ones at one time.

Research in Naturopathy

In view of increasing role of Naturopathy to intervene in various psychosomatic and lifestyle disorders, the scope of research to establish the efficacy of Naturopathy is also increasing. Currently, an exploration of potential of this system is approached at various premier Indian research institutions of modern medicine and also by some Naturopathy Hospitals.

Research is a determined and disciplined activity aiming at answering a particular question [21]. It is a challenging work requiring a great sum of efforts and dedication. The priority of research in naturopathy system is required to be decided as per the needs in reference to its limitations and expectations [14]. Bhole has categorized a few potential areas where research in the field of yoga can be undertaken. These areas are - Philosophical-literary research,

Educational research, Experimental research, Clinical and applied research and experiential research [21]. A further exploration to these areas may be done as under-

1. Standardization of Naturopathy treatments/techniques/modalities/procedures
2. Standardization of Naturopathy Hospitals
3. Research studies related to important National Health & Family welfare Programmes /National Rural Health Mission (NRHM)
4. Preventive Role of Naturopathy
5. Research studies with reference to promotion of positive health
6. Research studies on various folk/tribal community oriented health practices
7. Research on maintenance of good physical and mental practices (GPMP)
8. Survey on specific issues relating to Naturopathy
9. Research studies on vanishing folk/tribal health/medical practices
10. Research on ways of holistic personality development
11. Research on importance of food remedies used in houses as home remedy for prevention and treatment of various diseases
12. Study on Traditional Indian lifestyle and its importance/usefulness in combating various disorders which are the outcome of modern lifestyle
13. Research on Role of Naturopathy in School Health Care, Women Health Care, Geriatric Health Care & Aging
14. Research on Fasting as a tool for the management of various disorders
15. Research on the efficacy of Naturopathy in management of lifestyle disorders
16. Research to study the mechanism behind Naturopathy procedures
17. Research on the role of Naturopathy as an add on therapy/adjuvant therapy in the management of lifestyle disorders
18. Survey study on the attitude of physicians with reference to Naturopathy
19. Survey study on the level of awareness among the people regarding Naturopathy
20. Survey study on the perception of patients visiting Naturopathy hospitals for use of Naturopathy
21. Research on nutritional aspects

Rastogi and Murthy [14] have shown an inclination of patients towards non-pharmacological and non-invasive therapies of Yoga & Naturopathy for various acute and chronic disorders of common existence [14]. Some conditions which require a mention in this category include stress related ailments, irritable bowel syndrome, bronchial asthma, diabetes, rheumatoid arthritis, coronary artery disease, computer related health problems, insomnia, epilepsy, skin disorders, ulcerative colitis, osteoarthritis, gout and cancer.

Stress related ailments like anxiety neurosis, depression and hypertension are having a high prevalence these days. Studies revealed that these can be effectively managed by the techniques of Yoga & Naturopathy i.e. relaxation, pranayama, yoga nidra and water therapy.

Conclusion

The scientific development of a system primarily depends upon the findings of scientific studies conducted through a good protocol and methodology. Selection of various parameters and intervention programme therefore required to be designed carefully in consultation of experienced investigator and subject experts. The mechanism of working of intervention programme may be demonstrated clearly by the researchers. A research oriented scientific approach to establish the system of naturopathy is therefore, required urgently. Though various trials to study the efficacy of naturopathy have been made, a lot of work is still required to explore the potentials of this system for bringing an ultimate and dependable cure from their ambit. Rigorous clinical trials are required to affirm the possible role of naturopathy in management of various disorders.

Set backs

Lack of specific guidelines, improperly designed protocols, poor research methodologies and lack of trained man power are some of the limitations which act as the main set back in developing naturopathy system as the scientific ones.

References

1. (2005) Yogic & Naturopathic treatment for Common Ailment. CCRYN publication, New Delhi, India.

2. (2009) Yoga & Naturopathy. CCRYN publication, New Delhi, India.

3. Rastogi R (2001) An Introduction to Naturopathy. Asha Prakashan, Agra, India.

4. Lindlahr H (1990) Philosophy and Practice of Nature Cure. Sat Sahitya Sahayogi Sangh, Hyderabad, AP, India.

5. (2008) Concepts of Yoga & Naturopathy. CCRYN publication, New Delhi, India.

6. Stange R (2006) Naturopathic dietary treatment in functional disorders. MMW Fortschr Med 148: 34-36.

7. Douglass JM, Rasgon IM, Fleiss PM, Schmidt RD, Peters SN, et al. (1985) Effects of a raw food diet on hypertension and obesity. South Med J 78: 841-844.

8. Varady KA, Hellerstein MK (2007) Alternate-day fasting and chronic disease prevention: a review of human and animal trials. Am J Clin Nutr 86: 7-13.

9. Bostan B, Sen U, Güneş T, Sahin SA, Sen C, et al. (2010) Comparison of intra-articular hyaluronic acid injections and mud-pack therapy in the treatment of knee osteoarthritis. Acta Orthop Traumatol Turc 44: 42-47.

10. Lindlahr H (1995) Practice of Natural Therapeutics. Sat Sahitya Sahayogi Sangh, Hyderabad, AP, India.

11. Manjunath NK, Telles S (2006) Therapeutic Application of a Cold Chest Pack in Bronchial Asthma. W J Med Sci 1: 18-20.

12. Lämås K, Lindholm L, Engström B, Jacobsson C (2010) Abdominal massage for people with constipation: a cost utility analysis. J Adv Nurs 66: 1719-1729.

13. Rastogi R (2010) Walk can do a lot. Nisargopachar Varta 2: 15-17.

14. Rastogi R, Murthy BTC (2008) Scientific Research in Naturopathy and Yoga: Which way do we need to go? Inference from a Demographic Study. J Res Educ Indian Med 14: 33-40.

15. Sampson W, Vaughn L (2000) Science Meets Alternative Medicine: What the Evidence Says About Unconventional Treatments. Prometheus Books, Amherst, NY, USA.

16. Rastogi R, Murthy BT, Vinudha (2009) Non-pharmacological management of nasal polyp: a case report. Indian J Physiol Pharmacol 53: 380-382.

17. Rastogi S, Ranjana, Rastogi R (2007) Jala Neti application in acute rhino sinusitis. Indian Journal of traditional knowledge 6: 324-327.

18. Rastogi S, Alias A (2001) Management of chronic venous insufficiency with hydrotherapy. Cardiology today 5: 244.

19. Rastogi R (2011) Naturopathic and Yogic intervention in the Management of Coronary Artery Disease. Light on Ayurveda Journal 10: 49-54.

20. Vaidya NV, Bhole MV (2004) Helping yourself towards Zero backache: A holistic approach to backache and Yoga. Lokmanya Medical Research Centre, Pune, India.

21. (2008) Research Methodology in Naturopathy & Yoga. CCRYN publication, New Delhi, India.

12

Evaluation of the Safety and Efficacy of Complete Care Herbal Toothpaste in Controlling Dental Plaque, Gingival Bleeding and Periodontal Diseases

Madhumitha Mazumdar[1], Aritra Chatterjee[2], Swapan Mazumdar[3], Chandrika Mahendra[4] and Prahlad S Patki5*

[1]Head, Dept of Oral Medicine, Diagnosis & Radiology, Dr R. Ahmed Dental College& Hospital, Kolkota-14
[2]PG Scholar,Dept of Oral Medicine, Diagnosis & Radiology, Dr R. Ahmed Dental College& Hospital, Kolkota-14
[3]Consultant Orthodontist, Southern Dental Clinic, Kolkota
[4]Formulation Development, The Himalaya Drug Company, Makali, Bangalore
[5]Head- Medical services & Clinical trials, R&D Center, The Himalaya Drug Company, Makali, Bangalore

Abstract

Aim: The aim of the study is evaluation of safety and efficacy of complete Care Herbal Toothpaste in controlling dental plaque, gingival bleeding and periodontal diseases.

Materials and methods: A hundred subjects of both sex with dental plaque and other dental problems in the age group of 18-60 years, who willing gave informed written consent, were included in the study. All the subjects were given Complete Care Herbal Toothpaste and advised to brush the teeth twice daily for 6 weeks and to come for follow up visits at 2nd week, 4th week and 6th week. Improvement in plaque index, oral hygiene status and gingival index was evaluated in these patients.

Results: Ninety-two out of hundred subjects who were included in the trial completed till the six weeks of follow-up, there was significance of $p<0.05$ reduction in gingival index, plaque index, bleeding index and overall response in individuals with plaque. No clinically significant adverse reactions, were reported or observed, during the entire study period and overall compliance to the treatment was excellent. Therefore, Complete Care Herbal Toothpaste is effective and safe against gingivitis, plaque, bleeding of gums and other oral problems.

Conclusion: The effectiveness of Complete Care Herbal Toothpaste was evaluated in subjects with dental problems. At the end of the study, Complete Care Herbal Toothpaste showed significant reduction in gingival index, plaque index, bleeding index and overall improvement towards the oral problems of the subjects included in the study. A significant symptomatic relief was seen after treatment for 6 weeks with Complete Care Herbal Toothpaste. No clinically significant adverse reactions, were reported or observed, during the entire study period and overall compliance to the treatment was good.

Keywords: Plaque; Gingival index; Bleeding index; Complete care toothpaste

Introduction

Dental plaque is a soft, non- mineralised, microbial biofilm that consists of complex communities of bacterial species that reside on tooth surfaces or soft tissues and play an important role in oral and dental diseases. Regular removal of the plaque is, therefore, essential and has been the cornerstone of disease prevention [1,2]. Dental plaque accumulates on and adheres to teeth, restorations and prosthetic appliances in the mouth. Dental plaque is composed of salivary glycoproteins, bacteria (cocci, bacilli and filamentous forms) and their metabolic end-products arranged in matrix of extracellular material. Clinically, thick layers of dental plaque appear as yellowish or grey deposits which can be only removed mechanically. Dental plaque is classified according to its location on the tooth in relation to the gingival margin, into supra-gingival plaque which is located above the gingival margin, and is visible in the oral cavity and sub-gingival plaque which is located below the gingival margin.

There are three major stages in plaque formation with the microbial aggregation increasing in complexity over time. The first stage is the pellicle formation or acquired saliva pellicle which is a thin, bacteria free, pellicle that protects the surface of the tooth by regulating the mineral ions exchanged between the tooth and saliva. It is formed rapidly after tooth cleaning by selective absorption of glycoproteins from saliva. The second stage is the initial colonisation which occurs within minutes to hours after the pellicle is deposited and it refers to the stage where the pellicle is populated with bacteria. These bacteria are predominantly gram-positive facultative (*Streptococcus sanguis, oralis and mitis and Actinomyces viscosus*). Initially, there are a few plaque deposits which increase with time. The last stage is the development of complex flora or plaque maturation where the early supra-gingival plaque changes from simple gram-positive coccal bacteria to a complex flora with gram-positive and gram-negative rods and spirochetes.

The presence of gram-positive bacteria enhances the colonisation of other species such as the gram-negative rods by co-aggregation. Plaque reaches the mature stage after 7 to14 days and becomes relatively stable around the 21st day. However, this is only a simple description of the bacterial composition of plaque. Location and rate of plaque formation present a broad variability between individuals as these factors are influenced by the oral hygiene habits, diet, saliva composition and the flow rate of each person. Smoking, calculus, overhanging restorations, malocclusions, and local factors such as enamel hypoplasia, cervical root resorption and cracks in the enamel, may also favour plaque accumulation. The term *Materia alba* refers to the visible yellow/white soft deposits formed by the combination between bacterial deposits and epithelial cells that can be removed by rinsing off with

***Corresponding author:** Pralhad S Patki, M.D, Head - Medical Services & Clinical Trials R&D Center, The Himalaya Drug Company, Bangalore-562 123, India
E-mail: dr.patki@himalayahealthcare.com

water. Calculus is formed by calcium phosphate and consists of the mineralised bacterial plaque. Calculus is classified depending on its location on the tooth. Supra-gingival calculus is usually located near to the opening ducts of the salivary glands; its surface is porous and presents a yellow-white appearance which can adopt a darker colour by extrinsic staining in consequence of smoking, consumption of red wine and tea (tannins) and the application of agents such as chlorhexidine. Sub-gingival calculus has a green-black colour and it is firmly attached to the root of the tooth making necessary to use scaling instruments for its removal.

Daily interproximal plaque control is not a common behaviour [3]. However, the removal of plaque from interdental surfaces remains an important life-long objective for dental patients. A common problem with all interdental cleaning aids is patient dexterity and motivation. Additional oral hygiene aids have been developed in an attempt to augment the effect of tooth brushing on reducing interdental plaque [4].

For plaque control methods to be effective in preventing caries they one can: remove all plaque; reduce plaque levels below the threshold for disease; and alter plaque pathogenicity. Possible approaches might therefore include: mechanical removal of plaque; the use of antimicrobial drugs either locally or systemically; alteration in plaque biochemistry; prevention of bacterial attachment to the tooth surface; and alteration of plaque ecology. Within the limits of this review, evidence for mechanical and chemical plaque control measures having effects on caries will, be considered.

For personal oral hygiene, tooth brushing is not only the most common cleaning method, but the brush is also a most valuable vehicle for the delivery of fluoride-containing toothpastes to the teeth, with well-established benefits to caries prevention [5]. However, whether the mechanical action of brushing provides additional benefit is doubted by many researchers in the field [6,7]. Only a few attempts have been made to incorporate compounds which might inhibit plaque and prevent dental disease. Even in those cases where potential antiplaque or antimicrobial compounds have been placed into toothpastes, little or no evidence has been produced to support a beneficial effect. Presently available toothpastes can, in terms of hours, prevent the regrowth of plaque at the gingival margin [8], Furthermore, the limited effects of some toothpastes on plaque regrowth measured over several days have been demonstrated [9]. A qualitative effect of toothpastes on plaque, mediated through an antibacterial action of toothpastes, also must be questioned, as both in vitro and in vivo studies have shown extremely limited antimicrobial and plaque inhibitory activity of toothpastes by comparison to the known antiplaque agent chlorhexidine [9,10]. Chemical antiplaque agents, whether used alone or delivered by a toothbrush, could offer an alternative or adjunctive approach to the control of dental caries. To date, most successes have been achieved with those which exert an antimicrobial action.

The presentation of toothpaste based on herbal ingredients that processes strong anti-inflammatory, antioxidant, and antiplaque activity with adequate balance of all essentials that ensure proper oral hygiene has been incorporated in the Complete Care Herbal toothpaste by Himalaya. It not only protects the teeth from bacteria but acts through its unique antioxidant formulation acts on various toxins to help maintain healthy teeth and gums.

Materials and Methods

This was an open label phase II clinical trial on subjects with dental plaque, gingival bleeding and periodontal diseases conducted at Dept., of Oral Medicine, Diagnosis & Radiology, Dr. R. Ahmed Dental College & Hospital, Kolkata, from 2nd July 2012 to 30th October 2012, after getting an approval of the institutional ethics committee. Subjects who opted for treatment were informed of voluntary nature of trial and written consent was obtained. Complete Care Herbal Toothpaste Contains Extracts of *Punica granatum*, *Zanthoxylum alatum*, *Acacia Arabica*, *Triphala*, *Embelia ribes*, *Vitex negundo*, *Salvadora persica*, *Acacia farnesiana*, *Acacia catechu*, *Mimusops elengi*, *Trachyspermum ammi* and *Azadirachta indica*.

Study procedure

A hundred subjects of either sex aged between 18-60 years presenting with plaque and some other oral problems, who voluntarily gave written informed consent were included in the study. All the subjects included in the study were having various dental problems like dental plaque, gum bleeding, sensitivity, bad breath and other associated dental problems. All the subjects were given the Complete Care Herbal Toothpaste and advised to brush the teeth twice daily for 6 weeks. The subjects were advised to resort to only Complete Care Herbal Toothpaste and not to use any other form of dental formulation, mouthwashes or toothpaste for their oral problems. The criteria for evaluation will be the signs and symptoms were plaque index, gingival index, bleeding index and overall response. Subjects will be evaluated at the interval of 2 weeks for a period of 6 weeks.

The Demographic data of subjects on entry is tabulated in (Table 1).

Inclusion criteria

Hundred subjects of either sex with dental plaque, gingival bleeding and periodontal disease from the age group of 18-60 years and subjects are willing to give a written informed consent and follow the schedule and who has not participated in a similar investigation in past four weeks were enrolled in the study.

Exclusion criteria

Individuals below eighteen years, pre-existing systemic disease necessitating long-term medications, genetic disorder, endocrinal disorders, subjects with history or present condition of allergic response to any cosmetic/pharmaceutical products, toiletries or its components or ingredients in the test products and those who were not willing to give informed consent, were excluded from the study. Pregnant and lactating women were also excluded from the study.

Dosage On day 1, all the subjects were given the Complete Care Herbal Toothpaste and advised to brush the teeth twice daily for 6 weeks and to come for follow up visits at 2nd week , 4th week and 6th week. The subjects were advised to resort to only Complete Care Herbal Toothpaste and not to use any other form of denitrifies or mouth washes.

Parameter	Complete Care Herbal Toothpaste
Age (years)(mean ± SD)	25.43 ± 5.2
Weight in Kg (mean ± SD)	62.70 ± 6.9
Sex ratio (M:F)	32:68
Diet (Veg/Nonveg)	49/51
H/o smoking	05
H/o alcohol consumption	03
H/o Plaque (years)	1.8 ± 1.2

Table 1: Demographic data of subjects on entry (n=100).

Follow-up and assessment

All 100 subjects were reviewed for a period of 6 weeks at 2 weeks interval and at each follow-up visit, they were enquired about the frequency of brushing and use on all days and overall compliance to the treatment. Clinical assessment of dental and oral condition was done objectively (by the investigator) and also subjectively (by subject). Thorough examination was done at intervals of 2 weeks for 6 weeks. At every check- up the clinical response to the Dental condition, any adverse events and subject compliance was assessed. All the subjects were questioned for any untoward effects of the medications for irritation, burning sensation, peeling of the mucosal membrane.

Plaque index was scored on all four surfaces (buccal, lingual, mesical, and distal) of six representative teeth (16, 12, 24, 44, 32, 36). The mean index was calculated by dividing the sum of number from scale by the total number of sites scored within the mouth.

Bleeding index was measured by guiding probe through the gingival sulcus in the first and third quadrants from the buccal aspect and in the second and fourth quadrant from the oral aspect.

Gingival index was scored on the buccal marginal gingiva of the Ramfjord teeth. By summing the individual GBI scores and dividing that sum by the number of sites graded for each subject. All the indices will be evaluated using a visual analogue score of 0-3. The score for the assessment will be nil - 0, mild - 1, moderate - 2, and severe - 3. All the adverse events, either reported or observed by the subjects, were recorded with information about severity, date of onset, duration, and action taken regarding the study drug. Relation of adverse events to study medication was predefined as "Unrelated" (a reaction that does not follow a reasonable temporal sequence from the administration of the drug), "Possible" (follows a known response pattern to the suspected drug, but could have been produced by the subject's clinical state or other modes of therapy administered to the subject), and "Probable" (follows a known response pattern to the suspected drug that could not be reasonably explained by the known characteristics of the subject's clinical state). Subjects were allowed to voluntarily withdraw from the study, if they had experienced serious discomfort during the study or sustained serious clinical events requiring specific treatment. For subjects withdrawing from the study, efforts were made to ascertain the reason for dropout.

Primary and secondary endpoints

The predefined primary efficacy endpoints were reduction in plaque index, gingival index, bleeding index and overall response.

The predefined secondary endpoints were no adverse effects assessed by incidence of adverse events and subject compliance to the therapy.

Adverse events

None of the subjects had reported adverse effect (Table 2) and ninety two out of hundred subjects completed the study.

Eight subjects withdrew from the study. For subjects withdrawing from the study, efforts were made to ascertain the reason for dropout. Non-compliance (defined as failure to take less than 80% of the medication) was not regarded as treatment failure, and reasons for non-compliance were noted.

Statistical analysis

The values are expressed as Mean ± SD. Statistical analysis was performed by "Paired 't' Test" using GraphPad Prism, Version 4.03 for windows, Graphpad Software, San Diego, California, USA. www. graphpad.com.

Results

Ninety two out of hundred subjects successfully completed six weeks of clinical study. The results with respect to the criteria were showed as below (Table 3). Plaque index showed a significant linear decrease from baseline value to 2nd week that is 1.86 ± 0.23 to 1.31 ± 0.41 and later from week 4 to week 6 from 0.86 ± 0.36 to 0.55 ± 0.29 (Figure 1), gingival index also showed a good reduction rate from baseline value of 2.08 ± 0.31 to 1.11 ± 0.36. With Complete Care toothpaste it reduced to 0.72 ± 0.28 at 4 weeks. With continued use, gingival index score further reduced to 0.51 ± 0.29 at the end of 6 weeks with a significance of $p<0.05$ as compared to at entry values at the end of week 6 (Figure 2), the bleeding index also showed a reduction from 2.59 ± 0.33 to 0.79 ± 0.51 with a significance $p<0.05$ as compared as compared to one entry values (Figure 3). But the overall response with respect to the above indices towards the formulation showed a significant decrease from 2.35 ± 0.39 at the end of week 2 to 0.80 ± 0.69 at the end of week 6 (Figure 4). Plaque index, gingival index, bleeding index and overall response showed of significance of $p<0.05$ at 6 weeks as compared to on

Signs & Symptoms	Days of application			
	Initial	Week 2	Week 4	Week 6
Irritation	0.00 ± 0.00	0.00 ± 0.00	0.00 ± 0.00	0.00 ± 0.00
Burning sensation	0.00 ± 0.00	0.00 ± 0.00	0.00 ± 0.00	0.00 ± 0.00
Soreness or ulcer in the mouth	0.00 ± 0.00	0.00 ± 0.00	0.00 ± 0.00	0.00 ± 0.00

Values are expressed in mean ±SD.

Table 2: Safety Evaluation of Complete Care Herbal Toothpaste (n=92).

Parameter	Days of application			
	On entry	Week 2	Week 4	Week 6
Plaque index	1.86 ± 0.23	1.31 ± 0.41	0.86 ± 0.36	0.55 ± 0.29*
Gingival index	2.08 ± 0.31	1.11 ± 0.36	0.72 ± 0.28	0.51 ± 0.29*
Bleeding index	2.59 ± 0.33	2.00 ± 0.28	1.69 ± 0.18	0.79 ± 0.51*
Overall response	2.35 ± 0.39	2.01 ± 0.29	1.46 ± 0.74	0.80 ± 0.69*

p<0.05 as compared to the on entry values

Table 3: Effect of Complete Care Herbal Toothpaste on the following parameters.

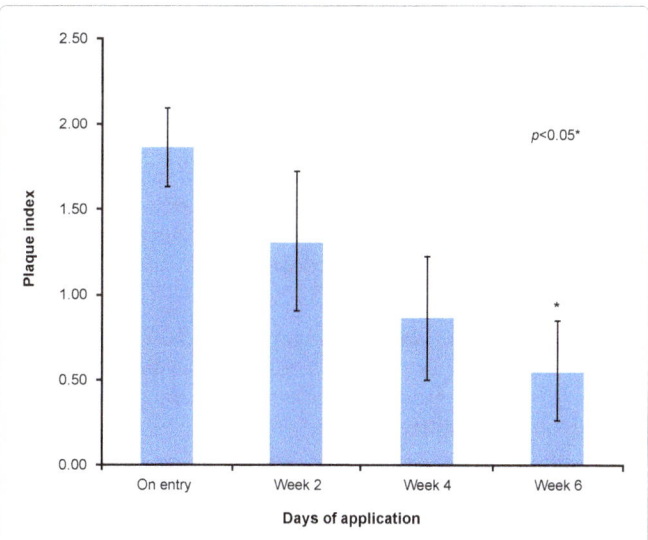

Figure 1: Effect of Complete Care Herbal Toothpaste on the Plaque index.

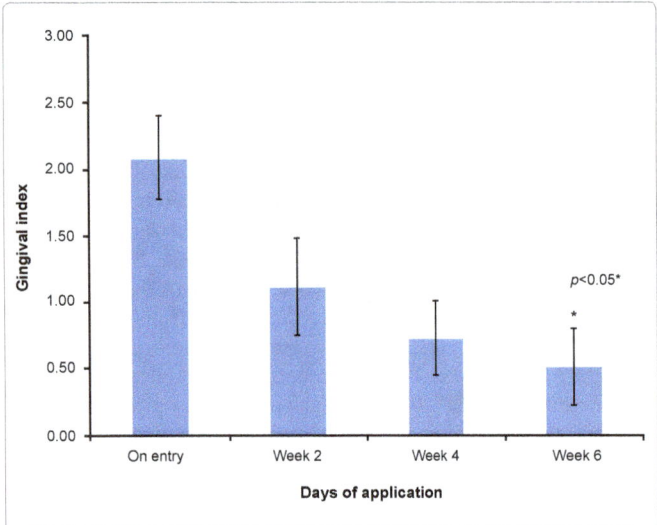

Figure 2: Effect of Complete Care Herbal Toothpaste on the Gingival index.

entry values. Thus, significant symptomatic relief was observed after 6 weeks of treatment with Complete Care Herbal Toothpaste. The results in this clinical trial indicate that Complete Care Herbal Toothpaste is effective agent in subjects with dental plaque.

Discussion

Complete Care Herbal Toothpaste has earlier undergone safety studies in healthy volunteers. Present study was carried out to evaluate the efficacy of Complete Care Herbal Toothpaste in dental plaque, gingival bleeding and periodontal diseases. Results have indicated significant improvement in plaque index, gingival index, bleeding index and overall response. The efficacy as evident by antiplaque activity could be attributed to antimicrobial properties of *Punica granatum, Zanthoxylum alatum, Acacia arabica,* Triphala, *Vitex negundo, Salvadora persica, Mimusops elengi, Trachyspermum ammi, Azadirachta indica.* Complete Care Herbal Toothpaste, in addition has shown anti-gingivitis activity which we believe could be due to antioxidant properties of ingredients of this novel dentifrice. Studies in literature have indicated that medications having anti-oxidant efficacy neutralizes free radicals. Several views advocating the development of antioxidant based drugs have provided optimistic points in rationalizing the development for the treatment of these agents act as scavengers, helping to prevent cell and tissue damage that could lead to cellular damage and disease [11] Potential mechanisms for periodontal tissue destruction by ROS could be as follows [12].

a) *Punica granatum:* Topical applications of Pomegranate (*Punica granatum*) have been found to be particularly effective for controlling oral inflammation, as well as bacterial and fungal counts in periodontal disease. Numerous in vitro studies demonstrate the antimicrobial activity of pomegranate extracts [13].

b) *Zanthoxylum alatum:* Synonym: *Zanthoxylum armatum* Fruit of *Zanthoxylum Armatum* are used to cure toothache and other diseases of teeth. The plant possesses antioxidant, anti- inflammatory, antimicrobial and antifungal activities [14].

c) *Acacia arabica: Acacia arabica* stem bark is considered as an astringent and credited with the antimicrobial activity [15].

d) Triphala (*Terminalia chebula:Terminalia belerica:Emblica officinalis*):

Triphala has potent antioxidant and antimicrobial activity and inhibited the growth of *S. mutans,* gram positive cocci, involved in plaque formation when it adsorbed to the tooth surface. The extract of Triphala is an effective agent to treat dental carries and to prevent the formation of dental plaques [16].

e) *Embelia ribes: Embelia ribes* is reported to possess antioxidant, anti-inflammatory and analgesic properties. Embelin, a major constituent of Embelia ribes represents a promising lead compound for designing a new class of analgesic and anti-inflammatory [17].

f) *Vitex negundo: Vitex negundo* possess numerous biological activities proved by many experimental studies. Anti- microbial and anti-inflammatory activity of *Vitex negundo* has been successfully demonstrated through various experimental studies [18].

g) *Salvadora persica: Salvadora persica L.* has been reported to have anti- microbial, anti-plaque, analgesic, anti-inflammatory, and astringent activities. It has great medicinal use in the treatment of toothache [19].

h) *Acacia farnesiana:* Because of its effective astringent and anti-

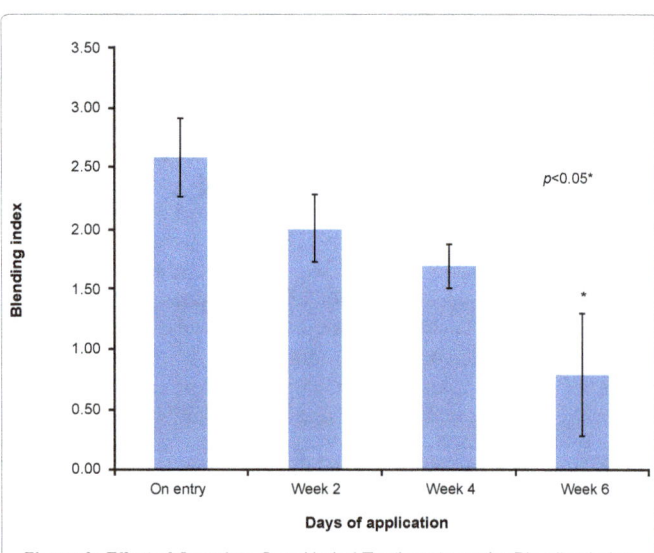

Figure 3: Effect of Complete Care Herbal Toothpaste on the Bleeding index.

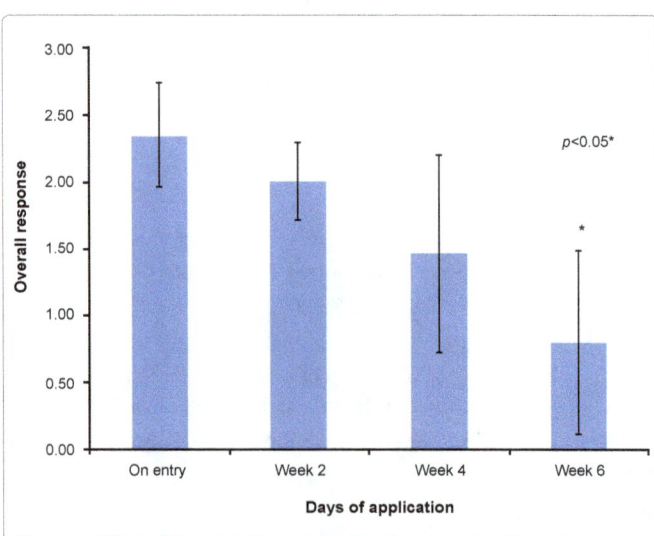

Figure 4: Effect of Complete Care Herbal Toothpaste on the Overall response.

inflammatory properties of *Acacia farnesiana* bark, it is beneficial in the dental conditions such as swollen gums and dental caries [20].

i) Acacia catechu: *Acacia catechu* has been credited with the properties such as antibacterial, anti- inflammatory, antioxidant and astringent, which may be useful in dental conditions [21].

j) Mimusops elengi: Studies have shown that *Mimusops elengi* or some part of its phytochemicals possess analgesic, anti-inflammatory, antimicrobial, antioxidant which is highly beneficial in oral conditions like Gingival bleeding [22].

k) Trachyspermum ammi: *T. ammi's* extracts especially ethanol, n-hexane showed significant antimicrobial potential against all pathogens [23] and reported with the analgesic activity [24] which may be beneficial in the oral conditions such as toothache .

l) Azadirachta indica: Synonym: *Melia azadirachta* Bark extract of *Azadirachta indica* has been reported with the antimicrobial property, which may be used in oral care preparations [25].

The efficacy of the Complete Care Herbal Toothpaste can be attributed to the synergistic activity of the potent herbs which have analgesic, antimicrobial property, astringent and anti-inflammatory property.

Conclusion

The Present clinical study clearly showed that Complete Care Herbal Toothpaste is effective in relieving the severity of plaque, gingivitis, gum bleeding etc. A significant relief was observed in all the dental signs after 6 weeks of treatment with Complete Care Herbal Toothpaste. No clinically significant adverse reaction, was reported or observed, during the entire study period and overall compliance to the treatment was satisfactory. Complete Care Herbal Toothpaste, with its unique selection of herbal ingredients, has been specially developed to make teeth and gums strong which have analgesic, antimicrobial property, astringent and anti- inflammatory property which takes care of inflammatory condition. Complete Care Herbal Toothpaste not only protects from germs producing dental plaque, but also has antioxidants that help in improvement of gum health.

Therefore, it may be concluded that Complete Care Herbal Toothpaste is effective and safe to use in the prevention and management of dental plaques and other common dental problems including gingival bleeding and periodontal diseases.

References

1. Marsh PD (2005) Dental plaque: biological significance of a biofilm and community life-style. J ClinPeriodontol 32: 7-15.

2. Overman PR (2000) Biofilm: a new view of plaque. J Contemp Dent Pract 1: 18-29.

3. Frascella JA, Fernández P, Gilbert RD, Cugini M (2000) A randomized, clinical evaluation of the safety and efficacy of a novel oral irrigator. Am J Dent 13: 55-58.

4. Warren PR, Chater BV (1996) An overview of established interdental cleaning methods. J Clin Dent 7: 65-69.

5. Murray JJ (1982) Fluorides in caries prevention (Dental Practitioner Handbook No.20) Bristol: John Wright 60-90

6. Sheiham A (1977) Prevention and control of Periodontal disease. International conference on research into the biology of periodontal disease. University of Illinois309-368.

7. Frandsen A (1985) State of the Science Paper: Mechanical Oral Hygiene Practices in Dental Plaque control measures and Oral Hygiene Practices Workshop. Bethesda Maryland, USA.

8. Stean H, Forward GC (1980) Measurement of plaque growth following toothbrushing. Community Dent Oral Epidemiol 8: 420-423.

9. Addy M, Willis L, Moran J (1983) Effect of toothpaste rinses compared with chlorhexidine on plaque formation during a 4-day period. J ClinPeriodontol 10: 89-99.

10. Moran J, Addy M (1984) The antibacterial properties of some commercially available toothpastes in vitro. Br Dent J 156: 175-178.

11. Carnelio S, Khan SA, Rodrigues G (2008) Definite, probable or dubious: antioxidants trilogy in clinical dentistry. Br Dent J 204: 29-32.

12. Lakshmi SS, Mythili R (2011) Indian Journal of Multidisciplinary Dentistry 1: 140-146

13. Jurenka JS (2008) Therapeutic applications of pomegranate (Punicagranatum L.): a review. Altern Med Rev 13: 128-144.

14. Mehta DK, Bhandari A, Satti NK, Singh S, Das R,et al. (2012) In-Vivo and In-Vitro Antioxidant Potential of Fruits of Zanthoxylumarmatum D.C, Research Article. JPharmRes5: 2031-2034.

15. Saurabh Rajvaidhya, Nagori BP, Singh GK, Dubey BK, Prashant Desai, et al. (2012) A Review on Acacia Arabica - An Indian Medicinal Plant. IJPSR 3: 1995-2005.

16. Jagadish L, Anand Kumar VK, Kaviyarasan V (2009) Effect of Triphala on dental bio-film. Indian Journal of Science and Technology 2: 30-33.

17. Mahendran S, Badami S, Ravi S, Thippeswamy BS, Veerapur VP (2011) Synthesis and evaluation of analgesic and anti-inflammatory activities of most active free radical scavenging derivatives of embelin-A structure-activity relationship. Chem Pharm Bull (Tokyo) 59: 913-919.

18. Vishal R Tandon (2005) Medicinal uses and biological acivities of Vitexnegundo: Reveiew article. Natural product radiance 4:162-165.

19. Verma Rajesh, Purohit Suresh, Bhandari Anil, Kumar Brijesh, Priyanka P (2009) Salvadora Persica L (Tooth Brush Tree): A Review. J Pharma Res 2: 1809-1812.

20. Rajkumar MH, Sringeswara AN, Rajanna MD (2011) Ex-Situ Conservation of Medicinal Plants at University of Agricultural Sciences, Bangalore, Karnataka: Recent Research in Science and Technology 3: 21- 27.

21. Borde VU, Pangrikar PP, Tekale SU (2011) Gallic Acid in Ayurvedic Herbs and Formulations. Recent Research in Science and Technology 3: 51-54.

22. Prasad V Kadam, Kavita N Yadav, Ramesh S Deoda, Rakesh S Shivatare, Manohar J Patil (2012) Mimusopselengi: A Review on Ethnobotany, Phytochemical and Pharmacological Profile. Journal of Pharmacognosy and Phytochemistry 1: 71-81.

23. Shabnam Javed, Ahmad Ali Shahid, Muhammad Saleem Haider, Aysha Umeera, Rauf Ahmad, et al. (2012) Nutritional, phytochemical potential and pharmacological evaluation of Nigella Sativa (Kalonji) and TrachyspermumAmmi (Ajwain). Journal of Medicinal Plants Research 6: 768-775.

24. Anonymous. The Ayurvedic Pharmacopoeia of India. Ministry of Health & FW. Department of AYUSH. Govt of India. New Delhi. Part I. Vol VI.343-345.

25. Tara E Gottschalck, John E Bailey (2009) International Cosmetic Ingredient Dictionary and handbook.

13

Cisplatin-Induced Ovarian Cytotoxicity and the Modulating Role of Aqueous Zest Extract of Citrus *limonium* (AZECL) in Rat Models

Akunna GG[1]*, Nwafor J[1], Egwu OA[1], Ezemagu UK[1], Obaje G[1], Adepoju LH[1] and Akingbade AM[2]

[1]*Department of Anatomy, Federal University Ndufu-Alike Ikwo (FUNAI), Ebonyi State, Nigeria*
[2]*Department of Anatomy, Afe Babalola University, Ado Ekiti, Nigeria*

Abstract

Cisplatin is a prominent member of the effective broad-spectrum antitumor drugs. However, its clinical usage is restricted due to some adverse side effects, such as testiculototoxicity, hepatotoxicity and nephrotoxicity. The aim of this study is to evaluate the effect of Aqueous Zest Extract of *Citrus limonium* (AZECL) on the ovary of female Wistar rat treated with Cisplatin. Twenty adult female Wistar rats were divided into four groups (A-D) containing five rats each. Group A rats served as negative control and were treated orally with 2.5 ml/kg body weight of normal saline, group B rats served as positive control group and were treated intraperitoneally with a single dose of 10 mg/kg body weight of Cisplatin, group C rats were treated orally with 50 mg/kg body weight of AZECL and group D rats were treated intraperitoneally with a single dose of 10 mg/kg body weight of Cisplatin and two weeks later treated orally with 50 mg/kg body weight of AZECL. Result showed a significant ($p<0.01$) decrease in primary follicles, secondary follicles, graafian follicles and a significant ($p<0.01$) increase in atretic follicles, PAS positive reaction and reduction in the total carbohydrate contents of the stromal cells in the positive control group. Also there was a significant ($p<0.05$) decrease in the activity level of FSH, LH and a significant ($p<0.05$) increase in Malondialdehyde when compared to rats in group A and C. The group post-treated with the extract had remarkable normalization of the histo-morphometric, histochemical and biochemical parameters when compared to the positive control group. Aqueous zests extract of *C. limonium* has a curative effect on cisplatin-induced cytotoxicity on the ovary.

Keywords: *Citrus limonum* zest; Cisplatin; Ovary; Histo-morphometry

Introduction

Cisplatin is a chemotherapeutic agent used for the treatment of a wide variety of cancers. Cisplatin have been implicated in premature ovarian failure, changes in the estrous cycle, increased follicular apoptosis, and a reduction in the number of Anti-Mullerian Hormone (AMH) secreting follicles among several women undergoing chemotherapy [1,2]. Ovarian failure is attributed to the inability of primordial follicular cells to regenerate [3]. Cisplatin treatment has also been associated with conditions such as nephrotoxicity, neurotoxicity, and reproductive toxicity among others [4].

Lipid peroxidation, mitochondrial damage, and DNA injury has been associated with increased generation of Reactive Oxygen Species (ROS), a major mechanism pathway for cisplatin-induced toxicity [5-9].

Citrus limonium (Lemon) is an important food source of the plant family Rutaceae. Generally, antibacterial, antifungal, antidiabetic, anticancer and antiviral activities of citrus flavonoids have been shown [10-12]. Peel, flowers and leaves of *Citrus aurantium* have been employed in minimizing central nervous system disorders in traditional medicine [13]. Flavonoids, a major phytochemical in *citrus* fruits has been shown to act as direct antioxidants and free radical scavengers together with modulating enzymatic activities and inhibiting cell proliferation. It has also been reported that fiber of citrus fruit contains bioactive compounds, such as ascorbic acid. In this study, we aimed to investigate modulating role effect of AZECL on the ovary of female Wistar rat treated with anticancer agent Cisplatin. We believed that AZECL will attenuate cisplatin-induced toxicities by reducing number of atretic follicules, lipid peroxidation by measures of malondialdehyde, total carbohydrate contents of the stromal cells through PAS positive reactions and increase in activity level of FSH, LH.

Materials and Methods

Plant materials

Plant source and identification: Fresh lemon fruits (*Citrus limonum*) were obtained from a farmland, identified and authenticated at the Department of Plant Science and Biotechnology, Faculty of Science, Ebonyi state University.

Preparation of aqueous zest extract of *Citrus limonum*: Lemon fruits were peeled with a zester or grater [14]. The zests were rinsed in clean water and dried at room temperature for about 2 weeks. It was grinded and reduced to a powdered form.

Calculated amount of volume of distilled water and powdered sample were mixed and the mixture was allowed to stand for 30 min before filtration. The mixture was then centrifuged and supernatant were collected, cleaned of particles by suction filtration using Whatmann no 1. Filter paper and cellulose filter paper. The extracts was then concentrated to dryness in vacuum at 40°C using a rotary evaporator and stored in a desiccator. Fresh solution of the different extract was then prepared in normal saline as vehicle when required [15,16].

Phytochemical analysis of the extracts: The phytochemical analysis to determine the presence of Alkaloids, Flavonoids, Saponins and Tannins was done as describe by Akunna et al. [16]

Animals

Twenty female Wistar rats (mature) weighing 100-150 g were obtained from Department of Pharmacology, Faculty of Pharmacy, University of Nigeria Nsukka (UNN).

*Corresponding author: Akunna GG, Department of Anatomy, Faculty of Basic Medical Sciences, Federal University Ndufu-Alike Ikwo (FUNAI), Ebonyi State, Nigeria
E-mail: ggakunna@gmail.com, gabriel.akunna@funai.edu.ng

The animals acclimatize for 2 weeks and were fed freely on standard commercial mouse cubes from Federal University Ndufu-Alike Ikwo (FUNAI).

Constant environmental condition were maintained (12 h light-12 h dark and 24°C ± 30°C). The weights of the animals were estimated using an electronic analytical and precision balance (PA, 4102).

Permission from the departmental ethical committee on animal research was gotten before the start of the experiment.

Experimental procedures involving the animals and their care were conducted in conformity with International, National and institutional guidelines for the care of laboratory animals in Biomedical Research and Use of Laboratory Animals in Biomedical Research as promulgated by the Canadian Council of Animal Care.

Animal groupings and treatments

This study was conducted in four (A, B, C and D) undisturbed cages. Twenty female rats were divided into four groups of five rats each. Group A rats served as the negative control group and were treated with 5 ml/kg body weight of normal saline daily for 3 weeks. Group B rats served as positive control and were treated intraperitoneally with a single dose of 10 mg/kg body weight of Cisplatin. Group C rats were treated orally with 50 mg/kg body weight of AZECL per day for 3 weeks while Group D rats were treated with a single dose of 10 mg/kg body weight of cisplatin and 10 days later were orally treated with 50 mg/kg body weight of AZECL per day for 11 days.

Animal sacrifice and sample collection

The rats were weighed and sacrificed by cervical dislocation. Blood samples were collected from the heart of each rat immediately after sacrifice with the aid of a 21G needle mounted on a 5 mL syringe (Hindustan Syringes and Medical Devices Ltd., Faridabad, India). This was inserted into the heart based on prior palpation of the apex beat. At least about 5 ml of blood was aspirated after which the thoracic cage was opened to allow direct access and more blood collected under adequate direct visualization of the heart. The blood obtained into tubes containing 2% sodium oxalate and centrifuged (3000 rpm for 10 min) accordingly using a table top centrifuge (P/C 03) and the serum extracted. The abdominal cavity was opened up through a midline abdominal incision and the ovaries were excised and one of the ovaries from each animal was fixed in Bouin's fluid for histomorphometric analysis. Serum and the remaining ovary homogenate of each animal were stored at -25°C for biochemical assays.

Determination of biochemical parameters

Serum hormonal assays-Luteinizing Hormone (LH), Follicle Stimulating Hormone (FSH) and progesterone (PROG). The assays were done according to the procedure adapted by Amballi et al. [17]. Briefly, one aliquot of each centrifuged specimen was taken at a time, to avoid repeated freezing and thawing, and the samples were analyzed for hormone estimation using Enzyme Immunoassay (EIA), according to the World Health Organization (WHO) matched reagent programme protocol (manual) for EIA kits (protocol/version of December 1998 for LH, FSH). Serum progesterone was determined by ELISA using MAP LAB PLUS (Biochemical systems international, RM 2060) according to the manufacturer's direction.

Estimation of lipid peroxidation (Malondialdehyde)

Lipid peroxidation in the ovarian tissue was estimated colorimetrically by thiobarbituric acid reactive substances (TBARS) method of Buege and Aust as described by Saalu [18]. It was expressed as nmol/mg protein.

Tissue preparation for histology and histochemistry

The fixed tissues were processed for histological and histochemical analysis as described by Akunna et al. [19]. Sections were stained with H&E and Periodic Acid-Schiff (PAS) reaction with hematoxylin counterstaining for histological and histochemical study respectively. The slides were viewed under a research microscope connected to a computer monitor for qualitative and quantitative evaluation.

Morphometric analysis

Ovarian follicles were identified and classified as described by Peters and Natty [20] while atretic follicles were identified following morphological criteria described by Greenwald and Roy [21].

Statistical Analysis

The results gotten from this study were expressed as mean ± SD of different groups. The differences between the mean values were evaluated by ANOVA followed by Student's "t" test using SPSS (version 20).

Results

Results of phytochemical analysis

We observed the presence of saponins, tannins and flavonoids, with tannins constituting the highest while Saponin was noted to be the lowest. Alkaloids were not detected in the extract as shown in Table 1.

Body Weight of Rats

The results of the body weight were outline. This result showed a progressive increase in body weight of rats used in this experiment throughout the period of study. However, there was a non-significant ($p > 0.05$) decrease in body weight of the animals in group B at 2nd week of administration as shown in Table 2.

Histomorphometry of the Ovary

The morphology of the ovaries was verified on the following: Primary follicles, secondary follicles, graffian follicles and atretic follicles (Table 3). Results showed a significant ($p < 0.01$) decrease in primary follicles, secondary follicles, graffian follicles and a significant ($p < 0.01$) increase in atretic follicles of rats treated with cisplatin-alone (group B). The rats in group C had geometric values comparable to that of the negative control group. There was a significant ($p < 0.05$) increase in primary follicles, secondary follicles and graftable fian follicles in rats

Parameters	Citrus limone	mg/g
Saponin	+ve	0.81 ± 0.00
Tannins	+ve	47.0 ± 31.05
Alkaloids	-ve	-
Flavonoids	+ve	11.4 ± 33.05

Table 1: Phytochemical constituents of AZECL.

Treatment Groups	Initial Weight	Weight 1	Weight 2	Weight 3
Group A	113.4 ± 8.3	127.8 ± 9.9	136.6 ± 10.7	146.0 ± 11.1
Group B	131.0 ± 18.6	145.0 ± 21.1	143.7 ± 10.2	145.6 ± 8.1
Group C	118.0 ± 13.5	125.4 ± 14.7	127.0 ± 17.1	128.7 ± 17.7
Group D	110.4 ± 14.5	117.8 ± 14.9	124.6 ± 14.3	125.0 ± 16.3

P>0.05 (There were no significant differences between the weights)

Table 2: Effect of cisplatin and AZECL on body weights (g) of female Wistar rats.

post-treated with AZECL (group D) and a significant (p<0.01) decrease in atretic follicles when compared to the rats treated with only cisplatin (group B).

Histochemical Observations

Total carbohydrates

Examination of ovary of control rats revealed that the germinal epithelial cells and the stromal cells showed a slight PAS positive reaction. The ovum of primary, secondary and Graafian follicles showed a moderate reactivity while the cytoplasm of their granulosa was slightly stained. The Zona pellucida encircling the oocyte in the different types of the follicles had a marked reaction. The corona radiata and the theca folliculi showed slightly positive PAS-reaction whereas the antrum of the follicles was negatively stained. The luteal cells of the corpora lutea appeared slightly reactive with PAS-reaction. The core of the atretic follicles showed a moderate PAS-positive reaction. Examination of ovary of rats treated with cisplatin and AZECL showed reduction in the total carbohydrate contents of the stromal cells, the ovum of primary, secondary and Graafian follicles compared with those of cisplatin alone treated animals (Figures 1-8).

Biochemical Results

The effect of cisplatin and AZECL on the three main female reproductive hormones namely FSH, LH and PROG activities and MDA levels were verified as shown in Table 4.

Treatment Groups	Primary Follicles	Secondary Follicles	Graffian Follicles	Atretic Follicles
Group A	10.2 ± 2.1	5.8 ± 0.8	4.2 ± 0.4	5.0 ± 0.7
Group B	4.0 ± 0.7**	2.4 ± 0.5**	1.8 ± 0.4**	21.8 ± 3.2**
Group C	10.6 ± 1.8	6.2 ± 0.8	4.4 ± 0.5	5.2 ± 0.8
Group D	7.8 ± 1.6a	4.4 ± 0.5a	4.2 ± 0.4a	11.2 ± 1.6aa

*,**Represent significant increases or decreases at p<0.05 and (p<0.01) respectively when compared to negative control (Group A)
a,aaRepresent significant increases or decreases at p<0.05 and (p<0.01) respectively when compared to group C Values are means ± SD; n=5 in each group.

Table 3: Effect of cisplatin and AZECL on primary follicles, secondary follicles, graffian follicles and atretic follicles of female Wistar rats.

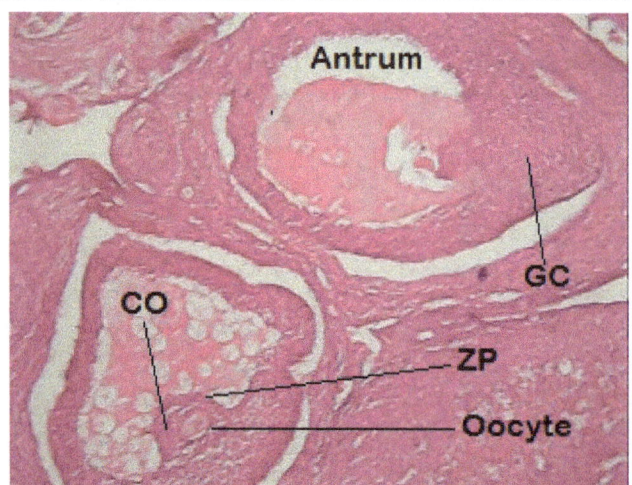

Figure 1: Cross-section of the ovary negative control rats (2.5 ml/kg body weight of normal saline). Slide showing the Antrum, Zona pellucida, Oocyte, Cumulus Oophorus (CO) and Granulosa Cells (GC). Stain: Haematoxylin and Eosin; Magnification: 400X.

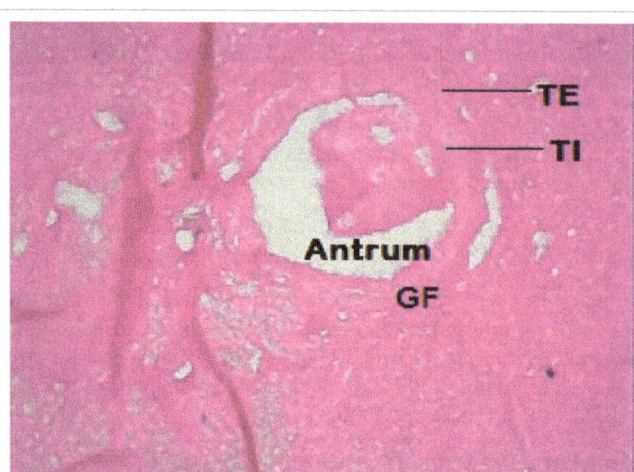

Figure 2: Cross-section of the ovary of negative control rats (2.5 ml/kg body weight of normal saline). Slide showing the Antrum, Graffian Follicles (GF), Theca Interna (TI), Theca Externa (TE), Stain: PAS; Magnification: 400X.

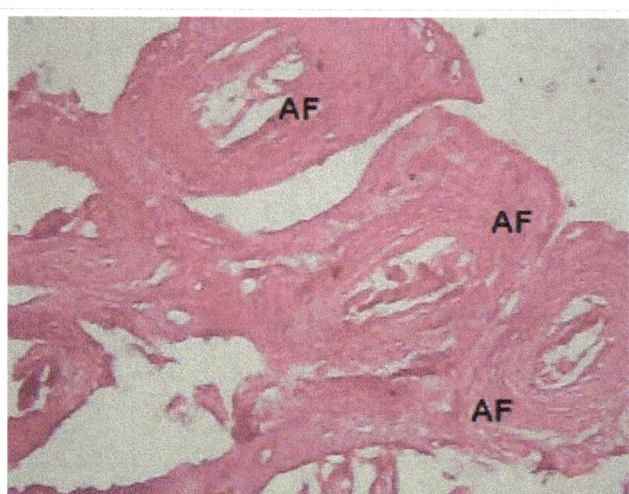

Figure 3: Cross-section of the ovary of positive control rats (10 mg/kg). Slide showing Atretic Follicles (AF) and some blood vessels. Stain: Haematoxylin and Eosin; Magnification: 400X.

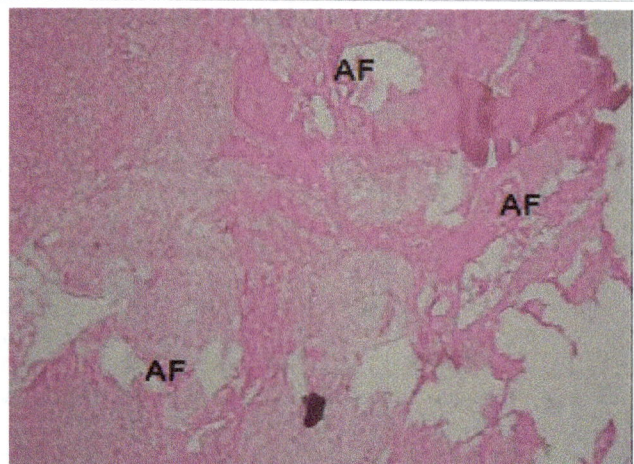

Figure 4: Cross-section of the ovary of positive control rats (10 mg/kg). Slide showing the Atretic Follicles (AF) and corpus lithium. Stain: PAS; Magnification: 400X.

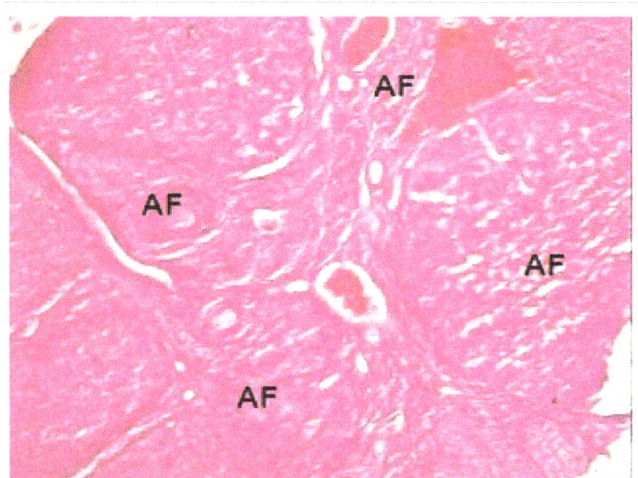

Figure 5: Cross-section of the ovary of rat treated with AZECL alone (50 mg/kg). Slide showing the Atretic Follicles (AF). Stain: Haematoxylin and Eosin; Magnification: 400X.

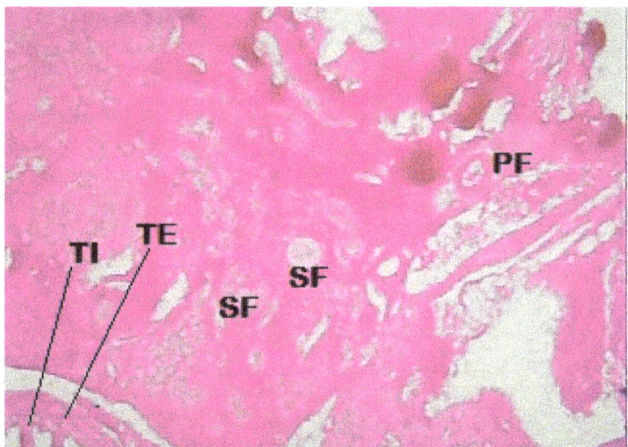

Figure 6: Cross-section of the ovary of rat treated with AZECL alone (50 mg/kg). Slide showing the Theca Interna (TI), Theca Externa (TE), Primary follicles, secondary follicles. Stain: PAS; Magnification: 400X.

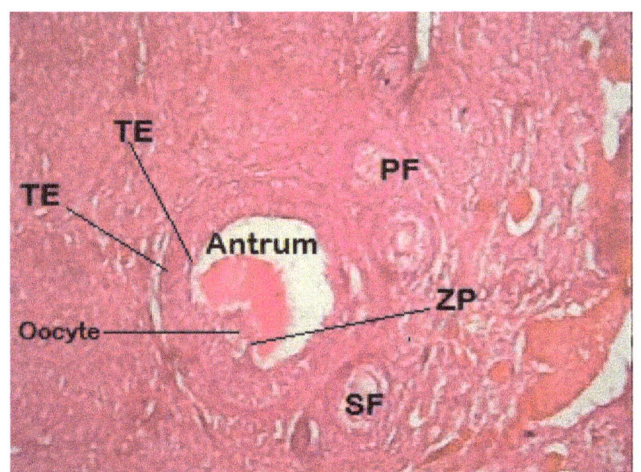

Figure 7: Cross-section of the ovary of rats post-treated with AZECL (10 mg/kg of Cisplatin+50 mg/kg of AZECL). Slide showing Antrum, Theca Externa (TE), Oocyte, Primary Follicles (PF), Secondary Follicles (SF) and Zona pellucid (ZP). Stain: Haematoxylin and Eosin; Magnification: 400X.

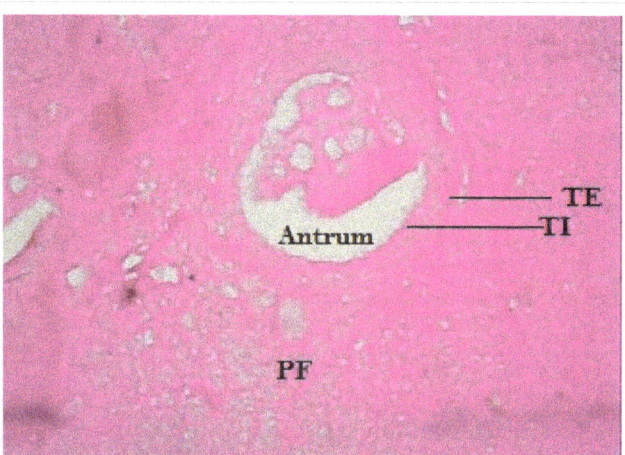

Figure 8: Cross-section of the ovary of rats post-treated with AZECL (10 mg/kg of Cisplatin+50 mg/kg of AZECL). Slide showing the Antrum, Theca Interna (TI), Theca Externa (TE) and Primary Follicles (PF). Stain: PAS; Magnification: 400X.

The rats treated with cisplatin alone had a significant ($p<0.05$) decrease in the level of FSH, LH and a significant ($p<0.01$) decrease in the activity level of PROG when compared with those of the negative control.

The rats in group C had a fluctuation in the level of FSH, LH and PROG but geometric values comparable to that of rats in group A. There was a significant ($p<0.05$) improvement in the activity level of FSH, LH and PROG in rats post-treated with the extract (group D) rats when compared to rats in group B. In the level of MDA the animals in group B showed a significant ($p<0.01$) increase when compared to animals in group A while the animals in group D showed a significant ($p<0.05$) decrease in the level of MDA when compared to animals in group B.

Discussion

General considerations

The use of cisplatin has been reduced due to severe cytotoxic side effects [22-24]. Due to elevated mitotic activities, gonads are one of the main targets [25].

Chemotherapy treatment has long been associated with premature ovarian failure and infertility in premenopausal patients. It is often assumed that chemotherapy drugs directly damage oocytes in the primordial follicle reserve and that it is this loss that leads to premature ovarian failure [26,27].

Animal-based researches have improved our understanding the underlying processes and a way forward to restoring the reproductive potential [28-34].

Gross Anatomical Parameters

In this study, the results show a progressive increase in body mass of experimental models throughout the duration of the study. Nevertheless, there exists a non-significant decrease in body weight of the animals in group B at 2nd week of administration. Our results in this regard were not in line with that of Atessahin et al. This could mean that the experimental animals have not passed their active growth phase or that the feeding habit was increased as a result of cisplatin toxicity [35,36].

Although Saalu et al.; Akunna and Ogunmodede; Akunna; Akunna and Saalu [32-40]; Akunna et al. [39-41]; Akingbade et al. [42]; Malarvizhi and Mathur [43], Setchell [44] and Creasy [45] have

Treatment Groups	FSH (mIU/ml)	LH (mIU/ml)	PROG (ng/ml)	MDA (nmol/mg)
Group A	3.8 ± 0.2	2.3 ± 0.11	51.8 ± 0.7	0.5 ± 0.07
Group B	1.9 ± 0.03*	0.7 ± 0.09*	30.6 ± 0.8**	3.8 ± 0.12**
Group C	3.2 ± 0.16	2.5 ± 0.06	50.3 ± 1.4	0.5 ± 0.03
Group D	2.4 ± 0.77	1.5 ± 0.07	37.8 ± 5.1	2.7 ± 0.5*

*,**Represent significant increases or decreases at p<0.05 and *p*<0.01 respectively, when compared to negative control (Group A). Values are means ± SD; n=5 in each group

Table 4: Biochemical results.

associated gonadal weight to infertility, it is important to state at this juncture that we couldn't determine the weight of the ovary because of the surrounding fats and adipose tissue which may influence the results.

The Morphological Effects

From our study, the follicular count showed a significant decrease in primary follicles, secondary follicles, graffian follicles and a significant (p<0.01) increase in atretic follicles of rats in group B when compared to the corresponding control (Group A). Data here are consistent with these findings, showing an increase in unhealthy follicles, and a reduction in total follicle number, following treatment with Cisplatin [27,46].

According to Perez [47], mice exposed to chemotherapeutic agents displayed apoptosis of granulosa cells in primordial follicles. Meirow [26] also evaluated human ovarian slices post-cisplatin exposure *in vitro* and his reports were consistent with that of Perez [48]. Our results were also in line with these findings as revealed by the impaired integrity of the surrounding granulosa layer in most of the follicles examined and significantly reduced number of primordial cells in cisplatin alone treated rats. Of course the damaging effects of cisplatin on ovarian follicles have been previously reported [49,50]. Yucebilgin et al. [1] reported a significantly damage primordial follicles in rats after a single dose of cisplatin (5 mg/kg) and paclitaxel (7.5 mg/kg) [1]. The geometric results in our study are in line with other reports on cisplatin-induced injury [51,52].

Histochemical results showed that rats treated with cisplatin alone had an increase in carbohydrate content when compared to the negative control as shown by histochemistry. The increased carbohydrate contents may be due to disturbance in carbohydrate metabolism. A significant increase in both blood glucose and liver glycogen in experimental animals have been reported.

The biochemical effects

The ovarian toxicity recorded in this study might be due to increase in lipid peroxidation resulting from the toxicity of cisplatin or its metabolite as shown previously in our laboratory [53]. Mathews [54] reported that the damage occurred in the cell membrane by hydroxyl radicals induced oxidation. This could also explain the marked degeneration, atrophied ovary and decrease number of viable follicles reported in this study which are in line with several reports [23,25,55-57].

Oxidative stress, a condition of an imbalance between free radicals and antioxidant defense system, is an important factor in the pathogenesis system that has high content of polyunsaturated membrane lipid [58]. Recent study indicated that cisplatin led to neurotoxic effects in human and animals via induction of lipid peroxidation [59]. Our present work showed that cisplatin produced a significant increase in MDA level that induced lipid peroxidation in the brain tissues accompanied with suppression in SOD activity [60]. On the other hand, therapeutic effects of cisplatin based on the interaction with DNA in the cell, preventing proliferation and inducing apoptosis in tumor cells. According to Mukhopadhyay et al. [61]; cisplatin induced mitochondrial ROS generation triggered inflammatory response, cell death and ovarian dysfunction.

It has also been suggested that cisplatin is able to generate reactive oxygen species by inducing glucose-6-phosphate dehydrogenase and hexokinase activity and inhibit the activity of antioxidant enzyme in tissue such as SOD, CAT, and GSH-Px [62].

MDA, an aldehyde product of lipid peroxidation, is commonly used as a marker of oxidative stress in cells and in the present study; we observed a significant increase in ovary MDA levels in cisplatin-alone treated. Our result is line with that of Atasayar et al. [63].

The rat models post-treated with AZECL had remarkable normalization of these parameters. Due to abundant phytochemicals in plants, they have been utilized for various ailments traditionally and cisplatin induced toxicity [64,65]. Improved ovarian histology and function post-antioxidants treatment has been reported severally [66,67].

In this study, we observed a significant decrease (p<0.05) in the level of FSH, LH and PROG in rat treated with cisplatin. FSH stimulates the growth and maturation of ovarian follicles by acting directly on the receptors which are located on the granulosa cells. As indicated in our study, the reduction in the levels of FSH by the cisplatin might have hampered folliculogenesis and delayed maturation of the follicle in the pre-ovulatory phase. It is also likely that that cisplatin might have had effect on the hypothalamus since the secretion of FSH is regulated by the hypothalamus through gonadotropic releasing hormone secreted.

It has been indicated that LH release surges at the proestrus stage initiates ovulation. Hence any substance capable of preventing the release of LH could interfere with ovulation by decreasing the number of mature follicles [68]. The group of rat that where post treated with AZECL had a significant (p<0.05) improvement in the level LH. Alkaloids and flavonoids from plants have been shown to reduce plasma concentrations of LH, estradiol and FSH [69]. Therefore, the presence of these phytochemicals (flavonoids) in AZECL in may account in part for the improvements observed in our study.

The decreased level of MDA after AZECL treatment may be a defense mechanism against oxygen free radical damage. Concerning the effect of *Citrus limonum*, when animals treated with cisplatin followed by AZECL marked improvement in the histological picture of ovary and the number of healthy follicles was seen as compared with ovary of animals treated with cisplatin alone.

Plants such as *Zingiber officinale, Hibiscus sabdariffa* and *Curcuma longa* have been reported to reduce CIS-induced toxicity [70-74].

The curative potential of AZECL might be attributed to these active molecules individually or synergistically indirectly through pituitary-gonadal axis or directly by sensitizing the follicular receptors to the available gonadotrophins. Also, the reduction in follicular atresia by AZECL may be due to availability of extra ovarian regulators, the gonadotrophins (FSH and LH). The active substances in the AZECL might have stimulated follicular growth in the ovaries by interfering at the level of receptors and mRNA expression of these intra ovarian and intra follicular regulating factors. Post-treatment with AZECL could have attenuated the cisplatin ovarian toxicity through a reduction of free radicals.

Conclusion

This study has demonstrated that post-treatment with aqueous zest extract of *Citrus limonum* containing powerful antioxidant vitamins and citrus bioflavonoids exerted a potent protective activity against cisplatin-induced morphological and biochemical impairment of the ovary of Wistar rats.

Limitation of the Study

We couldn't isolate the active ingredients from AZECL hence structural elucidation was out of the picture. This could have provided more insight into the possible mechanism of action of AZECL.

References

1. Yucebilgin MS, Terek MC, Ozsaran A (2004) Effect of chemotherapy on primordial follicular reserve of rat: an animal model of premature ovarian failure and infertility. Aust N Z J Obstet Gynaecol 44: 6-9.

2. Yeh J, Kim SB, Peresie J (2011) Reproductive toxic effects of cisplatin and its modulation by the antioxidant sodium 2-mercaptoethanesulfate (Mesna) in female Rats. Reprod Biol Insights 5: 17-27.

3. Jeruss JS, Woodruff KT (2009) Preservation of fertility in patients with cancer. N Engl J Med 360: 858-911.

4. Boulikas T, Vougiouka M (2003) Cisplatin and platinum drugs at the molecular level. Oncol Rep 10: 1663-1682.

5. Deavall DG, Martin AE, Horner MJ, Roberts R (2012) Drug-induced oxidative stress and toxicity. J Toxicol 2012: 645460.

6. Saalu LC, Oyewopo AO, Enye LA, Ogunlade B, Akunna GG, et al. (2012) The hepato-rejuvinative and hepato-toxic capabilities of *Citrus paradisi* Macfad fruit juice in Rattus Norvegicus. Afr J Pharm Pharmacol 14: 1056-1063.

7. Ogunlade B, Akunna GG, Fatoba OO, Ayeni OJ, Adegoke AA, et al. (2012) Aqueous extract of vernonia amygdalina protects against alcohol-induced hepatotoxicity in Wistar Rats. World J Young Res 2: 70-77.

8. Ogunlade B, Saalu LC, Ogunmodede OS, Akunna GG, Adeeyo OA, et al. (2012) The salutary role of *Allium cepa* extract on the liver histology, liver oxidative status and liver marker enzymes of rabbits submitted to alcohol-induced toxicity. J Lipid Res 2: 67-81.

9. Ogunmodede OS, Saalu LC, Ogunlade B, Akunna GG, Oyewopo OA et al. (2012) An Evaluation of the Hypoglycemic, Antioxidant and Hepatoprotective Potentials of Onion (*Allium* cepa L.) on Alloxan-induced Diabetic Rabbits. Environ Toxicol Pharmacol 8: 21-29.

10. Kawaii S, Tomono Y, Katase E, Ogawa K, Yano M, et al. (2000) Quantitative study of flavonoids in leaves of Citrus plants. J Agric Food Chem 48: 3865-3871.

11. Burt SA (2004) Essential oils: their antibacterial properties and potential applications in foods: a review. Inter J Food Microbiol 94: 223-253.

12. Ortuno A, Baidez A, Gomez P, Arcas CM, Porras I, et al. (2006) Citrus paradise and *Citrus sinensis* flavonoids: Their influence in the defence mechanism against *Penicillium digitatum*. Food Chem 98: 351-358.

13. Pultrini AM, Galindo LA, Costa M (2006) Effects of the essential oil from L. in experimental anxiety models in mice. Life Sci 78: 1720-1725.

14. Liogier HA (1990) Plantas medicinales de Puerto Ricoydel Caribe. San Juan, Puerto Rico p: 566.

15. Akunna GG, Saalu LC, Ogunlade B, Akingbade AM (2013) Tackling infertility with medicinal plant. Planta Med 1: 93-105.

16. Asuquo OR, Edet AG, Mesembe O, Atanghwo JI (2010) Ethanolic extracts of *Vernonia amygdalina* and *Ocimum gratissimum* enhance testicular improvement in diabetic Wistar rats. Internet J Altern Med.

17. Amballi AA, Dada OA, Adeleye AO, Jide S (2007) Evaluation of the determination of reference ranges for reproductive hormones (prolactin, FSH, LH, and testosterone) using enzyme immuno assay method. Sci Res Essays 2: 135-138.

18. Saalu LC (2012) The hepato-protective potentials of *Moringa oleifera* leaf extract on alcohol-induced hepato-toxicity in Wistar rat. Am J Biotechnol Mol Sci 2: 6-14.

19. Akunna GG, Obikili EN, Anyanwu EG, Esom AE (2017) Protective and curative role of citrus sinensis peel in cadmium-induced testicular and spermatic damage: a morphometric and immunohistochemical evaluation using monoclonal antibodies against Ki-67 and proliferating cell nuclear antigen. Eur J Anat 21: 19-30

20. Peters H, Natty KP (1980) The ovary: A correlation of strucure and function in Mammals. Granda Publishing, London, Toronto, Sydney and New York.

21. Greenwald GS, Roy SK (1994) Follicular development and its control. In the physiology of reproduction (2nd edn.). Raven Press Ltd., NY, USA.

22. Cohen SM, Lippard SJ (2001) Cisplatin: from DNA damage to cancer chemotherapy. Prog Nucleic Acid Res 67: 93-130.

23. Victoria C, Fuertes AM, Castilla J, Alonso C, Quevedo C, et al. (2007) Biochemical mechanisms of cisplatin cytotoxicity. Anticancer Agents Med Chem 7: 3-18.

24. Noori S, Yeow S, Ziauddin SW, Xin FM, Tran H, et al. (2008) Cisplatin enhances the antitumor effect of tumor necrosis factor-related apoptosis-inducing ligand gene therapy via recruitment of the mitochondria-dependent death signaling pathway. Cancer Gene Ther 15: 356-370.

25. Atessahin AI, Karahan G, Turk S, Yilmaz S, Ceribasi AO, et al. (2006) Protective role of lycopene on cisplatin induced changes in sperm characteristics, testicular damage and oxidative stress in rats. Reprod Toxicol 21: 42-47.

26. Meirow D (2000) Reproduction post-chemotherapy in young cancer patients. Mol Cell Endocrinol 169: 123-131.

27. Lopes M, Anderson G, Spears (2013) Cisplatin and doxorubicin induce distinct mechanisms of ovarian follicle loss, imatinib provides selective protection only against cisplatin. J Pone 8: 701-717.

28. Akingbade MA, Saalu LC, Oyebanji OO, Oyeniran AD, Akande OO, et al. (2014) Rhodinol-based incence testiculotoxicity in Albino rats: Testicular histology, Spermatogenic and Biochemical Evaluations. J Pharmacol Toxicol 9: 68-81.

29. Ogunlade B (2013) Haematological indices and splenic histo-architecture of Wistar rat treated with aniline: supplementary role of *Moringa oleifera* leave extracts. Int J Biotechnol Allied Field 1: 136-144.

30. Ogunlade B (2013) Highly active antiretroviral therapy: effects on foetal parameters heaematological indices and the histomorphology of the liver of the dams. Orient J Sci Res 2: 1

31. Saalu LC (2013) The Comparison of three experimental rat Varicocele models: Their effects on Histomorphometry, Spermiogram and Oxidative Status. J Exp Clin Anat 12: 22-30.

32. Saalu LC, Akuna GG, Enye LA (2013) Pathophysiology of varicocele: Evidences for oxidative stress as a mechanism pathway. Eur J Anat 17: 82-91.

33. Saalu LC, Akunna GG, Ogunmodede OS (2013) Evidences for deleterous role of free radicals in experimental varicocele using animal model. Br J Med Med Res 3: 1125-1143.

34. Akunna GG (2016) Spermiographic, 2 and 3-dimensional quantitative analysis of testicular tissues of rat submitted to citrus paradisi waste extract and cisplatin-induced cytotoxicity. Int J Cancer Res 12: 176-187.

35. Akunna GG (2011) Effect of two Nigerian made perfumes on the liver of adult Wister rat. J Med Sci 11: 220-225.

36. Akunna GG, Ogunmodede OS (2012) *Laurus nobilis* extract preserves testicular functions in cryptorchid Rat. World J Life Sci Med 2: 91.

37. Akunna GG (2012) Ameliorating effect of *Moringa oleifera* leaf extract on chromium-induced testicular toxicity in rat. World J Life Sci Med Res 2: 20-26.

38. Akunna GG, Saalu LC (2013) Anti-fertility role of allethrin based-mosquito coil on animal models. Int J Biol Pharm Allied Sci 2: 192-207.

39. Akunna GG (2014) Spermatotoxicity in animal models exposed to fragrance components. J Med Sci 14: 46-50.

40. Akunna GG, Akingbade AM, Faeji CO, Oni OI, Akande OO (2016) Reactive oxygen species generation could be a causative factor for perfume–induced testicular toxicity in male rat. Intl J Med Health Res 2: 28-34.

41. Akunna GG, Saalu LC, Ogunlade B (2015) Histo-morphometric evidences for testicular derangement in animal models submitted to chronic and sub-chronic inhalation of fragrance. Am J Res Commun 3: 85-101.

42. Akingbade AM, Akunna GG, Faeji CO (2015) Histomorphometric and spermatogenic evaluation of musk based-incense induced testisculotoxicity in adult Albino rats. Sch J App Med Sci 3: 2111-2117.

43. Malarvizhi D, Mathur PP (1995) Effect of cisplatin on physiological status of normal rat testis. Indian J Exp Biol 33: 281-283.

44. Setchell BP (1998) Anatomy, vasculature, innervations and fluids of the male reproductive tract. New York, USA pp: 753-836.

45. Creasy DM (2003) Evaluation of testicular toxicology: A synopsis and discussion of the recommendations proposed by the society of toxicologic pathology. Birth Defects Res B Dev Reprod Toxicol 68: 408-415.

46. Shugaba AI, Asala AS, Gambo IM, Mohammed BM (2012) The effects of physical and oxidative stress on the ovary of the female Wistar rat. An Int J Life Sci Chem 29: 326-335.

47. Perez GI (2000) Identification of potassium-dependent and-independent components of the apoptotic machinery in mouse ovarian germ cells and granulose cells. Biol Reprod 63: 1358-1369.

48. Perez GI (1997) Apoptosis-associated signaling pathways are required for chemotherapy-mediated female germ cell destruction. Nat Med 3: 1228-1232.

49. Yeh JB, Kim B, Liang YJ, Peresie J (2006) Müllerian inhibiting substance as a novel biomarker of cisplatin-induced ovarian damage. Biochem Biophys Res Commun 348: 337-344.

50. Ozcelik B, Turkyilmaz C, Ozgun MT, Serin IS, Batukan C (2010) Prevention of paclitaxel and cisplatin induced ovarian damage in rats by a gonadotropin-releasing hormone agonist. Fertil Steril 93: 1609-1614.

51. Nakai M (1995) Deformation of the rat Sertoli cell by oral administration of carbendazim (methyl 2-benzimidazole carbamate). J Androl 16: 410-416.

52. Narayana K (2005) The antiviral drug ribavirin reversibly affects the reproductive parameters in the male Wistar rat. Folia Morphol 64: 65-71.

53. Akunna GG (2013) Pyrethroid-based insecticide induces testicular toxicity via oxidative pathway: study suggest. Oriental J Sci Res 2: 1.

54. Mathews CK (2000) Electron transport, oxidative phosphorylation and oxygen metabolism. Virginia 3: 523-557.

55. Scholzen T, Gerdes J (2000) The Ki-67 protein: from the known and the unknown. J Cell Physiol 182: 311-322.

56. Zhang X (2001) Cisplatin-induced germ cell apoptosis in mouse testes. Arch Androl 46: 43-49.

57. Ferrara D (2006) Acute and long-term effects of in utero exposure of rats to di(n-butyl) phthalate on testicular germ cell development and proliferation. Endocrinol 147: 5352-5362.

58. Boekelheide K, Schoenfeld HA, Hall SJ, Weng CC, Shetty G, et al. (2005) Gonadotropin-releasing hormone antagonist (Cetrorelix) therapy fails to protect nonhuman primates (Macaca arctoides) from radiation-induced spermatogenic failure. J Androl 26: 222-234.

59. Acar N, Berdeaux O, Grégoire S, Cabaret S, Martine L, et al. (2012) Lipid composition of human eye: Are red blood cells a good mirror of retinal and optic nerve fatty acid? PLoS ONE 7: e35102.

60. Kamisli S, Ciftci O, Kaya K, Cetin A, Kamisli O, et al. (2013) Hesperidin protects brain and sciatic nerve tissues against cisplatin-induced oxidative, histological and electromyographical side effects in rats. Toxicol Ind Health 31: 841-851.

61. Mukhopadhyay P, Horváth B, Zsengellér Z, Zielonka J, Tanchian G, et al. (2011) Mitochondrial-targeted antioxidants represent a promising approach for prevention of cisplatin-induced nephropathy. Free Radic Biol Med 52: 497-506.

62. Naziroglu M, Simsek M, Simsek H, Aydilek N, Ozcan Z, et al. (2004) The effects of hormone replacement therapy combined with vitamin C and E antioxidants level and lipid profiles in postmenopausal woman with type 2 Diabetes. Clin Chem Acta 344: 63-71.

63. Atasayar S, Orhan H, Gürel B, Girgin G, Özgüneş H, et al. (2009) Preventive effect of aminoguanidine compared to vitamin E and C on cisplatin-induced nephrotoxicity in rats. Exp Toxicol Pathol 61: 23-32.

64. Yang HS, Han DK, Kim JR, Sim JC (2006) Effects of alpha- tocopherol on cadmium-induced toxicity in rat testis and spermatogenesis. J Korean Med Sci 21: 445-451.

65. Azu OO, Duru FIO, Osinubi AA, Noronha CC, Elesha SO, et al. (2010) Protective agent, Kigelia Africana fruit extract, against cisplatin-induced kidney oxidant injury in Sprague–Dawley rats. Asian J Pharma Clin Res 3: 84-88.

66. Peng SJ, Lu RK, Yu LH (1997) Effect of Semen cuacutae, Rhizoma curculiginis, Radix morindae, Officinalis on human spermatozoa's motility and membrane function in vitro. Zhongguo Zhong Xi Yi Jie He Za Zhi 17: 145-147.

67. Lirdi LC, Stumpp T, Sasso-Cerri E, Miraglia SM (2008) Amifostine protective effect on cisplatin-treated rat testis. Anat Rec Hoboken 291: 797-808.

68. Benie T, Duval J, Thieulant ML (2003) Effect of some traditional plant extracts on rat oestrous cycle compared with clomid. Phytother Res 17: 748-755.

69. Amin A, Hamza A (2006) Effects of ginger and roselle on cisplatininduced reproductive toxicity in rats. Asian J Androl 8: 607-612.

70. Yüce A, Atessahin A, Ceribas AO, Aksakal M (2007) Ellagic acid prevents cisplatin-induced oxidative stress in liver and heart tissue of rats. Basic Clin Pharmacol Toxicol 101: 345-349.

71. Ilbey YO, Ozbek E, Cekmen M (2009) Protective effect of curcumin in cisplatininduced oxidative injury in rat testis: mitogen-activated protein kinase and nuclear factor-kappa B signaling pathways. Hum Reprod 24: 1717-1725.

72. Amin A, Ghoneim MD, Syam MI, Daoud S (2012) Neural network assessment of herbal protection against chemotherapeutic-induced reproductive toxicity. Theor Biol Med Model 24: 1.

73. Vernet P, Aitken RJ, Drevet JR (2004) Antioxidant strategies in the epididymis. Mol Cell Endocrinol 216: 31-39.

74. Kalender Y, Yel M (2005) Doxorubicin hepatotoxicity and hepatic free radical metabolism in rats. The effects of vitamin E and catechin. Toxicology 209: 39-45.

14

Determination of Chronic Disease Origin Using Time Reversal Computations

Jahangir A. Satti*

Department of Radiation Oncology, Albany Medical College, 43 New Scotland Ave, MC 95, Albany, NY 12208-3478, USA

Abstract

All chronic inflammatory processes in a living organism pass through a series of biological stages to form tumors. This is similar to a natural effort to repair a chronic wound. Sometimes, the origin of metastasized tumors cannot be located with our conventional biomedical and biochemical tools. However, each tumor has a specific growth rate based on an individual's health status. The tumor growth rate can be calculated from the CT scan information taken at different time intervals. Then one can determine the tumor's initiation time at cellular level with the help of growth rate parameters. A time reversal mathematical model has been proposed to determine the initiation time of a tumor. This model can be used to estimate the origin of some tumors for better treatment planning in chronic diseases. Since cancer is not a local malady the holistic approach is required to analyze the possible root cause of this degenerative disease.

Keywords: Chronic; Diseases; cancer; CT

Background Introduction

Studies indicate that about 45% Americans entered the 21st century carrying chronic diseases with them. About 61 million among these patients had multiple chronic conditions [1]. The chronic diseases consume 78% of the health spending budget in the USA. The majority of victims suffering from chronic diseases fall in the age group of 65 and older.

It has also been reported that 85% of our seniors are suffering from chronic diseases while 62% have multiple chronic conditions.

Female patients have more chronic conditions than male population. About 46% white and 37% black have reported chronic conditions in some research studies. But the chronic conditions almost equally affect different income classes across the board (41% poor, 46% near poor, 44% low income, 43% middle income, and 44% high income). According to another, study the cost of chronic diseases amounted to $277 billion in the USA during 2003 fiscal year. The lost in productivity due to chronic diseases during the same period reached one trillion dollars. The news about chronic diseases at global level is also alarming. According to the World Health Organization (WHO) report, 59% of deaths and 46% of the global burden of diseases are attributed to chronic maladies [2]. The lack of resources, infrastructure and know-how of conventional therapies make it impossible to deliver meaningful health benefits to a great majority of patients in the developing world [3-5]. As most of the populace resides in the countryside, any conventional medical facility is mostly inaccessible to them anyway. There is an urgent need to explore alternative methods to combat chronic diseases at an early stage throughout the world [6].

Historically homeopathy has prided itself in dealing with the chronic diseases since its early days. The epitome of chronic diseases philosophy in homeopathy was authored by Hahnemann himself almost two hundred years ago [7]. While dealing with chronic diseases, he was forced to challenge some of his own earlier theses about medicine. Hahnemann's dramatic departure from classical homeopathic philosophy was primarily because of the complex nature of chronic diseases. First, he introduced the name "disease" as the title of his new book "Chronic Diseases". But in his earlier philosophy of similia, he vehemently rejected to label any sickness with the word disease [8]. Second, he coined the term "anti" i.e., anti-miasmatic, anti psoric, etc. This was in direct contradiction with his original philosophy

of "homeo", the hallmark of his new system of medicine popularly known as homeopathy. Third, Hahnemann advocated the alternation of medicines in stubborn chronic cases. But he strictly accentuated about single remedy in his prior philosophy in the "Organon of Medicine". Fourth, the strengths of drugs were also revised though he claimed that drugs get highly energetic with his regular centesimal succession. Fifth, the dominant factor in chronic diseases was miasma. The vital force was not any more the sole contender in guaranteeing health. The role of miasma can be elucidated from the fact that Hahnemann mentioned it about one hundred times in his book Chronic Diseases. The word vital force is barely mentioned about a dozen times in the same manuscript. The word vital force is mentioned over 200 times and miasma about 50 times in the Organon of Medicine. In nutshell, the nature of chronic diseases even forced Hahnemann to abandon his original philosophy and venture on to a different course. This also shows the level of complications embedded in chronic diseases and the time required in setting back the convoluted biological evolutionary processes to their original course. Unfortunately, there were no serious efforts after Hahnemann to address the nature of chronic diseases in depth on scientific lines [9].

Cancer is mostly referred as an ulcer in Hahnemann's works. Today, cancer is considered as the most deadly disease among chronic maladies. It formed merely 3% of the total disease burden at the turn of the last century. Just in one hundred years cancer has affected almost 45% of the patients in the United States alone. Subclinical chronic inflammations, mostly from suppressed diseases, eventually lead to tumor formations. Organs consisting on parallel sub functional units, such as liver, lung and kidneys may breed tumors for years without any observable signs or symptoms. Cancerous cells from these sites

---

*Corresponding author: Jahangir A. Satti, Department of Radiation Oncology, Albany Medical College, 43 New Scotland Ave, MC 95, Albany, NY 12208-3478, USA, E-mail: DrJSatti@Gmail.Com

dislodge and migrate through circulatory systems to distant parts of the body. For instance tumors found in brain mostly originate in lung [10]. The chemotherapy is limited in treating brain tumors because of the limitations of blood-brain barrier. Brain tumors are mostly treated with radiation and surgical techniques for local control. The combined applications of these marvelous clinical techniques could not extend the survival time beyond one year [11].

Even with combined whole brain radiation therapy and stereotactic radiosurgery (SRS), the median survival rate was only 11 months [12]. Survival rate for patients suffering from brain cancers is much better than patients suffering from brain tumors [13-17]. It has been reported that when the cancer origin was liver, the poor patients had not even time to get treated as their conditions deteriorated quickly [18]. There is also a tumor spread from Non-Small Cell Lung Cancer (NSCLC) to other organs such as lymph nodes, pleura, brain, liver, bone, pericardium, and renal system [19]. Furthermore, there can also be some rare cases when tumor spread to brain occurs from endometrial carcinomas [20]. The prominent cancer that spreads to other organs originates in lung [21]. Intracranial metastases are mostly from lung, breast, renal and skin i.e., melanoma origin. It has also been found that about 70% intracranial lesions are located within the brain parenchyma, the rest involves the pachymeningeal envelopes. Intracranial metastasis makes up to 17% of all brain tumors [22]. However, only 15% patients die due to brain metastasis [23]. Leptomeningeal metastases have origins in leukemia, lymphoma and breast carcinoma but these are rare. Computed Tomography (CT) scanning is state of the art technology to acquire appropriate information about site, size, and morphological metastasis of the brain tumors.

It has been suggested that a holistic approach, in addition to local treatment, may well enhance the quality and length of lives for cancer patients [24]. Such a treatment plan needs comprehensive information about a cancer patient. Since cancer masks the most of the conventional symptoms, there is a need to plan an elaborate strategy to evaluate cancer as a chronic disease. For instance, researchers have found that they could not find significant differences in tumor distribution between symptomatic and asymptomatic patients in non-small cell lung cancer with brain metastasis [25]. An alternative solution to this problem is to trace out the possible root of a tumor. A mathematical model has been developed to estimate the possible initiation time of a tumor. A physician can use this model to investigate the patient's medical history.

Materials and Methods

Different models have been in use to estimate the tumor growth rate [26,27]. Meanwhile different techniques have also emerged to utilized Computed Tomography (CT) information to determine tumor volume [28]. These volume growth rates can be generalized for particular kind of tumors as it varies from patient to patient [29-30]. Some otherwise healthy individuals may have very slow growing tumor while patients suffering with multiple chronic diseases have accelerated growth rate. It is possible to determine growth rate for an individual based on tumor volume at two different points of time. The following model can be used to individualized patients when two different scans are compared over time. Mühe et. al. have reported that among different patients, the doubling time varied as between 50 days and 860 days in squamous cell carcinoma's, 22 day to 2098 days among soft tissue sarcoma, 15 days to 2798 days among sarcoma of bone etc. [31]. So the case of chronic diseases is highly individualized among patient though suffering from the same type of cancer. Hence, an approach based on individual patient is required to analyze the case in a holistic manner.

Estimating the roots of chronic diseases

Change in tumor volume, V, with time can be defined as,

$$\frac{dV}{dt} = \eta V$$

Where η is growth rate constant for a particular tumor.

$$\frac{dV}{V} = \eta dt \tag{A}$$

Suppose the initial volume of tumor is V_1 at time t_1 and as tumor grows its volume at time t_2 reaches V_2. Integrating equation (A)

$$\int_{V1}^{V2} \frac{dV}{V} = \eta \int_{t1}^{t2} dt$$

$$\ln\left(\frac{V_2}{V_1}\right) = \eta\left(t_2 - t_1\right) = \eta\Delta t \tag{B}$$

Taking exponential on both sides

$$V_2 = V_1 e^{\eta\left(t_2 - t_1\right)} = V_1 e^{\eta\Delta t} \tag{C}$$

Equation (B) can also be rearranged as,

$$\eta = \frac{Ln\left(\dfrac{V_2}{V_1}\right)}{\left(t_2 - t_1\right)} \tag{D}$$

Or

$$\Delta t = \left(t_2 - t_1\right) = \frac{Ln\left(\dfrac{V_2}{V_1}\right)}{\eta} \tag{E}$$

Suppose $\Delta t = \tau$ is the time when tumor volume doubles from volume V1 to V2 i.e. ($V_2 = 2V_1$), then we have from equation (E)

$$\tau = \frac{Ln(2)}{\eta} \quad \text{Or} \quad \eta = \frac{0.693}{\tau}$$

Using the value of η in equation (D) and after rearrangement

$$\tau = \frac{0.693\left(t_2 - t_1\right)}{Ln\left(\dfrac{V_2}{V_1}\right)} = \frac{0.693t}{Ln\left(\dfrac{V_2}{V_1}\right)} \tag{F}$$

Or

$$V_2 = V_1 e^{\frac{0.693\left(t_2 - t_1\right)}{\tau}} = V_1 e^{\frac{0.693t}{\tau}}$$

$$Ln\left(\frac{V_2}{V_1}\right) = \frac{0.693\left(t_2 - t_1\right)}{\tau} = \frac{0.693t}{\tau} \tag{G}$$

Example1

If the initial volume of a tumor was measured to be 1.23 cm³ and after 14 months, the tumor size is 1.45cm³. What would be the doubling time τ for this tumor?

Solution: using equation (F) we can estimate the doubling time

$$\tau = \frac{0.693 \times 14}{Ln\left(\dfrac{1.45}{1.23}\right)} = \frac{9.702}{0.16455} = 58.96\, Months$$

So from above calculation we figure out the doubling rate of this tumor is ~ 59 months, which is almost 5 years. This is an example of very slow growing tumor, such as Prostate.

Example 2

Using images as shown in figure 1A and 1B, if the tumor growth rate is $\tau = 5 months$ and the current volume measured through CT scan is ~3 mm³. Suppose the volume of single cell for such cancer is 10 μm^3 when the initial cancer started?

Solution: using equation (F)

The radius of tumor cell, r=5 μm

The volume $V_1 = \dfrac{4}{3}\pi r^3 = 5.236 \times 10^{-16}$ m³.

$$\tau = \dfrac{0.693 \times t}{Ln\left(\dfrac{V_2}{V_1}\right)}$$

After rearrangement

$$t = \dfrac{\tau \times Ln\left(\dfrac{V_2}{V_1}\right)}{0.693}$$

$$t = \dfrac{5 \times Ln\left(\dfrac{3 \times 10^{-9}}{5.24 x 10^{-16}}\right)}{0.693} = \dfrac{5 \times 15.56}{0.693}$$

$t = 112.3 Months$ or over 9 years.

Check with the patient what happened 9 years ago in his/her medical history tries to locate the root of diseases in that region

Conclusion and Discussion

The use of toxic drugs, continuous exposure to environmental particulates, inhibitions of evolutionary biological processes, suppressions of infectious diseases and administration of hormones form the root causes of chronic maladies. These prolonged external assaults initiate necrotic foci in the biological systems. Most of these necrotic centers release chemical signals during subsequent repair processes. In reaction the affected system produces localized

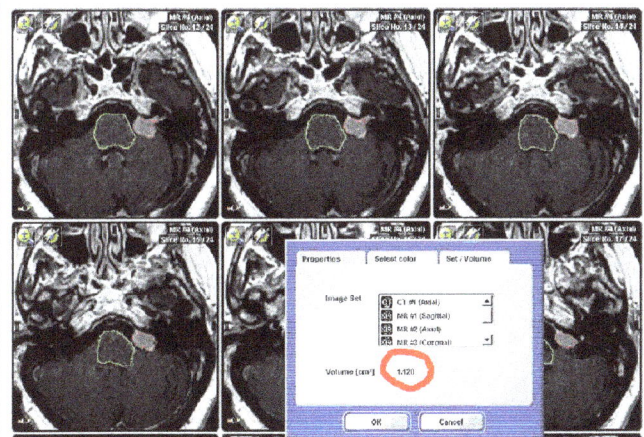

Figure 1a: The contouring of Acoustic Neuroma of the right side of a patient. The tumor volumes are computed by the software. This is a teaching example and may not be clinically valid.

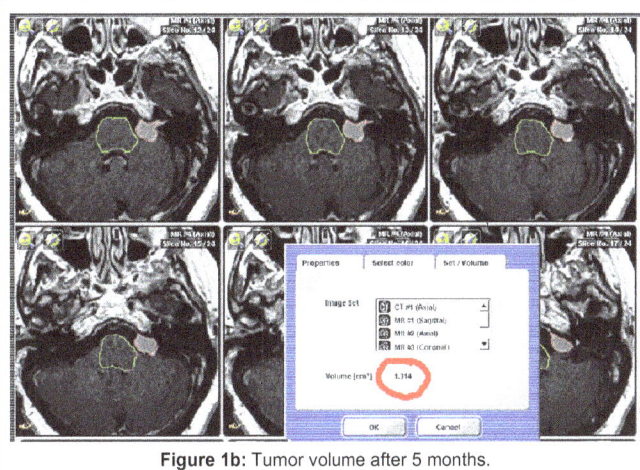

Figure 1b: Tumor volume after 5 months.

inflammation. Such inflammatory processes resemble chronic wounds that never heal. Using the above information a physician can explore the medical history of the patient. In the above case, the physician can inquire what happened 9 years ago. Since most cancers arise from chronic diseases, it would be prudent to heal the system at the root level. Almost all the local controls in cancers are limited and patients die soon after they are treated. It will be advisable for patients to have alternative therapy for chronic conditions along with conventional medicine. Caution must be observed that all tumors do not grow exponentially. It is true especially with breast/prostate tumors and in laboratory animals where the subject is otherwise healthy. However, tumors involving the deterioration of the entire system grow exponentially. Again one must keep in mind that estimating tumor volume is subjective and two experts may not agree or even one expert at two different occasions may come up with different results. Automated computer based imaging tools may be more reliable in assessing the tumor volume.

Acknowledgement

Thanks are due to Waseem Khan Raja of Tuft University for typing mathematical equations.

Conflict of Interest

No financial involvement with any person or organization is related to this study.

References

1. Anderson G, Horvarth J (2004) The growing burden of chronic disease in America. Public Health Report 119: 263-270.

2. WHO (2008) http://www.who.int/dietphysicalactivity/publications/facts/chronic/en/

3. Bosanquet N, Sikora K (2004) The economics of cancer care in the UK. Lancet Oncol 5: 568-574.

4. Chirikos TN (2002) Cancer economics: on variations in the costs of treating cancer. Cancer Control 9: 59-66.

5. Tassinari D, Poggi B, Fantini M, Tamburini E, Nicoletti S, et al. (2006) Cost–opportunity analysis in clinical oncology: from the "wild far-west" to a correct integration of the disciplines, avoiding the "war of the worlds", letters to the editor. Ann. Oncol 17: 876-877.

6. Satti JA The emerging low dose therapy for advanced cancer. Dose-Response International (to appear)

7. Hahnemann S (1962) The Chronic Diseases. Masood Publishers. Lahore, Pakistan.

8. Hahnemann S (1962) Organon of Medicine. Masood Publishers. Lahore, Pakistan.

9. Tyler ML (1939) Cancer. The Homoeopathic Recorder 8.

10. Fokas E, Engenhart-Cabillic R, Daniilidis K, Rose F, An H-X (2007) Metastasis: the seed and the soil theory gains identity. Cancer Metastasis Rev 26: 705-715.

11. Lagerwaard FJ, Levendag PC, Nowak PJ, Eijkenboom WM, Hansens PE, et al (1999) Identification of prognostic factors in patients with brain metastases: a review of 1292 patient. Int J of Radiat Oncol Biol.Phys 43: 795-803.

12. Kondziolka D, Patel A, Lunsford LD, Kassam A, Flickinger JC (1999) Stereotactic radiosurgery plus whole brain radiotherapy versus radiotherapy alone for patients with multiple brain metastases. Int J Radiat Oncol Biol Phys 45: 427-34.

13. Farng KT, Chang KP, Wong TT, Guo WY, Ho DM (1999) Pediatric intracranial germinoma treated with chemotherapy alone. Zhonghua Yi Xue Za Zhi (Taipei) 62: 859-866.

14. Zhang R, Zhou L (1999) Medulloblastoma. Chin Med J (Engl) 112: 297-301.

15. Kellie SJ, Boyce H, Dunkel IJ, Diez B, Rosenblum M et al (2004) Intensive cisplatin and cyclophosphamide-based chemotherapy without radiotherapy for intracranial germinomas: failure of a primary chemotherapy approach. Pediatr Blood Cancer 43: 126-133.

16. Puzzilli F, Ruggeri A, Mastronardi L, Di Stefano D, Lunardi P (1998) Long-term survival in cerebral glioblastoma. Case report and critical review of the literature. Tumori 84: 69-74.

17. Xue H, Horwitz JR, Smith MB, Lally KP, Black CT, et al (1995) Malignant solid tumors in neonates: a 40-year review. J Pediatr Surg 30: 543-545.

18. Chang L, Chen YL, Kao MC (2004) Intracranial metastasis of hepatocellular carcinoma: review of 45 cases. Surg Neurol 62: 172-177.

19. Stenbygaard LE, Sorenson JB, Larsen H, Dombernowsky P (1999) Metastatic pattern in non-resectable non-small cell lung cancer. Acta Oncol 38: 993-998.

20. Martinez-Manas RM, Brell M, Rumia J, Ferrer E (1998) Brain metastasis in endometrial carcinoma. Gynecol Oncol 70: 282-284.

21. Cheong TH, Wang YT, Poh SC, Thung JL (1989) Carcinoma of the lung with metastasis to skeletal muscles. Singapore Med J 30: 605-606.

22. Boccardo F, Comelli G, De Menech R, Mina G, Zanardi S (1984) Natural history and staging of brain metastases. Minerva Med 75: 1369-1378.

23. Wakelee HA, Bernardo P, Johnson DH, Schiller JH (2006) Changes in the natural history of nonsmall cell lung cancer (NSCLC) – comparison of outcomes and characteristics in patients with advanced NSCLC entered in Eastern Cooperative Oncology Group trials before and after 1990. Cancer 106: 2208-2217.

24. Nguyen DX, Bos PD, Massagne J (2009) Metastasis: from dissemination to organ-specific colonization. Nature Reviews Cancer 9: 274-285.

25. Hi AA, Digumarthy SR, Temel JS, Halpern EF, Kuester LB, et al. (2006) Does initial strategy or tumor histology better identify asymptomatic brain metastasis in patients with non-small cell lung cancer? J. Thorac Oncol 1: 205-210.

26. Collins VP, Loeffler RK, Tivey H (1956) Observations on growth rates of human tumors. Am J Roentgenol Radium Ther Nucl Med 76: 988-1000.

27. Schwartz M (1961) A biomathematical approach to clinical tumor growth Cancer. 14: 1272–1294.

28. Beriman RS, Beck JW, Korobkin M, Glenny R, Akwari OE, et al (1982) Volume determinations using computed tomography. AJR 138: 329-333.

29. Winer-Muram HT, Jennings SG, Tarver RD, Aisen AM, Tann M, et al (2002) Volumetric growth rate of stage I lung cancer prior to treatment: Serial CT Scanning. Radiology 223: 798-805.

30. Mehrara E, Forssell-Aronsson E, Ahlman H, Bernhardt P (2007) Specific growth rate versus doubling time for quantitative characterization of tumor growth rate. Cancer Res 67: 3970-3975.

31. E. Muhe, F.P. Gall, B. Angermann (1981) Are Growth Rates of Tumors of Any Clinical Importance? Medical and Pediatric Oncology 9: 35-40.

15

Effectiveness of Leech Therapy in *Gambhira Vata-Rakta* (Acute Gout)

Ashok Kumar Panda* and Saroj Kumar Debnath

Department of Ayurveda Research, Ayurveda Regional Research Institute - A unit of CCRAS, Department of AYUSH, Government of India, Gangtok, Sikkim, India

Abstract

Bloodletting is a mainstay of *Panchakarma* therapy as per Susruta. Leech therapy has been indicated as means of bloodletting for both types of *Vata-rakta* where pain, burning and redness found as per *Charaka chikitsa*. Medical science has enormous leaps in terms of diagnosis and treatment yet there is renewed interest in leech therapy among modern as well as traditional medicine practitioners. Most of studies of leech therapy are found for plastic surgery and pain reduction in osteo- arthritis. US, FDA also approves leech therapy as tool of skin graft. Therefore, we conducted a non randomized controlled pilot study in between June 2011 to Sep 2011 to assess the efficacy of leech therapy in *Gambhira Vatarakta* as diagnosed as acute Gout. Twelve patients (eight male and four female) with a mean age of 47 (9) years were treated with two - four leeches for seven days with a follow up to four weeks. Another 10 patents those were not willing for leech therapy was treated with tropical Diclofenac sodium gel for 7 days as control. The mean length of blood socking is 32 (5) minute. The mean quantity of blood sucked by Individual leech per suck is 6 (2) ml. In comparison with control, leech application led to rapid relief of pain and swelling immediate after the detachment of leech. Most significant clinical improvement was noted after 14 days and slightly reduction of serum uric acid were also noted after three weeks of treatment. 90% Patient described the initial leech therapy as a painless and two patients had mild to moderate itching but no local infection was noted in treated group. Our study was limited to small sample size but it had remarkable treatment effect. Larger randomized control trial should be undertaken to study the safety and efficacy of leech therapy in acute gout.

Keywords: Leech; Bloodletting; Ayurveda; Acute; Gout; Patients

Introduction

Rakamokshyana (Bloodletting) is an ancient procedure that was utilized in Ayurveda in the setting of a humoral and pathological concept as a general treatment for all ailments, as well as during the middle ages primarily as a remedy for the treatment of inflammatory and infectious diseases by other traditional medicines of world. The general population was convinced of the efficacy of this treatment for centuries, even requesting it on occasion on a prophylactic basis. Leech has been used from ancient days in Grace, Roma and Arabian countries. Susruta (1000 BC) and Charak (600-200 BC) are two sages from India to describe about leech therapy whereas western literature mentioned about Themison (80-40 BC) – a pupil of Asclepiads is the first person to describe about leech therapy [1].

Leech is an Anglo-Saxon word derived from "Loece" meaning "to heal" and the oldest therapeutic book about leech is leechdom [2]. Leech is an: "aquatic worm with a flattened body, tapering toward each end, and terminating in circular flattened discs, the hinder one being the larger of the two. It swims with a vertical undulating motion, and moves when out of water by means of these discs or suckers, fastening itself first by one and then by the other, and alternately stretching out and contracting its body. The mouth is placed in the center of the anterior disc, and furnished with three cartilaginous lens-shaped jaws at the entrance of the alimentary canal. These jaws are lined at their edges with fine, sharp teeth, and meet so as to make a triangular incision in the flesh. The head is furnished with small, raised points, supposed by some to be eyes. Leech belongs to the Phylum Annelida family of fresh-water parasitic invertebrates [3]. It was noticed that leech bites continued to bleed after the leech was withdrawn. This phenomenon was finally explained in 1884 when John Berry Hay croft, a Birmingham chemist, discovered an anticoagulant, called "hirudin", that the leech injected into the blood, which kept the capillaries flowing [4].

The resurgence of Leech therapy in treatment of hypertension, migraines, phlebitis, varicose veins, arthritis, hemorrhoids, and ovarian cysts were introduced in Russia after 1990's [5,6]. In the United States, plastic surgeons use them to drain blood from wounds after limb or tissue reattachment [7,8]. Some Indian clinical trials of leech therapy in Osteoarthritis, Frostbite, Hypertension, Migraine are in Progress from Unani Research Council [9]. Recent research also supports leech use in relieving pain in patients with osteoarthritis of the knee, as well as in treating purpura fulminans, periorbital hematoma, sublingual hematoma, systemic lupus erythematous, and ear infection [10].

The prevalence of Gout is now as high as 12.6% may due to increased frequency of obesity and hypertension. Monosodium urate crystal is the active constituent for acute inflammatory reaction in Gout [11]. Colchine, corticosteroid and NSAID are the choices of drugs in acute gout with their proven adverse effect [12]. Leech therapy has been indicated as means of bloodletting for both types of *Vata-rakta* where pain, burning and redness found as per *Charaka chikitsa* [13,14]. Some Chinese evidences of Bloodletting in Gout with Cupping and herbal medicinal are there with significant result [15]. Some traditional healers of Sikkim have been practicing leech therapy in acute gout also [16]. But no clinical studies available on leech therapy in acute gout except some review. Therefore, we conducted a non randomized Controlled pilot study in between June 2011 to Sep 2011 to assess the efficacy of leech therapy in *Gambhira Vatarakta* as diagnosed as acute Gout.

*Corresponding author: Ashok Kumar panda, Department of Ayurveda Research, Ayurveda Regional Research Institute - A unit of CCRAS, Department of AYUSH, Government of India, Gangtok, Sikkim, India
E-mail: akpanda_06@yahoo.co.in

Patients and Methods

We recruited 22 patients of acute gout from the OPD of our Institute by preset exclusion and inclusion criteria. An informed consent was obtained from all participants in the study and all patients were informed about 2-4 leech application. The patients were male and nonpregnant women in between the age of 18-60 years were included in the study based on the American College of Rheumatology 1980 classification criteria [17]. The major exclusion criteria were treatment with anticoagulants, haemorrhagic disorders, treated with western medication and preexisting arterial insufficiency. The patients were treated with two - four leeches in the affected area for seven days with a follow up to four weeks. Leech (*Hirudo medicinalis*) was used for the treatment after identified by local zoologist and conformed from literature [18]. The leech were attached, monitored and detach as per the published recommendations [19]. Eligible patients also had at least 1 CBC, blood chemistry, and urinalysis performed within 1 year prior to trial, the results of which revealed no abnormalities that would contraindicate treatment with either study medication.

Efficacy & Safety Evaluation

The primary outcome (0-7 days) was measured by pain intensity in the index joint by Visual analogous scale (VAS) i.e. 0= no pain & 10= extremely painful on D0, immediately after therapy for 7 days daily with a fellow up for 28 days.

The secondary outcome i.e. tenderness (0–3-point scale), and swelling (0–3-point scale) are also assessed. The patient's and investigator's global assessments of response to therapy (0 = excellent; 4 = poor) and the investigator's assessments of study joint tenderness (0 = no pain; 3 = patient states there is pain, winces, and then withdraws), swelling (0 = none; 3 = bulging beyond the joint margins), and erythema (present, absent, or not assessable) were conducted on day0, immediately after therapy for 7 days daily with a fellow up for 28 days. The patients were advised for visit if problem arise in between. The serum uric acid was measured on D0, D1, D4, D8, D14, D21 and D28. The outcome of safety measured by patient's and investigator's global response to treatment with any adverse effect was observed during the therapy and observed period.

Observations and Results

Total 22 patients were recruited in the study and man patient 14 (64%) are dominant in the study with more educated people 16 (73%) are attracted to this Ayurveda therapy (Table 1). All the patients have the classical symptoms of acute gout but elevated uric acid observed in only 10 (83.33%) in leech therapy group and 7 (70%) in control group. Presence of trophy is very less in both the groups. Polyarticular joint pain was found in maximum patients. The most affected joint was great toes in both the groups (Table 2).

We attached the leech by griping in dry gauze to the site or by placing a drop of glucose on desired site. We noticed that some time leech migrate from one site to another. 90% Patient described the initial leech therapy as a painless. The mean feeding time was 32(5) minute. The mean quantity of blood sucked by Individual leech per suck is 6(2) ml. Three patients had mild to moderate itching and Bleeding from the site of application was seen in 2 patients and was easily managed with compressive dressings. No other complications or infections were noted.

The mean changes in primary outcome i.e. Pain (VAS) was significantly reduced immediate after the leech therapy and completely disappear in 28 days, whereas pain in control group was poorly reduced and reappeared after the cessation of application of Diclofenac gel in the affected area (Table 3). The secondary outcomes were also assessed by the patient's and investigators global assessment to response to the therapy, tenderness, swelling and noting erythema in leech and control groups. Leech group was responded well even after the cessation of treatment but control group had reappeared the symptoms after the cessation of treatment (Table 4,5). The primary and secondary endpoints were also compared in trial and control group and significant response was observed in trial group compared to control group (Table 6).

Discussion

A seven days course of leech therapy was effective in relieving pain, tender, swelling, erythema in acute gout and the effect was intact up to 28 days of observed period. These types of pain relieving effect was also observed in other randomized control studies in the treatment of Osteoarthritis and epicondylitis [20,21].

The saliva of leeches contains a variety of substances such as hirudin, hyaluronidase, histamine-like vasodilators, collagenase, inhibitors of kallikrein and superoxide production, and poorly characterised anaesthetic and analgesic compounds [22,23]. Therefore, a regional analgesic and antiphlogistic effect by these substances enforced by hyaluronidase as well as counter-irritation might be possible. Leeches might be considered as an additional option in the therapeutic approach to acute Gout. Our study was limited to small sample size but it has remarkable treatment effect. Larger randomized control trial should be undertaken to study the safety and efficacy of leech therapy in acute gout.

Variables	Test group	Control Group	Total
No of patients	12	10	22
Percentage of Male	8(66.66%)	6(60%)	14(64%)
Mean age in Years	47(9)	50(10)	
Percentage of Educated person (above matric)	9(75%)	7(70%)	16(73%)
Duration of diseases	8.1(6.2)	7.3(4.5)	7.9(4.9)
Monoarticular joint pain	5	4	09
Polyarticular	7	6	13
Metatarsophalangeal (foot)	3	3	6
Ankle	2	2	4
Knee	1	1	2
Great toe proximal interphalangeal joint	6	4	10
Others	0	0	0

Table 1: Patient's demographic variables of studied 22 patients.

Clinical variables	Test group	Control group
Pain in Joint	12	10
Swelling of the joints	12	10
Joints of limited mobility	12	12
Redness of Joint	11	10
Elevated uric acid	10	07
Presence of Trophy	03	02

Table 2: Clinical variables of studied 22 patients.

Group	Baseline	Day1	Day4	Day8	Day14	Day21	Day28
Leech (n=12)	7.6	3.4	2.3.	1.4	1.0	1.0	1.0
Diclofenac gel (n=10)	6.4	5.8	4.8	4.0	6.0	6.0	6.0

Table 3: Mean changes in the primary outcome (Pain Score-VAS) in different duration of treatment in Studied & Control group.

Assessment Scale	Day0	Day1	Day4	Day8	Day14	Day21	Day28
Patient global assessment to response to therapy (0-4)	NA	2.26	1.06	0.86	0.86	0.56	0.56
Investigator's global assessment of response to therapy (0–4 scale)	NA	2.16	1.02	0.72	0.72	0.34	0.34
Study joint tenderness (0–3 scale)	2.56	2.24	1.16	0.84	0.84	0.20	0.20
Study joint swelling (0–3 scale)	2.58	2.26	1.16	0.34	0.34	0.20	0.20
Study of Erythema	p	p	p	A	A	A	A

Table 4: Mean changes in secondary outcome in leech therapy group (n=12).

Assessment Scale	Day0	Day1	Day4	Day8	Day14	Day21	Day28
Patient global assessment to response to therapy (0-4)	NA	1.06	1.16	1.26	0.96	0.96	0.96
Investigator's global assessment of response to therapy (0–4 scale)	NA	0.98	0.62	0.48	0.72	0.72	0.92
Study joint tenderness (0–3 scale)	2.46	2.46	2.36	1.88	2.64	2.64	2.64
Study joint swelling (0–3 scale)	2.34	2.16	2.16	1.84	2.34	2.34	2.34
Study of Erythema	p	p	p	A	p	p	p

Table 5: Mean changes in secondary outcome in control group (n=10).

Assessment Scale	Baseline mean	Treatment Mean	P value	REMARK
Pain Scale Leech Group Control group	7.6 6.4	1.0 6.0		
Patient global assessment to response to therapy (0-4) Leech Group Control group	NA NA	0.56 0.96		
Investigator's global assessment of response to therapy (0–4 scale) Leech Group Control group	NA NA	0.34 0.92		
Study joint tenderness (0–3 scale) Leech Group Control group	2.56 2.46	0.20 2.64		
Study joint swelling (0–3 scale) Leech Group Control group	2.58 2.34	0.20 2.34		
Study of Erythema Leech Group Control group	P P	A P		

Table 6: Mean change in the primary and secondary end points from baseline in both studied and Control Groups.

References

1. Garrison FH (1929) An introduction to the history of medicine with medical chronology, suggestions for study and bibliographic data. (4thedn), W.B. Saunders Company, Philadelphia.

2. Davis AB, Appel T (1979) Bloodletting instruments in the National Museum of History and Technology.

3. Seigworth GR (1980) Bloodletting over the centuries. N Y State J Med 80: 2022-2028.

4. Whitaker IS, Rao J, Izadi D, Butler PE (2004) Historical Article: Hirudo medicinalis: ancient origins of, and trends in the use of medicinal leeches throughout history. Br J Oral Maxillofac Surg 42: 133-137.

5. Abdelgabar AM, Bhowmick BK (2003) The return of the leech. Int J Clin Pract 57: 103-105.

6. Eldor A, Orevi M, Rigbi M (1996) The role of the leech in medical therapeutics. Blood Rev 10: 201-209.

7. Whitaker IS, Izadi D, Oliver DW, Monteath G, Butler PE (2004) Hirudo Medicinalis and the plastic surgeon. Br J Plast Surg 57: 348-353.

8. Mumcuoglu KY, Pidhorz C, Cohen R, Ofek A, Lipton HA (2007) The use of the medicinal leech, Hirudo medicinalis, in the reconstructive plastic surgery. The Internet Journal of Plastic Surgery 4: 12.

9. http://www.news24.com/World/News/Thumbs-up-for-leech-therapy-20050824

10. Michalsen A, Klotz S, Lüdtke R, Moebus S, Spahn G, et al. (2003) Effectiveness of leech therapy in osteoarthritis of the knee: a randomized, controlled trial. Ann Intern Med 139:724-730.

11. Panda A.K, Misra S (2009) Prevalence and Clinical Profile of Gout. J Hill Res 22: 37-38.

12. Smith HS, Bracken D, Smith JM (2011) Gout: current insights and future perspectives. J Pain 12: 1113-1129.

13. http://ancientayurved.org/blog/view/id_4348/title_Rationality-of-Jalaukavcharan-Leech-Therapy-in/

14. Pandey KN, Chaturvedi GN. Charak Samhita. "Vidyotini" Comm.

15. Zhang SJ, Liu JP, He KQ (2010) Treatment of acute gouty arthritis by blood-letting cupping plus herbal medicine. J Tradit Chin Med 30: 18-20.

16. Panda AK, Misra S (2010) Health traditions of Sikkim Himalaya. J Ayurveda Integr Med 1: 183-189.

17. Wallace SL, Robinson H, Masi AT, Decker JL, McCarty DJ, et al. (1977) Preliminary criteria for the classification of the acute arthritis of primary gout. Arthritis Rheum 20: 895-900.

18. Trontelj P, Utevsky SY (2005) Celebrity with a neglected taxonomy: molecular systematics of the medicinal leech (genus Hirudo). Mol Phylogenet Evol 34: 616-624.

19. Singh AP (2010) Medicinal leech therapy (hirudotherapy): a brief overview. Complement Ther Clin Pract 16: 213-215.

20. Andereya S, Stanzel S, Maus U, Mueller-Rath R, Mumme T, et al. (2008) Assessment of leech therapy for knee osteoarthritis: a randomized study. Acta Orthop 79: 235-243.

21. Backer M, Ludtke R, Afra D, Cesur O, Langhorst J, et al. (2011) Effectiveness of Leech Therapy in Chronic Lateral Epicondylitis: A Randomized Controlled Trial. Clin J Pain. 27: 442-447.

22. Rigbi M, Levy H, Iraqi F, Teitelbaum M, Orevi M, et al. (1987) The saliva of the medicinal leech Hirudo medicinalis--I. Biochemical characterization of the high molecular weight fraction. Comp Biochem Physiol B 87: 567-573.

23. Orevi M, Rigbi M, Hy-Am E, Matzner Y, Eldor A (1992) A potent inhibitor of platelet activating factor from the saliva of the leech Hirudo medicinalis. Prostaglandins 43: 483-495.

24. Rubin BR, Burton R, Navarra S, Antigua J, Londoño J, et al. (2004) Efficacy and safety profile of treatment with etoricoxib 120 mg once daily compared with indomethacin 50 mg three times daily in acute gout: a randomized controlled trial. Arthritis Rheum 50: 598-606.

16

Acupuncturists in Primary Health Care: Knowing to Legitimate and to Expand

Leandra Andréia de Sousa[1,2]*, Gláucia Tamburu Braghetto[1], Jéssica Oliveira Pigari[1] and Maria José Bistafa Pereira[1]

[1]*Ribeirão Preto College of Nursing (EERP/USP), University of São Paulo, Ribeirão Preto, Brazil*
[2]*Avenida dos Bandeirantes, Campus Universitário, Monte Alegre, Ribeirão Preto, SP, Brazil*

Abstract

The present research takes a different approach to acupuncture. While most researches have studied aspects related to the treatments and effects of acupuncture use, which undoubtedly are of great importance, we are dedicated to studying aspects related to health policies 1. Therefore, we take Primary Health Care as a research field for acupuncture and other alternative and complementary medicines, which are denominated in Brazil, of Integrative and Complementary Practices.

Acupuncture is the fastest growing therapy in the world, including encouragement and recommendations from the World Health Organization for its inclusion in public health systems. In order for acupuncture to be offered in public health systems it is essential to have acupuncturists in sufficient quality and quantity, another aspect that is also discussed by WHO.

Given the relevance of these considerations, in this research, we seeked to map and identify the professionals specialized in acupuncture and who are interested in exercising the offer of this therapeutic practice in Primary Health Care. For this, we seeked to identify the number of acupuncturists; Describe socio-demographic profile of acupuncturists; Identify the different formations in acupuncture; to identify the interest and availability of acupuncturist professionals in acupuncture in primary health care services.

In order to collect data, we prepared a questionnaire and submitted it to a process for validating the appearance and semantics of the content, carried out by five judges with higher education in the health area, specialization in acupuncture and experience in Primary Health Care, which favored the accuracy of the instrument. Only after the validation by the judges the questionnaire was applied to the participants of the research in the online and printed format.

Keywords: Acupuncture; Legitimate; Socio-demographic

Introduction

The growing worldwide interest in inserting acupuncture in primary health care requires that national and international health authorities seek ways to ensure safety in their use. One of the aspects that the World Health Organization draws attention to is the importance of professional training for the practice of acupuncture, especially in countries where Western medicine 'is the sole basis of the national health system [1,2].

Although the offer of acupuncture and other alternative and complementary medicines, called integrative and complementary practices in Primary Health Care in Brazil, are greatly encouraged by the WHO [1-3], has been expanding and has been happening for decades in different countries, there are still some needs in the process of implementation in regard to the available human resources for the practice of acupuncture [1,2]. In Brazil, such needs are evidenced by several difficulties, especially the low percentage of acupuncturists who work in public health services and because there is no formal work contract for acupuncturists in these services. However, there is interest among professionals to specialize in acupuncture and most of them are interested in acting in Primary Health Care services as an acupuncturist [4].

In the Brazilian context, there are still neither institutions nor actors in sufficient number that are at the same time well established and linked to integrative and complementary practices such as acupuncture and other medical rationalities, converging to the ideals of the Unified Health System, of health promotion and of health care integrality, and being immediately *"partners to be recognized and valued as references"* [5] for integrative and complementary practices and other medical rationalities [4].

A recent study shows that, although there are health professionals with specialization in acupuncture in the municipal public health network, there is no survey on the quantity of them, on which services they work and if they have an interest in acupuncture in Primary Health Care Health. There is good acceptance and demand from the population for acupuncture; however, because of the scarce amount of acupuncturists, the waiting list of people for this care is continuously growing [5].

The hiring of more acupuncturists is not yet a priority in the agenda of decisions of the health manager. Thus, the specific position for this hiring in the institutional personnel framework has not yet been given, either due to administrative, financial difficulties or health care model. So, the supply is restricted and the population is without this access [5]. The incorporation of either unconventional practices or alternative and complementary medicines into national health systems, with new conceptions of the health-disease process, of the care and of the cure themselves depend on the conjuncture of central or local governments, social demand and political pressure in their favor [6]. All these issues have an impact on the expansion and strengthening of the acupuncture offer and, consequently, on the National Policy on Integrative and Complementary Practices (created in 2016) in the Unified Health System [7]. In this perspective, it is worth highlighting that the Integrative and Complementary Practices starts from the premise that acupuncture can be exercised in a multiprofessional

*Corresponding author: Leandra Andréia de Sousa, Avenida dos Bandeirantes, Campus Universitário, Monte Alegre, Ribeirão Preto, SP, Brazil
E-mail: leandra.sousa@usp.br, sousa.leandra2015@gmail.com

manner by the professional categories present in the Unified Health System, and in consonance with the level of attention [8]. This premise favors the broadening of the acupuncture practices. It is also important to mention that currently several professional councils recognize acupuncture as specialty [7], among them the physical therapy, nursing, occupational therapy, biomedicine, pharmacy, naturology, medicine and others. In addition, it is emphasized that the World Health Organization presents guidelines and recommendations for basic training according to the different professional categories [1]. In view of this diversity of training possibilities, and also considering that in the context of the study, the Municipal Health Department adopted only medical professionals for acupuncture care, we questioned: how many university-level professionals working in the Health Units of the Unified Health System, has specialization in acupuncture, considering the recommendations of WHO and the National Policy on Integrative and Complementary Practices?

Aims of the Survey

Based on these considerations, it is necessary to map and identify the professionals specialized in acupuncture and who have an interest in exercising the offer of this therapeutic practice in the Primary Health Care in the public health services network at the municipal level. Besides this, these were also the objectives of this investigation: To identify the amount of acupuncturists; to describe socio-demographic profile of acupuncturists; to identify training in acupuncture; and to identify the interest of acupuncturist professionals in acupuncture.

Materials and Methods

This is a descriptive study with a quantitative approach.

Place of Study

The study was carried out in the health units of the Primary Health Care Network at the municipal level, from June to July 2015. This health care network is organized into five health districts that are: the northern district, the eastern district, the central district, the southern district and the western district, consisting of one Emergency Care Unit, four Districtal Basic Health Units, 26 Basic Health Units and 14 Family Health Units, which serve about 604,682 people [9]. There are several types of employment relationships within the framework of health professionals in this network. For this study, considering this variety of professional relationships and also considering the different levels of health care assistance, for this research only the health units of the primary level of care were included, regarding that the professionals have a municipal employment relationship, hired by contest. Thus, the total of units that participated in this study, according to health districts was: 12 units of the northern district, 6 units of the eastern district, 5 units of the central district, 4 units of the southern district and 12 units of the western district, totaling 39 health units.

Participants

In order to select the participants of the research, the inclusion criteria were defined as: to be a professional with a municipal employment relationship (hired by the City Hall); to work in the Primary Health Care Network of the Municipal Health Department; to exercise a contracted function requiring a higher education level; to work in the units participating in this study, described in the previous item. Participants who did not meet the inclusion criteria were excluded from the study. For example, participants who were on vacation, leave or who were not present at the health unit during the period of data collection and those who refused to participate. Professionals working in more than one health unit answered the questionnaire only once. Thus, the study included 156 participants.

Data Collection

In order to collect the data, we used the questionnaire, both in online format and in printed format, composed of three parts. In the first part of this questionnaire were the identification data, university education, position that the subject currently exercised in the public service and its duration. In the second part of the questionnaire were the data referring to the specialization in Integrative and Complementary Practices, requesting that it was specified if the answer was yes and whether or not there was an interest in carrying out a specialization in some of the types of Integrative and Complementary Practices. For those who did not have a specialization in acupuncture, the questionnaire was closed. However, for those with a specialization in acupuncture, there was the third part of the questionnaire, containing questions, whose objective was to identify the acupuncture specialization, whether the practitioner was currently practicing acupuncture and about the interest in acting in the different services of Primary Health Care as an acupuncturist. The collection was carried out in July 2015.

Questionnaire Validation Process

This questionnaire was submitted to a validation process for the appearance and semantics of the content [10]. To this end, it counted with the participation of five judges with higher education in the area of health, specialization in acupuncture and experience of the professional practice in Primary Health Care, from different regions of the country. We first made phone calls to the judges to explain the research and invite them to participate in the questionnaire validation. Subsequently, we sent by e-mail the Informed Consent Form and the questionnaire for validation by the judges. For each question listed, we asked judges to assess the content for clarity, objectivity, organization, easy reading and understandable content. We accepted the suggestions of the questions regarding age and working time, providing the answers in intervals of years, as suggested by the judges, and in the question about specialization, we accepted the suggestion to write "Integrative and Complementary Practices" instead of keeping only the acronym "ICP". The validation process favored the accuracy of the instrument. Only after the validation by the judges was the questionnaire applied to the participants of the research.

Application of the Questionnaire

The questionnaire was sent in the online format, by email, to all health units in the municipality, making it accessible to all professionals participating in the survey. Online questionnaires have many advantages for those who fill them and for the researcher, such as speed, convenience and cost reduction. However, in spite of these advantages, there was a low adherence of the professionals, generating little participation in the questionnaire in the online format (less than 8%), even when the researchers contacted the unit managers explaining the importance, encouraging participation and resending the questionnaire. This was a difficulty for the researchers.

Faced with this obstacle, the researchers opted for a second alternative: to do the questionnaire in printed format and to go personally to the health units to apply it to professionals. The average time to answer the questionnaire ranged from three to 5 min. This experience showed that there is not yet an established habit for the participation in research questionnaires in the online format, and the presence of the researcher or research technicians applying the questionnaire made a significant difference for the participants' adherence to the research. During the visits at the health units, the managers reported the updated staff group of each unit, describing the quantity of them who were hired, the quantity of them who were on vacation or maternity leave. From this description, it was expected the participation of 266 professionals. However, considering the professionals who were on vacation and health/maternity leave, the total number of professionals was 186.

Of these 186 participants, 141 answered the printed questionnaires that were distributed in the health units, which corresponds to 75.8%. As participation is voluntary and not compulsory, among the 45 individuals who did not respond to the questionnaire, which corresponds to 24.2%, the justifications alleged for non-participation were lack of interest, lack of time and overwork.

Considering the number of questionnaires printed and online answered, respectively, 141 and 15, the total number of participants that took part in this study was 156. That is, 90.4% answered the printed questionnaire and 9.6% answered the online questionnaire.

It is worth emphasizing that the process of validation of the questionnaire by the judges was fundamental to make it clearer and, consequently, faster to be answered by the interviewees. This was undoubtedly a positive aspect in this research development. Nevertheless, the online questionnaire has not yet proved to be a productive data collection instrument. We believe there is a need to change people's habits to increase acceptance and adherence to respond online questionnaires, by the easiness itself. There is also time gain mainly related to the application of the online questionnaire in relation to the printed questionnaire.

After the collection, a descriptive statistical analysis of the data was performed.

Ethical Procedures

The study was approved by the Ethics Committee of the University of São Paulo at Ribeirão Preto College of Nursing under no. 897.644/2014, according to the ethical standards required by National Health Council Resolution n. 466/2012. Since the research involved human beings, the study took place after every participant signed the Informed Consent Term.

Discussion

Acupuncturists sociodemographic profile

Of the 156 participants of this study, 106 are female, corresponding to 67.9% and 50 males, which is equivalent to 32.1% of the total participants. It is noted that the participation of females is twice as large as the participation of males.

Regarding the participants' age range, 36 (23.1%) reported being between 50 and 54 years old; 33 (21.1%) reported being between 55 and 60 years old; 20 (12.8%), between 45 and 49; 18 (11.5%), between 35 and 39 years old; 15 (9.6%), between 30 and 34 years old; 13(8.3%), between 40 and 44 years old; 11 (7.1%) reported being over 60 years old and 10 (6.4%) reported being between the ages of 25 and 29. It can be concluded that the majority of the participants in the present study are between 50 and 54 years old. Regarding university education, 66 (42.3%) are physicians, 42 (26.9%) are nurses, 33 (21.1%) are dentists, 9 (5.8%) are pharmacists, 2 (1.2%) speech therapists, 2 (1.2%) psychologists and 2 participants (1.2%) did not identify their university education. It is identified that among the total of interviewees, medical and nursing studies predominated, respectively.

Acupuncture training

Regarding integrative and complementary practices, we consider as specializations acupuncture, homeopathy, herbal medicine/phytotherapy, thermalism/crenotherapy and anthroposophic medicine, both contemplated by the National Policy of Integrative and Complementary Practices in the Unified Health System. When questioned if they had a specialization in Integrative and Complementary Practices, 139 participants, which corresponds to 89.1%, reported that they did not have any specialization in Integrative and Complementary Practices while 17, which is equivalent to 10.9%, refers having a specialization in one or more of the Integrative and Complementary Practices. This analysis led us to raise some questions: Does the high number of professionals without specialization in Integrative and Complementary Practices mean that there is "no interest" in these practices or does it mean lack of knowledge about Integrative and Complementary Practices?

Of the 17 participants with some specialization in Integrative and Complementary Practices, eight (47%) have specialization in homeopathy, five (29.4%) have specialization in acupuncture, two (11.7%) have specialization in acupuncture and homeopathy and 1 (5.8%) in herbal medicine/phytotherapy. According to the questionnaire, one participant (5.8%) was attending a specialization in phytotherapy.

Regarding the interest or not of specializing in Integrative and Complementary Practices, 55.2% (79 subjects) reported not having interest in any specialization in Integrative and Complementary Practices. In contrast, 44.8% (64 participants) referred having interest in doing some specialization in Integrative and Complementary Practices. It is observed that almost half of the subjects are interested in performing some specialization in Integrative and Complementary Practices, and from these:

- 39% are interested in specializing in acupuncture;

- 15.6% are interested in specializing in herbal medicine/phytotherapy;

- 11% are interested in specializing in acupuncture and herbal medicine/phytotherapy;

- 4.7% are interested in specializing in acupuncture and homeopathy;

- 4.7% are interested in specializing in homeopathy and herbal medicine/phytotherapy;

- 3.1% are interested in specializing in homeopathy;

- 3.1% are interested in specializing in anthroposophic medicine;

- 3.1% are interested in specializing in anthroposophic medicine and herbal medicine/phytotherapy;

- 4.5% are interested in specializing in three or more Integrative and Complementary Practices;

- 1.5% are interested in specializing in some Integrative and Complementary Practices, however, without preferences, and 9.4% scored no response.

The considerable percentage of participants (39%) interested in specializing in Integrative and Complementary Practices/acupuncture is noteworthy.

Interest and availability of acupuncturists in practicing acupuncture

Of the six interviewees who have a specialization in acupuncture, five are interested in working as an acupuncturist in the health units of primary health care, corresponding to 83.3%; and one (16.7%) has no interest. Of the 83.3% of acupuncturists interested in working as acupuncturists in health units of primary health care, 60% reported availability in the morning and 40% did not mention the availability. It is worth mentioning an interesting data according to the questionnaire, which shows that a respondent with acupuncture specialization acts as an acupuncturist in the health unit but is not formally hired as an acupuncturist.

The study shows the low percentage of acupuncturists working in public health services and reveals that there is no formal working contract as acupuncturists in these services. However, there is interest among professionals in doing acupuncture specialization and most of them are interested in acting in Primary Health Care services as an acupuncturist.

Conclusion and Recommendations

Acupuncture is the fastest growing therapy in the world, including encouragement and recommendations from the World Health Organization for its inclusion in public health systems. In order for acupuncture to be offered in public health systems, it is essential to have acupuncturists in sufficient quality and quantity, another aspect that is also discussed by WHO. Given the relevance of these considerations, in this research, we sought to map and identify the professionals specialized in acupuncture and who are interested in providing the offer of this therapeutic practice in Primary Health Care. For this, we sought to identify the number of acupuncturists; to describe socio-demographic profile of acupuncturists; to identify the different formations in acupuncture; to identify the interest and availability of acupuncturist professionals in acupuncture in primary health care services. This survey contributed to increase the possibility of re-shaping the staff and increasing acupuncturists in primary health care, meeting the pent-up demand and thus broadening and strengthening the offer of acupuncture. This strategy can also contribute to the health services of primary health care in different countries to articulate and trigger viable strategies for the implantation and implementation of acupuncture and other integrative and complementary practices in their different contexts and realities. It is recommended that the Primary Health Care services review the structure of their work contracts, formally inserting acupuncturists and other professionals with training in other integrative and complementary practices, thus materializing the legitimacy of these health professionals. It is also recommended that acupuncturists, who are interested in acting as acupuncturists in the Primary Health Care services, should express this interest and, together with the managers, seek strategies to formally institute this specialty within the framework of professionals in the Primary Health Care services, legitimating it. Acupuncture and other integrative and complementary practices can contribute to change the logic of the medical-care model focused on complaint and prompt care, since acupuncture not only favors treatment and recovery but also emphasizes the promotion of health and prevention of diseases, potentializing the materialization of the assistance integrality, of health as rightly and strengthening the health systems through primary health care. We defend health as a right, and above all, we argue that people have the right to choose the therapy they want to take care of their health and their illness. Therefore, we understand that acupuncture

and other Integrative and Complementary Practices should be offered in the different health services of Primary Health Care. And, for this therapeutic option to be assured, it is fundamental that Primary Health Care services have such professionals. We believe that this research may contribute to other research aimed at implanting or expanding acupuncture and other integrative and complementary practices in the different health systems of Primary Health Care, pointing out specific human needs. Therefore, identifying practitioners of integrative and complementary practices in Primary Health Care, knowing their training and interest, is essential, since it is from this identification that it will be possible to make a concrete plan to implant or to expand the offer of acupuncture and other therapeutic approaches within the health systems of Primary Health Care.

Acknowledgments

The authors would like to acknowledge José Renato Gatto Júnior, doctorate student at the University of São Paulo, Postgraduation Program of Psychiatric Nursing, for the translation of this article.

References

1. http://www.who.int/medicines/publications/traditional/trm_strategy14_23/en/

2. http://apps.who.int/medicinedocs/pdf/s4932s/s4932s.pdf

3. OMS (1978) Primary health care. Report of the International Conference on Primary Health Care Alma-Ata. Genebra: Orgnización Mundial de la Salud.

4. Tesser CD (2009) Complementary practices, medical rationalities and health promotion: few contributions explored. Cadernos de Saúde Pública, Rio de Janeiro 25: 1732-1742.

5. Sousa LA (2014) Acupuncture in SUS-reality and perspectives. Ribeirão Preto: EERP-USP.

6. Galhardi WMP, Barros NF, Leite-Mor ACMB (2013) The knowledge of municipal health managers on the National Policy on Integrative and Complementary Practice and its influence on the offer of homeopathy in the local Unified Health System. Ciênc Saúde Coletiva 18: 213-220.

7. Ministério da Saúde, Gabinete do Ministro (2006) Ordinance No. 971 National Policy on Integrative and Complementary Practices in the Unified Health System-SUS Approves the National Policy on Integrative and Complementary Practices (PNPIC) in the Unified Health System. Official Journal of the Union, Brasília, DF, Seção I pp: 20-25.

8. Ministry of Health (2008) Secretariat of Health Care. Department of Basic Attention. National Policy on Integrative and Complementary Practices in SUS: PNPIC: access expansion. Brasília, DF (Series B. Basic Texts of Health).

9. https://www.ribeiraopreto.sp.gov.br/ssaude/pdf/pms-rp-2014-2017.pdf

10. Reis RA (2008) Specific module for health related quality of life assessment for children and adolescents living with hearing loss-ViDA. Tese EERP-USP 153: 84-94.

17

Effect of Serially Diluted Drug *Digitalis purpurea* on Modulation of Anesthetized Consciousness of Indian *Bufomelanostictus*

Anup Sharma[1]* and Bulbul Purkait[2]

[1]*Indian Institute of Technology, Kharagpur, India*
[2]*Department of Biochemistry, Midnapur Medical College and Hospital, Midnapore, India*

Abstract

Concept prevails amongst believers that serially diluted drugs do not produce any side effect. The modus operandi of the serially diluted drugs is through neural network. The practitioners of different systems of medicine with paradigmatic differences use the same drug substance in different dilution to treat patients with contrary clinical conditions, *Digitalis purpurea* is one such drug. The present work describes the effect of ultra-diluted drug *Digitalis purpurea* and Digoxin on modulation of Diethyl ether induced anesthesia in Indian *Bufomelanostictus*. Diethyl ether and rectified spirit (also used as diluent for ultra-dilution) are used as controls in this experimental work. In this preliminary study, it is found that the reflex and anesthetic action of *Digitalis purpurea* 200 is similar to rectified spirit probably because of the simple dilution of the active ingredient. *Digitalis purpurea* 30 was found to be more effective than rectified spirit. *Digitalis purpurea* 30 produced the longest period of anesthesia while Digoxin reduced duration of anesthesia. Both *Digitalis purpurea* 6 and Rectified spirit were effective for almost same duration. The ultra-diluted drug samples and digoxin were further analyzed by Cyclic Voltammetry and Fluorescence spectroscopy which establishes the cause and effect relationship.

Keywords: Serial dilution; Anesthesia; Unconsciousness; Reflex; Fluorescence; Cyclic voltammetry

Abbreviations: CV: Cyclic Voltammetry; DP: *Digitalis purpurea*; GC: Glassy Carbon; IBM: Indian *Bufomelanostictus;* Rec-Spirit: Rectified Spirit

Introduction

Digitalis purpurea (DP) had been used since 1785 by Erasmus Darwin and William Withering for dropsy, and pulmonary consumption [1]. Hahnemann used it around 1803. Practitioners of prevalent system of medicines used it for various purposes as like beautification, poison arrow (BC 1500), arrhythmia and many other diseases. DP has been used, in varying concentration / dilution by practitioners of different systems of medicine with paradigmatic differences to treat the patients for clinical conditions expressed in contrary to each other. Digoxin (Figure 1) the purified derivative of DP is used in modern medicine to treat patients with increased cardiac rate. On the contrary in homeopathic system DP is used in ultra-dilution to treat patients with decreased cardiac rate [2]. Such uses of medicines as *Digitalis* have given birth to inter/intra systems conflict affecting pharmacological standard and safety. These were the motivations to carry out a systematic study of the effect of serially diluted DP and Digoxin which is aderivative of DP used in allopathic system of medicine [3].

Out of about thirty known organic compounds that DP contains predominantly 5-7 are medicinally active components such as digoxin, digitoxigenin, digoxigenin and saponins. Observations related to response obtained from serially diluted drugs [4-7] motivated us to find out the competence of Ultra-diluted drug DP to alter neurological signals in susceptible animal IBM. Humans and mammals were known to be susceptible to Digitalis. However, their effects on other species such as amphibians (specifically IBM) have not been reported. Digitalis-like poisoning has been reported with the skin-extract of IBM [8]. DP, even in serial dilutions, is known to have produced unconsciousness, fainting and confusion in humans [2].

Anything more dilute than micro volume (10^{-6}) i.e. as a concentration of one micro-liter or micro-gram of solute in one liter of solvent is considered as 'ultra-diluted'. The saturated extractof DP in rectified spirit -water mixture and its serial dilutions prepared as per India Homeopathic Pharmacopoeia, which are available commercially, were used in the experiment.

Diethyl ether was used as General anesthetic agent in order to induce unconsciousness in IBM. Diethyl ether, which has high water and lipid solubility, provides only mild euphoria but excellent anesthesia. It may produce unconsciousness, analgesia, amnesia, immobility and hemodynamicresponses (in response to noxious stimulation). Known toxicological effect [9] of Diethyl ether at various concentrations (between 71,600 ppm and 192,500 ppm ethyl ether by volume) on animals like monkeys, rabbits, mice,ratshave been described by The National Institute for Occupational Safety and Health (NIOSH), Centers for Disease Control and Prevention.

The molecular mechanisms related to the brain structure and circuitry involved in the anesthetic loss of consciousness is unknown in spite of about more than a century long research by Meyer (1899) and Overton (1901). Diethyl ether inhibits alcohol dehydrogenase, and thus slows down alcohol metabolism. Diethyl ether can act as a hydrogen bond acceptor but not a donor [10].

Anesthetic Diethyl ether and rectified spirit used as diluent for preparation of ultra-diluted DP were used as controls.

IBM was chosen for the experiment, on the basis of preliminary studies conducted in our laboratory, suggesting that IBM are susceptible to DP, rectified spirit, Inj. Digoxin, and ether.

Fluorescence spectroscopy and cyclic voltammetry were carried out on the experimental drug samples to get the possible cause and effect relationship.

***Corresponding author:** Anupsharma, Indian Institute of Technology, Kharagpur -721302, India, E-mail: sharma_anup@yahoo.com

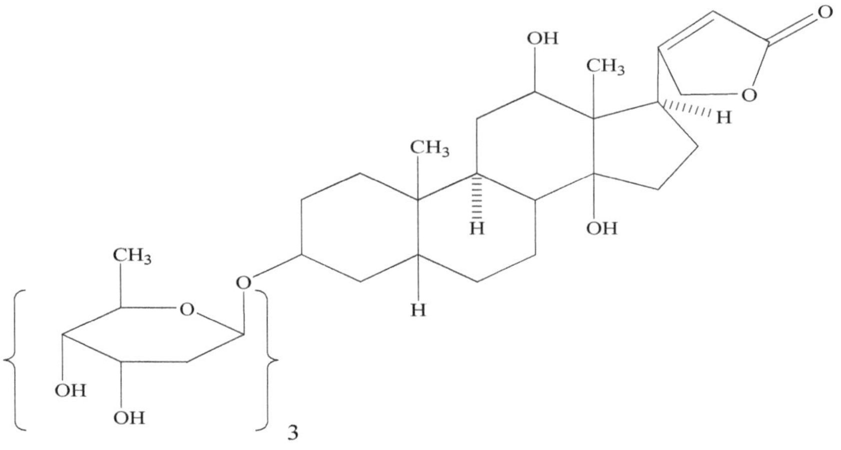

Figure 1: Structure of Digitalis.

Methodology

The institutional ethical committee for research on humans and animals in Indian Institute of Technology, Kharagpur, India (IEC), granted necessary clearance to carry out the research and along with AYUSH (Government of India) provided the infrastructure for the purpose. A veterinary surgeon was also engaged to give guidance on all the aspects of animal facility, care, and animal research. Dedicated electrical earthing was installed in the animal house and in the entire laboratory.

Diethyl Ether ($C_4H_{10}O$, M=74.12 g/mol; 1l=0.71 kg) manufactured by Merck was used for inducing inhalation anesthesia. Rectified Spirit (aqueous ethanol 91.4%) was acquired from Bengal Chemicals and Pharmaceuticals, India. The solvent/diluent was manufactured without any other inclusions such as acetone. In all experimental procedures, the solvent used (even for rinsing of glassware etc.) was ethanol. A thorough cleansing and rinsing of glassware, trays, cuvette, hands etc., were done with ethanol only, before and immediately after each reading. Homeopathic drugs *Digitalis purpurea* Q or θ (Batch no. 6725 of September 2005), *Digitalis purpurea* 6, *Digitalis purpurea* 30, and *Digitalis purpurea* 200, (all Batch of June 2005) and the solvent were procured from the authorized manufacturer M/s Hahnemann Publishing Company, Kolkata, India.

Inj. Digoxin, 25 mg/ml, (Batch of June 2005) manufactured by Samarth Pharma was used. Glass double distilled water was used in the experiment.

Animals, procured from authorized vendors, were screened for general health, injury marks, and heart conditions using highly sensitive cardio phonic stethoscope. Acclimatization of IBM was carried out for about 10 days in an animal house. Sufficient water and recommended feed, not known to have medicinal influence, was provided. They were made familiar to human presence and contact, cotton and electrodes. Experimental animals- IBM were washed with water to reduce skin impedance and remove interfering substance like hellebrigenin, secretions, excretions, dust etc. Inhalation anesthesia was given to the animal till complete flaccidity of muscle of hind limbs and loss of reflexes to mechanical stimuli were achieved. Specially designed Ag/AgCl electrodes to suit the limbs of the animals were attached to recognize digital signals on slightest muscular movement of the animal. Total duration of anesthesia / absence of reflex were noticed. To avoid anything like bias all the experiments were randomly carried out by three experts / trained personnel.

Two batches of animals were taken as control. One batch (n= 25) was treated with diethyl ether only. Second batch of control (n=27) was treated with diethyl ether followed by rectified spirit, which was used as diluent in the experimental homeopathic drugs. Deep ether anesthesia was induced in 10 IBMs. Rest of the anesthetized animals were individually treated randomly with intraperitoneal injection, using Insulin syringes, with either 0.5 ml of *Digitalis purpurea* θ (n=21) or *Digitalis purpurea* 6 (n=33) or *Digitalis purpurea* 30 (n=21) or *Digitalis purpurea200* (n=25) or Digoxin (n=14). Since the effect of Digoxinis well documented, restricted numbers of animals were used for observations after administration of Digoxin. Out of these, two animals died after giving rectified spirit, one animal died after *Digitalis purpurea* θ, one animal died after *Digitalis purpurea* 30, four animals died after giving deep anesthesia, two animals died after giving Digoxin. Since the death rate of animals was very high with deep anesthesia, experiment with deep ether anesthesia was discontinued. Average duration of anesthesia produced by the drugs in each IBM was recorded (Figure 2).

Statistical basis for the sample size was determined by using various software, which include, SPSS 12, Excel, SAS, and SQL. Opinion of masters of statistics, bio-statistics, veterinarians, epidemiologist, mathematicians, planners, and designers, researchers was sought in this context. ANOVA was done to compare the duration of anesthesia produced by each drug. Since there were problems of retrieval of some data, the sample size also got truncated. The outliers were removed and some data that the program could not correctly interpret were also removed as if they never existed.

Cyclic voltammetry

Electrochemical measurements were performed using two-compartment three-electrode cell with a polycrystalline Au working electrode (2 mm diameter, BAS, USA), a Pt wire auxiliary electrode and Ag/AgCl (3 M NaCl) reference electrode. Cyclic voltammograms were recorded using a computer controlled CHI643B electrochemical analyzer attached with a Faraday cage/picoampere booster (CH Instruments, Austin, TX). The geometrical surface area of 0.031 cm² was cleaned electrochemically by cycling the potential between - 0.2 and 1.5 V in 0.25 M H_2SO_4 at the scan rate of 10 V/s for~10 min until the characteristic cyclic voltammogram for a clean Au electrode was obtained for use as working electrode. The GC electrode was used directly after sonication.

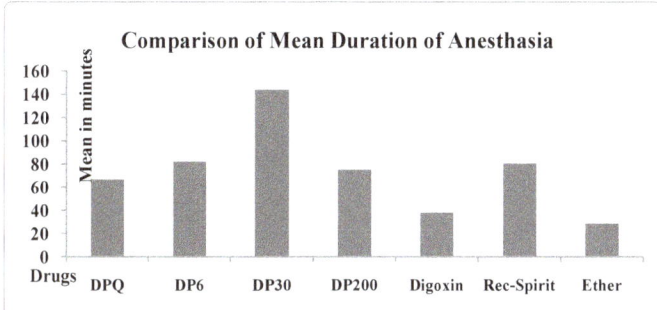

Figure 2: Comparison of Average duration of anesthesia produced by the drugs on IBM.

The voltammograms using *Digitalis purpurea* θ, 6, 12, 30, and 200 dilutions and Digoxin were obtained using bare Au electrodes and GC electrodes at pH 11, and scan rate of 100mV/s (Figures 3-5). Although voltammetric measurements of saturated extracts of the drug DP θ were carried out, for constraints attempt to detect the upper limit could not be carried out.

Fluorescence spectroscopy

The absorption and fluorescence spectra were measured using a Shimadzu (model no: UV-1601) spectrophotometer and a Spex-Fluorolog-3 (model no.FL3-11) spectrofluorimeter. The spectra with possible interpretation and analysis obtained for different dilutions of *Digitalis purpurea* θ, 6, 30, and 200 are given herein below along with the obtained relevant emission spectra shown in (Figure 6). Fluorescence spectroscopy was carried out to detect the presence of *Digitalis purpurea* and Digoxin-like compounds in serial ultra-dilutions for comparison of the components of *Digitalis purpurea*, which is having intrinsic fluorescence. The fluorescence is likely to be due to α, β-unsaturated lactone present in the compound. The compound is known to be hydrophobic in nature, but the sugar moiety attached to the compound changes its solubility. Fluorimetric method is unsuitable due to inner filter effect in the solutions at saturated concentrations.

Result and Discussion

Time taken by the animals to get anesthetized was variable.Time taken to inject the drug in an animal immediately after anesthesia was about less than half a minute. Graphical representation of result is given in (Figure 2). Comparisons of mean duration of anesthesia, in minutes, are shown in (Table 1). Response of Digoxin is in accordance with its known ability to shorten duration of anesthesia. Rectified spirit and Diethyl ether are proven anesthetics. There may be a combined effect of the DP and the alcohol that increases the anesthetic effect. With Digoxin alone the duration of anesthesia reduces. It is also observed that DP θ, which contains concentrated proportion of medicinally active ingredients, also reduces the duration of anesthesia (Figure 2).

Ether as a single chemical substance can achieve all the actions considered important for general anesthesia. By themselves, there are many other ways of correlating anesthetic effects; limitation of the work does not permit elaboration of the same.

Any relationship to the processes involving the CNS, which lead to unconsciousness, remains unknown. One of the possible explanations given on the matter is by the generalized Lipid hypothesis. General anesthetics do not totally inhibit neuronal functions while abolishing consciousness. It has also been suggested that the site of anesthetic inhibition of motor response may be in the spinal cord [11]. The consciousness aspect related to subtypes of receptor, voltage-gated ion

channels, and the intercellular connection of central nervous system is still unknown. Manfred E Wolf reported "General anesthetic-induced inhibition of voltage-gated calcium channel is not only important in the pre-synaptic actions of anesthetics, but also provides a possible explanation for general anesthetic-induced myocardial depression" [12]. The findings related to changes in heart conduction produced by Digoxin, and DP in various concentrations has been published [6].

Pair wise comparison of drug effectiveness, in producing period of anesthesia with respect to rectified spirit and Diethyl ether is given in (Tables 2 and 3). *Digitalis purpurea* 30 has produced the longest period of anesthesia and inhibition of reflex actions in IBM, while Digoxinhas reduced duration of anesthesia, and shortened duration of inhibition of reflex action. Both *Digitalis purpurea* 6 and Rectified spirit produced the same effectiveness in producing duration of anesthesia. Rectified spirit is more effective than DP θ. *Digitalis purpurea* 200 is similar to Rectified spirit in duration of anesthetic action and inhibition of action reflex.

The same network of sympathetic and parasympathetic nerves that produces effect on heart also seemingly modulates unconsciousness and suppression of reflex action. These ultra-diluted drugs increase the duration of unconsciousness, and suppress reflex action, but the neural correlates of these are unknown [6]. The consciousness aspect is still unknown with regard to subtypes of receptor, and voltage gated ion channels, and the intercellular connection of central nervous system. However, the most important question regarding the modus operandi of the ultra-diluted drugs remains unresolved. This work may be a small step forward to open more opportunities for further research.

Cyclic voltammetry

(Figure 3) shows voltammetric (gold electrode) pattern of Digoxin and DP 200 are similar for which oxidation potential is at 0.32 V to 0.35 V. Though (a) and (b) have similar Voltammetric pattern but current intensity is higher in Digoxin (a) which does not contain ethanol at all. But in DP 200, Digoxin moiety is one the active ingredients but lower current intensity may be due to the dilution effect. (b) Is the Voltammetric response for the oxidation of ethanol and this peak pattern is similar to the literature data for ethanol oxidation by gold electrode. Basically DP 200 is nothing but the serial dilution of the plant extract in ethanol. For the clarification of the presence of digoxin moiety in plant extract, we have measured the Cyclic Voltammetry of DP 200 and only ethanol where concentration of ethanol is same

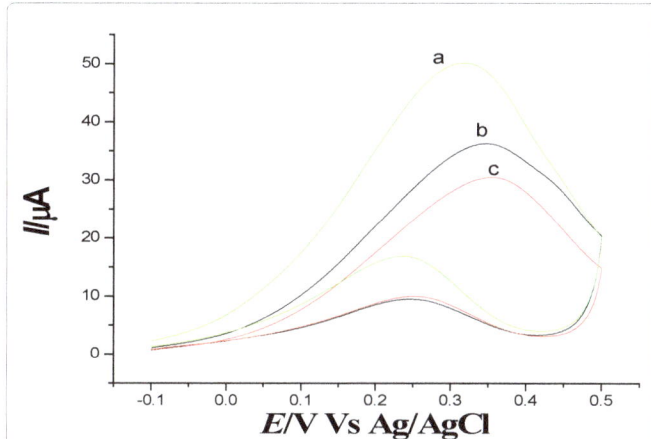

Figure 3: Voltammogram obtained (Au Electrode) for (a) Digoxin, (b) Digitalis purpurea 200, and (c) Ethanol sample interval (V) 0.001, Quite Time (s) 2, Sensitivity (A/V) 5e-6, scan rate (V/S) = 0.1.

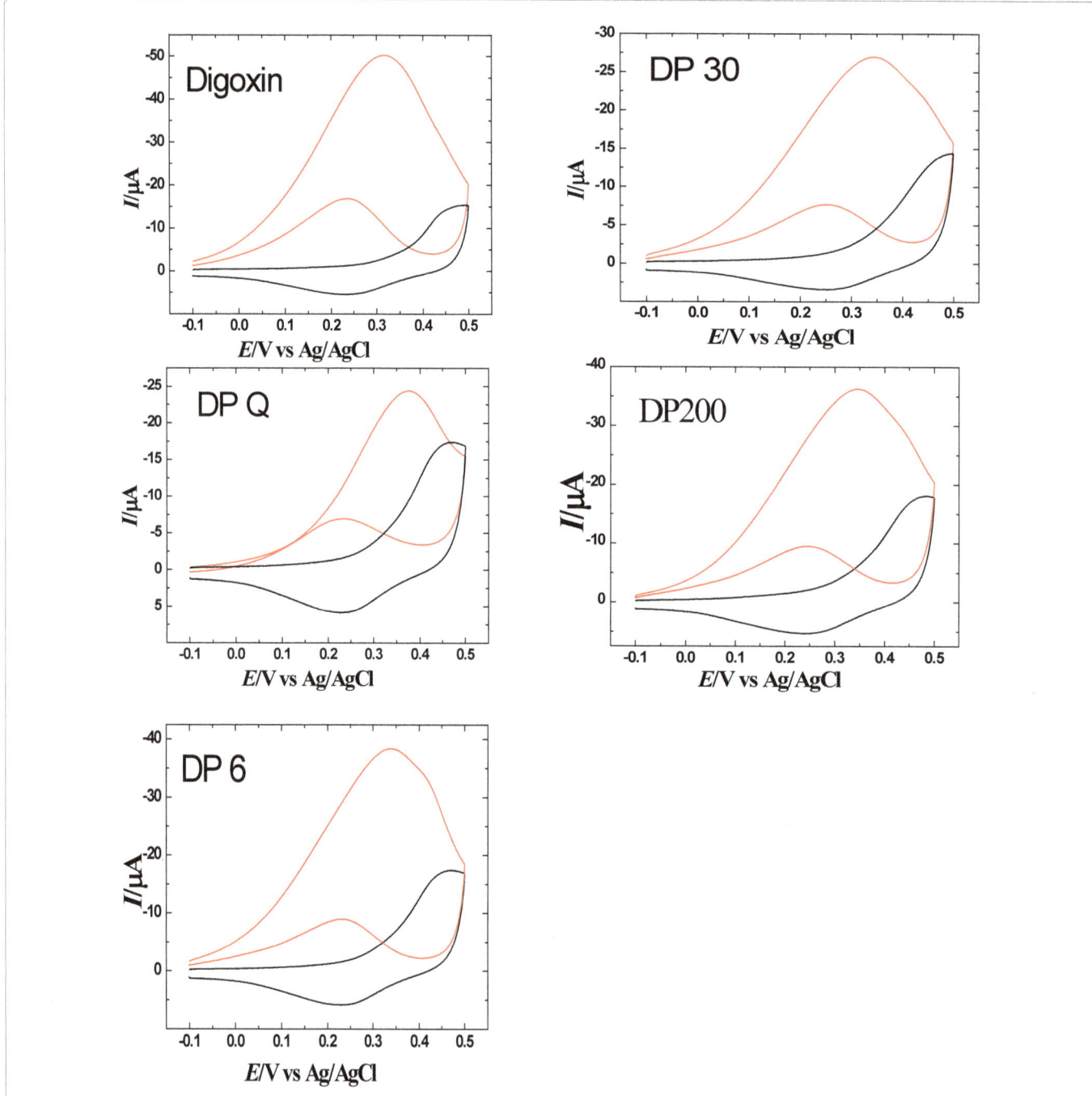

Figure 4: Cyclic voltammograms obtained for Digoxin, DP Q, DP 6, DP 30, DP 200, at Au electrode at pH – 11, and the corresponding black voltammograms are for bare Au electrode at same pH. Scan rate 100mV/s.

(91.4%). The observed higher current in DP 200 compared to the ethanol indicates digoxin moiety is expected to be present in the plant extract.

The voltammograms using *Digitalis purpurea* θ, 6, 12, 30, and 200 dilutions and Digoxin were obtained using bare Au Electrodes and GC at pH 11, and scan rate of 100mV/s (Figure 4 and 5) show characteristic difference. Corresponding black voltammograms are for bare Au / GC electrodes. For constraints attempt to detect the upper limit could not be carried out, although voltammetric measurements using saturated extracts of the drug were carried out.

These voltammograms clearly indicate the presence of redox pair showing distinct peak potentials, with gold (Au) electrode ~0.25 and 0.35 volt, while bare Au electrode showed presence of redox pair at ~0.35 and 0.45 volt. The same redox pair is seen with the pure medicinally active derivative Digoxin, which does not contain ethanol at all. Perfect reversible cyclic-voltammograms are obtained with the Au electrode. However, for glassy carbon (GC) and bare GC electrodes, reversible cyclic plots are not observed. Interestingly, for both Au and bare Au cases we get the same potential separation for the cathodic and anodic peaks. The CV indicates presence of the peak at the same level as that of purest *Digitalis purpurea* medicinal derivative Digoxin

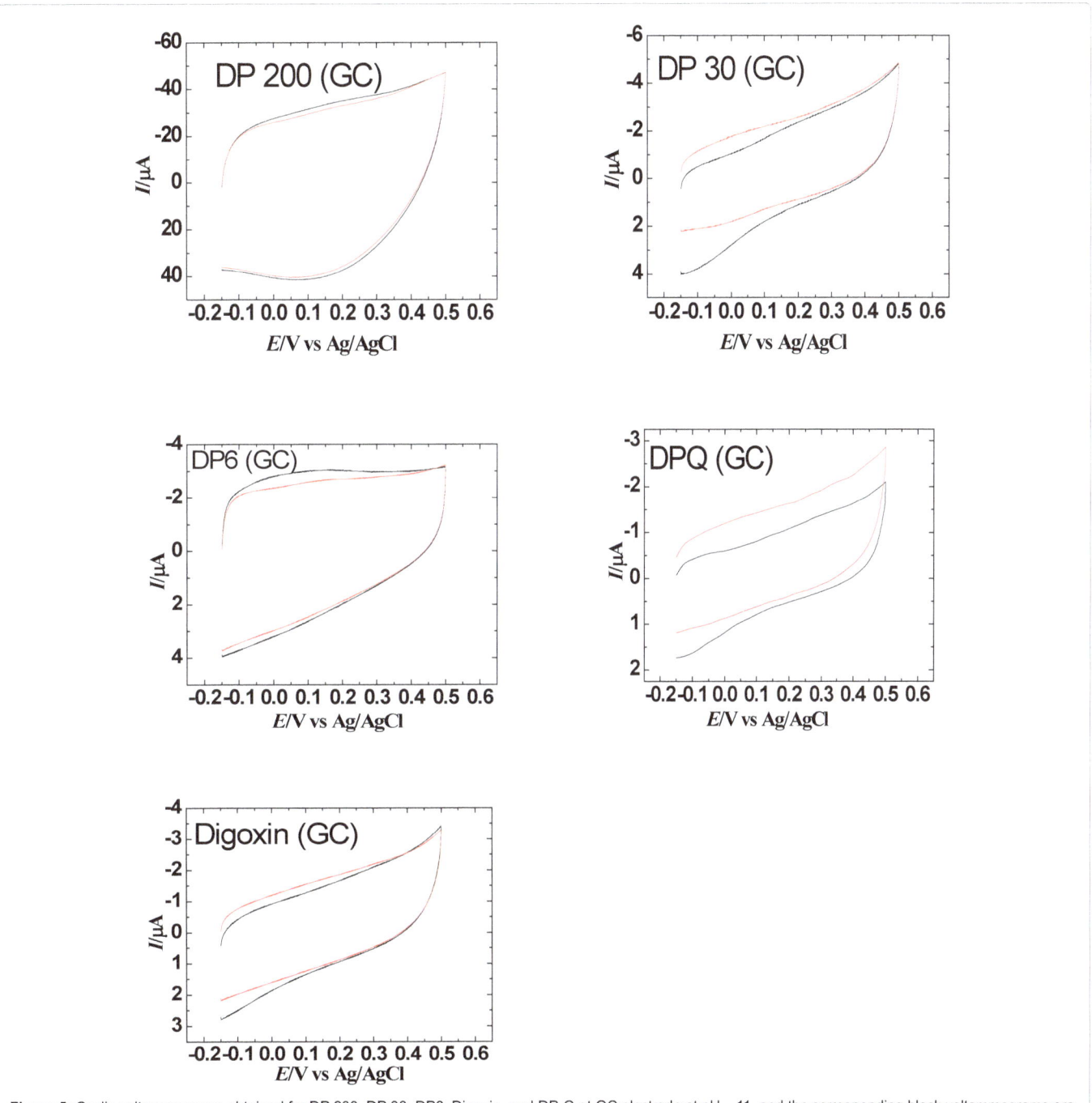

Figure 5: Cyclic voltammograms obtained for DP 200, DP 30, DP6, Digoxin, and DP-Q at GC electrode at pH – 11, and the corresponding black voltammograms are for bare GC electrode at same pH. Scan rate 100mV/s.

and is ascertainable in serial ultra-dilutions. This indicates presence of Digoxin-like substance in the ultra-diluted samples of the drug. As the structure in (Figure 1) indicates the five-member moiety containing α,β-unsaturated lactone is responsible for accepting one electron during reduction in the CV.

Emission spectra

The spectra with possible interpretation and analysis obtained for different dilutions of *Digitalis purpurea* θ, 6, 30, and 200 are given herein below along with the obtained relevant emission spectra shown in (Figure 6). Fluorescence spectroscopy was carried out to detect the presence of *Digitalis purpurea* and Digoxin-like compounds in serial ultra-dilutions for comparison of the components of *Digitalis purpurea*, which is having intrinsic fluorescence. It has been observed that U-V absorption maxima for the same substance are at 255 nm. It is in corroboration to the finding of the research group [5,13].

The fluorescence spectrum of the compound was taken at different dilution in aqueous ethanol. Fluorimetric method is unsuitable due to inner filter effect in the solutions at saturated concentrations. In all the emission studies, the samples were excited at 255 nm. The emission spectra of different dilutions are shown as C, D, E, and purest medicinally active ingredient Digoxin is shown as B in (Figure 6).

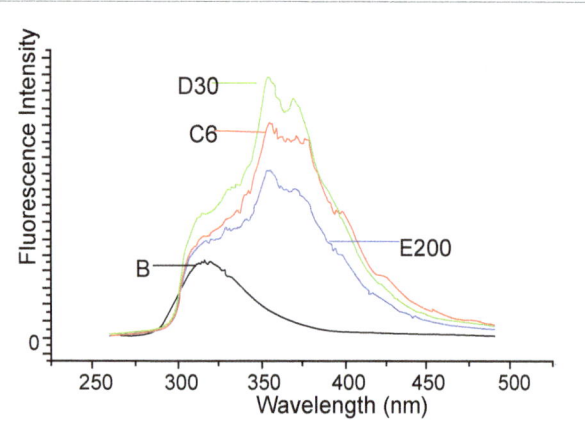

Figure 6: Emission spectra obtained by Analytical Fluorescence spectroscopy of *Digitalis purpurea* derivative *Digoxin* (B) showing emission maxima at 318 nm showing a relative intensity of 4.5x10⁶. C6 = *Digitalis purpurea* 6 having emission maxima 357 nm and 374 nm showing a relative intensity of 13x10⁶ and 12x10⁶. D30 = *Digitalis purpurea*30 emission maxima 357 nm and 374 nm showing a relative intensity 16x10⁶ and 14.5x10⁶. E200 = *Digitalis purpurea* 200, emission maxima 357 nm and 374 nm showing a relative intensity ~10x10⁶ and 9 x10⁶.

Drug	No. of Sample (n)	Sample Mean ($\bar{Y}$)	Sample S.D. (S or σ) ±	Student - t Distribution 95% Confidence interval for μ is
DP 200	25	69	28	69 ± 11.56
DP 30	20	138	69	138 ± 32.29
DP 6	33	76	29	76 ± 9.89
DP θ	20	53	28	53 ± 13.10
Digoxin	12	33	17	33 ± 10.80
Rectified spirit	25	74	51	74 ± 21.05
Ether	25	29	12	29 ± 4.95

Table 1: Probability distribution of period of anesthesia of various samples.

These Fluorescence spectra revealed that Digoxincomponent shows a structure less fluorescence with emission maxima at 318 nm with a relative intensity of $4.5×10^6$. The serial sequential dilution of the natural product at 6c, 30c and 200c levels of dilution show emission maxima at 318 nm rather than the structured emission as observed with purest digitalis. The emission spectra of *Digitalis purpurea* 6 is structure less emission found to be modified with a semi-structured emission with maxima at 357 nm and 374 nm and further a shoulder at about 318 nm remained which could be due to the original Digoxin. The appearance of additional bands at 357 and 374 nm may be ascribed to loss of self-quenching or dissociation of component substance due to serial dilution and these bands showed an increase in intensity with subsequent dilutions up to a certain level.

Conclusion

The reflex and anesthetic action of *Digitalis purpurea* 200 is similar to Rectified spirit probably because of the simple dilution of the active ingredient. *Digitalis purpurea* 30 was found to be more effective than Rectified spirit. *Digitalis purpurea* 30 produced the longest period of anesthesia while Digoxin reduced duration of anesthesia. Both *Digitalis purpurea* 6 and Rectified spirit are effective for almost same duration. It seems to be the probable effect of segregation, purification, and isolation by serial dilution of the drug *Digitalis purpurea*. To conclude it may be said that probably ethanol soluble ultra-diluted drugs may modulate anesthesia, and it requires further experimentation.

The CV and Analytical Fluorimetry indicate presence of the peak

at the same level as that of the purest *Digitalis purpurea* medicinal derivative Digoxin and are ascertainable in serial ultra-dilutions. This indicates presence of Digoxin-like substance in the ultra-diluted samples of the drug. CV and Analytical Fluorimetry also reveal that the process of serial ultra-dilution of natural organic-drugs involves phenomenon like partial segregations and purification

Cyclic Voltammetry (CV) and Analytical Fluirimetry (optical spectroscopy) both can be used to identify *Digitalis purpurea* and its derivatives, even in ultra-diluted solutions.

Limitations of the study

It is laboratory based Randomized Control Trial. This study has several limitations. There are some other components, which are naturally present in *Digitalis purpurea* and show different activities. Inclusion could not be made of the presence of other predictors of anesthesia and variability analysis. More than one statistical method of interpretation that represents this work has been included. Other than anesthesia studies of associated parameters are also included. Clinical conditions are too many, only a few examples could be cited in the text. For confines of the article non-parametrical statistical analysis was not conducted. Medicinally active ingredients of ultra-diluted drugs are difficult to detect analytically in laboratory. Ultra-diluted drug is not detectable in biological specimen, bringing limits to the design of the research. Commercially available medicines were only tried. Inference could be drawn only about the quality of the commercially manufactured drug. Studies conducted on albino rats, rabbits to monitor the effect of ultra-diluted drugs in producing anesthesia, is not included in this paper as it is noticed that anesthetic effect, Heart rate, heart conduction of these animals are not comparable with humans, in spite of their genetic proximity. The amount of knowledge relating to nervous system, nerve conduction, anesthesia, and drugs is so vast that it is not possible to encompass the same within the confines of the present work.

The drug DP θ was not diluted for improved physicochemical analytical studies; such dilutions are not found in commercial circulation.

Future scope

This study opens up a vast research area for exploration of non-invasive *in vivo* study of ultra-diluted drugs. The results obtained even in dilutions have characteristic findings, and the techniques/methodologies cited in this dissertation may be used as a tool for identification, quality assessment, toxicological analysis, and point-of-care analysis for other homeopathic drugs. Further study for physicochemical analysis of mother tinctures (θ) may be conducted. These findings also open up the scope for assessment of clinical toxicity that may be produced by the drugs in dilutions. These methods can be used for characterization / standardization of sensitive ultra-diluted organic substances. It remains to be seen if there appears any change of configuration, dilution, and effectiveness caused by ultra-dilution and agitation, which may be correlated by CV and fluorescence data. Further analysis of fluorophores and CV of the drug DP and Digoxin may provide an in-depth understanding of the components that can bring changes in biological system. It is envisaged that fine-tuning of the anesthetized unconsciousness may become possible without any side effect of drugs like Digitalis or similar ones.

Conflict of Interests

No known conflict of interests exists.

Pair: Effectiveness Comparison	Mean of drug substance= μ_1	Variance of drug substance = S_1^2	Mean of control substance = μ_2	Variance of control substance= S_2^2	Pooled estimate of the common variance s²	Value of 't' to test the hypothesis is	$\mu_1 > \mu_2$ or $\mu_1 = \mu_2$ Comments
DP200 Vs. Rectified spirit	DP200 = 69	DP200 = 784	Rectified spirit = 74	Rectified spirit = 2601	70.52 (s = 8.39)	2.10	't' is not large enough to reject $H_0 : \mu_1 = \mu_2$. It cannot be said that alternative hypothesis is true i.e. $\mu_1 > \mu_2$. Treatment resembles each other. Hence, DP200 is almost same as Rectified spirit.
DP30 Vs. Rectified spirit	DP30 =138	DP30 = 4761	Rectified spirit = 74	Rectified spirit =2601	171.21 (s = 13.08)	16.30	Single tail test has been carried out for t_{50} (95% confidence interval) for d.f.=43 i.e. inference = 1.645. Therefore, $\mu_1 > \mu_2$, DP30 is more effective than Rectified spirit.
DP 6 Vs. Rectified spirit	DP6 = 76	DP6 = 841	Mean of RECTSP = 74	RECT SP= 2601	61.46 (s = 7.84)	0.96	Single tail test has been carried out for t_{05} (95% confidence interval) for d.f.=56 i.e. inference = 1.645. *Either both are same effective* or result is inconclusive.
DP θ Vs. Rectified spirit	DPQ = 53	DP θ = 784	Rectified spirit = 74	Rectified spirit = 2601	78.72 (s = 8.87)	7.89	Single tail test has been carried out for $\mu_2 > \mu_1$ (95% confidence interval) for d.f. =43 i.e. inference = 1.645. 't' is large enough to reject the null hypothesis. So $\mu_2 > \mu_1$ i.e. Rectified spirit is more effective than DP θ.
DIGOXIN vs.Rectified spirit	DIGOXIN = 33	DIGOXIN= 289	Rectified spirit = 74	Rectified spirit = 2601	82.57 (s =9.08)	12.86	Single tail test has been carried out for t_{50} (95% confidence interval) for d.f.=35 i.e. inf. = 1.645 't' is large enough to reject the null hypothesis. So, alternative hypothesis is true i.e. $\mu_2 > \mu_1$. Hence, Rectified spirit is more effective than Digoxin.

Table 2: Pair wise comparison of drug effectiveness, in producing period of anesthesia with respect to Rectified spirit.

Pair :Effectiveness Comparison	Mean of drug substance = μ_1	Variance of drug substance = S_1^2	Mean of control substance = μ2	Variance of control substance = S_2^2	Pooled estimate of the common variance = s2	Value of 't' to test the hypothesis is	$\mu_1 > \mu_2$ or $\mu_1 = \mu2$ Comments
Ether Vs Rectified spirit	Ether = 29	Ether = 144	Rectified spirit = 74	Rectified spirit = 2601	57.18 S= 7.56	21.04	Single tail test has been carried out for t_{50} (95% confidence interval) for d.f.=48 i.e. inf. = 1.645 Observed t is large enough to reject the null hypothesis. So, alternative hypothesis is true i.e. $\mu_2 > \mu_1$. Hence, Rectified spirit is more effective than ether.
DP200 vs. Ether	DP200 = 69	DP200 = 784	Ether = 29	Ether = 144	19.33 (s =4.39)	32.26	Single tail test has been carried out for t_{50} (95% confidence interval) for d.f.=48 i.e. inf. = 1.645. Observed t is large enough to reject the null hypothesis. $\mu_1 > \mu_2$ i.e. DP200 is more effective than ether.
DP6 vs Ether	DP6 = 76	DP6 = 841	Ether = 29	Ether = 144	17.59 (s= 4.19)	42.34	Single tail test has been carried out for t_{50} (95% confidence interval) for d.f.=56 i.e. inf. = 1.645.Observed t is large enough to reject the null hypothesis. So, alternative hypothesis is true i.e. $\mu_1 > \mu_2$. Hence, DP6 is more effective than ether.
DP30 vs. Ether	DP30 = 138	DP30 = S_1^2 = 4761	Ether = 29	Ether = 144	114.06 (s = 10.68)	34.06	Single tail test has been carried out for t_{50} (95% confidence interval) for d.f.=43 i.e. inf. = 1.645. Observed t is large enough to reject the null hypothesis. So, alternative hypothesis is true i.e. $\mu_1 > \mu_2$. Hence DP30 is more effective than ether.
DP θvs Ether	DP θ = 53	DP θ = 784	Ether = 29	Ether = 144	21.58 (s = 4.64)	32.37	Single tail test has been carried out for t_{05} (95% confidence interval) for d.f.=43 i.e. inf. = 1.645. Observed t is large enough to reject the null hypothesis. So, alternative hypothesis is true i.e. $\mu_1 > \mu_2$. DP θ is more effective than ether.
Digoxin vs. Ether	DIGOXIN = 33	DIGOXIN = 289	Ether = 29	Ether = 144	12.37 (s = 3.51)	3.25	Single tail test has been carried out for t_{50} (95% confidence interval) for d.f.=35 i.e. inf. = 1.645. Observed t is not large enough to reject the null hypothesis. At the same time we cannot say alternative hypothesis is true i.e. $\mu_1 > \mu_2$. Treatment is very much resembles to each other. Hence, Digoxin is complementary to ether.
Rectified spirit vs. Ether	Ether = 29	Ether = 144	Rectified spirit = 74	Rectified spirit = 2601	57.18 (s = 7.56)	21.04	Single tail test has been carried out for t_{50} (95% confidence interval) for d.f.=48 i.e. inf. = 1.645. Observed t is large enough to reject the null hypothesis. So, alternative hypothesis is true i.e. $\mu_2 > \mu_1$. Hence, Rectified spirit is more effective than ether

Table 3: Pair wise comparison of drug effectiveness, in producing period of anesthesia with respect to Diethyl ether.

Acknowledgment

Thankfully acknowledge support extended by Prof C. R. Raj, Prof NilmoniSarkar, Prof M. Halder, Prof. A. Roy, Prof. I. Chakraborty, Dr. Ramendra Sundar Dey, Dr. Sudip Chakraborty, Dr. A. B. Bera, and Dr. Sudip Chakraborty, Dr. B. Bhattacharya, IIT Kharagpur, AYUSH.

References

1. Medical Transactions (1785) Volume 3. Transaction XVI. Published by the College of Physicians, London.

2. Herring C (1997) Guiding Symptoms of our Materia Medica (1st edn). Jain Publishers Pvt Ltd. New Delhi, India.

3. Roden DM (2001) The pharmacological basis of therapeutics. McGraw Hill, New York, USA.

4. Sharma A, Thakur AK, Purkait B (2010) Identification of medicinally active ingredients in ultradiluted Digitalis purpurea: FTIR and Raman spectroscopic studies. Med Chem Res 19: 643-651.

5. Sharma A, Purkait. B, 2009. Energy in Commercially Available ultra-diluted Natural Cardiotropic Drug Digitalis purpurea: An UV Spectroscopic Study. Research Journal of Pharmcology 3: 58-62.

6. Sharma A, Purkait B (2013) Quality Assessment of Serially Ultradiluted and Agitated Drug Digitalis purpurea by Emission Spectroscopy and Clinical Analysis of Its Effect on the Heart Rate of Indian Bufo melanostictus. Journal of Pharmaceutics.

7. Sharma A, Purkait B (2012) Identification of Medicinally Active Ingredient in Ultradiluted Digitalis purpurea : Fluorescence Spectroscopic and Cyclic-Voltammetric Study. Journal of Analytical Methods in Chemistry.

8. Kwan T, Paiusco AD, Kohl L (1992) Digitalis toxicity caused by toad venom. Chest 102: 949-950.

9. http://www.osha.gov/SLTC/healthguidelines/ethylether/recognition.html

10. Douglas ER and Robert JC (2002) The Role of Electrostatic Interactions in Governing Anesthetic Action on the Torpedo Nicotinic Acetylcholine Receptor. Anesthesia and Analgesia 95: 356-361.

11. Rampil IJ (1994) Anesthetic potency is not altered after hypothermic spinal cord transection in rats. Anesthesiology 80: 606-610.

12. Thomas RE (1996) Medical chemistry and drug discovery, (6th Edn) Wiley-Inter science publication. New York, USA.

13. Lindholm P, Gullbo J, Claeson P, Göransson U, Johansson S, et al. (2002) Selective cytotoxicity evaluation in anticancer drug screening of fractionated plant extracts. J Biomol Screen 7: 333-340.

18

Treatments of Lung Diseases by Treating Liver, Kidney and Spleen with Kampo Medicines or Traditional Chinese Medicines

Hijikata Y*

Toyodo Hijikata Clinic, 567-0031 Kasuga 3-11-29 Ibaraki, Osaka, Japan

Abstract

Background: Chronic lung diseases can be treated successfully, by applying five phases theory to the symptoms of lung disease results for 3 situations: (1) excessive Liver qi injures Lung qi (rebellion) (相侮or反侮), (2) Kidney deprives Lung qi through engendering route (child deprives mother qi; Kidney: child, Lung: mother) (相生), (3) Spleen deprives Lung qi through engendering route (Spleen: mother, Lung: child (相生). Preventing lung disease then requires one or more of the following approaches: (1) restraining Liver qi (sometimes with supporting Lung qi), (2) giving qi to Kidney so it will not take qi from Lung, and (3) giving qi to Spleen so it will not take qi from Lung.

Objectives: Applying Kampo or Traditional Chinese Medicine (TCM), can cure patients with pulmonary disease by restoring Lung qi in the following ways: (1) suppressing hyperactive Liver qi, (2) decreasing Lung qi stolen by Kidney through engendering Lung-Kidney route through supplementation of Kidney qi, (3) decreasing Lung qi stolen by Spleen through engendering Spleen-Lung route, through supplementation of Spleen qi.

Methods: In one case, author prescribed formulas like Jia-wei-shao-yao-san (加味逍遥散), gan-mai-da-zao-tang (廿麦大棗湯) or Si-ni-san (四逆散) and others to soothe Liver to stop rebellion from Liver to Lung. In second case, author prescribed a Kidney-tonic formula like Ba-wei-di-huang-wan (八味地黄丸) so the Kidney would not deprive Lung qi. In the final case, the author prescribed a spleen-tonic formula like Chuan-si-jun-zi-tang (喘四君子湯) to give qi to Spleen so the Spleen would not deprive qi from Lung.

Results: In all three cases, lung symptoms such as cough, high susceptibility to colds and wheezing disappeared by prescribing the respective Kampo formulas mentioned above.

Conclusions: Symptoms like cough, wheezing and user susceptibility caused by Liver rebellion Lung were prevented by soothing Liver with Jia-wei-shao-yao-san and gan-mai-da-zao-tang. In the Kidney invades Lung case, giving Qi to Kidney with Ba-wei-di-huang-wan resulted in recovery from Lung trouble. In Spleen invades Lung case, spleen-tonic formula, Chuan-si-jun-zi-tang cured the Lung disease.

Discussion: Lung diseases are cured: (1) by restraining Liver qi with soothing Liver formula, (2) supplementing Kidney qi with warming Kidney formula and (3) supplementing Spleen qi-tonic formula so as not to deprive Lung qi. These findings suggest that in the Liver rebellion Lung, Lung qi is shunted from Lung to Kidney or from Lung to Spleen through the engendering route and that five phases theory has a physiologic regulatory correlate worthy of further investigation.

Keywords: Kampo; Traditional Chinese medicine (TCM); Lung disease; Chronic; Chinese medicine; Kidney disease

Introduction

The author reported about Five phases theory and the application to the treatment of various diseases [1,2]. According to this five phases theory, we can treat lung diseases as reported below.

As shown in Figure 1, the five viscera, Lung, Kidney, Liver, Heart and Spleen (→Lung) have engendering relationships. Engendering denotes right side viscera nurtures, or transmits the Qi to next left side viscera. Furthermore, the five viscera, Lung, Liver, Spleen, Kidney, Heart (→Lung), have the restraining relations between opposite two viscera.

Restraining denotes the principle one viscus restrains the opposite side viscus to keep within normal condition of whole body (Figure 1).

When the restraining viscus (such as Liver) gets excessive power, so-called overwhelm occurs. Overwhelms is an abnormal, excessive restraint. This happens in two cases. First, it may occur when one viscus (such as Liver) becomes excessively powerful and so overwhelms the corresponding viscus (Spleen). Second, the corresponding viscus (Such as Spleen) becomes too weak the former viscus (Liver) overwhelms Spleen. But one viscus (such as Liver) becomes excessively powerful, it not only overwhelm the corresponding viscus (spleen) but also

excessively restrains Lung to an opposite direction from Liver to Lung which is called rebellion, causing Lung disease. In this situation, Lung not only can't restrain Liver, but also is injured by Liver's excessive rebellion against Lung (Figure 2). We often meet with the pathology Liver rebellions Lung. (Figure 2)

When Lung diseases are not cured with prescriptions primarily for Lung, we must consider the Lung related viscera in five phase theory that is Spleen, Kidney regarding engendering relations, and Liver for rebellion.

We sometimes encounter chronic refractory lung diseases that are not cured with a series of therapeutic Kampo or Traditional Chinese Medicine (TCM) for pulmonary diseases. These treatments

---

*Corresponding author: Hijikata Y, Toyodo Hijikata Clinic, 567-0031 Kasuga 3-11-29 Ibaraki, Osaka, Japan
E-mail: hijikata@hcn.zaq.ne.jp

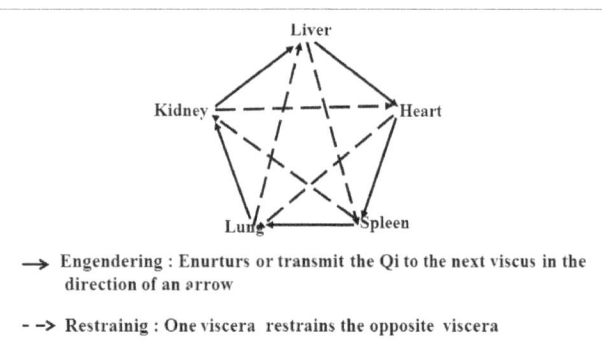

→ **Engendering** : Enurturs or transmit the Qi to the next viscus in the direction of an arrow

- -→ **Restrainig** : One viscera restrains the opposite viscera

Figure1: Engendering and restraining among five viscera work to keep normal physiology of the body.

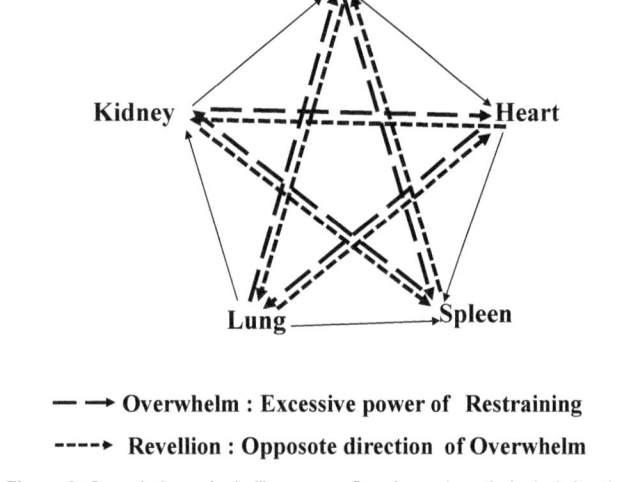

— → **Overwhelm : Excessive power of Restraining**

- - - → **Revellion : Opposote direction of Overwhelm**

Figure 2: Overwhelm and rebellion among five viscera in pathological situation.

include xiao-qing-long-tang (小青竜湯), qing-fei-tang (清肺湯), ma-xing-gan-shi-tang (麻杏甘石湯) ge-gen-tang (葛根湯) as well as prescriptions including chai-fu (柴胡) such as si-ni-san (四逆散), Shen-bi-tang (神秘湯) and so on.

In these cases, some medicines selected based on five element theory, sometimes dramatically works as described below.

Main three causes for intractable Lung diseases are shown below.

1. The lengthening of Liver qi stagnation produced by continuing stressful state, leads to rebelling of Liver against Lung followed by the appearance of incurable pulmonary diseases due to Liver fire invading Lung. This situation is sometimes accompanied by gastrointestinal symptoms as well. Because lengthening of Liver qi stagnation, not only rebell Lung but also overwhelm Spleen especially in cases with weak Spleen (Figure 3).

2. The chronicity of Kidney qi deficiency leads to Lung qi deficiency. Because Kidney steals qi from Lung through the engendering route between Kidney and Lung. By supplementing Kidney qi, the volume of Lung qi stolen by Kidney, followed by an improvement in pulmonary diseases (Figure 4).

3. The chronicity of Spleen qi deficiency leads to Lung qi deficiency. Because Spleen steals qi from Lung through the engendering route

between Spleen and Lung. By supplementing Spleen qi, the volume of Lung qi stolen by Spleen decreases followed by an improvement in pulmonary diseases. When Spleen qi is very small, overwhelming from Liver to Spleen may happen but omitted here.

(We omit discussion of the relationship between Heart and Lung in spite of quite familiar relations of Heart and Lung because they are routinely treated with conventional therapies). Diagnosis of diseases of patients is carried out based on conventional medicines, traditional Chinese medicines (TCM) or Kampo Medicines.

Cases above mentioned in (1): Rebellion of Liver against Lung

Liver fire invading Lung (Simultaneous Liver and Lung disease through restraining route) successfully treated clinical cases were reported below.

Case 1-1: This case was written more than 200 years ago in Japanese literature which was translated into English below [3].

"Mr Tokumi an elderly male living in Nagasaki prefecture, had been suffering from empyema. He had been treated by various doctors for more than 3 years in vain. He wished to be treated by Dr Tokaku Wada who lived in Kyoto, because he was hoping to begin a new job far from his residence at the time. Dr Wada diagnosed Mr Tokumi's disease as being derived from his mental distress and accepted his request to treat him because he had successfully treated many similar cases.

Chief complaint: Dirty running snot with empyema.

Identification: Lengthy Liver qi stagnation (Liver miasma) caused Lung disease (Liver fire invading the lung through rebellion route between Liver and Lung). (In conventional medicine, empyema).

Treatment: Pacify Liver qi to decreases rebellion from Liver to Lung.

Prescription: Two or three doses daily decoction of modified si-ni-san (四逆散) together with wu-zhu-yu (呉茱萸) and mu-li (牡蛎).

Result: The patient's symptom had disappeared by the time he arrived at Shinagawa after departure from Kyoto for Edo (Tokyo) on foot.

Discussion: Dr Tokaku Wada diagnosed Mr Tokumi's symptoms as having originated due to lengthy Liver qi stagnation with mental conflicts. The diagnosis was also suspected due to uncomfortable fullness of abdominal muscle in hypochondrium which is one of the results of accumulated Liver qi stagnation (miasma). With the additional effect of wu-zhu-yu to warm gallbladder meridian which will support good circulation around nose and mu-li to decrease snivel, si-ni-san worked to pacify Liver qi and there by decrease the rebellion from Liver to Lung. This was followed by an improvement in Lung symptom, specifically the cessation of "Dirty running snot" stopped.

Case 1-2: A 52-year-old Japanese female (height, 161 cm weight, 62 kg) (Figure 5).

Chief complaint: Hot flashes, chronic cough, palpitations, shortness of breath.

Present history: Since she had a lot of psychological stress, she suffered particularly from, allergic rhinitis, hay fever, nasal congestion and dry coughs. Her menstruation got irregular, and she became quick of temper and suffered flushing of the soles and palms, night sweats, excessive dreaming, uneasiness, depilation and fragile nails. She had

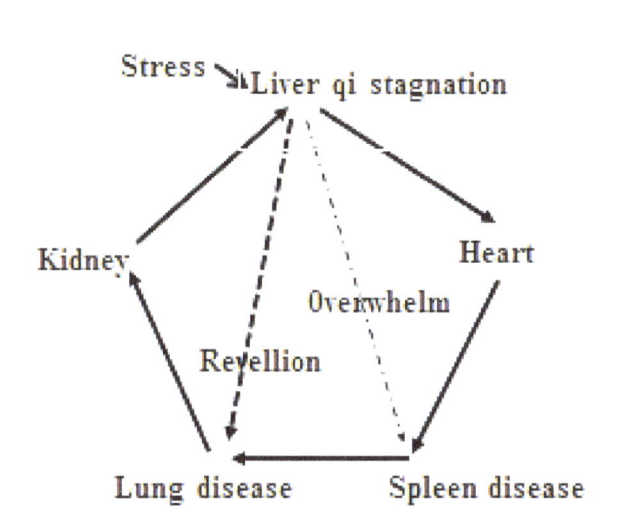

Figure 3: Pathological situation of Lung produced by rebellion from Liver against Lung.

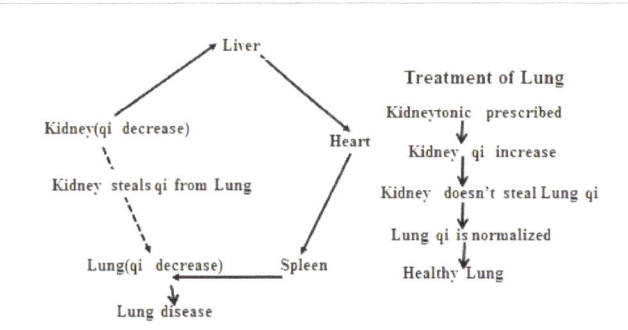

Figure 4: The chronicity of Kidney qi deficiency leads to Lung qi deficiency followed by Lung disease.

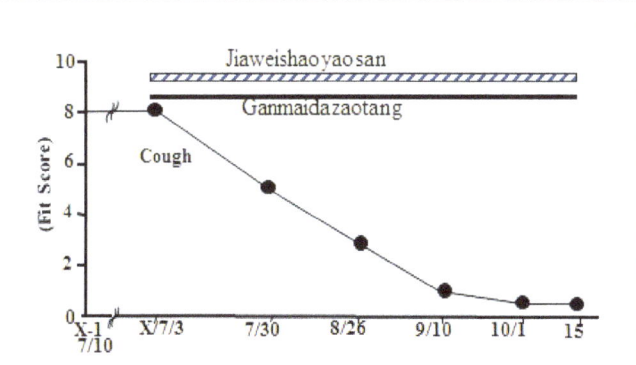

Figure 5: Case 1-2. A 52-year-old Japanese female (Rebelling of Liver against Lung).

also been suffering from sensitivity to cold, chilblains during winter, and feels distress on rainy days and her digestive system was not working properly due to greasy food. In spite of modern medicines, her condition didn't improve at all. Coldness, rainy days and fatty food worsened her digestive condition.

Past history: She had been abused by school teachers and friends and she had been in depressive state. She had suffered from tonsillitis,

hay fever, nasal congestion and dry coughs. She had been a habitual drinker.

Family history: The patient's mother had been bedridden due to rheumatic diseases more than 30 years. Father had senile dementia and her younger sister has rheumatism.

States praesens: Tongue body: red/slightly dark, fistura all over the body. Tongue coating is thick and white. Puls: strongly pressed her pulse feel week, and 78 beat/min, Blood Pressure: 130/76 mmHg. Abdominal muscle: fullness and tenderness of the hypochondrium.

Identification: Liver impacts Heart. Liver rebels against Lung. Yin deficiency with yang hyperactivity. In conventional medicine, she was diagnosed as autonomic imbalance.

Treatment: Soothe Liver to stop the rebellion from Liver to Lung. Tranquilize the Heart

Prescription: Jia-wei-shao-yao-san (加味逍遥散 TJ-24:7.5 g/day) Gan-mai-da-zao-tang (甘麦大棗湯 TJ-72: 7.5 g/day) TJ means the product of Tsumura Co.

Result: Twenty days after beginning her prescriptions, her nasal obstruction and mental stress improved (VAS: 10→5). After 39 days, her cough disappeared. She became quite relaxed and told me jia-wei-shao-yao-san had worked for her nagging cough. Panic attacks rarely appeared except in response to terrible events.

Discussion: The patient had many stressing factors which caused an accumulation of Liver qi, "Liver miasma" overflow. Because of the rebellion of Liver to Lung, her cough continued. Jia-wei-shao-yao-san soothed Liver and Gan-mai-da-zao-tang tranquilized Heart which helped to soothe Liver.

Case 1-3: A 54 year- old Japanese female (height, 162 cm. weight, 62 kg) (Figure 6).

Chief Complaint: Dyspnea, cough and heavy stomach with increasing need to care for her parents.

Present history: With the patient's increasing responsibilities for her parents' care, her dyspnea and cough gradually increased. Treatments by the respiratory division of a hospital did not work. She didn't sweat during exercise in the summer. Dull arbitrarily positioned headache, shoulder stiffness, difficulty in sleeping, light tinnitus, heavy stomach, belching gas, bruising long-standing heart beat connected with stomach condition and susceptibility to cold. She likes warm foods and cooling caused diarrhea. She has two children.

Past history: The patient suffered from alopecia areata in her 20s and during pregnancy and had severe menstrual cramps. Atopic dermatitis with onset in her 40s.

Family history: The patient's father suffered a ruptured aortic aneurysm and lung cancer successfully resected at age 74. Her mother also suffered from lung cancer with onset at age 78 and successfully resected.

States presens: Pale red tongue body with thin white fur. Swelling of the sublingual collateral vessels. Pulse: 63 per min, irregular, fine, slippery, weak. String like left guan puls. Slight fullness of the hypochondrium. Blood pressure (BP) of 116/58 mmHg.

Identification: Liver qi depression with blood stasis. Liver rebellions against Lung. Liver overwhelms spleen. In conventional medicine, diagnosed as asthma bronchitis.

Treatment: Sooth liver and clear lung. tonify heart and fortify spleen.

Prescription: Modified Zhi-gan-cao-tang (炙甘草湯)] combined with Xiong-gui-tiao-xue-yin (芎帰調血飲):Zhi-can-cao (炙甘草)3, Gan-jian (乾姜)1, Gui-zhi (桂枝)3, Ma-zi-ren (麻子仁)3, Ren-shen (人参)3, Da-zao (大棗)3, Di-huang (地黄)6, Mai-men-dong (麦門冬)6, E-jiao (阿膠)2, Chai-fu (柴胡)2, Xiang-Fuzi (香附子)2, U-yao (烏薬)2, Chen-pi (陳皮)2, Chuan-xiong (川芎)2, Yi-mu-cao (益母草)1.5, Mu-dan-pi (牡丹皮)2,Huang-qi (黄耆)3, Bai-shu (白朮)2, Fu-ling (茯苓)2 (Numeral: g/day).

Result: At 13 days after starting her prescription, the patient's dyspnea and cough disappeared, and her palpitations decreased. She continued to take the same prescription. At 86 days after starting herbal medicines, her good condition continued with this treatment After 1 year, she began taking half portions, and after 2 years began to use the medicines only when her condition was bad. Overworking sometimes brings on palpitations but the patient's cough and dyspnea have so far not returned.

Discussion: The patient's weak irregular pulse (Heart qi deficiency) continued since long before the onset of her current symptoms this time and she notes that episode of irregular pulse synchronize with digestive function. Accordingly, a Heart qi deficiency will not be the primary reason for aggravation of her asthma-like symptoms. Furthermore her chief complaints with her increasing responsibility for her parents' care, reflecting Liver qi depression followed by Liver rebellions against Lung and overwhelming Spleen.

In Xiong-gui-tiao-xue-yin, Chai-fu, Xiang-Fuzi, U-yao, Chen-pi will soothe Liver, regulate qi, inhibit the rebellion against Lung, and block Liver from overwhelming Spleen. Chuan-xiong, Yi-mu-cao and Mu-dan-pi will resolve blood stasis and improve circulating.

Cases above mentioned in (2): Kidney qi deficiency leads to Lung qi deficiency

Case 2-1: A 56-year- old Japanese female (height, 153 cm. weight, 55 kg).

Chief complaint: Fatigue and difficulty in expiration with wheezing after improvement of a common cold.

States presens: Pulse: 70 per minute: slippery, stringlike, BP: 116/74 mmHg, Tongue body: teeth-marked and slightly dark. Sublingual collateral vessels: dark and swelling, Tongue fur:thick, slightly yellowish. Celiopathy:tenderness of the hypochondrium.

Present illness: As a medical doctor, the patient leads a stressful life which often causes diarrhea with stress. She took bu-zhong-yi-qi-tang '(補中益気湯) and Jia-wei-xiao-yao-sang (加味逍遥散) and routinely wore a belly band to warm her body. On June 2, she got a common cold with a temperature 38.5°C after overworking. This was followed by a cough with wheezing, diarrhea and fatigue. She took Qin-fei-tang (清肺湯) and an antibiotic. Two days later, only her cough had improved.

Identification: Liver qi depression with blood stagnation lung qi deficiency kidney yang deficiency in conventional medicine, asthma bronchitis.

Treatment: Tonic Kidney yang with Lu-rong (鹿茸).

Results: As no improvement was observed, on the next day, she changed to another antibiotic and herbal medicines, Mai-men-dong-tang (麦門冬湯) together with Jie-geng (桔梗) and Xuan-shen (玄参). With the newly applied medications which did not work, so author diagnosed she had Kidney Yang deficiency. Author added 鹿茸 (lurong) to tonic Kidney yang, next day her wheezing and diarrhea disappeared and continued 鹿茸 one more day and stopped without recurrence.

Discussion: As no improvement was observed with herbs for Lung, the author diagnosed her condition as Kidney yang deficiency because she had been very sensitive to cold so far. The author prescribed 鹿茸 which worked dramatically which will mean Qi stolen from Lung by Kidney must be decreased which would lead to an disappearance of wheezing which is a symbol of Lung yang deficiency.

Case 2-2: A 60-year-old Japanese female (height, 160 cm. weight, 48 kg) (Figure 7).

Chief complaint: Too frequent catching common colds

States presens: Puls: slightly slippery, weak. 72 per minute, BP: 120/62 mmHg, Tongue body: Pale red. Sublingual vessels: slightly dark and swelling, Tongue fur: slightly Celiopathy: Slight tenderness of hypochondrium.

Present illness: If the patient took Ge-gen-tang (葛根湯) upon catching a cold, she improved quickly, but a few days later she would again catch cold and this pattern repeated.

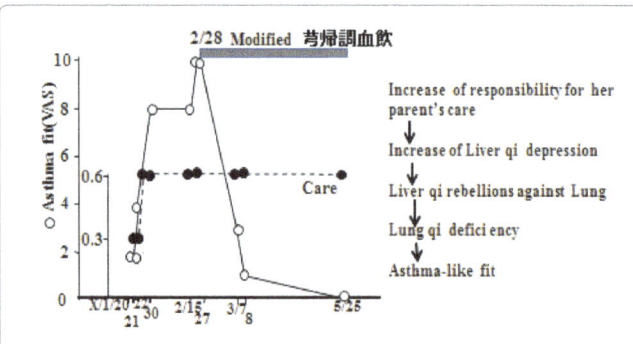

Figure 6: Case 1-3. A 60-year-old Japanese female (Rebelling of Liver against Lung).

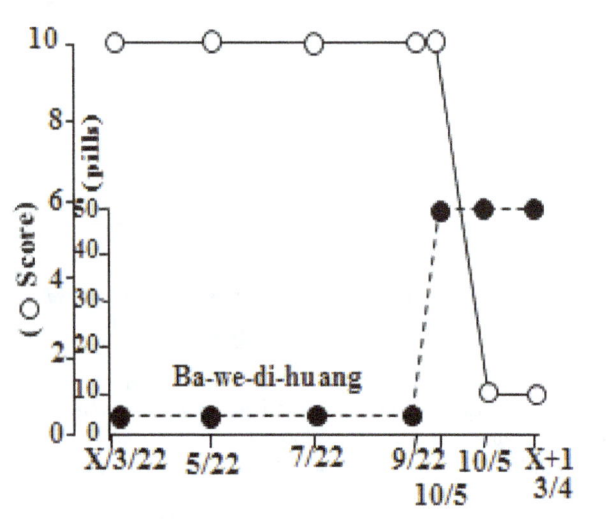

Figure 7: Case 2-2. A 60-year-old Japanese female Kidney qi deficiency leads to Lung qi deficiency score 10: She caught cold very often.

Past history: With dysmenorrhea a total hysterectomy was carried out when the patient was 40 years old. She has a cold-sensitive constitution and lacks physical strength. During childhood, she had empyema which was successfully treated with herbal medicine.

Family history: Her mother suffered from an adrenal tumor and died from breast cancer at 93 years old.

Identification: Kidney Qi deficiency. Kidney deprives Lung qi.

Treatment: Tonic Kidney for it not to deprive Lung qi.

Prescription: Ba-wei-di-huang-wan (八味地黄丸) (her intake was increased to 30 pills per day from 5 pills per day).

Result: Since starting increased vol of Ba-wei-di-huang-wan until the time of her visit to my clinic 5 months later, the patient never caught cold.

Discussion: In spite of the absence of obvious symptom of Kidney qi deficiency, increase of intake of Kidney tonic 八味地黄丸 dramatically worked. Her Kidney qi deficiency may have existed from her birth. Because she hated coldness, she is apt to take 10 cups of Japanese hot tea every day and she lacks physical strength which means she has had Kidney qi deficiency with her increasing age. This deficiency has progressed to frequent catching cold.

In this case, I felt enough volume is necessary to obtain necessary cure.

Cases above mentioned in (3): The Spleen qi deficiency leads to Lung qi deficiency

Case 3-1: A 42 year-old Japanese female (height: 163 cm, weight: 42 kg)

Chief complaint: Overeating and fatty food intake caused expiratory dyspnea.

States presens: Slightly slippery and string like. 66 per minute. BP: 116/72 mmHg, Tongue body: pale red, tooth-marked with thin fur. Sublingual vessels: slightly dark.

Present illness and Past history: During summer and autumn, the patient experienced fits related to her chief complaint, sometimes stress has evoked asthmatic fits (Liver rebellion against Lung).

Family history: The patient's mother had hypertension, her younger brother suffered from asthma during childhood, and her grand

farther had asthma which disappeared when he stopped smoking.

Identification: Spleen (mother) deprives Lung (child) qi. In conventional medicine, diagnosed as asthma bronchitis.

Treatment: Tonic Spleen so that Spleen doesn't deprive Lung qi.

Prescription: Chuan-si-jun-zi-tang {喘四君子湯：Ren-shen (人参)2, Hou-po (厚朴)2, Su-zi (蘇子)2, Chen-pi (陳皮)2, Fu-ling (茯苓)4, Dang-gui (当帰)4, Bai-shu (白朮)4, Suo-sha (縮砂)1, Mu-xiang (木香)1, Shen-xiang (沈香)1, Gan-cao (甘草)1, Sang-bai-pi (桑柏皮)1.5, added with Fu-zi (附子)1, Rou-gui (肉桂)2, Shan-zha-zi (山査子)2, and Tau-ren (桃仁)2.

Result: At 22 days after intake of the above prescription, the patient's fits decreased. At 85 days she reported that the level of her fits had decreased from 10 to 3 on the VAS scale. At 144 days, her fits occurred only after overeating and then disappeared as she continued to follow the same prescription.

Discussion: Despite the patient's good appetite, it was only when she had heavy food, that she suffered asthmatic fits. This means that when she has heavy food, a Spleen qi deficiency is produced. Her symptoms decreased with a spleen qi-tonic containing herbs like 喘四君子湯 probably because Lung qi stolen by Spleen through the engendering route was diminished.

Addendum Cases

One male (34 years old) with asthma bronchitis improved with the administration of Liu-jun-zi-tang (六君子湯) or Bu-zhong-yi-qi tang (補中益気湯) [4]. The present results suggest that in the context of the five-phase theory, a Spleen-tonic prescription worked for Lung disease probably because Lung qi is supplied by a Spleen-tonic prescription worked for Lung diseases probably because Lung qi is supplied by Spleen tonic prescriptions like 六君子湯 or 補中益気湯 through the Lung-Spleen engendering route.

References

1. Hijikita Y (2011) Application of "five elements theory for treating diseases in Chinese medicine. Intec web Org Croatia 3: 45-78.

2. Kuang H (2014) Recent advances in theories and practice of Chinese medicine. Intechweb Org Croatia pp: 504

3. Modern Kampo medicine complication Meichoshuppan (1986) Lectures of Treatments with Kampo Medicines near the window by the Japanese banana trees (3rd ed.) pp: 283-285.

4. Fujihara J (2003) Spleentonic Kampo medicines worked for Asthma with qi deficiency in both Spleen and Lung. Kampo no Rinsho 50: 1142-1143.

19

Invitro Evaluation of *Centratherum anthelminticum* Seeds for Antinephrolithiatic Activity

Varsha J. Galani* and Rital R. Panchal

M.Pharm (Pharmacology), A. R. College of Pharmacy & G. H. Patel Institute of Pharmacy, Gujarat, India

Abstract

Antinephrolithiatic activity of 70% methanolic extract of *Centratherum anthelminticum* seeds (CAE) was evaluated *in vitro* on nucleation and aggregation of calcium oxalate crystallization. Calcium oxalate crystallization was induced by the addition of 0.01 M sodium oxalate solution in synthetic urine. The effect of CAE (100, 200, 300, 400, 600, 800 and 1000 µg/ml) was studied by the measurement of turbidity in presence or absence of extract at 620 nm of a spectrophotometer. The rates of nucleation and aggregation were evaluated by comparing the turbidity of a control system with that of one exposed to the extract. Crystals in the urine were also analysed by light microscopy. From photomicrograph, it is confirmed that CAE inhibited the nucleation of calcium oxalate crystals, decreasing their number and size. Also percentage inhibition of crystals aggregation increased as the concentration of CAE increased. The results of the present study indicated that 70% methanolic extract of *C. anthelminticum* seeds has the higher capacity to inhibit the crystal formation and aggregation. These suggested possible antinephrolithiatic activity of *C. anthelminticum* seeds against calcium oxalate stones.

Keywords: Anti- nephrolithiatic activity; *Centratherum anthelminticum* (L) kuntze; Calcium oxalate

Introduction

Urolithiasis denotes presence of one or more stone in any location within the urinary tract, is one of the oldest and wide spread diseases known to man [1]. It is a serious, debilitating problem in all societies throughout the world, affecting approximately. 12% of the population and men are three times more prone than women [2]. It is more prevalent between the ages of 20 and 40 in both sexes [3]. The overall probability of forming stones differs in various parts of the world, and is estimated at 1–5% in Asia, 5–9% in Europe, and 13% in North America. The recurrence rate of renal stones is approximately 75% in a 20-year span [4]. Etiology is multifactorial and is strongly related to dietary lifestyle habits or practices [5]. The most common (more than 80%) renal stones are calculi of calcium oxalate crystals followed by uric acid, struvite cystine and other stones [6,7].

The crystallization of the calcium oxalate begins with increased urinary supersaturation, with the subsequent formation of the solid crystalline particles within the urinary tract. This is followed by nucleation, by which stone-forming salts in supersaturated urinary solution coalesce in to clusters that then increase in size by the addition of new constituents [8]. These crystals then grow and aggregate with other crystals in solution, and are ultimately retained and accumulated in the kidney [9]. Renal injury promotes crystal retention and the development of a stone nidus on the renal papillary surface, and further supports crystal nucleation at lower supersaturation levels [10]. Therefore, levels of urinary supersaturation correlate with the type of stone formed, and reducing supersaturation is effective in preventing stone recurrence. Therefore, if this progression of crystallization can be prevented, then lithiasis could also be prevented.

The stone formation requires supersaturated urine which also depends on urinary pH, ionic strength, solute concentration and complexions. Various substances in the body have an effect on one or more of the above processes, thereby influencing a person's ability to promote or prevent stone formation [8].

Management of stone disease depends on the size and location of the stones. Stones larger than 5 mm or stones that fail to pass through should be treated by some interventional procedures such as extracorporeal shock wave lithotripsy (ESWL), ureteroscopy (URS), or percutaneous nephrolithotomy (PNL) [11]. The recent treatment procedures are very costly for common man as well as recurrence of kidney stone and numbers of side effects are associated with these procedures [12]. Hence, search for new antinephrolithiatic drugs from natural sources assumed greater importance as herbal drugs are cost effective and they confer lesser side effects.

Traditional herbal medicines provide many opportunities for the development of potential therapeutic drugs, in the form of either extracts alone, in combination with other herbs, or in the form of phytochemical compounds isolated from them. There are several reports related to anti-crystallization compounds extracted from medicinal plants.

Centratherum anthelminticum (L.) Kuntze (compositae), commonly known as Kaligiri. It is highly reputed in Hindu medicine as remedy for leucoderma and other skin diseases. The seeds have a hot sharp taste, acrid, astringent to the bowels, anthelmintic and cure ulcers. The seeds are used as purgative, for asthma, kidney troubles and hiccough, applied in inflammatory swelling, remove blood from liver, good for sores and itching of the eyes. In Punjab, it is considered as antipyretic. The seeds are also credited with tonic, stomachic, and diuretic properties [13,14]. Different organic solvent and aqueous extracts of these seeds were scientifically evaluated for antifilarial, antibacterial, larvicidal, antiviral, antifungal, anticancer, anthelmintic, antidiabetic, antioxidant, analgesic, antipyretic, anti-inflammatory, diuretic, wound healing activities [15]. There is no scientific evidence

*Corresponding author: Varsha J. Galani, M. Pharmacy, Ph.D, Department of Pharmacology, A. R. College of Pharmacy & G. H. Patel Institute of Pharmacy, 388120-Vallabh Vidyanagar, Gujarat, India
E-mail: vrp173@yahoo.com

regarding nephroprotective action of this plant. Based on that, aim of the present study is to evaluate nephroprotective activity of *Centratherum anthelminticum* using *in vitro* experimental models of nephrolithiasis.

Materials and Methods

Preparation of extract

Dried seeds of *Centratherum anthelminticum* were procured from Anand Agriculture University, Anand. Plant material was authentified by Dr. Jina Patel, Department of Botany, Gujarat University, Ahmedabad. The voucher specimen (Authentication reference number: RRP/CA-1/7/ARGH -11-13) was deposited at the pharmacognosy department of our institute. The seeds were air-dried and ground to fine powder. About 0.5 kg powdered sample was defatted with petroleum ether (40-60°C). The remaining part was extracted with (70:30) methanol and water by cold maceration for 4 days with frequent shaking. (Yield -11.49% w/w). Hydromethanolic extract after evaporating the solvent, was dried under vacuum and stored in an air-tight container at 4°C. The dried extract was dissolved in distilled water and used for further study.

Preliminary phytochemical screening

The qualitative chemical investigation of hydroalcoholic extract was carried out to check the presence of various phytoconstituents [16].

Preparation of synthetic urine: The artificial urine was prepared according to the method of Burns and Finlayson [17] and had the following composition: sodium chloride 105.5 mmol/l, sodium phosphate 32.3 mmol/l, sodium citrate 3.21 mmol/l, magnesium sulfate 3.85 mmol/l, sodium sulfate 16.95 mmol/l, potassium chloride 63.7 mmol/l, calcium chloride 4.5 mmol/l, sodium oxalate 0.32 mmol/l, ammonium hydroxide 17.9 mmol/l, and ammonium chloride 0.0028 mmol/l. The synthetic urine was prepared fresh each day and pH adjusted to 6.0.

Experimental protocol: The classical model for the study of oxalate crystallization was chosen because of its simplicity and satisfactory reproducibility. According method reported by Sasikala et al. [18] which involves crystallization without inhibitors and with it, in order to assess the inhibiting capacity of test material used was suitably modified for the study.

Nucleation assay: The inhibitory activity of the extracts on the nucleation of calcium oxalate crystals was determined by a spectrophotometric assay [19]. Solution of calcium chloride and sodium oxalate were prepared at the final concentrations of 5 mmol/l and 7.5 mmol/l respectively in a buffer containing Tris 0.05 mol/l and NaCl 0.15 mol/l at pH 6.5. 950 µl of calcium chloride solution mixed with 100 µl of herb extracts at the different concentrations (100 µg/ml to 1000 µg/ml). Crystallization was started by adding 950 µl of sodium oxalate solution. The temperature was maintained at 37°C. The rate of nucleation was determined by comparing the induction time of crystals (time of appearance of crystals that reached a critical size and thus became optically detectable) in the presence of the extract and that of the control with no extract. The absorbance (optical density) was recorded at 620 nm using spectrophotometer (Shimadzu). The growth of crystals was expected due to the following reaction:

$$CaCl_2 + Na_2C_2O_4 \rightarrow CaC_2O_4 + 2NaCl$$

Aggregation assay: The method used was similar to that described by Atmani and Khan [20] with some minor modifications. Calcium oxalate crystals were prepared by mixing calcium chloride and sodium oxalate at 50 mmol/l. Both solutions were equilibrated to 60°C in a water bath for 1 hour and then cooled to 37°C overnight. The crystals were harvested by centrifugation and then evaporated at 37°C. Calcium oxalate crystals were used at a final concentration of 0.8 mg/ml, buffered with Tris 0.05 mol/l and NaCl 0.15 mol/l at pH 6.5. The absorbance (optical density) was recorded at 620 nm spectrophotometer (Shimadzu). Experiments were conducted at 37°C in the absence or presence of the plant extract. The percentage aggregation inhibition rate (Ir) was then calculated by comparing the turbidity in the presence of the extract with that obtained in the control using following formula:

$$Ir = \left(1 - \frac{\text{Turbidity of sample}}{\text{Turbidity of control}}\right) \times 100$$

Results

The in vitro inhibitory effect of CAE on various phases of calcium oxalate crystallization was determined by the time course of turbidity measured in synthetic urine at extract concentrations of 100, 200, 400, 600, 800 and 1000 µg/ml. Incubating the metastable solutions of Ca^{+2} and oxalate without extract resulted in the formation of bipyramid calcium oxalate crystals (Figure 1A). The respective crystals, observed under the light microscope (100×), in solutions incubated with CAE at 100 – 1000 µg/ml are shown in Figures 1B-G. CAE also caused a morphological change in calcium oxalate crystals, which was not fully grown as bipyramid calcium oxalate crystals that were inhibited in nucleation phase. The optical density decreased with the increase in concentration of CAE indicating that decreased the nucleation of calcium oxalate particles (Table 1). The optical density was highest (0.931) of positive control i.e. in the absence of herb extract and it was lowest (0.654) at the highest concentration of CAE (1000 µg/ml). The crystals formed in the presence of CAE were less than that in the control, showing that crystals were less aggregated. As shown in Table 2, the percent inhibited aggregation associated with the CAE at concentration of 100 µg/ml was found to be 57.96 while percent was maximum i.e. 70.04 at highest concentration of CAE (1000 µg/ml).

Discussion

Kidney stone function is a complex process that results from a succession of several physico-chemical events including supersaturation, nucleation, growth, aggregation and retention within renal tubules [21]. Thus if supersaturation or later steps in crystallization can be prevented, then lithiasis should be avoided. Nucleation is the formation of a solid crystal phase in a solution. It is an essential step in renal stone formation [22]. The main findings of the present study were that CAE inhibited the crystallization by inhibiting nucleation of calcium oxalate in solution; less and smaller particles were formed with increasing concentrations of the CAE. The results of the nucleation assay confirmed that the extract contained nucleation-preventing agents. The limiting factors in stone formation could be those processes that affect crystal growth, because particles may become large enough to occlude the urinary tract, leading to stone formation [23]. The herb extracts may contain substances that inhibit the growth of calcium oxalate crystals. This property of plants may be important in preventing the growth of kidney stone. Aggregation may be an important factor in the genesis of stones [24]. Crystal aggregation is the most critical step, as it occurs very rapidly and has a considerable effect on particle size, and aggregated crystals are commonly found in urine and renal stones [25]. Recurrent calcium stone formers excrete clusters of crystals in the urine, caused by aggregation, also named agglomeration, whereas urine from normal people contains mainly single crystals

[24]. Again, percentage inhibition of crystals aggregation increased as the concentration of CAE increased indicating antinephrolithiatic activity. The efficacy of most herbal remedies is attributed to various active principles, in combination. Results of phytochemical screening showed the presence of carbohydrates, proteins, saponins, flavanoids,

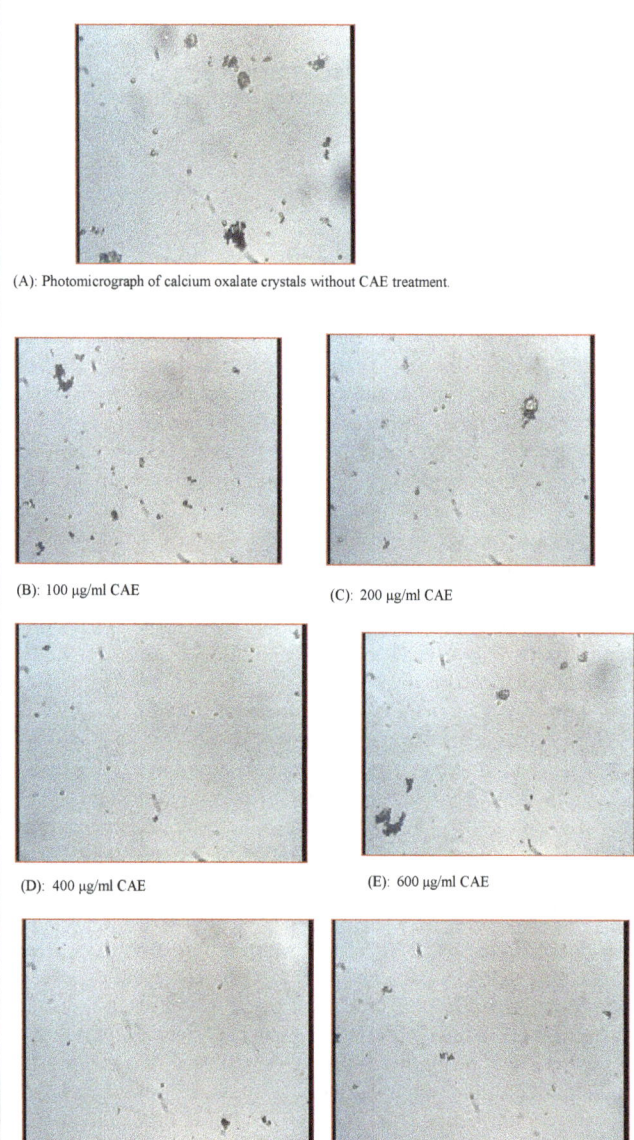

(A): Photomicrograph of calcium oxalate crystals without CAE treatment.

(B): 100 µg/ml CAE

(C): 200 µg/ml CAE

(D): 400 µg/ml CAE

(E): 600 µg/ml CAE

(F): 800 µg/ml CAE

(G): 1000 µg/ml CAE

Figure 1: (B-G) Photomicrograph of calcium oxalate crystals with of *C. anthelminticum* seeds (CAE) treatment.

Concentration (µg/ml) of CAE	Absorbance (620 nm)
Control	0.931
100	0.909
200	0.898
400	0.855
600	0.808
800	0.785
1000	0.654

Table 1: Effect of *C. Anthelminticum* seeds (CAE) on nucleation of calcium oxalate crystals.

Concentration (µg/ml) of CAE	% Inhibition
100	57.96
200	59.62
400	59.98
600	60.04
800	62.04
1000	70.04

Table 2: Effect of *C. Anthelminticum* seeds (CAE) on aggregation of calcium oxalate crystals.

tannins and polyphenols in the seeds. Saponins are known to have anti-crystallisation properties by disaggregating the suspension of mucoproteins, the promoters of crystallization [26]. Antiurolithiatic activities also have been attributed to triterpenes, lupeol [27] and polyphenolic compound like quercetin [28]. It is therefore probable that the components that are present in abundance in the extract might exert their action directly on the calcium oxalate crystallization.

In conclusion, 70% methanolic extract of *Centratherum anthelminticum* seeds (CAE) have inhibitory effect on the nucleation and aggregation of calcium oxalate crystallization in vitro. Thus, this scientific evidence may rationalize the traditional use of *Centratherum anthelminticum* seeds for the treatment of nephrolithiasis. However, a detailed preclinical and clinical study is required to establish the use of plant as antinephrolithiatic agent.

References

1. Prasad KVSRG, Sujatha D, Bharti K (2007) Herbal drugs in urolithiasis - A review. Pharmacog Rev 1: 175-178.

2. Grover PK, Kim DS, Ryall RL (2002) The effect of seed crystals of hydroxyapatite and brushite on the crystallization of calcium oxalate in undiluted human urine in vitro: implications for urinary stone pathogenesis. Mol Med 8: 200-209.

3. Worcester EM, Coe FL (2008) Nephrolithiasis. Prim Care 35: 369-391.

4. Abbagani S, Gundimeda SD, Varre S, Ponnala D, Mundluru HP (2010) Kidney stone disease. Etiology and evaluation. Int J Appl Biol Pharm Tech 1: 175-182.

5. Taylor EN, Stampfer MJ, Curhan GC (2005) Obesity, weight gain, and the risk of kidney stones. JAMA 293: 455-462.

6. Daudon M, Bader CA, Jungers P (1993) Urinary calculi: review of classification methods and correlations with etiology. Scanning Microsc 7: 1081-1104.

7. Bangash K, Shigri F, Jamal A, Anwar K (2011) Spectrum of renal stones composition; chemical analysis of renal stones. Int J Pathology 9: 63-66.

8. Basavaraj DR, Biyani CS, Browning AJ, Cartledge JJ (2007) The role of urinary kidney stone inhibitors and promoters in the pathogenesis of calcium containing renal stones. EAU-EBU Update Series 5: 126-136.

9. Kok DJ, Papapolous SE, Bijovet OL (1990) Crystal agglomeration is a major element in calcium oxalate urinary stone formation. Kidney Int 37: 51-56.

10. Fasano JM, Khan SR (2001) Intratubular crystallization of calcium oxalate in the presence of membrane vesicles: an in vitro study. Kidney Int 59: 169-178.

11. Coll DM, Varanelli MJ, Smith RC (2002) Relationship of spontaneous passage of ureteral calculi to stone size and location as revealed by unenhanced helical CT. AJR Am J Roentgenol 178: 101-103.

12. Nabi G, Downey P, Keeley F, Watson G, McClinton S (2007) Extracorporeal shock wave lithotripsy (ESWL) versus ureteroscopic management for ureteric calculi. Cochrane Database Syst Rev.

13. Kirtikar KR, Basu BD, ICS (1981) Indian medicinal plants. (2ndedn), Lalit Mohan Basu, Allahabad, India.

14. Chopra RN, Chopra IC, Handa KL, Kapur LD (1994) Indigenous Drugs of India. (1stedn), Dhur DK of Academic Publisher, Calcutta, India.

15. Paydar M, Moharam BA, Wong YL, Looi CY, Wong WF, et al. (2013) *Centratherum anthelminticum* (L.) Kuntze a potential medicinal plant with pleiotropic pharmacological and biological activities. Int J Pharmacol 9: 211-226.

16. Kokate CK (1994) Practical Pharmacognosy. (4thedn), Vallabh prakashan, New Delhi, India.

17. Burns JR, Finlayson B (1980) Changes in calcium oxalate crystal, morphology as a function of concentration. Invest Urol 18: 174-177.

18. Sasikala V, Radha SR, Vijayakumari B (2013) *In vitro* evaluation of *Rotula aquatica* Lour. for antiurolithiatic activity. J Pharmacy Res 6: 378-382.

19. Patel PK, Patel MA, Vyas BA, Shah DR, Gandhi TR (2012) Antiurolithiatic activity of saponin rich fraction from the fruits of *Solanum xanthocarpum* Schrad. & Wendl. (Solanaceae) against ethylene glycol induced urolithiasis in rats. J Ethnopharmacol 144: 160-170.

20. Atmani F, Khan SR (2000) Effects of an extract from *Herniaria hirsuta* on calcium oxalate crystallization *in vitro*. BJU Int 85: 621-625.

21. Khan SR (1997) Interactions between stone forming calcific crystals and macromolecules. Urol Int 59: 59-71.

22. Finlayson B (1978) Physicochemical aspects of urolithiasis. Kidney Int 13: 344-360.

23. Chaudhary A, Singla SK, Tandon C (2010) *In vitro* evaluation of *Terminalia arjuna* on calcium phosphate and calcium oxalate crystallization. Indian J Pharmaceutical Sci 72: 340-345.

24. Fleisch H (1978) Inhibitors and promoters of stone formation. Kidney Int 13: 361-371.

25. Masao T (2008) Mechanism of calcium oxalate renal stone formation and renal tubular cell injury. Int J Urol 15: 115-120.

26. Gurocak S, Kupeli B (2006) Consumption of historical and current phytotherapeutic agents for urolithiasis: a critical review. J Urol 176: 450-455.

27. Anand R, Patnaik GK, Kulshreshtha DK, Dhawan BN (1994) Antiurolithiatic activity of lupeol, the active constituent isolated from *Crateva nurvala*. Phytother Res 8: 417-421.

28. Park HK, Jeong BC, Sung M, Park M, Choi EY, et al. (2008) Reduction of oxidative stress in cultured renal tubular cells and preventive effects on renal stone formation by the bioflavonoid quercetin. J Urol 179: 1620-1626.

20

Incidence of Zeeq-un-Nafas Shoabi (Bronchial Asthma) in Individuals of Different Temperaments

Jamal Akhtar[1], Abid Ali Ansari[2]*, Nazema Farhin[3] and Rasheed HMA[4]

[1]Lecturer, Department of Kulliyat, Hakeem Abdul Hameed Unani Medical College, Eidgah road, Dewas (MP), India
[2]Professor & Head Department of Kulliyat, HMS, Unani medical College, Sadashivnagar, Tumkur, Karnataka, India
[3]Department of Kulliyat, Govt. Nizamia Tibbi College, Hyderabad-(AP), India
[4]Professor & Head Department of Kulliyat, Govt. Nizamia Tibbi College, Hyderabad (AP), India

Abstract

Aims and objectives: To know the incidence of *Zeequn Nafas* (Bronchial Asthma) in the patients of different temperaments at Govt. Nizamia General Hospital and College, Charminar, Hyderabad, Andhra Pradesh.

Methodology: Ninety (90) individuals of both the sexes were included in the study between the ages of 20 to 60 years. The duration of the study was 4 months. The eligible individuals were selected randomly on the basis of clinical symptoms, examinations and who were taking bronchodilator drugs. Then their temperaments were assessed by the pre-structured proforma based on *Ajnas-e-Ashra*. To assess the amount of fat in the body "*Slim Guide Skin fold caliper*" was used to measure the skin fold thickness at biceps between the proximal end of radius bone and acromion process. To assess the amount of muscle (Lahm), mid upper arm circumference is measured with tailors tape. Lastly on the basis of total score of *Ajnas-e-Ashra* (10 determinants), a particular *Mizaj* was assigned to the patient.

Results: The study revealed that 40% have *Balghami* (Phlegmatic) temperament, 34% have *Damvi* temperament (Sanguineous) temperament followed by 15 % in *Safravi* (Choleric) and lowest in *Saudavi* (Melancholic) individuals respectively.

Conclusion: On the basis of above results it can be concluded that this disease is more common in *Balghami Mizaj* persons Females are found to be more prone to develop this disease.

Keywords: *Zeequn Nafas;* Bronchial Asthma; *Mizaj; Balghami* (Phlegmatic); Mid upper arm circumference (MUAC); Prevalence

Introduction

Asthma is a common chronic inflammatory disease of the lungs, which shows the symptoms of cough, wheeze, chest tightness and shortness of breath. The number of people with asthma continues to grow. Current estimates suggest that 300 million people worldwide suffer from Bronchial Asthma and in addition 100 million may be diagnosed with Bronchial Asthma by 2025. The strongest risk factors of asthma are allergens such as house dust, mites in bedding, pollens, smoking and chemical irritants etc. This disease may also triggers by cold air, extreme emotion, anger or fear and physical exercise. Delay in diagnosis avoidance triggers may lead to tightening of airway which can be a life threatening condition. Increase in prevalence of such diseases demand their early detection which not only controls the disease but also prevents from other complications. Proper diet, safety measures and change of environment is essential in terms of their benefits which is better than medication [1-3].

This disease is very well recognized since ancient times in Unani system of medicine. Various ancient Unani Scholars and Physicians have use different Arabic terms like *Rabu* (short inspiration and prolonged expiration) [4], *Buhar, Damma, Intesab Nafas* and *Zeequn Nafas* under the caption of bronchial asthma. They also described the etiopathological factors, clinical features, types, and various complications of bronchial asthma that are presented in detail in their concerning treatises [5-8].

As per Unani theory, *Mizaj* (Temperament) is an important pillar and plays a major role whether it is a temperament of any person, drug, or season. Diagnosis and treatment of disease mainly depends on the concept of temperament. Every person from birth is endowed with a unique *Mizaj* (temperament) which represents his healthy state. Health and fitness stays as long as the temperament is in its balanced state and any alteration from normal indicates the disease. Environmental factors *(Asbabe Sitta Zaruriya and Asbabe Ghair Zaruriya)* are mainly responsible for change in normal *Mizaj* (temperament) and occurrence of the disease. Controlling these external factors and maintaining the normal *Mizaj* of a person is an important step in treating the disease in Unani theory. The predisposition towards a disease mainly depends on the *Mizaj* (temperament) such that the incidence of a particular disease will be more in a particular temperament when compared to different temperaments in different phases of their lives. Therefore, the present study was planned with an objective to know the incidence of Asthma *(Zeequn Nafas)* in the patients of different temperaments, So that, awareness of temperament and factors responsible for its alteration can be prevented and controlled to greater extent by providing specific preventive measures.

Keeping these points into consideration, this study was conducted in the patients attending Govt. Nizamia General Hospital and College, Charminar, Hyderabad, Andhra Pradesh.

Methodology

The study was conducted at our Door Patient section of Govt.

---

*Corresponding author: Abid Ali Ansari, Professor & Head Department of Kulliyat, HMS, Unani medical College, Sadashivnagar, Tumkur, Karnataka, India
E-mail: abid_ali1996@yahoo.in

Nizamia General Hospital and College, Charminar, Hyderabad, Andhra Pradesh during the period of Oct 2011 to Jan 2012. Ninety (90) individuals of both the sexes were included in the study between the ages of 20 to 60 years. The eligible individuals were selected randomly on the basis of clinical symptoms, examinations and who were taking Bronchodilator drugs such Asthalin, Theoasthalin or Inhaler. Then their temperaments were assessed by the pre-structured Proforma based on *Ajnas-e-Ashra*.

In addition, two arbitrary parameters were devised to assess the *Mizaj*; to assess the amount of fat in the body *"Slim Guide Skin fold caliper"* is used to measure the skin fold thickness at biceps between the proximal end of radius bone and acromion process. Findings obtained by the instrument were calculated and presented in a mean and standard deviation (SD). To assess the amount of Muscle (Lahm), mid upper arm circumference is measured with tailors tape and presented as mean and Standard deviation (SD) (Figure 1). Lastly on the basis of total score of *Ajnas-e-Ashra* (10 determinants) (Table 1), a particular *Mizaj* was assigned to the patient.

Result and Discussion

According to Unani concept everything in this universe has their own specific *mizaj* (temperament). Every individual has specific temperament even drug and disease have their own specific temperament. According to Unani System of Medicine the management of any disease depends upon the diagnosis of disease. In diagnosis sign, symptom, laboratory findings and *mizaj* play an important role. So the temperament determination is very important in Unani System of Medicine for characterizing a person normal state, as well as the nature of disease.

A maximum number of 40 (44.44%) patients were found *Balghami Mizaj* followed by *Damvi* 34 (37.77%), *Safravi* 15 (16.66%) & *Saudavi Mizaj* 1 (1.11%) respectively (Figure 2 and Table 2). The result clearly indicated that maximum number of the asthmatic patients was *Balghami mizaj* and Unani philosophers also indicated that *Balghami mizaj* patients are at greater risk of *Zeequn Nafas*. Due to the scarcity of previous study in this direction, concurrent inference cannot be drawn but present study shows that *Balghami Mizaj* individuals are more prone to develop *Zeequn Nafas* (asthma). Distributions of Male and Female individuals according to temperament were also noticed (Figure 3 and Table 3). In the present study number of *Balghami mizaj* more in Females than Males. Females are more *Balghami* than Males due to sedentary life and indoor resters. Hence in the present study incidence of *Zeequn Nafas* were maximum in Females as American

S.no	Parameters	Damvi	Balghami	Safravi	Saudavi
1.	Malmas(Touch)	Warm, soft	Cold, soft	Warm, dry	Cold, dry
2.	Lahm wa Shahm (Built) a)Mid arm Circumference	Muscular	Fatty& Broad	Muscular &Thin	Lean
	b)Skin fold Thickness				
3.	Sha'ar (Hair) a)Structure	Thick, Straight	Thin, Straight	Thick, Curly	Thin, Curly
	b) Color	Blackish	Brownish	Black	Brown &White
	d)Growth & distribution	Rapid & Average	Slow & Scanty	Rapid & Profuse	Excessive
4.	Laun-e-badan (Complexion)	Reddish	Whitish(pale)	Yellowish	Blackish
5.	Haiyat-e-Aza a)Physique	Muscular	Fatty	Slim	Lean & Thin
	b)Blood Vessels	Mild Prominent	Not Prominent	More Prominent	Narrow
6.	Kaifiat-e-Inf'al a)Well Tolerance	Dryness	Heat	Cold	Dampness
	b)Blood Vessels	Spring	Summer	Winter	Autumn
7.	Afal-e-Aza a)Appetite	Normal	Less	Increased	False
	b)Digestion	Average	Poor	Strong	Irregular
	c)Physical activity	Average	Lazy & Dull	Hyperactive	Decreased
8.	Fuzlaat-e-Bad a)Stool	Semi solid Brownish	Constipated Whitish	Loose yellowish	Solid Blackish
9.	Naum-wa-Yaqzah a)Sleep	Average	Excessive	Less	Less & disrupted
	b)Sleep Duration/ Day				
10.	Inf'alat-e-Nafsania a)Memory	Good, Long term Retention	Good, can't retain for long time	Not good, short term	Not good but excellent retention
	b)Emotions	Normal	Calm, Quiet	Angry	Nervous
	c)Dreams	Blood red objects	White cold objects	Fiery red or yellow object	Fearful black object

Table 1: Ajnas-e-Ashrah (10 determinants).

Lung Association "Trends in Asthma Morbidity and Mortality" Epidemiology and Statics Unit Research and Program Services Division, July 2011, indicated that the asthma is more common in Females [8]. Distribution of individuals according to Mid Upper arm circumference (MUAC) and temperament in Mean and Standard deviation is shown in Figure 4 and Table 4, which shows that maximum mean of Mid upper arm circumference is found in *Balghami Mizaj* individuals of both the gender i.e., Males (29.5 ± 2.9 cm) and Females (28.8 ± 3.5 cm) followed by *Damvi* and *Safravi Mizaj* individuals. This clearly indicated that the patients of *Zeequn Nafas* are more in overweight or obese. Overweight or obesity comes due to deposition of *Balghami* matter in the body which is greater risk to develop Asthma. *Balgham* are deposited in the body more easily due to sedentary life. There is no previous study in this regard. But in Unani literature *Samne Mufrat* (Obese) individuals are at greater risk to develop *Balghami Amraz* (Diseases). Skin fold thickness are also suggestive of overweight and obesity, obesity are significantly related to asthma as indicated in Anne E. Dixon, et al. a study published in An Official American Thoracic

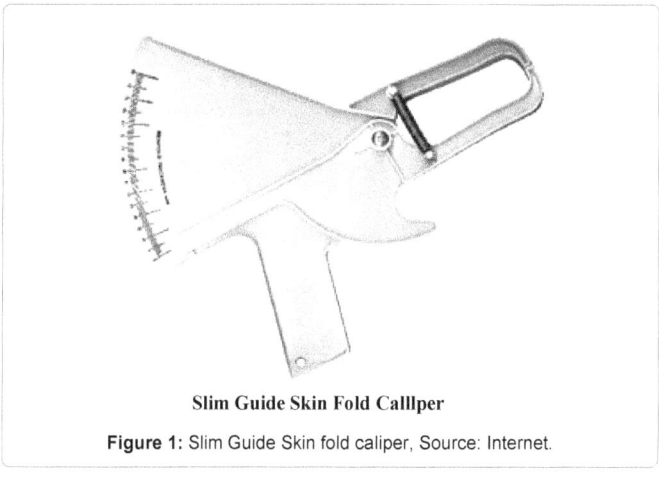

Slim Guide Skin Fold Calliper

Figure 1: Slim Guide Skin fold caliper, Source: Internet.

Society Workshop Report: Obesity and Asthma [9]. In the present study skin fold thickness are found maximum in *Balghami Mizaj* of both sexes as indicated in Figure 5 and Table 5.

Conclusion

In light of above discussion it can be concluded that Balghami *Mizaj* individuals are more prone to develop asthma. Further large scale study is needed for more precise result and community based

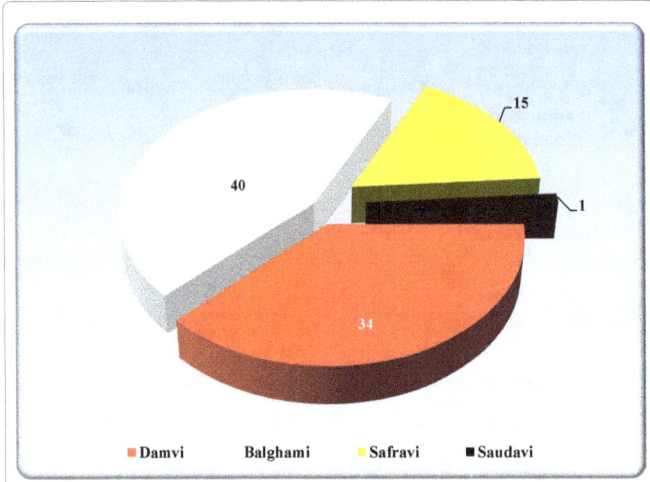

Figure 2: Distribution of Individuals according to temperament.

Temperaments	Frequency	Percentage (%)
Damvi	34	37.77
Balghami	40	44.44
Safravi	15	16.66
Saudavi	01	1.11
Total	90	100

Table 2: Distribution of individuals according to temperament.

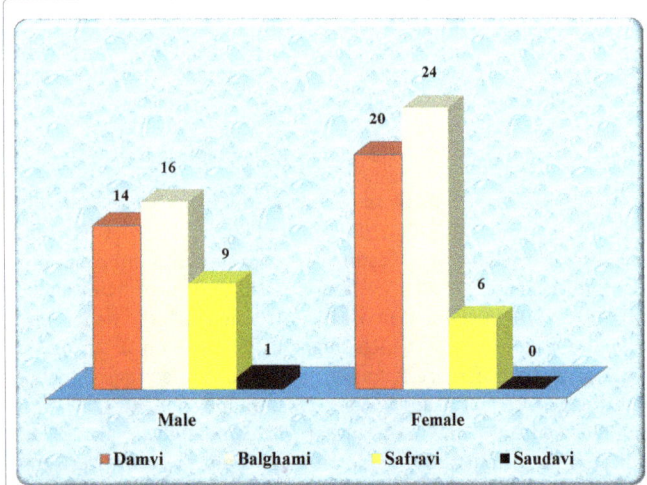

Figure 3: Distribution of male & female individuals according to temperament.

Sex	Damvi	Balghmi	Safravi	Saudavi	Total
Male	14	16	9	1	40
Female	20	24	6	0	50
Total	34	40	15	1	90

Table 3: Distribution of Male & Female Individuals according to Temperament.

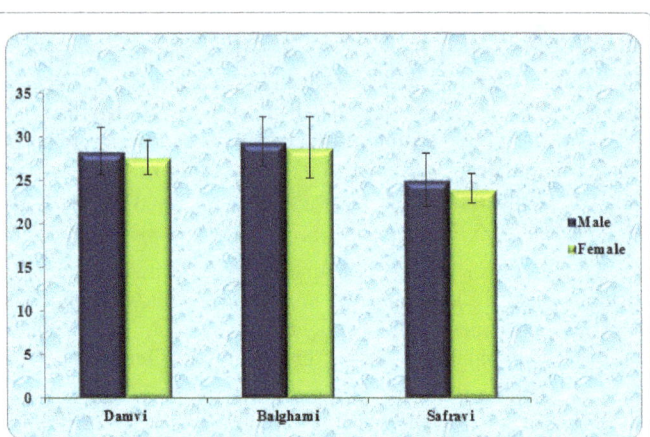

Figure 4: Distribution of individuals according to mid arm circumference and temperament.

Temperament	Mid arm Circumference					
	Male			Female		
	Frequency	Range	Mean ± SD	Frequency	Range	Mean ± SD
Damvi	14	24-36	28.4 ± 2.7	20	25-32	27.7 ± 2.0
Balghami	16	26-34	29.5 ± 2.9	24	20-34	28.8 ± 3.5
Safravi	9	19-31	25.1 ± 3.1	6	22-26	24.1 ± 1.7
Saudavi	1	28	-	0	-	-

Table 4: Distribution of individuals according to mid arm circumference and temperament.

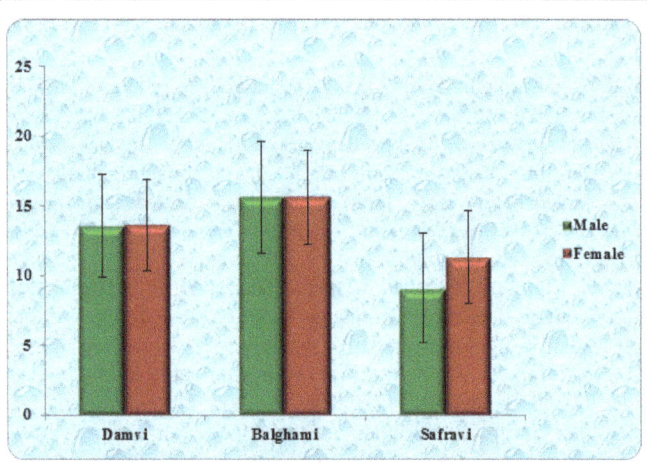

Figure 5: Distributions of individuals according to skin fold thickness and temperament.

Temperament	Skin fold Thickness					
	Male			Female		
	Frequency	Range	Mean ± SD	Frequency	Range	Mean ± SD
Damvi	14	10-19	13.57 ± 3.7	20	7-20	13.65 ± 3.3
Balghami	16	10-20	15.6 ± 4.0	24	8-20	15.62 ± 3.4
Safravi	9	15-16	9.1 ± 3.9	6	8-18	11.33 ± 3.3
Saudavi	1	-	-	0	-	-

Table 5: Distributions of individuals according to Skin fold Thickness and Temperament.

survey are also required for temperamental assessment to provide primary prevention.

Acknowledgement

Authors are deeply indebted to Dr. Arifuddin, Principal, Government Nizamia

Tibbi College, Charminar, Hyderabad for providing necessary facilities for this study. Authors are also highly thankful to Dr. H. M. A. Rasheed, HOD, P.G Department of Kulliyat Government Nizamia Tibbi College, Charminar, Hyderabad, for his supervision and kind co-operation during the study period.

References

1. Kumar P, Clarks M (2009) Clinical Medicine (7thedn), Saunders Elsevier Publication, Philadelphia, USA.

2. Bijanzadeh M, Mahesh PA, Ramachandra NB (2011) An understanding of the genetics basis of asthma, Indian J Med Res 134: 149-161.

3. Yeatts K, Sly P, Shore S, Weiss S, Martinez F, et al. (2006) A brief targeted review of susceptibility factors, environmental exposures, asthma incidence, and recommendations for future asthma incidence research. Environ Health Perspect 114: 634-640.

4. Tabri R (2010) *"Firdausul Hikmat"* Urdu Translation, Idara Kitabul Shifa, 2075,Kucha chelan, New Delhi, India: 195-196.

5. Ibn-sina (2007)*"Al-Qanoon-fi-Tib"*(Vol 3), Idara Kitab-us-Shifa, 2075,Kucha chelan, Daryagunj,New Delhi, India: 279

6. Ismael Jurjani (2010) *"Zakhera Khuwarzim Shahi"*, Urdu translation by Hadi Hussain Khan, Idara Kitab ul-Shifa, New Delhi, India: 257-258.

7. Auz Kirmani, Alama Burhanuddin (Vol 2) "*Shahra-e-Asbab*"Urdu Translation by Alama Kabiruddin, Faisal brothers, Deoband, Delhi, India: 451-454.

8. American Lung Association (2011) "Trends in Asthma Morbidity and Mortality" Epidemiology and Statics Unit Research and Program Services Division.

9. Dixon AE, Holguin F, Sood A, Salome CM, Pratley RE, et al. (2010) An Official American Thoracic Society Workshop Report: obesity and asthma, Proc Am Thorac Soc 7: 325-335.

21

The Effects of Homeopathic Medicines on Reducing the Symptoms of Anxiety and Depression: Randomized, Double Blind and Placebo Controlled

Mandana Bagherian*, Adis Keraskian Mojembari and Mohammad Hakami

Department of Psychology, Karaj Branch, Islamic Azad University, Karaj, Iran

Abstract

Background: Anxiety and depression are two of the most prevalence psychological disorders in the world.

Objective: This study investigates the effects of homeopathic medicine on reducing the symptoms of anxiety and depression.

Method: According to the procedure, thirty patients (twenty female and ten male) with the mean age of 45 (range 22-67) were selected randomly and classified in two experimental and controlling groups. The patients were evaluated based on Beck Depression Inventory (BDI) and Spielberger State-Trait Anxiety Inventory (STAI)-Y. The Pretest – posttest, and follow-up pattern was designed, homeopathic remedies were used and analysis of covariance with repeated measures is used for data analysis.

Results: Findings depict significant differences ($P<0.01$) between two stages of intervention and sustaining of this effectiveness is shown in following-up procedure.

Conclusion: These findings suggest that homeopathic therapy can be used as an effective method to treat anxiety and depression disorders.

Keywords: Anxiety; Beck depression Inventory; Depression; Homeopathy; Spielberger stat-Trait anxiety inventory

Introduction

Anxiety is the most prevalent psychological disorder around the world, which is rated in the first place of mental diseases. Women are engaged twice more than me [1]. According to DSM-5, anxiety is an unreasonable inner anguish or discomfort that can be easily diagnosed from fear which is determined from external reasons. Fear is an emotional response to real or perceived imminent threat, whereas anxiety is an anticipation of future threat. It is associated with physiological agitation and excitement in which the patient is supposed to escape from those situations or stay with imposed tremendous suffering [2].

Depression is also one of the most disabling disorders and as well as anxiety, there is a double rate outbreak among women [1]. DSM-5 classifies depression as a mood disorder that illustrates itself in sadness, aggression and guilty feelings. This derangement is often followed by joylessness; some physiological changes such as, sleep rhythm disorder and appetite decreasing or increasing; suicidal thoughts accompanied by somatic and cognitive changes that significantly affect the individual's capacity of function.

As a natural holistic therapy, homeopathy can significantly reduce symptoms of anxiety and depression. This science is founded by Samuel Hahnemann, German physician (1755-1843) who found that natural remedies by the time that they are potentized can cure natural diseases based on the similar symptoms [3].

Two stages in homeopathic treatment are considerable. One is case taking and other is choosing a simillimum, means similar remedy. The case tacking stage plays a vital role to diagnose patient's disease and find the appropriate remedy. Approaching patient heeling requires taking a picture from all levels of human being, such as physical, mental and emotional. It means that the totality of symptoms should be recorded by a homeopath, even the least important ones. No items should be neglected [4]. For more insurance, a questionnaire can be beneficial.

Furthermore, the patient's relatives are a great to help complete the patient image [5]. The second stage is to find the best remedy according to the patient's report. Remedies are originated from any natural sources or materials in the nature. Each substance which can make some symptoms in healthful person is potential to destroy those very symptoms in sick one On the other hand, each substance has some effects on human body, and patients who have those symptoms similar to them, will be cured by getting pointing substance. There are two processes to provide homeopathic remedies: dilution and shacking. Dilution is used for reclining toxic effects and omitting side effects of substances. As these dilutions proceed in several scales, Decimal, Centesimal and other potencies, they can provide a range of doses utilized for different purposes. Shacking is used to make the remedies dynamic [5].

The differentiation feature between homeopathy and other medicines is following the holistic principles. Focusing on the patient instead of the disease, considering a patient as a whole, eliminating the fundamental reasons of the diseases verses omitting symptoms, restoring health to all levels of body and preserving it by enhancing defense mechanism; and the last but not the least, using natural remedies which will not put harmful effects on body, obviously, make homeopathy more powerful than the other routine therapies.

*Corresponding author: Bagherian M, Department of Psychology, Karaj Branch, Islamic Azad University, Karaj, Iran
E-mail: waghuladehema@gmail.com

Therefore, while the patient's chief complaints are under treatment, other symptoms will be also cured [5].

One of the fundamental ideas about the homeopathic remedy is that a remedy is curative when it is prescribed on the basis of patient's deepest level of experience and his or her vital sensation. At that level, there is an energy that corresponds to something non-human, something which is like a plant, mineral or animal. It seems like nonsense. It is as if there are two songs playing inside the same person: the human part, which is supposed to be there, and the non-human which isn't. The song of the remedy will express itself with the language of its kingdom: plant sensitivity, mineral structure, or animal survival. It will express itself precisely as the song of the substance [6].

The philosophy of homeopathy is to find what is curable in disease. The answer will appear when the physician has knowledge about the real nature of the patient. To reach this goal, all of the patient's symptoms in all levels of human body should be taken, so, after that the crucial reasons of diseases will be revealed. Afterwards, removing the disease with restoring health, the very aim of homeopathy, will happen [7,8].

Homeopathy can be used for treatment of psychological disorders such as anxiety and depression. Moreover, some studies have shown the homeopathic effectiveness on other psychological abnormalities, such as PTSD, acute stress disorder, and Trauma [9]. Many psychiatric problems can be relieved by homeopathic therapy in clinical approaches. A study results claimed that in many clinical findings homeopathy can cure schizophrenia, autism, OCD, agoraphobia, suicidal depression, hysteria, sleep disorders as well [3]. Some studies of case analysis have shown the curative effects of homeopathic remedies for fears and phobia [10].

Although, many researches have been conducted conversely, more comprehensible investigations are necessary. A research acknowledged that homeopathic remedies have significant effects on depression. To find this result, they chose 30 patients randomly from 162 participants examined by self-report long-term questionnaire that has shown depression. They divided into two experimental and control groups and they were monitored for 6 to 12 months after intervention [11]. Another research demonstrated that homeopathic remedy can treat major depression. They worked on 228 patients randomized in 2 groups, experimental group which took homeopathic remedy and control group which took placebo [12]. One study that used homeopathic – complex remedy to treat anxiety and sleep disorders [13]. One research that has been done for Over- the- Counter- drugs (OTC) for the treatment of mood and anxiety disorders found that Herbal drugs and Homeopathic formulations which were used most frequently than the others are so beneficial for depression, anxiety, and sleep disorders. This investigation was done by 690 German pharmacists, using OTC drugs, about 12 costumers per day [8]. Another research has done based on the Characteristics, associated with use of homeopathic drugs for psychiatric symptoms in general population. They worked on 36,785 persons participating in the Mental Health Survey in general population. The result has shown the significant reducing in psychiatric symptoms [14].

The research question is: "Can Homeopathy reduce the symptoms of anxiety and depression?"

Method

Design

This search is a quasi- experimental survey, which is done in pretest post-test with following-up stages. Statistical pattern is analysis of covariance with repeated measures. This present study includes three stages: first assessment of patients in the baseline. Participants were evaluated by related questionnaires at the first phase of research, so, anxiety and depression rates were determined. In the second stage appropriate remedy was prescribed for them according to homeopathic principles. The third one was monitoring and following-up the patients to show the effects of intervention on corresponding groups.

Participants

The 30 patients were sampled from whom that referred to the Homeopathic Center in Iran, Tehran since November 2013 to April 2014. The trial using 2×2 factorial designs with 16 weeks of study duration per patient was performed. Patients were randomized to one of the two groups: 1) Homeopathic group, 2) Placebo group. During the first visit, patients who had anxiety and depression treated by classical homeopathic remedy (constitutional therapy) 30C potencies and for control group, placebo was prescribed. This trial was performed in double blind study.

Materials

Homeopathy questionnaire: According to the homeopathic laws, finding an appropriate remedy especially in classical approach needs taking a comprehensive picture of patient which involved totality of the symptoms in all levels of human beings. This questionnaire designed to reach this goal and for the patients, who are not interested in talking about some symptoms or suffers from lack of memory, so they can write those [14].

Emotional assessment instruments: The anxiety was measured by using State-Trait Anxiety Inventory (STAI-Y) including 20 anxiety symptoms that patients show complementary, and 20 anxiety symptoms which participants depict frequently. Scores ranges between (20-80), with the higher score indicating great anxiety in two mentioned states. This test has good internal consistency (.74) and test-retest reliability (88) and (93) for state anxiety and (92) and (94) for trait anxiety) [6].

The depression levels of participants were measured using Depression Inventory (BDI) including 21 depression symptoms that participants rated for that moment. Scores ranges between"14-63", with the higher score indicating great depression. The internal consistency is (86) and test-retest reliability is (93) [15].

Homeopathic intervention: As it · was mentioned before, homeopathic medicines were used in constitutional way to relief patients' anxiety and depression. All remedies are prepared in homeopathic way, well-potentized and are used only in 30- potency according to classical approach. Single dose method with monitoring is prescribed.

Procedures

The given sample was categorized in gender and marital status; homeopathic group: 10 women, 5 men, case history, and placebo group: 10 women, 5 men, and case history. Patients took remedy in the first visit and they were followed up for 16 weeks and all the symptoms and clinical signs were controlled. The patients should have been examined by inventories each section and the numbers of their anxiety and depression were caught. Each patient had the rights to participate and they could leave it as soon as they decided. The 30C potencies of homeopathic remedies in constitutional approach were prescribed. Written informed consent was obtained from all patients. And after the end of the research, the entire control group was treated by homeopathic remedy.

Results

Baseline characteristics

Mean number and standard deviation of depression and anxiety (state and trait) in two groups experimental and control), during pretest, posttest and follow-up, has shown in Table 1.To find the effects of homeopathic remedies on reducing anxiety (state and trait) and depression symptoms, analysis covariance with repeated measures has been used. According to homoscedasticy for depression [$F_{(1,28)}$=0.542, p=0.468] , state anxiety [$F_{(1,28)}$=0.787, p=0.383] and trait anxiety [$F_{(1,28)}$=2.403, p=0.132]; linear relationship between pretest-posttest depression [$F_{(1,26)}$=98.321, p<0.01] and state anxiety[$F_{(1,26)}$=70.371, p<0.01] and trait anxiety [$F_{(1,26)}$=68.440, p<0.01] numbers ; and regression slope for depression [$F_{(1,26)}$=1.699, p=0.204] ,state anxiety [$F_{(1,26)}$=1.470, p=0.236] and trait anxiety [$F_{(1,26)}$=1.226, p=0.278] are equal; the results of analysis and ANOVA analysis for depression and anxiety(state and trait) numbers are shown in Table 2.

Anxiety and depression measures

The results of ANCOVA (Table 2) show the significant differences between modified post-tests of two groups (experimental and control). In other hand:

- The average of depression post-test in experimental group after elimination of pretest effect (16.81) was lower than the average of post-test in control group after elimination of pretest effect (29.6).

- The average of state anxiety post-test in experimental group after elimination of pretest effect (52.71) was lower than the average of posttest in control group after elimination of pretest effect (60.96).

- The average of trait anxiety post-test in experimental group after elimination of pretest effect (45.38) was lower than the

average of post-test in control group after elimination of pretest effect (60.55).

These findings show the effectiveness of homeopathic therapy to decrease anxiety and depression symptoms.

To assess the stability of effectiveness of homeopathy to reduce anxiety and depression, variance analysis with repeated measurement has been used. The results were shown in Table 3, with normal multivariate data distribution, the summery of analysis and variance analysis with repeated measurement, and the comparison of 3- time measurements of variables in experimental group.

Stability of effectiveness

According to the findings of variance analysis and two by two comparisons of mean numbers in this research results show that (Table 3) the effect of homeopathic therapy in reducing anxiety and depression symptoms has stability.

Discussion

According to the statistical findings, homeopathic remedies can reduce anxiety and depression symptoms dramatically. Many previous researches have shown this effect and confirmed obtained results. Although more researches show the odd ratio of homeopathic therapy in treating psychological abnormalities, some others have the opposite consequences that are considerable. For discussing about the approving homeopathic effects and talking about for and against concepts, researchers preferred to review other researchers' findings. Initially, it should be mentioned that one study showed seriously that the effects of homeopathic remedies were accurate and those were not just placebo effects [16]. Some of researches have shown that homeopathic remedies can cure anxiety and sleep disorders, and their findings are aligned with this very research [17]; some studies reported that the homeopathic medicines are useful to cure social anxiety, panic disorder and manic

variable	group	n	pretest		posttest		Follow-up	
			M	SD	M	SD	M	SD
depression	E	15	33.13	6.42	18.00	4.69	13.33	5.27
	C	15	29.87	9.78	27.87	8.18	26.87	8.99
State anxiety	E	15	64.27	7.62	53.93	6.53	46.00	8.61
	C	15	61.40	8.68	59.73	9.50	59.13	9.81
Trait anxiety	E	15	65.47	7.70	48.47	7.67	43.40	8.02
	C	15	59.27	10.54	57.47	12.90	57.87	13.09

$**P<0.01$

Table 1: Mean number for each condition during pretest, posttest and follow-up and standard deviation of depression and state-trait anxiety.

Dependent Variable: post test	Source	Sum of Squares	df	Mean Square	F	Partial Eta Squared
Depression	Covariate	1025.785	1	1025.785		
	Fixed Factor (E-C)	1081.601	1	1081.601	132.773 **	0.832
	Error	219.949	27	8.146		
	Corrected Total	1975.867	29			
State anxiety	Covariate	1357.618	1	1357.618		
	Fixed Factor (E-C)	493.532	1	4393.532	26.531**	0.496
	Error	502.249	27	18.602		
	Corrected Total	2112.167	29			
Trait anxiety	Covariate	2365.107	1	2365.107		
	Fixed Factor (E-C)	1540.426	1	1540.726	52.767**	0.662
	Error	788.360	27	29.199		
	Corrected Total	3760.967	29			

$**P<0.01$

Table 2: The results of analysis and covariance analysis.

variable	Mauchly's test of sphericity			Repeated Measure		Two by two comparison results
	Mauchly's W	$X^2_{(df=2)}$	Greenhouse-Geisser Epsilon	df	F	
Depression	0.796	2.962	0.831	2,28	151.771 **	pre-test>post-test>follow-up
State anxiety	0.556	7.637*	0.692	1.38,19.39	72.844 **	pre-test>post-test>follow-up
Trait anxiety	0.301	15.624**	0.588	1.18,16.48	172.501 **	pre-test>post-test>follow-up

*$P<0.05$, **$P<0.01$

Table 3: Analysis and variance analysis with repetitive measurements for experimental group.

depression [5,18], which is similar to the result of the research; one research confirmed the capability of homeopathic treatment in medical sciences [15]. This finding shows alignment with this research; a recent study has acknowledged the effects of homeopathy in mood disorders and anxiety that is aligned with current research [10]; in one study that used constitutional homeopathic intervention to cure psychological disorders especially anxiety, depicted the effects of homeopathic remedies on curing those disorders. Researchers reported that women, youngsters and well-educated people showed higher effects [7]; a study resulted that homeopathy can cure depression [1]. This finding has alignment with this present research; findings of some researchers have the same results. The other research reported that homeopathic therapy has significant effects on insomnia [19-25]. All of these mentioned researches have shown the power of homeopathic remedies to treat psychological disorders such as anxiety, depression and others; while, some findings report that it doesn't have any significant effect on mood and psychological disturbances.

In a recent study, homeopathic remedies were used for patients who suffered from cancer. Although this intervention had many significant consequences in reducing clinical symptoms, it didn't have the same effects on fatigue, anxiety, depression and mood disturbances of those patients [8]. On the other hand, one study acknowledged that the combined odd ratio for the 89 studies entered into the main meta-analysis was 2.45 in favor of homeopathy, the odds ratio was 1.66 and the corrected for publication bias was 1.78 [16].

The question is why some findings have shown that homeopathy doesn't have significant effects on mental and emotional state. To answer, we should mention that homeopathy has some principles that must be considered during intervention [9]. If these rules are neglected, the results are changed. So, it can be resulted that, in some cases, disrespecting these rules, may lead in differences in those findings. These rules are [1] patients should know about homeopathy and remedy and their diseases prognosis as well [2] they should change their lives and remove barriers [3] patients have to know about their exiting and sustaining causes to omit obstacles and change their life style [4] homeopath should do without judgment or bias and just record patients symptoms [5] simillimum remedy should be prescribed [6] remedies must be well-made and well-potentized [7] the doses and potencies of homeopathic remedies should be taken correctly [9,23-27].

References

1. Sadock BJ, Sadock VA, Kaplan HI (2007) Kaplan & Sadock's Synopsis of psychiatry behavioral sciences. (Translated by Farzin Rezai, 2012).

2. American Psychiatric Association (2013) Diagnostic and statistical manual of mental disorders, fifth edition, American psychiatric publishing.

3. Johannes K, Zee VDH (2009) Homeopathy and mental health care. Home links.

4. Vithoulkas G (2012) Talks on classical homeopathy. B.Jain.

5. Groth-Marnt G (2003) Handbook of psychological assessment. (Translated by Sharifi HP & Nikh khoo MR, 2012).

6. Naude FD, Couchman SM, Maharaj A (2010) Chronic primary insomnia: Efficacy of homeopathic simillimum. Homeopathy. 99: 63-68.

7. Hahnemann S (1989) Organon of medicine. Berkeley international university press.

8. Hamann J, Lind K, Schweiger HD, Kusmakow O, Forstl J (2014) Over-the-Counter-Drugs for treatment of mood and anxiety disorders-The view of German pharmacists. Georg Thieme Verlag KG Stuttgart.

9. Chappell, Peter (2003) Emotional healing with homeopathy- treating the effects of trauma. North Atlantic books.

10. Guethlin C, Walach H, Naumann J, Bartsch HH, Rostock M (2010) Characteristics of cancer patients using homeopathy compared with those in conventional care: a cross-sectional study. Ann Oncol 21: 1094-1099.

11. Viksveen P, Relton C (2014) Depression treated by homeopaths: A study protocol for a pragmatic cohort multiple randomized controlled trial. Homeopathy. 103: 147-152.

12. Adler C, Kruger S, Teut M, Ludtke R, Schutzler L, et al. (2013) Homeopathy for depression: a randomized, partially double-blind, placebo-controlled, four-armed study (DEP-HOM). Plos one. 8: e74537.

13. Montanaro F, Coppola L (2013) Effect of a homeopathic-complex medicine on state and trait anxiety and sleep disorders: a retrospective observational study. Homeopathy. 102: 254-261.

14. Grolleau A, Begaud B, Verdoux H (2013) Characteristics associated with use of homeopathic drugs for psychiatric symptoms in the general population. Homeopathy 102: 254-261.

15. Bucher JN, Mineka S, Hooley J (2007) Abnormal psychology. (Translated by Mohammadi YS, 2012).

16. Davidson JR, Morrison RM, Shore J, Davidson RT, Bedayn G (2012) Homeopathic treatment of depression and anxiety. Altern the Health Med 3: 46-49.

17. Kent TJ (1921) Lectures on homeopathic Materia Medica. B. Jain publishers.

18. Kent TJ (2002) The art and science of homeopathic medicine. Dover.

19. Kent TJ (2006) Lectures on philosophy. Berkeley international university press.

20. Lert F, Grimaldi-Bensouda L, Rouillon F, Massol J, Guillemot D, et al. (2012) Characteristics of patents consulting their regular primary care physician according to their prescribing preferences for homeopathy and complementary medicine. Homeopathy103: 51-57.

21. Linde K, Clausius N, Ramirez G, Melchart D, and et al. (1997) Are the clinical effects of homeopathy placebo effects: a meta-analysis of placebo controlled trials. The Lancet Journal. 350: 834-843.

22. Morrison R, Herrick N (2012) Psychiatric disorders with relevant remedies for anxiety, fear & phobia. Bjain press.

23. Sankran R (2007) Sensation refined. Homeopathic medical publishers.

24. Schmidt JM (2014) New approaches within the history and theory of medicine and their relevance for homeopathy. Homeopathy 103: 153-159.

25. Shang A , Huwiter-Muntener K , Nartey L, Juni P, Dorig S, Sterne JA, et al. (2005) Are the clinical effects of homeopathy placebo effects: Comparative study of placebo-controlled trials of homeopathy and allopathy. The Lancet. 366: 726-732.

26. Swayne J (2000) International dictionary of homeopathy. Churchill livingstone.

27. Vithoulkas G, Van Woensel E (2010) Levels of health. International academy of classical homeopathy.

22

HIV/AIDS Education in Traditional Indian Systems of Medicine: Faculty Perspectives

Jayagowri Sastry[1]*, Vineeta Deshmukh[2], Vijay Dhoiphode[3], Asmita Wele[4], Manisha Solanki[5], Farha Rizwan[6], Amita Gupta[7] and Anita Shankar[8]

[1]Head, Department of Clinical Research & Development, Shrimati Kashibai Navale Medical College and General Hospital (SKNMC-GH), Pune, India
[2]Bharatiya Sanskriti Darshan Trust's Ayurved Hospital and Research Center, Pune, India
[3]Tilak Ayurved Mahavidyalaya, Pune, India
[4]Bharati Vidyapeeth College of Ayurved, Pune, India
[5]Dhondumama Sathe Homeopathic Medical College, Pune, India
[6]ZVM Unani Medical College, Azam Campus, Pune, India
[7]Johns Hopkins School of Medicine, USA
[8]Johns Hopkins School of Public Health, USA

Abstract

Background and objective: There are over 500 colleges within the Indian System of Medicine and Homeopathy (ISM & H) that includes Ayurveda, Yoga and Naturopathy, Unani, Siddha and Homeopathy (AYUSH). Therapies from AYUSH are widely utilized throughout India for both acute and chronic illnesses and may be an important source of care for HIV-infected individuals. This qualitative study documents faculty perspectives within AYUSH institutions of higher learning to understand how the etiology, diagnosis and treatment of HIV/AIDS is taught within their curriculum.

Methods: Thirty-three faculty and student informants from five AYUSH institutions in Pune and one College of Siddha in Chennai were interviewed from June 2009-August 2010. Topics included etiology, pathogenesis, diagnostics, treatment and management of HIV/AIDS within each system.

Results: Thematic analysis revealed that although generally biomedical textbooks were used to provide the background training on HIV/AIDS and diagnostics, the pathogenesis and symptomatology allowed the disease entity to fit into established disease concepts within the relevant AYUSH system. Each AYUSH system viewed HIV as an amalgam of conditions and abnormal lifestyles leading to the disease. In general, in AYUSH, there was greater reference to religion and a moral component in disease management and prevention. Faculty from Ayurveda, Unani and Siddha faculty stressed the need for positive health promotion through lifestyle changes in diet and adherence to healthful daily routines. AYUSH faculty believed in referring patients to biomedicine for antiretroviral therapy (ART), although indicated that alternative treatments may be provided in addition to ART.

Conclusions: There is no formal inclusion of AYUSH treatments within the national Indian HIV health policy, yet AYUSH practitioners exceed that of medical doctors. Greater efforts are needed to identify areas of collaboration between experts in biomedicine and AYUSH medical systems in India.

Keywords: Complementary and alternative medicine & HIV/AIDS; HIV/AIDS; HIV/AIDS teaching; Indian traditional medicine; Traditional medicine; ISM&H

Introduction

In India, HIV-infected individuals face numerous challenges in their search for treatments. Currently, western allopathic medicine (hereinafter 'biomedicine') offers antiretroviral therapy (ART) for HIV/AIDS and associated co-morbidities that have prolonged survival and improved quality of life [1-3]. Estimates of ART coverage are between 39%-54% and significant numbers of HIV-infected individuals continue to explore alternative treatment options due to ART toxicities, resistance and associated expenditures [4-7]. The Indian System of Medicine and Homeopathy includes multiple medical systems as Ayurveda, Yoga and Naturopathy, Unani, Siddha, and Homeopathy (AYUSH) and has existed for centuries before the rise of biomedicine. While there is a dearth of current data available, it is estimated that almost 65% of India's rural population uses AYUSH for primary health care [8] and 70%–80% of the general population uses AYUSH at some point [9-11]. In recent years the numbers of registered AYUSH practitioners have begun to decline (after experiencing a peak in 2010) but are still roughly equal to the number of biomedical doctors at over 600,000 for the country [12-14].

In areas of medical innovation and expertise, it is generally accepted that academic institutions are most likely to have consolidated, reviewed and tested the most effective approaches to healing. Institutes of higher learning for AYUSH are well established throughout India, with over 254 Ayurvedic medical colleges, 185 Homeopathic colleges, nearly 40 Unani colleges and 7 Siddha colleges [15]. The objective of this paper is to document the role of AYUSH for HIV/AIDS in India from the perspectives of faculty and students within a sample of institutions of higher learning.

Methods

Study design

Qualitative methods were used to interview 26 faculty and 7

*Corresponding author: Jayagowri Sastry, Department of Clinical Research & Development, Shrimati Kashibai Navale Medical College and General Hospital (SKNMC-GH), 49/1, Off Westerly Bypass Highway, Narhe (Ambegaon), Pune 411041, India
E-mail: gowsas@gmail.com, gowrisastry@skhnmcgh.org

students from five AYUSH institutions in Pune, Maharashtra (three Ayurvedic, one Homeopathic and one Unani College) and one Siddha College in Chennai, Tamil Nadu. The 33 key informants were from a range of departments and included department heads, professors, lecturers and students with at least two years of learning. The faculty and students were chosen based on their knowledge of HIV/AIDS education or clinical exposure to HIV-infected patients.

All interviews were conducted by trained data collectors using structured discussion guides and written consent was obtained from all respondents. Interviews were taped if prior consent was obtained. Interview guides were prepared for each branch of alternate medicine after several consultations with the collaborating AYUSH faculty from Pune.

Period

Data collection was purposive and carried out between June 2009 and August 2010 in Pune and Chennai, India with the following number of interviews: Ayurveda: 11 faculty and 3 student; Homeopathy: 9 faculty and 1 student; Unani: 5 faculty and 1 student and Siddha: 1 faculty and 2 student. If there was difficulty in understanding certain concepts at the time of transcription, participants were contacted for a second interview to seek clarifications. Translated transcripts were used for analysis from these interviews. Secondary data such as course plans, syllabi, degree programs, textbooks, etc. were also reviewed.

Data processing and analysis

Every interview was read twice and a summary of its salient points made along with the background information of the respondent. Using these summaries, a master list of codes was drawn up separately for each alternate system of medicine. Coding of the interviews and qualitative data analysis was done manually by two coders. Reliability testing was done on 10% of the interviews and discrepancies were reviewed and resolved through discussion. Data were coded, codes were grouped into categories and emerging themes were then identified iteratively following the general principles of grounded theory [16]. Results are presented as broad themes related to the relationship between biomedicine and AYUSH as well as specific data on the nature of the teachings of HIV/AIDS within AYUSH.

Ethical approval for study

This study was approved by the HMSC and the ethical committees of BJ Medical College and Sassoon General Hospitals, Pune, India, YRG Foundation IRB, Chennai, India and the Johns Hopkins IRB, USA.

Results

The role of biomedicine in AYUSH is central in the teaching of HIV/AIDS

There has been intention to integrate biomedicine within AYUSH in India by teaching the principles of the former to the graduates of AYUSH and vice versa [17]. AYUSH systems are required by the national government to cover certain 'biomedical concepts' including cell biology, germ theory and immunology. In addition, many students of Ayurveda and Unani intern for about six months, at a biomedical hospital. Ayurvedic and Unani practitioners are fully licensed to practice and prescribe medicines both from Ayurveda/Unani and biomedicine.

Respondents confirmed that students are given a background in the biomedical understanding of HIV, including modes of transmission,

pathogenesis and prevention. However, they emphasized that this information was to supplement the specific AYUSH conceptualizations of HIV infection, so that students can have a fundamental grasp of the principles of biomedicine in order to function effectively in India's modern medical system. HIV is a new disease and is therefore not mentioned in any of the classic texts on which these systems are based and none of these systems utilize the concepts of infection and germ theory to explain the etiology of specific diseases. While students are taught the basics of biomedical therapy, patients are advised to visit a biomedical physician for ART.

Ayurvedic principles for the treatment and management of HIV

Explanation of HIV etiology: In Ayurveda, the concept of AIDS falls under decreased immunity by disturbances in *dhatu, dosha, Agni* (biological energy system of the body responsible for transformation as the various enzymes present in the elementary canal, liver and the tissue cells that helps with all kinds of metabolic and digestive activity of the body), and *mala* (waste products). The *dhatu*, responsible for overall process of regeneration of all the tissues in the body (governs or controls phenomena of cell reproduction), is also co-related with the pathogenesis of HIV/AIDS. In the case of HIV the initial imbalance in the body is thought to come from improper sexual behavior that oversteps the normal guidelines established in the Ayurvedic treatises.

Improper sex that oversteps the guidelines of *brahmacharya* is defined as 1) sex with too many partners, promiscuity 2) sex without urge 3) sex with an inappropriate partner (such as a commercial sex worker) and unnatural sex (such as between two men). There is also the concept of "*Sadvartan*" (good behavior) that is taught to first, second and third year students.

Diagnostic tools and treatment: The Ayurvedic diagnostic approach is independent of a patient's HIV status and does not depend on laboratory tests or imaging. It consists of patient's history and physical exam from which a practitioner infers the state of the *doshas, dhatu* and *Agni* in a patient. Then, along with medicine, the patient is counseled about the "*Aahar*" (diet), so that many follow "*Pathya*" (Things we should eat that would be helpful to our constitution) and "*Apathya*" (Things we should avoid eating as they could be harmful to our constitution) diet. Patients are also told about "*Vihar*" (behavior, movement).

Relevant curriculum: Most faculties expressed that Ayurveda has expanded to include newer or emerging infections such as HIV and AIDS that are generally discussed for two or three lectures. Students are taught the diagnosis, clinical features, treatment and management of the disease using both biomedicine and Ayurvedic principles in their undergraduate years.

Unani principles for the treatment and management of HIV

HIV etiology: Before HIV was properly understood among Unani physicians, it was considered an *Amraz-e-Zohriya* (Peeth), a venereal disease. *Zohriya* translates as backside, since HIV was originally a disease of homosexual men and hence this disease was placed in this category.

The Unani faculty generally accepts the biomedical model of HIV etiology as the correct way to interpret disease causation. The term *Qillat-e-Manaat* (immunity power) was in use long before the discovery of the immune system or the development of germ theory, and was originally used to simply denote someone who seemed to get sick more than was normal. When dealing with HIV in the present day, many Unani physicians (hakims) will send patients for a laboratory test of CD[4+] counts and then will use the results as a more quantitative indicator of the patient's *Qillat-e-Manaat*. Faculty indicated that Unani attaches a negative moral appraisal to all sexually transmitted infections (STI) and considers them a punishment for improper sexual behavior.

Diagnostic tools and treatment: Unani students are taught to fit HIV into the humoral theory of disease. Most of the Unani physicians agree that imbalance of the humor blood causes HIV infection; however, the symptoms a patient presents will determine particular diagnosis and treatment and may differ by individual. Additional supports include: 1) Cupping (*Hijama*) given to alleviate pain 2) *Maqqavi Aza-e-Raeesa advia* tonics to support vital organs and immunity and 3) *Ilaj-bil-giza* special diet therapy.

Relevant curriculum: HIV is included in the curriculum during the pathology course, first when the students discuss the etiology of the cold, wet temperament (*balgham*) with which HIV is usually associated, and when students discuss immunity problems or *Qillat-e-Manaat*. There is also time set aside to address HIV as a specific disease. This is done from a biomedical approach, and then again from a Unani approach as part of the section on STIs. Students learn about the Unani concept of pathology, based around the theory of four humors and an individual's temperament. In general, HIV is usually associated with a switch in a person's temperament towards one that is colder and wetter, more phlegmatic, as patients usually present with cough and cold.

Siddha principles for the treatment and management of HIV

HIV etiology: HIV is taught as "*vettai noi*" or '*theivu noi*'. From the original Siddha literature, *Theivu Noi* "will make our body to give up all good cells". This disease will make the body "like a dry tree". Other names mentioned are: "*vellai noi, mega noi*". "*Vellai*" is white discharge and "*mega noi*" is an STI. Faculties also mention male and female genital disorders of 21 types, most of which are caused due to wrong diet and excessive sex causing depletion of *prana* (life force). By stating this, Siddha medicine does not mean to judge people or make a moral stand but it is argued that meaningless sex depletes a person emotionally, physically and spiritually. It emphasized that the fundamental concept of the body's immunity is heavily depleted by excess indulgence as stated by the Siddhars. Siddhars have evaluated that Azhal thathu (same as dhatu) is responsible for the defense of the body.

Diagnostic tools and treatment: In response to general treatment for HIV that includes other chronic illnesses, a faculty detailed that a primary treatment includes *Rasa Gandhi Melugu*, a mercury preparation with some additional 40 drugs. Other drugs like Kodiveli, (*Plumbago zeylanica Linn*, belonging to the family Plumbaginaceae), Panaivellam (palm jaggery), Garlic, Sukku (dry ginger), *Melagu* (wax), and *Thippili* (Indian long pepper or piperum longum) are also added to that so it comes into a form of *melugu*. Rasam means mercury and Kandhagam means sulphur that is used as broad spectrum antibiotic. The need to enhance immunity in the body, through diet and medication was also stressed.

Relevant curriculum: There is no specific place for the teaching of HIV in the Siddha curriculum. However, there is a special out-patient department for HIV-infected persons and students are taken to observe the wards. Undergraduate students are usually taught the basics about HIV in their final year. Mostly the focus is on prevention, since that is thought more important than understanding what is needed for a cure. For example, adolescents are counseled practice abstinence to focus on

their career since HIV "will spoil the future". Use of condom and clean needles is also mentioned.

Homeopathic principles for the treatment and management of HIV

HIV etiology: The concept of HIV etiology is the same in homeopathy and biomedicine except that infection occurs when the vital force is weakened. The faculty interviewed identified the major difference between homeopathy and biomedicine as different approach to treatment, rather than different explanations of biological phenomena. Homeopaths place emphasis on the supposed miasm (susceptible constitutional types) when treating a patient, and will identify the miasm based on the symptoms that are presenting at the time, rather than on the diagnosis of a particular disease such as HIV. HIV is considered a mixed miasm disease, with different miasms presenting at different times depending on the characteristics of the patient.

Diagnostic tools and treatment: Homeopaths use both case histories and biomedical laboratory tests to track the progress of HIV treatment. There is no such homeopathic medicine "for" HIV. The prescription of medications is based only on a patient's presenting symptoms, not on the presence of the virus. The strength of the vital force or the susceptibility governs whether a person will contract HIV, when and how opportunistic infections will manifest, and when a patient will progress from HIV to AIDS.

Relevant curriculum: Most of the information students receive about the conceptualization and management of HIV under the AYUSH systems comes from their professors' own understanding, journal articles, booklets published by faculty members and websites or are interpreted from the AYUSH reference books. In Homeopathy, HIV is formally discussed under the section for skin and venereal diseases. Students learn the pathology of HIV from a biomedical perspective. The clinical features of HIV are discussed in the subject of Medicine, including presenting symptoms, etiology, common complications and aspects of prevention.

'Morality' and 'class' of society and HIV in India

One interesting finding that emerged during the in-depth interviews from all the examined medical systems was the 'moral' and religious association with HIV and its spread. According to one Ayurvedic respondent, an important way to way to reduce HIV "is imparting education about moral values." When asked about preventive measures used in their field, a Homeopath says: "basic ethics, condom" When asked if an entity such as HIV or AIDS exists in Unani: "This entire thing (HIV) is in Unani, it is sexually transmitted, it is there, and if it is done with the wrong female or male, 80% people gets that who does wrong. We have gonorrhea, syphilis in the main diseases here and we correlate it with this and according to that, and it is a punishment to that person that he cannot save his life".

Discussion

A growing number of studies have investigated the role of AYUSH for HIV/AIDS [6,18-23] but few have examined AYUSH educators understanding of HIV/AIDS [24] despite the fact that AYUSH practitioners nearly equal that of biomedical doctors.

The proportion of HIV-infected adults who access traditional medicines in developing countries is estimated to be very high [6,7,21,22,25]. Across all AYUSH systems, biomedical concepts were central to the teaching and discussion of HIV/AIDS. While each

AYUSH system begins with grounding in biomedical theory and treatment, these concepts are placed within the larger construct of their specific medical tradition. AYUSH systems teach students about HIV/AIDS using biomedical texts and tools diagnostics but have found a place in their own texts to support the causation and treatment of the various symptoms that are manifested in HIV-infected individuals.

The systematic nature of learning and practice in each AYUSH tradition differs from what has been reported elsewhere where HIV is a significant public health issue [26]. However, the curriculum on HIV/AIDS with AYUSH institutions is still developing and relies in large part on the faculty efforts to incorporate this information in their training.

Each AYUSH system focuses on understanding a deeper root cause of disease that exposes patients to infection or disorder, generally referred to as "vital force" that leave a person susceptible to disease. Although treating disease in the biomedical sense may ameliorate symptoms, it does nothing to correct the vital force itself and therefore does not address the true cause of illness, leaving the patient open to relapse or future infection [27]. While vital force many be considered generally by the biomedical community to correspond to the strength of the immune system, vital force is much more encompassing with respect to the overall health of the person and includes both body and mind. This more holistic view of the body thus lends itself to public health directives that include an array of moral and lifestyle choices.

The idea of moral or lifestyle choices that have led to the vital force imbalance is not for the purpose of condemning individuals who are ill; on the contrary, it is designed to help ameliorate the spread of illness and disease due to risky health behaviors. However, due to the language used to discuss these issues, it is likely that the biomedical public health community will have the concern of moral judgment and discriminatory actions that may result. In addition, while no faculty expressed the relationship between health and religion, the links between living a 'moral' life according to ancient teachings remain.

On the other hand, the integral nature of AYUSH traditions to consider both mind and body as well as clear directives for lifestyle choices may be more effective for patients to understand, manage and treatment their ailments. The long history of Indian medical traditions, dietary suggestions, and lifestyle directives are well imbedded in much of Indian culture. The biomedical public health community could certainly benefit from this more holistic approach. Based on faculty reports, there are many AYUSH treatments that appear to demonstrate positive impacts on individuals infected with HIV. For example, Rasa Gandhi Melugu, which is used effectively in Siddha medicine is widely available in both powder and pill form. There is evidence of limited efforts to examine potential Ayurvedic, Homeopathic and Siddha medicines [23,28-31] and considerable financial and management support is still needed to conduct systematic research.

Limitations and Conclusions

While this study has been able to elucidate some important aspects of the role of AYUSH systems for the management and treatment of HIV/AIDS in India, there are still several limitations. Primarily, we investigated only a few AYUSH institutions in Maharashtra state and 1 Siddha institution in Tamil Nadu. However, we believe that this study is the first of its kind to examine AYUSH traditions from the perspective of the faculty and students from institutions of higher learning. Moreover, all the Colleges of Indian Systems of Medicine are affiliated to various Universities in the Country. These Colleges are following the minimum standards of education and Curricula

and Syllabi, prescribed by Central Council. Revision and updating the Curriculum and Syllabus is a regular process and CCIM aims to achieve quality education and best standards for ISM students.

Additional research is needed to examine specific formulations that hold promise of enhanced immunity and possible interactions between traditional formulations and ART. Further, AYUSH's holistic approach that focuses on improved lifestyle and dietary choices may be an important complement to existing biomedical treatments. Greater efforts are needed to identify areas of collaboration between experts in biomedicine and AYUSH systems in India.

Acknowledgments

The authors would like to thank the Samueli Institute, Alexandria, VA, USA for funding this study. They would also like to gratefully acknowledge the contributions of Ms. Neelam Joshi, Pune, Ms. Gayathri and Mr. S. Sibi of YR Gaitonde Center for AIDS Research & Education (YRG), Chennai, India, Ms.Khyati Gupta Medical Student Albert Einstein College of Medicine, Beth Israel Medical Center, USA and Ms. Katherine Kentoffio Medical Student, Harvard Medical School USA for their help with data collection, and all the participant faculty and students.

Disclosure Statements

This study was funded by the Samueli Institute, Alexandria, VA, USA. The funders participated in the study design. They did not participate in data collection, analysis, interpretation or publication. Jayagowri Sastry used to receive funding from the NIH until 2011. Amita Gupta receives funding from US NIH, WHO and Gilead Foundation. Anita Shankar receives funding from the US NIH. None of the other authors had any actual or potential conflict of interest including any financial, personal or other relationships with other people or organizations within three years of beginning the work submitted.

References

1. Morineau G, Vun MC, Barennes H, Wolf RC, Song N, et al. (2009) Survival and quality of life among HIV-positive people on antiretroviral therapy in Cambodia. AIDS Patient Care STDS 23: 669-677.

2. Matida LH, Ramos Jr AN, Heukelbach J, Sañudo A, Succi RC, et al. (2011) Improving survival in children with AIDS in Brazil: results of the second national study, 1999-2002. Cad Saude Publica 27: 93-103.

3. Stover J, Korenromp EL, Blakley M, Komatsu R, Viisainen K, et al. (2011) Long-term costs and health impact of continued global fund support for antiretroviral therapy. PLoS One 6: 21048.

4. Littlewood RA, Vanable PA (2008) Complementary and alternative medicine use among HIV-positive people: research synthesis and implications for HIV care. AIDS Care 20: 1002-1018.

5. Bishop FL, Yardley L, Lewith GT (2007) A systematic review of beliefs involved in the use of complementary and alternative medicine. Journal of Health Psychology 12: 851-867.

6. Chomat AM, Wilson IB, Wanke CA, Selvakumar A, John KR, et al. (2009) Knowledge, beliefs, and health care practices relating to treatment of HIV in Vellore, India. AIDS Patient Care STDS 23: 477-484.

7. Peltzer K, Preez NF, Ramlagan S, Fomundam H (2008) Use of traditional complementary and alternative medicine for HIV patients in KwaZulu-Natal, South Africa. BMC Public Health 8: 255.

8. World Health Organization (2002) WHO Traditional Medicine Strategy 2002-2005. Geneva.

9. http://www.who.int/mediacentre/factsheets/fs134/en/.

10. Khare RS (1996) Dava, Daktar, and Dua: Anthropology of practiced medicine in India. Social Science & Medicine 43: 837-848.

11. Arnold D (1996) The rise of western medicine in India. Lancet 348: 1075-1078.

12. http://indianmedicine.nic.in/writereaddata/linkimages/7545557388-Medical_Manpower.pdf.

13. http://www.mciindia.org/tools/announcement/MCI_booklet.pdf.

14. http://mohfw.nic.in/WriteReadData/l892s/9457038092AnnualReporthealth.pdf.

15. AYUSH (2010) Department of AYUSH, Ministry of Health and Family Welfare. Government of India.

16. Glaser B, Strauss A (1967) The Discovery of Grounded Theory: Strategies for Qualitative Research. Aldine publishing company, Chicago.

17. Sharma DC (2001) India to promote integration of traditional and modern medicine. Lancet 358: 1524.

18. Fritts M, Crawford CC, Quibell D, Gupta A, Jonas WB, et al. (2008) Traditional Indian medicine and homeopathy for HIV/AIDS: a review of the literature. AIDS Res Ther 5: 25.

19. Chaudhury R (2002) HIV/Aids and Traditional Medicine: A Journey to Dialogue. (1stedn), Alpha Science International Ltd, New Delhi.

20. Ramchandani SR, Mehta SH, Saple DG, Vaidya SB, Pandey VP, et al. (2007) Knowledge, attitudes, and practices of antiretroviral therapy among HIV-infected adults attending private and public clinics in India. AIDS Patient Care STDS 21: 129-142.

21. Torri MC (2013) Perceptions of the use of complementary therapy and Siddha medicine among rural patients with HIV/AIDS: a case study from India. Int J Health Plann Manage 28: 63-84.

22. Bhalerao MS, Bolshete PM, Swar BD, Bangera TA, Kolhe VR, et al. (2013) Use of and satisfaction with complementary and alternative medicine in four chronic diseases: A cross-sectional study from India. Natl Med J India 26: 75-78.

23. Somarathna KI, Chandola HM, Ravishankar B, Pandya KN, Attanayake AM (2010) A short-term intervention trial on HIV positive patients using a Sri Lankan classical rasayana drug-Ranahamsa Rasayanaya. Ayu 31: 197-204.

24. Nyamathi A, Singh VP, Lowe A, Taneja D, Khurana A, et al. (2008) Knowledge and attitudes about HIV/AIDS among homoeopathic practitioners and educators in India. Evid Based Complement and Alternat Med 5: 221-225.

25. Kisangau D, Lyaruu H, Hosea K, Joseph C (2007) Use of traditional medicines in the management of HIV/AIDS opportunistic infections in Tanzania: a case in the Bukoba rural district. J Ethnobiol Ethnomed 3: 24-27.

26. Mngqundaniso N, Peltzer K (2008) Traditional healers and nurses: a qualitative study on their role on sexually transmitted infections including HIV and AIDS in KwaZulu-Natal, South Africa. Afr J Tradit Complement Altern Med 5: 380-386.

27. Sankaran R (1991) The Spirit of Homeopathy. Homeopathic Educational Services, New Delhi.

28. Chaudhury R (2001) A clinical protocol for the study of traditional medicine and human immunodeficiency virus-related illness. J Altern Complement Med 7: 553-566.

29. Ullman D (2003) Controlled clinical trials evaluating the homeopathic treatment of people with human immunodeficiency virus or acquired immune deficiency syndrome. J Altern Complement Med 9: 133-141.

30. Govindarajan R, Vijayakumar M, Pushpangadan P (2005) Antioxidant approach to disease management and the role of 'Rasayana' herbs of Ayurveda. J Ethnopharmacol 99: 165-178.

31. Mukherjee PK, Wahile A (2006) Integrated approaches towards drug development from Ayurveda and other Indian systems of medicine. J Ethnopharmacol 103: 25-35.

23

In Vitro Antimicrobial Activity of Crude Leaf Extracts from *Aloe secundiflora, Bulbine frutescens, Vernonia lasiopus* and *Tagetes minuta* against *Salmonella typhi*

Rachuonyo HO[1]*, Ogola PE[2], Arika WM[2], Nyamai DW[2] and Wambani JR[3]

[1]Department of Microbiology, Kenyatta University, Kenya
[2]Department of Biochemistry and Biotechnology, Kenyatta University, Kenya
[3]Department of Medical Laboratory Sciences, Kenyatta University, Kenya

Abstract

Four medicinal plants leaves were investigated to evaluate their antibacterial potential of the methanol extracts against *Salmonella typhi* by disc diffusion method. The methanol extract from *Aloe secundiflora* showed strong antibacterial activity against a clinical isolate of *Salmonella typhi* at low concentrations (5.5 mg/ml) as compared to *Bulbine frutescens* extract (8.8 mg/ml). The minimum inhibitory concentration ranged from 5 mg/ml - 9 mg/ml whereas the maximum bactericidal concentration range from 7 mg/ml - 11 mg/ml. The standard antibiotic used was ciprofloxacin (15 µg/ml) was used as a positive control while dimethyl sulphoxide and distilled water were used as the negative control. The extracts were preliminary screened for the presence of secondary metabolites to determine the presence of flavonoids, alkaloids, tannins and saponins. The results supported the use of the medicinal plants in the treatment of infections caused by *Salmonella typhi*.

Keywords: *Salmonella typhi*; Disc diffusion; Medicinal plants; Secondary metabolites; Methanol extract

Introduction

Medicinal plants have been identified and used throughout human history [1]. The use of medicinal plants (herbs) to treat diseases is almost universal among non-industrialized societies, and is often more affordable than purchasing expensive conventional drugs [2]. The genus Tagetes belongs to the Asteraceae family which presently comprises of 56 species, 27 biennials and 29 perennials. Tagetes species are grown all over the world as multipurpose plants [3]. Plant parts such as flowers and leaves have been known to contain flavonoids that are scavengers for free radicals which enhances the antimicrobial activity of the *Tagetes minuta* extracts [4]. Phytochemicals from the plant such as carotenoids have also been used in pharmacological preparations and they have been found to contain anti-aging and anti-cancer effects [5]. The plant extracts have been used in treating intestinal and stomach problems [6,7]. Aloes are perennial succulent xerophytes which develops water storage tissues in leaves to survive in areas with low or erratic rainfall [8]. Aloe extracts have been used for many centuries for their curative and therapeutic properties [9]. Extracts of Aloes especially its leaf gel have shown antibacterial activity by inhibiting the growth of both Gram negative bacteria and Gram positive bacteria [10]. *Aloe secundiflora* leaf components have been credited for antibacterial, antifungal and antiviral and antihelmintic medicinal properties [11]. *Aloe secundiflora* has been used in treating ailments including; chest problems, polio, malaria and stomach ache by herbalists in the Lake Victoria region [12]. Bulbine is a genus of plants in the family xanthorrhoeaceae and sub family asphodeloideae and its members are well known for their medicinal value [13]. Bulbine plant has been used for medicinal purposes in the early stages of the eighteen century by Dutch and British settlers of South Africa in treating various ailments [14]. The leaves of the plant have been used in the treatment of wound thought to be infected with bacterial pathogens and it has shown antibacterial properties [15]. Some of the species of the plant found in South Africa have been used for blood cleansing, treatment of ringworms and gravel rush by some local communities such as the Xhosa [14]. A decoction of bulbs and roots of some of the species has been used in the treatment of some of the venereal diseases in women and stomach upsets [16]. Vernonieae is a tribe which has about 1300 species and in the family Asteraceae (Compositae) which mostly contains herbaceous plants [17]. *Vernonia lasiopus* decoctions from the stems and leaves have been traditionally been used by herbalists in East Africa to treat, malaria, worms and gastrointestinal problems [18]. Its extracts have also been used in treating some of the sexually transmitted diseases in southern parts of Africa [19]. In this study the antimicrobial activity of the leaf extracts from the plants against clinical isolate of *Salmonella typhi* was tested and screened for the presence of phytochemicals.

Materials and Methods

Plant material collection

The fresh plant leaves of *Aloe secundiflora, Bulbine frutescens, Vernonia lasiopus* and *Tagetes minuta* were collected at Kenyatta University Arboretum. Voucher specimens were prepared and deposited in the university herbarium in Plant Sciences Department for future reference. The plants leaves were brought to the laboratory and thoroughly washed in running water to remove debris and dust particles and then rinsed using distilled water and finally air dried.

Preparation of plant extract

The air dried plants leaves were tause into powder and soaked in methanol for 72 h and placed in a Gallenkamp shaker at 65 revolutions per minute. The contents were homogenized and filtered using

*Corresponding author: Rachuonyo HO, Department of Microbiology, Kenyatta University, Kenya, E-mail: hibertrachuonyo@gmail.com

whatman filter paper no. 1. The filtrate was poured into a round bottom flask and concentrated using a vacuum evaporator and stored in a labelled amber glass bottle at room temperature away from light and heat before being used for antibacterial efficacy test.

Antimicrobial susceptibility testing

The microorganism used was clinical isolate of *Salmonella typhi* obtained from Kenyatta University Health Centre Laboratory, Nairobi. *Salmonella typhi* was tested against methanol extracts of *Tagetes minuta*, *Aloe secundiflora*, *Bulbine frutescens* and *Vernonia lasiopus*. *Salmonella typhi* inoculum was concentrated by comparing it with a 0.5 McFarland standard. Discs of 6 milliliters were prepared from whatman no.1 filter paper. The discs were sterilized by autoclaving. After sterilization the moisture discs were dried on hot air oven at 50°C [20]. The various solvent extracts discs prepared were impregnated with the extracts from the highest concentration of 1000 mg/ml to the lowest concentration of 1 mg/ml [21]. The antimicrobial efficacy test was carried out using Kirby Bauer method [22]. Muller Hinton agar was used in the spread plate technique where *Salmonella typhi* was spread using sterilized cotton wool swab and exposed to extracts impregnated discs in milligrams per microliter from *Aloe secundiflora*, *Tagetes minuta*, *Vernonia lasiopus* and *Bulbine frutescens*. The discs were placed with equal distance between them on agar plates inoculated with *Salmonella typhi*. Positive control discs contained ciprofloxacin (15 µg/ml) while negative control discs were impregnated with dimethyl sulphoxide and distilled water. The Petri dishes were incubated at 37°C for 24 h. Zones of inhibition formed were measured in millimetres and their average determined. The experiment was carried in duplicates and the diameter of zones of inhibition formed measured. Minimal Inhibitory Concentration (MIC) was determined using the broth tube method [23]. 100 µl of 250 mg/ml of methanol extract was added to 100 µl of sterile bacteriological peptone in the first well of the 96 well micro plates and mixed well with a micropipette. 100 µl of this dilution was transferred subsequently to wells two folding each dilution of the original extract. This was done to the extracts of *Aloe secundiflora*, *Bulbine frutescens*, *Vernonia lasiopus*, and *Tagetes minuta*. An inoculum of 100 µl (0.5 McFarland standards) of overnight clinical culture of *Salmonella typhi* was added in each of the wells. Triplicate of each micro plate were made and the procedure repeated. The plates were then incubated at 37°C for 24 h. After incubation 40 µl of 0.2 mg/µl of INT was added in each of the wells and the plates examined after an additional 60 minutes of incubation. Growth was indicated by a red colour (conversion of INT to formazan). The lowest concentration at which the colour was apparently invisible as compared to the next dilution was taken as the minimum inhibitory concentration [24]. Minimum bactericidal concentration (MBC) was determined by taking 100 µl of suspension from micro plate wells that demonstrated no growth and inoculated on agar plates. The plates were incubated at 37°C for 24 h. In the case where, there was no bacterial growth and value not greater than the minimum inhibitory concentration the concentration was used as the maximum bacterial concentration.

Phytochemical analysis

Presence of saponins, tannins, flavonoids and alkaloids in the crude extract were determined [25].

Tannins: Each of the extracts was weighed to 0.5 mg and dissolved in 1 ml of distilled water. Filtration was carried out after 2 ml of FeCl₃ was added. If there was presence of a blue or black precipitate then it indicated the presence of tannins.

Flavonoids: Each of the extracts was weighed to 0.5 mg and dissolved in 1 ml of ethanol and filtered. 2 ml of 1% HCl and magnesium ribbon was added to the filtrate. If there was formation of a pink or red colour it indicated the presence flavonoids.

Alkaloids: Each of the extracts was weighed to 0.5 mg and dissolved in 1 ml of methanol and filtered. 1% HCL was added to the filtrate and the solution heated. Mayor`s reagent was added drop wise and if there was formation of any colored precipitate it indicated the presence of alkaloids.

Saponins: Each of the extracts was weighed to 0.5 mg and dissolved in 1 ml of methanol and filtered. Distilled water was added and shaking done for a few minutes. If there was persistence frothing then it indicated the presence of saponins.

Results and Discussion

In this study the antibacterial activity of leaf extracts from *Tagetes minuta*, *Aloe secundiflora*, *Vernonia lasiopus* and *Bulbine frutescens* were evaluated against *Salmonella typhi*. Following methanolic extraction, the antibacterial activity of the extracts was determined by disc diffusion method. Table 1 presents the antimicrobial test of the plant extracts against *Salmonella typhi*. The results indicated that all the plants extracts were active against *Salmonella typhi*. The antimicrobial activity of these extracts varied greatly on Muller Hinton agar. The positive control used (Ciprofloxacin) produced significantly sized zones of inhibition of approximately 24 mm. However, the negative controls (dimethyl sulphoxide and distilled water) produced no zone of inhibitory. All the four extracts used showed good antibacterial activity with Aloe secundiflora showing the highest activity at low concentrations (MIC 5.5 mg/ml). Bulbine frutescens extract showed minimum activity (MIC 8.8 mg/ml).

The plant extracts were tested for the presence of secondary metabolites. Table 2 shows that all the methanolic leaf extracts from the plant had the four secondary metabolites being tested for.

The antimicrobial activity from the extracts against *Salmonella typhi* may be due to presence of saponins, alkaloids, tannins and flavonoid in the plant extracts; *Bulbine frutescens* [26]; *Vernonia lasiopus* [18]; *Aloe secundiflora* [20,27,28]; *Tagetes minuta* [29,30].

Plant extracts	MIC (mg/ml)	MBC (mg/ml)	Zone of Inhibition (mm)
Aloe secundiflora	5.5	7.3	16 ± 0.68
Vernonia lasiopus	5.6	7.5	13 ± 1.68
Tagetes minuta	6.1	8.2	17 ± 1.15
Bulbine frutescens	8.8	10.9	15 ± 0.15
+ve control	-	-	24
-ve control	-	-	-

Key: ± Standard error; **-ve control** (dimethyl sulphoxide and distilled water); **+ve control** (ciprofloxacin), **MIC:** Minimum Inhibitory Concentration; **MBC:** Maximum Inhibitory Concentration.

Table 1: Efficacy test of the plants leaf extracts against *Salmonella typhi*.

Plant extracts	Saponins	Tannins	Alkaloids	Flavonoids
Aloe secundiflora	+	+	+	+
Vernonia lasiopus	+	+	+	+
Bulbine frutescens	+	+	+	+
Tagetes minuta	+	+	+	+

Key: (+) present

Table 2: Phytochemical tests on the plant extracts.

Conclusion

In conclusion, the present study will help us to use these medicinal plants as a source of herbal medicine to treat different infectious diseases caused by *Salmonella typhi* and other gram negative bacterial pathogens. The extracts can also be used as raw material in the manufacturing of conventionally used drugs against pathogenic bacteria that have developed resistance against standard antibiotics. Further isolation of the specific bioactive compounds responsible for the antimicrobial activity will give us other natural resources that can be used in treating bacterial infections.

References

1. Lichterman BL (2004) Aspirin: The Story of a Wonder Drug. British Medical Journal 329: 1408.

2. Fabricant DS, Farnsworth NR (2001) The value of plants used in traditional medicine for drug discovery. Environmental Health Perspective 1: 69-75.

3. Soule JA (1993) *Tagetes minuta* A Potential New Herb from South America: New Crops. Proceedings of the New Crops Conference, pp. 649-654.

4. De las Rivas J (1989) Reversed-phase high performance liquid chromatographic separation of lutein and lutein fatty acid esters from marigold flower petal powder. Journal of Chromatography 464: 442-447.

5. Basile A, Sorbo S, Giordano S, Ricciardi L, Ferrara S, et al. (1992) Antimicrobial resistance of Shigella isolates in Bangladesh, 1983-1990: increasing frequency of strains multiply resistant to ampicillin, trimethoprim-sulfamethoxazole, and nalidixic acid. Journal of Clinical Infectious Diseases 14: 1055-1060.

6. Broussalis AM, Ferraro GE, Martino VS, Pinzon R, Coussio JD et al. (1999) Argentine plants as potential source of insecticidal compounds. Journal of ethno pharmacology 67: 219-223.

7. Tereschuk ML, Riera MVQ, Castro GR, Abdala LR (1997) Antimicrobial activity of Flavonoids from leaves of *Tagetes minuta*. Journal of Ethno pharmacology 56: 227-232.

8. Talmadge J, Chavez J, Jacobs L, Munger C, Chinnah T, et al. (2004) Fractionation of *Aloe vera L.* inner gel, purification and molecular profiling of activity. International Immuno pharmacology journal 4: 1757-1773.

9. Habeeb F, Shakir E, Bradbury F, Cameron P, Taravati MR et al. (1994) Effect of garlic on lead contents in chicken tissues. DTW 101: 157-158.

10. Ferro VA, Bradbury F, Cameron P, Shakir E, Rahman SR, et al. (2003) *In vitro* susceptibilities of *Shigella flexineri* and *Streptococcus pyrogenes* to inner gel of *Aloe barbadensis* Miller. Antimicrobial agents and chemotherapy 43: 1137-1139.

11. Kaingu F, Kibor A, Waihenya R, Shivairo R, Mungai L (2013) Efficacy of *Aloe secundiflora* Crude Extracts on *Ascaridia galli in vitro*. Sustainable Agriculture 2: 49-53.

12. Kigondu EVM, Rukunga GM, Keriko JM, Tonui WK, Gathitwa JW, et al. (2009) Anti-parasitic activity and cytotoxicity of selected medicinal plants from Kenya. Journal of ethno pharmacology 123: 504-509.

13. Acock JPH (1975) Veld types of South Africa. Memoirs of Botanical Survey of South Africa Botanical Research Institute, Pretoria.

14. Coopsamy RM, Magwa ML, Mayekiso B (2000) Proceedings: Science and Society University of Fort Hare, Bhisho, Eastern Cape, South Africa.

15. Kelmanson JE, Jager AK, Van Staden J (2000) Zulu medicinal plants with antibacterial activity. Journal of ethno pharmacology 69: 241-246.

16. Van Wyk BE (2008) A broad review of commercially important Southern African medicinal plants. Journal of ethno pharmacology 119: 342-355.

17. Keeleya SC (2007) A phylogeny of the "evil tribe" (Vernonieae: Compositae) reveals Old/New World long distance dispersal: support from separate and combined congruent datasets. Molecular Phylogenetics and Evolution 44: 89-103.

18. Kareru PG, Gachanja AN, Keriko J M, Kenji GM (2007) Antimicrobial activity of some medicinal plants used by herbalists in Eastern province, Kenya. African Journal of Traditional Complementary And alternative Medicine 5: 51-55.

19. Kambizi L, Afolayan AJ (2001) An ethno botanical study of plants used for the treatment of sexually transmitted diseases (Njovhera) in Guruve District, Zimbabwe. Journal of ethno pharmacology 77: 5-9.

20. Arunkumar S, Muthuselvam M (2009) Analysis of phytochemical constituents and antimicrobial activities of *Aloe vera* L. against clinical pathogens. World Journal of Agricultural Sciences 5: 572-576.

21. Joshua M, Ngonidzashe M, Bamusi S (2010) An evaluation of the antimicrobial activities of *Aloe barberdensis, A. chabaudii* and *A. arborescens* leaf extracts used in folk fore veterinary medicine in Zimbabwe. Journal of animal and veterinary advances 9: 2918-2923.

22. Newall CA, Anderson LA, Phillipson JD (1996) Herbal medicines. The pharmaceutical Press, London.

23. Eloff JN (1998) A sensitivity and quick microplate method to determine the minimal inhibition concentration of plant extracts for bacterial organisms. Medicinal plants journal 64: 711-713.

24. Rabe T, Mullholland D, Van Staden J (2002) Isolation and identification of antibacterial compounds from *Vernonia colorata* leaves. Journal of Ethnopharmacology 80: 91-94.

25. Parekh J, Nair R, Chanda S (2005) Preliminary screening of some folklore medicinal plants from Western India, for potential antimicrobial activity. Indian journal of pharmacology 37:406-409.

26. Yakubu MT, Afolayan AJ (2009) Effect of aqueous extract of *Bulbine natalensis* (Baker) stem on the sexual behaviour of male rats. International Journal of Andrology 32: 629-636.

27. Devaraj A, Karpagam T (2011) Evaluation of anti-inflammatory activity and analgesic effect of *Aloe vera* leaf extract in rats. International Research Journal of Pharmacy 2: 103-110.

28. Mariappan V, Shanthi G (2012) Antimicrobial and phytochemical analysis of *Aloe vera. L*. International Research Journal of Pharmacy 3: 158-161.

29. Irum S, Amjad H, Ummara WK, Mohammad MS (2010) Evaluating biological activities of the seed extracts from *Tagetes minuta* L. found in Northern Pakistan. Journal of medicinal plants research 4: 2108-2112.

30. Lubna T, Naeem K (2012) Antibacterial potential of crude leaf, fruit and flower extracts of *Tagetes minuta l*. Journal of Public Health and Biological Sciences 1: 74-78.

24

A Study on the Plants Used as *Chopachini*

Perera BPR*

Gampaha Wickramarachchi Ayurveda Institute, University of Kelaniya, Sri Lanka

Abstract

Chopachini/Dvipantaravacha or China root is used in many alternative systems of medicine. The plant, first mentioned in Bhavaprakasha in 16th century has been attributed to variety of scientific names in literature. A study was conducted to find out the plants that have been used as *Chopachini*. The study resulted in several varieties of genus Smilax as well as *Gynura paseudo-china* of family Asteraceae. *Smilax china* is native to China and Japan and could be the reason the plant is called "*Cheenaala*" in Sinhala. *Gynura pseudo-china* is native to Indonesia, Thailand, and China. Both the plants are used in venereal diseases in the traditional systems of medicine in their native countries but have not been scientifically proven to be effective for treating syphilis. Therefore, it is unclear whether the plant mentioned in Bhavaprakasha is *Smilax china* or *Gynura psuedo-china*. However, considering the medicinal properties, *Smilax china* qualifies to be used as *Chopachini/Dwipantaravacha*.

Keywords: *Chopachini*; Dwipantaravacha; *Smilax china; Gynura pseudochina;* China root

Introduction

Chopachini or *Dvipantaravacha* is an herbal ingredient used in Ayurveda and Indigenous medicine in Sri Lanka. In Ayurveda, the first reference to *Chopachini* is in Bhavaprakasha in 16th century. *Chopachini* is mentioned in the texts of Indigenous medicine in Sri Lanka such as *Vaidyaka Hasthasaraya*, but whether it has been used prior to 16th century is unclear. *Chopachini* is referred to as "*Cheena ala*", "*Seena ala*" or "*Ala beth*" within the indigenous system of medicine. In Ayurveda texts, it is sometimes referred to as *Madhusnuhi*. Evidently 4 species from the genus Smilax and *Gynura pseudochina* of family Asteraceae are used as *Chopachini* (Table 1). Among these, *Smilax china* is officially considered as the authentic identification as per The Wealth of India series [1]. This raises the question why a Gynura species has been used instead in some instances. In India, always a Smilax species has been used as *Chopachini* but in Sri Lanka use of *Gynura pseudochina* can be seen. According to "A checklist of flowering plants in Sri Lanka" only 3 Smilax species found in Sri Lanka and those are *S. perfoliata* (*Maha Kabarossa*), *S. zeylanica* (*Heen Kabarossa*) and *S.aspera*. Two Gynura species are found in Sri Lanka; *G. pseudochina* which is identified as *Chopachini* (*alabeth* in Sinhala) and *G. hispida* (*Hulantala*). All of these plant species have been called China root masking exactly what species was in use in the past.

Phiranga roga- syphilis

Chopachini or china root was renowned to be effective in the treatment of Syphilis and used extensively in various indigenous medical systems. The plant is indicated especially for *Phiranga roga*, a new disease that makes its first appearance in Bhavaprakasha. *Phiranga roga* was not found or has not reached to epidemic levels in India by the time the great Ayurveda treatises were written. Hence the authors were unaware of the disease. Syphilis began to raise its dreadful head in Europe in 1493 A.D [2] and was a new disease in Asia around 1500. *Phiranga roga* is Syphilis or Yaws that found its way to India with the with the first Portuguese fleet, in 1498, and by 1504/5 who had established themselves at Goa and some parts of India by early sixteenth century A.D [3]. Since then it has become a widely known was also used by the Maldivians. Portuguese were also held responsible for syphilis in Sri Lanka. The disease arrived in Canton between 1504 and 1506, about 15 years before the Portuguese established there. In 1505, or, according to another source, 1512, syphilis landed in Japan, where the disease was called Chinese ulcers, or Portuguese disease [3].

According to Van Linschoten, in India it was an everyday disease. It was cured with *Radix china* or *chinae* which, according to Jan Huyghen van Linschoten, who came to India in the 1580s, had not been introduced in India from China until 1535 [3]. He said that „the pox" was so common in China, that God had sent them Radix china. It is evident that a plant which the westerners called China root was used to treat the disease. Apart from the vague descriptions, no authentic information could be found about the plant used as China root. China root had sudorific (sweat inducing) properties [4]. It had been used in Asia as a panacea for many illnesses, including jaundice, leprosy and many other skin diseases. It was reportedly used as a cure for beriberi. Sudorifics were also used in Europe against syphilis from a syphilis, which according to contemporary medical opinion came from the West Indies, should be cured. In 1516, Portuguese arrived in China and many valuable Chinese products of vegetable origin were carried to Europe in the 16th Century, especially medicines. Among the latter China root was found in Europe, since about the year 1535. The emperor Charles V is reported to have been cured of gout by this drug [5].

The drug imported by westerners from China known as "China root", "China wood" or simple "China" is controversial. Many Smilax species are called China root and in European countries and in South America it is called Sarsaparilla. The original species, *Smilax aspera*, is found in above areas whereas other species are found in other parts of the world. Another celebrated species is *Smilax china* which is inhabited in China. Two species, *Smilax glabra* and *lancefolia* can be found in India and their roots are so similar to that of *Smilax china* that it is difficult to differentiate the species. A similar species is common in the southern part of North America and has been called *Smilax pseudo-china*, a name which is probably used to name more than one species. However, CRC world dictionary of medicinal plants and poisonous plants mentions that *Gynura pseudochina* as a source of china root [6].

---

*Corresponding author: Perera BPR, Gampaha Wickramarachchi Ayurveda Institute, University of Kelaniya, Sri Lanka
E-mail: bprperera@gmail.com

Source	Type	Species Used	Botanical Family
Srilanka Ayurveda Materia Madica	Book	*Smilax glabra*	Smilacaceae
Indian Materia Madica	Book	*Smilax china*	Smilacaceae
Deshiya Vaidya Shabda Koshaya	Book	*Gynura pseudochina*	Asteraceae
Medicinal Plants	Book (D.M.A, 2006)	*Gynura pseudochina*	
Evaluation of adaptogenic and anti-stress effects of Ranahamsa Rasayanaya-A Sri Lankan classical Rasayana drug on experimental animals	Research (Somarathna, 2010)	*Gynura pseudochina*	Asteraceae
Medicinal plants of Sikkim in Ayurvedic practice	Research (Panda,2007)	*Smilax lanceaefolia roxb*	Smilacaceae
In vitro studies of antimicrobial properties of extracts from unani medicinal plants	Research (Namra H,)2012	*Smilax glabra*	Smilacaceae
Demand and Supply of Medicinal Plants in India	Report (DK Ved,2007)	*Smilax glabra*	Smilacaceae
Ethno medicinally important plants of Pachmarhi region, Madhya Pradesh, India	Research (Mishra,2012)	*Smilax lanceifolia*	Smilacaceae
Nutritional assessment of some selected wild edible plants as a good source of mineral	Research (Shivprasad Mahadkar, 2012)	*Smilax zeylanica*	Smilacaceae
CRC World Dictionary of Medicinal and Poisonous Plants: Common Names Scientific Names, Eponyms, Synonyms, and Etymology (5 Volume Set)	(Quattrocchi, 2012)	*Gynura pseudochina*	
A Hand Book of the Flora of Ceylon	(Trimen, 1895)	*Gynura pseudochina*	

Table 1: The literature in recent history uses different scientific names for *Chopachini*. These differences range from variants within a genus to plant from different botanical families.

Gynura pseudochina extends from Sierra Leone eastwards through the Central African Republic and Ethiopia to Somalia and south to Malawi, Zambia and Angola. It also occurs in Sri Lanka, India, Bhutan, China, Myanmar, Thailand, Vietnam and Australia. It is cultivated in Java (Indonesia) and Peninsular Malaysia [7].

Chopachini or china root is also called *Dwipantaravacha* in Sanskrit and the name bears some significance. The word *Dvipantara* can be separated in to "*Dvipa*" and "*Antara*" with *Dvipa* meaning island and *antara* meaning in between or across. "*Dvipantara*" is historically used to denote Indonesia [7]. Indonesia has adopted the name during the time of King Hayam Wuruk the Majapahit Empire who ruled from 1331-1364, that is at the end of the 13th century. Therefore it is possible that material imported from the area has adopted the name *Dvipantara* and Bhavaprakasha which was written in 16th century mentioned it as *Dvipantaravacha*. According to India Major: Congratulatory volume Presented to J.Gonda, *Dwipantara* in old Javanese being either "Indonesia, the islands" as in Sanskrit or "the islands other than Java" [7]. *Gynura pseudochina* being extensively cultivated in Java and Indonesia might have been called *Dwipantaravacha* to denote its origin.

Garcia d"Orta, the First physician to the Portuguese Viceroy of India at Goa and a resident in India for 30 years gives an account of Indian spices and medicines in his book. The author mentions several Chinese drugs including *Radix chinae* and its medicinal virtues, stating that in China it is used for venereal and cutaneous diseases. China root become first known in India in A.D. 1535 through Chinese traders. The Chinese call the plant *Lampatam*. The latter name given by Garcia seems to be a corruption of long *Jan tu'an*, which according to the Chinese Herbal is *t'u fuling* or China root [5]. Miller-Martyn"s Dictionary mentions *Smilax pseudochina* stating that it occurs in China. It is frequently used instead of true China root. A small quantity of it, even in cold water tinges of a deep red, whereas the true root yields a light yellow brown [5].

This poses a question as to what plant is meant as *Dwipantaravacha* by *Bhavamishra*. However, according to many texts, China root is not a native of India and imported to India around A.D. 1535, is provided as a cure for Syphilis.

Indian Sanskrit texts mention characteristics of *Dwipantaravacha* or *Chopachini* as follows.

फ़्न्नम्म चिब्फ़िरुन्न सर्चिसुच्च् फेम्न्ज्ज्जन्चुज्जूझ् श्ज्झक्पहिर्ह्सिन्ज् स्च्जम्फिम्न्ज्जम्फ़ुम्य्

सर्झ्सिजम्न् ज्जब्न्जूं हिर्मि छ्जम्झम्न्जम्ह्न्ज्जि (Bhavaprakasha Haritakyadi Varga Sol 269)

-Dvipantaravacha is a bit bitter and of hot potency. It kindles digestive fire, alleviates *adhmana, shula,* and purifies *malas*. *Dvipantaravacha* is to be used in *vatavyadhi, apasmara, unmada, shula,* and especially in *Phiranga roga.*

Bhavaprakasha lacks description of the plant. The name *Dvipantaravacha* is mentioned in *Haritakyadi varga* in Bhavaprakasha whereas the name *Chopachini* is mentioned in the *Phirangadikara*. However there is no reference whether the two terms are synonymous other than the fact that they are indicated for *Phiranga roga.*

बित्ज्जूपिम्झम्गर्थे चोप्च्जम्न्जूंनी पृष्ज्जम्न्त्झुण प्रयोग (Bhavaprakasha Phirangadhikara 249) फुज्झम्झम्मम्ग्म्स चोंजबोर्ज्च छ्म्यूं सम्म्चिन्जेल्झी क्छ्त्म्च्च्चम्हन्न ल्झुम्न स्च्झम्जनम्म्न वझिल्झर्चि

सोम्झम्पइग्म्ज्स् स्म्म्न श्च्छम्न्म्ल् ज :Nsiss.slsun.:

The name *Chopachini* is used Shiva Nigantu and some information on identification has given saying it is like *Ashwagandha* (*Withania somnifera*). However, it is not clear as to what aspect of *Ahwagandha* the text is referring to. Whether it looks like *Withania somnifera* plant or whether it has an odor similar to the characteristic odor of the plant.

In Bhaishajya Rathnavali *Chopachini* is indicated for *Phiranga roga.*

चोंप्चींनी झन् न्झुग शाणामान ममर्ज्जिणम्प् ष्रिन्ड्ढ ल्झापिजल्झ्चय मझुप्ज्ज्णम्न त्यर्ज्जन्

Yogarathnakara indicates *Chopachini* for rejuvenation in *Chopachini paka*. Sahasrayoga also indicates it for rejuvenation but it uses the name *Mahusnuhi*.

In Siddha Bhaishajya Manimala *Chopachini* is indicated for *Sandhivata.*

जन्न्ज्जर्फर्छ्च्झील्ल्स्ज्जन्ल्झ झम्ग ल्झिफम्झम्छिन्ग्. जस्च्छ्ज्जम्न बैझिल्झी झि ड़िप्डी क्षर्जन :Bhaishajya Manimala 4479)

Smilax china

It is a common mountain plant, which sometimes climbs, but its stem is strong, hard and covered with spines. The leaves are large, round like hoof of a horse and shining. In the autumn it bears yellow flowers followed by red fruits. The root is very hard and is covered with bristle like hairs. A decoction which is sour and harsh is made of the root. It is a kind of shrub indigenous to China and Japan where it is called *Toojuh*. It is not grown in India although the china root is common in all the bazaars. It is believed that the root of *Smilax glabra* probably constitute part of the dried tuberous roots. It has long held the reputation of possessing properties allied to those of Sarsaparilla, which is the root of several species of Smilax indigenous to tropical America. The drug is imported from China to a considerable extent by coating steamers trading with Calcutta and Bombay" [8].

The same book gives the following description on *Dvipantaravacha*.

It is a kind of twining plant found in many parts of India. It is slightly bitter, stimulant, conductive of digestive fire and beneficial in Pains, Hysteria, Rheumatism, Insanity and pains in the body. It is especially alleviative of syphilis and mercurial poison". This description is similar to what is mentioned in Bhavaprakash, and could be a mere translation.

Smilax pseudochina

Smilax pseudochina is a climbing plant, having a spotted stem and the leaves which are not opposite, somewhat resemble large bamboo leaves, but are thicker, more glabourous and five or six inches long. The root somewhat resembles that of Smilax china, but is round and consist of a conglomeration of tubers, being found at varying depths in the ground. The flesh is very tender and can be eaten raw. Flesh could be either red or white. The latter is used in medicine. This is the principle substance known as China root, although *Pachyma, cocos* is also included under this name, and it is sometimes difficult to separate the two products or distinguish them on the market [8]. It is found on the market in the form of brown, irregular, nodulated, branching, tuberous roots, with wiry radicals of some length attached to them. The interior is white and starchy, and sweet to the taste, with patches of yellow near the surface. It can be used as food strengthening the body and assisting in keeping one awake on journeys prolonged into the night. It is regarded as tonic, astringent or corrective in diarrheas, and curative in ulcers and mercurial sores. But it is mainly used in Syphilitic difficulties, especially the secondary and tertiary manifestations. Dr Waring found the large tuberous roots of the Burmese variety, the *Smilax prolifera* of Roxburgh, very useful in the form of a decoction of the fresh root, in secondary Syphilis, cachexia and chronic skin diseases [8].

Smilax species also demonstrate pharmacological actions similar to those mentioned for *Chopachini*. It is anticonvulsant, testicular antioxidant (Saraswati, 2012) and useful in treating syphilis.

Gynura pseudochina

Gynura pseudochina is a perennial, erect, semi-succulent herb up to 130cm tall. Roots are tuberous, round or lobed, 2-6cm in diameter. Leaves are arranged in a rosette, simple, often shallowly lobed, petiole 0.3-3 cm long. Blade obovate, spatulate, and elliptical or ovate. Upper leaves are more dissected and smaller.

Flower is an inflorescence a camoanulate head, loosely racemosely or paniculately grouped, peduncle up to 4 cm long, inner involucral bracts13, 7-12 cm long. Corolla 10-13mm long. Yellow to red Fruit an achene, 3-4mm long [9]. *Gynura pseudochina* is extensively cultivated in Indonesia and is used in the indigenous medical system of the country. It is mentioned that the plant is used to treat various kinds of skin irritation, herpes infections, breast tumors and sore throat [10]. In Thailand, *Gynura pseudochina var hispida* (Thai name- *Wan Mahakaan*) is externally used as anti-itching, anti-inflammatory, and

anti-herpes virus. In Singapore, Malaysia and Indonesia the plant has been traditionally used as remedies for eruptive fever, rash, kidney diseases, migraine, constipation, hypertension, DM and Cancer [11]. *Gynura pseudochina* is used as a medicine in African continent as well. In northern Nigeria it is cultivated as a medicinal plant to treat fever. The fresh leaves are used for their demulcent property and leaf sap is applied to sore eyes. In Asia, leaves are used to reduce skin irritation caused by insect stings, pimples and bruises and to cure scabies and erysipelas. Leaves, stems and roots are variably accredited with haemostatic, antipyretic and vulnerary activity. Plant parts are used to regulate menstruation, to treat breast tumors, herpes infections and sore throats [2].

Modern findings

No study has been done to demonstrate the effectiveness of Smilax species or *Gynura pseudochina* against Syphilis. But *Gynura pseudochina* has an effect against herpes virus. But Smilax species have been proven to possess other properties of *Chopachini*. Traditionally Smilax species are being used for the treatment of epilepsy and scientifically the anti-epileptic property has been proven in two Smilax species, *Smilax china* and *Smilax zeylanica* which is the substitute of *Smilax china* used in Sri Lanka [12,13]. The study substantiates the use of *Smilax zeylanica* as an additional botanical source for the Ayurvedic drug *Chopachini* in the treatment of epilepsy. Another study has been carried out to demonstrate the anti-stress activity of *Smilax china* on male infertility in rats [14]. According to the study the aqueous extract of the tuber *Smilax china* has been reported to possess and anti-nociceptive activities in rats. However, other Smilax species also said to possess anti-inflammatory beneficial effects such as immuno-modulatory activity in the aqueous extract from the rhizome of *Smilax glabra* and anti-oxidant activity in the leaf extract of *Smilax excels*. Smilax china has also proven to have an anti-diabetic effect [12]. The available scientific data on Smilax china confirms the usage of *Chopachini* for *Apasmara* (epilepsy).

Gynura pseudochina has been proven to possess anti-cancer effect. In Thailand, *Gynura pseudochina var hispida* is externally used as anti-itching, anti-inflammatory and anti-herpes virus. In Singapore, Malaysia, and Indonesia, the plant has been traditionally used as remedies for eruptive fever, rash, kidney diseases, migraine, constipation, hypertension, diabetes mellitus, and cancer [14]. The results of the researches done on *Gynura pseudochina* do not confirm properties of *Dwipantaravacha* mentioned in Bhavaprakasha, but its practical usage in indigenous medicine justifies the properties; *shulaprashamana* (Pain relieving property), *mala shodhaka* (purifying excrement), and use in *Vata vyadhi* [15-25].

Discussion

When compared with the description in Bhavaprakasha, one cannot conclude what plant species is referred by *Chopachini*. In Bhavaprakasha, usually, for a single plant many synonyms which are suggestive of the appearance or other characteristics of the plant are given. The reason for lack of description of characteristic for *Dwipantaravacha* or synonyms could be due to this plant being foreign to the country. It is also possible that only the dried parts were exported to the country at that time. A vague description of the appearance of the plant is given on Shivadatta which was written much later than Bhavapakasha [26]. According to Shivadatta, *Dwipantaravacha* is similar to *Ashwagandha* (*Withania somnifera*). The Smilax species bears some resemblance to outward appearance of *Withania somnefera* in the fact that both plants bear bright red berry like fruits. The dried root, which is the parts used of both the species do not have any outward similarities. However, *Withania somnifera* is a shrub and Smilax is a perennial vine. Considering the resemblance with *Gynura pseudochina*, the only similarity that can be pointed out is that the leaves look somewhat similar and the musky odor of the root.

Available data suggests that few number of Smilax species including *Smilax china* and *Smilax glabra* are used as China root or *Dwipantaravacha*. Certain other species like *Smilax pseudochina* and *Smilax zeylanica* are also used as China root but they are more often used as substitutes. Apart of the Smilax species [27], *Gynura pseudochina* is also called as China root. Based on the available data conclusion cannot be drawn as to what species is meant by Bhavamistra as *Chopachini* nor does it reveal why *Gynura pseudochina* is called China root. However, according to the available data, *Smilax china* is more eligible to be used as *Chopachini* [28,29].

Recommendations

The effectiveness of *Smialx china* and *Gynura pseudochina* plants against *Treponema pallidum* is worth investigating.

Acknowledgement

The immense support from Dr. Danister L. Perera and Dr. Udaya Samarathunga is acknowledged.

References

1. Anonymous (1950) The wealth of India, Vol. VIII. New Delhi: Council of Scientific and Industrial Research, 365.

2. Sidkar JC (1982) Phirangíroga (syphillis) and its management as described in Vaidyaka Samgraka, an old Gujarati manuscript of an unknown author (18th century AD). Indian J Hist Sci 17: 132-153.

3. Madhavan V (2008) Antiepileptic activity of alcohol and aqueous extracts of roots and rhizomes of Smilax zeylanica linn, Pharmacologyonline, 3: 263-272.

4. Malalavidhane TS, Wickramasinghe SM, Jansz ER (2000) Oral hypoglycaemic activity of Ipomoea aquatica. J Ethnopharmacol 72: 293-298.

5. Boomgaard P (2007) Syphilis, Gonorrhoea, Leprosy and Yaws in the Indonesian Archipelago, 1500-1950, Journal of Humanities.

6. Panda AK (2007) Medicinal plants of Sikkim in Ayurvedic practice. Tadong, Gangtok (Sikkim): Regional Research Institute.

7. Davis JF (1848) The Chinese: A general description of the empire of China and its inhabitants, New York, 2: 543

8. Stuart G, Porter F Chinese materia medica (p. 410). Shanghai? Presbyterian Mission Press

9. Ved DK, Goraya GS (2007) Demand and Supply of Medicinal Plants in India. New Delhi: National Medicinal Plants Board.

10. Jacob Ensink PG (1972) India Maior: Congratulatory Volume Presented to J. Gonda. Brill Archive.

11. Quattrocchi U (2012) CRC World Dictionary of Medicinal and Poisonous Plants: Common Names, Scientific Names, Eponyms, Synonyms, and Etymology (5 Volume Set). CRC Press.

12. Bret Schneider E (1898) History of European Botanical Discoveries in China. Sampson Low, Marston and Company.

13. Dr. Duke's Phytochemical and Ethnobotanical Databases. Online Database (2014)

14. EJ Brill L (1972) India Major: Congratulatory Volume Presented to J Gonda (PG Jacob Ensink, Ed.) Netherlands: Brill Archive.

15. Bosch CH (2004) Gynura pseudochina (L.) DC. In: Grubben GJH, Denton OA (eds). PROTA 2: Vegetables/Légumes. [CD-ROM]. PROTA, Wageningen, Netherlands.

16. Grubben G (2004) Gynura pseudochina. In Vegetables (p. 309). Netherlands: Backhuys.

17. Gupta KN (1914) The Ayurvedic System of Medicine or Indian Indigenous Drugs and Plants.

18. Jarikasem S, Charuwichitratana S, Siritantikorn S, Chantratita W, Iskander M, et al. (2013) Ant herpetic Effects of Gynura procumbens. Evid Based Complement Alternat Med 2013: 394-865.

19. MV S (2011) Anti-stress activity of Smilax china on male infertility in rats. Bangalore: Nargund College of Pharmacy.

20. Namra H (2012) In Vitro Studies of Antimicrobial Properties of Extracts. International Journal of Pharma and Bio Sciences, 240-249.

21. Rao S (2005) Encyclopedia of Indian Medicine: Historical perspective. Bangalore: Ramadas Bhatkal.

22. Ray P (2004) History of Chemistry in Ancient and Medieval India. Varanasi: Chawkanha Krishnadas Academy.

23. Shivprasad Mahadkar SV (2012) Nutritional assessment of some selected wild edible plants as a good. Asian J Plant Sci Res, 2: 468-472.

24. Siriwatanametanon N, Fiebich BL, Efferth T, Prieto JM, Heinrich M (2010) Traditionally used Thai medicinal plants: in vitro anti-inflammatory, anticancer and antioxidant activities. J Ethnopharmacol 130: 196-207.

25. Somarathna KI, Chandola HM, Ravishankar B, Pandya KN, Attanayake AM, et al. (2010) Evaluation of adaptogenic and anti-stress effects of Ranahamsa Rasayanaya-A Sri Lankan classical Rasayana drug on experimental animals. Ayu 31: 88-92.

26. Trimen H (1895) A Hand-Book of the Flora of Ceylon (Vol. Part III). London: Dulau & Co.

27. Vijayalakshmi A, Ravichandiran V, Anbu J, Velraj M, Jayakumari S (2011) Anticonvulsant and neurotoxicity profile of the rhizome of Smilax china Linn. in mice. Indian J Pharmacol 43: 27-30.

28. Xu Y, Liang JY, Zou ZM (2008) Studies on chemical constituents of rhizomes of Smilax china. Zhongguo Zhong Yao Za Zhi 33: 2497-2499.

29. Yance D (2013) Adaptogens in medical herbalism: Elite herbs and natural compounds for mastering stress, aging, and chronic disease. Inner Traditions / Bear.

25

Valuable Assessment of Quality of PatoladiLepa: An Ayurvedic Paste

Kumaradharmasena LSP[1]*, Fernando PIPK[2], Arawwawala LDAM[2], Kamal S[1] and Peiris KPP[3]

[1]Department of Shalya Shalakya, Institute of Indigenous Medicine, University of Colombo, Rajagiriya, Sri Lanka
[2]Industrial Technology Institute, Bauddhaloka Mawatha, Colombo 07, Sri Lanka
[3]Gampaha Wickramarachchi Ayurveda Institute, University of Kelaniya, Sri Lanka

Abstract

More than one fourth of world population is suffering from dental caries. It is a burden to governments of both developed and developing countries as they have to spend lot of money on treatments for dental caries. PatoladiLepa is an Ayurvedic paste used for dental caries and it consists of 7 plant ingredients, rock salt and honey. The objective of the current research was to determine the organoleptic properties, pH value, total ash, water soluble ash, acid insoluble ash and heavy metals such as Arsenic (As) and Lead (Pb) in PatoladiLepa using standard protocols. Moreover, Thin Layer Chromatography (TLC) fingerprint was developed for the paste using dichloromethane, cyclohexane and methanol in a ratio of 20:6:0.4 v/v. According to the results, PatoladiLepa appeared to be semi solid, blackish brown with pungent taste. In addition, pH value, total ash, water soluble ash, acid insoluble ash were 5.8 ± 1 at 29°C, $12.1 \pm 0.0\%$ w/w, $1.8 \pm 0.0\%$ w/w and $0.24 \pm 0.0\%$ w/w respectively. As and Pb were not present in PatoladiLepa. In conclusion, quality control parameters were established for PatoladiLepa for the first time.

Keywords: PatoladiLepa; Physico-chemical parameters; TLC fingerprint

Introduction

The craniofacial complex allows us to speak, smile, kiss, touch, smell, taste, chew, and swallow and to cry out in pain. It provides protection against microbial infections and environmental threats. Oral diseases restrict activities at school, work and home causing millions of school and work hours to be lost each year the world over. Moreover, the psychosocial impact of these diseases significantly diminishes quality of life [1]. An awareness of dental diseases and there treatments are reveal under medical topics in historical records. Dental diseases include dental caries, developmental defects of enamel, dental erosion and periodontal disease. The main cause of tooth loss is dental caries and it is commonly known as cavities or tooth decay [2,3]. In the presence of sweet and sticky foods, acid-producing bacteria living in the oral environment and thereby caused dental caries [3]. More than one fourth of world population is suffering from dental caries. It is a burden to governments of both developed and developing countries as they have to spend lot of money on treatments for dental caries [4]. Dental caries affects both men and women in all races, socio-economic status and every age group and it leading to pain and discomfort [5,6].

Medicinal plants have considerable potential against dental diseases including dental caries [7]. Since time immoral, Ayurvedic physicians have successfully treated dental caries by using herbal based treatments. PatoladiLepa, is one of the medicated pastes prescribed in Datta [8] as a remedy for dental caries. It consists of 7 medicinal plants, rock salt and honey (Table 1). In this study, we have made an attempt to assess the quality of the PatoladiLepa according to standard protocols.

Materials and Methods

Herbarium sheets were prepared for plant ingredients listed in Table 1, and authenticated by the Senior Scientist, Botany Division and Quality Assurance and Standardization Division at Bandaranayaks Memorial Ayurvedic Research Institute, Nawinna, Maharagama, Sri Lanka.

Preparation of PatoladiLepa

PatoladiLepa was prepared according to the method described in Sharangadhara Samhita. Preparation of PatoladiLepa was carried out at Pharmacy, Institute of Indigenous Medicine, University of Colombo, and Rajagiriya, Sri Lanka. In brief, all the purified raw materials of PatoladiLepa, except honey, were grounded individually by using the pulverizer. The powder was passed through the No. 180 size sieve and fine powder was obtained. Equal amount of each ingredient was mixed and ground on a grinding stone with a little quantity of honey, till it gets soft and spreads evenly. The manufactured paste was stored in an air tight sterilized containers.

Establishment of quality control parameters for PatoladiLepa

Organoleptic properties and physico-chemical parameters of PatoladiLepa were evaluated. In addition, confirmation of raw materials in PatoladiLepa and phytochemical screening were done.

Organoleptic properties

Color, smell and appearance of PatoladiLepa were evaluated.

Physico-chemical parameters

Parameters such as pH, total ash, water soluble ash, acid insoluble ash, heavy metals of PatoladiLepa were investigated using standard techniques.

pH value

Paste (5 g) was mixed with water (45 ml) by using magnetic stir (IKA C-MAG HS10 Digital) for 1 h and observed the pH at 29°C by using a pH meter (Consort C533).

Total ash, acid insoluble ash and water soluble ash

Amounts of total ash, acid insoluble ash and water soluble ash in the PatoladiLepa was determined according to WHO [9] guidelines.

*Corresponding author: Dr. Kumaradharmasena LSP, Department of Shalya Shalakya, Institute of Indigenous Medicine, University of Colombo, Rajagiriya, Sri Lanka, E-mail: menuka@iti.lk

Heavy Metals

Presence or absence of Arsenic (As) and Lead (Pb) in the PatoladiLepa were determined according to the method described in AOAC guidelines [10].

Thin Layer Chromatography (TLC)

For ingredients: Ingredients of the drug in a ratio of 1:1 w/w were mixed, extracted into dichloromethane (20 ml) and filtered. This was repeated thrice and concentrated by using the rotavapor under vacuum pressure at 40°C.

PatoladiLepa: Paste (5.0 g) was dissolved in water (25 ml) and extracted into dichloromethane (20 ml) and filtered. This was repeated thrice and concentrated by using the rotavapor under vacuum pressure at 40°C.

Concentrated dichloromethane extracts of both ingredients and PatoladiLepa were spotted (5 μL from each) on a TLC plate (Silica gel GF254 pre- coated). TLC fingerprint was developed using dichloromethane, cyclohexane and methanol in a ratio of 20: 6: 0.4 v/v and observed under UV light (at both 254 nm and 366 nm). Finally, vanillin sulphate was sprayed on the TLC plate and heated at 110°C for 5 min.

Phytochemical screening: Presence or absence of alkaloids, polyphenols, flavonoids, steroids, saponins and tannins in PatoladiLepa was carried out as described by Yadav and Agarwala [11].

Results and Discussion

Plant based medicines are used for wide range of disease conditions in both humans and animals [12]. Non-availability of proper standards for herbal medicine is the major drawback in herbal medicine industry. Since the synthetic drugs are subjected to severe quality control, the plant products must also comply with the same quality standards [13]. This affects both physicians and patients and also face difficulties when promoting herbal medicine to Western countries [14].

However, in Sri Lanka, attempts have been taken to assess and establish the quality control parameters for herbal medicines such as Vipadikahara Grita Taila [15], Sarasvatha Choorna [16], Haridradi Ashcyotana [17], Dhanyamla [18] and Mustadi Taila [19]. In the present study, quality control parameters were established for PatoladiLepa which used as a remedy for dental caries. Organoleptic properties and physico-chemical parameters of PatoladiLepa were shown in Table 2.

The ash value was determined by 3 different methods, which measured total ash, acid insoluble ash, and water soluble ash. Acid insoluble ash measures the amount of silica or acid insoluble matter in the paste. Water soluble ash is the water soluble portion of the total ash. These ash values are important quantitative standards [20]. R_f values of standard mixture of raw materials and PatoladiLepa are shown in Table 3. According to the R_f values, it was revealed that all the plant ingredients which should be present in PatoladiLepa were present in the paste.

Phytochemical screening revealed the presence of polyphenols, flavonoids, steroids and tannins in PatoladiLepa. Secondary metabolites such as polyphenols, flavonoids, steroids and tannins have shown potent antimicrobial activity [21]. Therefore, presence of secondary metabolites in PatoladiLepa may play a key role when it is used as a remedy for dental caries. In addition, these secondary metabolites are act as nutraceuticals and may help to prevent diseases such as diabetes, cardiovascular diseases, etc. [22,23].

Ingredients	Parts of the plant
Trichosanthes cucumerina Linn.	Whole plant
Picrorrhiza kurrooa Benth.	Rhizome
Zingiber officinale Linn.	Rhizome
Piper nigram Linn.	Fruit
Piper longum Linn.	Fruit
*Cissampelos pareira*Linn.	Whole plant
Clerodendrum serratum Linn.	Root
Rock salt	N/A
Honey	N/A

Table 1: Ingredients of PatoladiLepa.

Organoleptic properties	
Colour	Blackish brown colour
Appearance	Semi solid
Taste	Pungent taste
Physico-chemical parameters	
pH value	5.8 ± 1 at 29°C
Colouring matter	Synthetic dyes were not present
Total ash	12.1 ± 0.0% w/w
Water soluble ash	1.8 ± 0.0% w/w
Acid insoluble ash	0.24 ± 0.0% w/w
Heavy metals (Pb, As)	Not detected

Table 2: Organoleptic properties and Physico-chemical parameters of Patoladilepa.

PatoladiLepa	Before spraying	0.02, 0.08, 0.30, 0.33, 0.38, 0.42, 0.47, 0.57, 0.82, 0.93
	After spraying	0.12, 0.29, 0.38, 0.42, 0.44, 0.57, 0.83, 0.92
Standard mixture of raw materials	Before spraying	0.12, 0.19, 0.29, 0.33, 0.38, 0.42, 0.47, 0.56, 0.82, 0.93
	After spraying	0.12, 0.29, 0.38, 0.42, 0.44, 0.57, 0.83, 0.92

Table 3: R_f values of PatoladiLepa and its standard mixture of plant ingredients.

Conclusion

Present study established the quality control parameters of PatoladiLepa for the first time and can be used as a reference.

References

1. WHO (1987) Prevention of Oral Diseases. World Health Organization publication, Geneva pp: 1-83.

2. Moynihan P, Petersen PE (2004) Diet, nutrition and the prevention of dental diseases. Pub Health Nutr 7: 201-226.

3. Harford J, Spencer J, Roberts-Thomson K (2003) Oral health. The health of Indigenous Australians, Oxford University Press, South Melbourne pp: 313-338.

4. http://www.rightdiagnosis.com/d/dental_caries/stats-country.htm

5. http://www.who.int/mediacentre/factsheets/fs318/en/

6. Cowson RA, Odell EW, Porter S (2002) Cowson's Essentials of Oral Pathology and Oral Medicine (7th edn.) London, Livingstone pp: 336-352.

7. Kelmanson JE, Jager AK, Staden J (2000) Zulu medicinal plants with antibacterial activity. J Ethnopharmacol 69: 241-246.

8. Datta C (1992) With Padarthaodhini Hindi Commentary. Publication of Chaukhamba Surbharati Prakashan, Varanasi.

9. WHO (2011) Noncommunicable Diseases. World Health Organization publication, Geneva.

10. AOAC International (2000) Official Methods of Analysis of AOAC International (17th edn.) Garthersburg, USA.

11. Yadav RNS, Agarwala M (2011) Phytochemical analysis of some medicinal plants. J Phytol 3: 10-14.

12. Cordell GA, Colvard MD (2007) Natural products in a world out-of-balance. Archive Organic Chem 5: 97-115.

13. Karlsen J (1991) Quality control and instrumental analysis of plant extracts. The medicinal plant industry, Publication of CRC press, USA pp: 99-105.

14. Hildreth J, Hrabeta-Robinson E, Applequist W, Betz J, Miller J (2007) Standard operating procedure for the collection and preparation of voucher plant specimens for use in the nutraceutical industry. Analyt Bioanal Chem 389: 13-17.

15. Hewageegana HGSP, Arawwawala LDAM, Fernando PIPK, Dhammarathana I, Ariyawansa HAS, et al. (2013) Standardization of Vipadikahara grita taila: An Ayurvedia medicated ouil for common skin diseases. Unique J Ayur Herb Med 1: 48-51.

16. Karunaratne TDN, Sugataratana K, Ariyawansa HAS, Silva HAD, Samarasingha K, et al. (2015) Standardization of Sarasvatha Choorna: Used as a remedy for dementia. Am J Clin Exp Med 3: 288-292.

17. Silva LDRD, Peiris A, Kamal SV, Jayaratne DLSM, Arawwawala LDAM (2015) Haridradi Ashcyotana: Quality assessment of a herbal eye drop. Int J Pharamaco Phytochem Res 7: 1096-1098.

18. Ranasinghe RLDS, Ediriweera ERHSS, Wasalamuni WADD, Arawwawala LDAM (2015) Assessment of quality of Dhanyamla: A fermented cereal used in Ayurveda. Brit J Pharma Res 8: 1-5.

19. Kumaradharmasena LSP, Arawwawala LDAM, Fernando PIPK, Peiris KPP, Kamal SV (2015) Quality assessment of Mustadi Taila: An Ayurvedic oil as remedy for dental caries (Krimi Danta). J Pharmacogn Phytochem 4: 21-24.

20. Singh MP, Sharma CS (2010) Pharmacognostical evaluation of Terminalia chebula fruits on different market samples. Int J Chem Res 2: 57-61.

21. Compean KL, Ynalvez RA (2014) Antimicrobial activity of plant secondary metabolites: A review. Res J Med Plants 8: 204-213.

22. Ciccone MM, Aquilino A, Cortese F, Scicchitano P, Sassara M, et al. (2010) Feasibility and effectiveness of a disease and care management model in the primary health care system for patients with heart failure and diabetes (Project Leonardo). Vascular Health Risk Manag 6: 297-305.

23. Ramaa CS, Shirode AR, Mundada AS, Kadam VJ (2006) Nutraceuticals-An emerging era in the treatment and prevention of cardiovascular diseases. Current Pharma Biotech 7: 15-23.

26

Contribution of Socio-Anthropology in Schistosomiasis Control - TAABO/ Côte d'Ivoire Experiment

Abe N'doumy Noël*

Anthropologist, Research-Teacher, Université Alassane Ouattara, Côte d'Ivoire

Abstract

Introduction: Schistosomiasis is the most common parasitic disease in the world after malaria. 85% of affected populations live in Africa. Clinical complications are many. WHO notes that on average 46 people die every hour of Schistosomiasis in the world. The health and economic impact of this epidemic appears indisputable. Several endemic foci are reported in Côte d'Ivoire. Most research work in relation to this is carried out from biomedical and geographical perspectives. Actually, how can you lead an effective program to control this epidemic if risk behaviours are ignored? This is the fundamental issue that justifies the scientific relevance of this study. Biomedical and geographical perspective cannot be the only way to propose a comprehensive and permanent solution. Failure to focus on issues involving risk factors associated with humans in this case, limits the effectiveness of such control. This is why it is important to involve socio-anthropology in order to establish a multidisciplinary field of Schistosomiasis control.

Methodology of Work: The study area is Taabo region, located in the centre of Côte d'Ivoire. The study area consists of five (5) sites: Ahondo, Bonikro, Léléblé, Taabo-village and Takohiri. This is a qualitative study. The survey population consists of key informants. Collection techniques are the same as a documentary research method, direct observation and group interviews with key informants.

Results: Physical characteristics : The physical environment of the region has a mixed character astride the savannah and forest. It is an area around the Bandama River large dam where a variety of surface water sources are found.

Schistosomiasis: Is not seen as a pathological fact a far as the community is concerned. Indeed, it is not considered a serious disease.

Human risk factors: Most human activities associated with water are carried out in the multitude of surface water sources. Moreover, the virtual absence of latrines in communities is an increased risk factor as regards contamination of the disease.

Social aetiology and parasitological treatment perception: Field data show a completely wrong aetiology based on a parasitological treatment that is not in line with reality.

Conclusion: The socio-anthropological study focused on lifestyle has actually highlighted the belief system of the observed populations, their way of life and their social practices that promote endemic Schistosomiasis. The interest of this study was to make these socio-anthropological findings available so that the communicative dimension of the control of the disease should consider them in its communication activities for behaviour change. This is one of the conditions for a more effective Schistosomiasis control.

Keywords: Anthropology; Health education; Community health; Schistosomiasis; Taboo

Introduction

Schistosomiasis is a parasitic infection caused by Schistosomia kind of worms. Schistosomiasis is the most common parasitic disease in the world after malaria. Its various forms are endemic in 76 countries. Of these, 42 are found in Africa. Moreover, of the 207 million people infected, 85% live in Africa. Parasites of the disease being common in freshwater, then the most at risk of contamination are farmers, fishermen and women who mainly carry out such activities as washing up clothes, etc., in there.

WHO notes that Schistosomiasis may cause some skin, cancer (bladder), cardiac and pulmonary (high blood pressure) complications; it may also cause infertility due to affected genitals. In addition, the Organisation notes that 46 people on average die every hour of Schistosomiasis in the world. As a result of this fact observed, the endemic Schistosomiasis has a real impact on the economy and health where it occurs. Therefore, to improve the socio-economic status and well-being of populations in endemic areas of this disease, studies and awareness actions have been implemented.

Côte d'Ivoire is no exception to this rule because a multitude of

endemic foci of Schistosomiasis have been listed in there, especially in the West [1], Centre [2], the Southeast [3], Southwest [4] etc.

Yet, an analysis of the facts shows that most research work carried out is driven by two major perspectives: biomedical perspective and geographical perspective. Biomedical perspective work is guided by several disciplines that are:

- Parasitology – aiming to detect Schistosome eggs in faeces and urine to confirm the presence or absence of Schistosomiasis.

- Epidemiology–describing patterns of disease distribution as

*Corresponding author: Abe N'doumy Noël, Anthropologist, Research-Teacher, Université Alassane Ouattara de Bouaké, Côte d'Ivoire
E-mail: ndoumyabe@yahoo.fr

per socio-demographic variables: sex, age, living environment, etc.

- Entomology – examining the life cycles of the disease vector.

Regarding the geographical work perspective, the focus is on natural factors, that is to say how variably, land use, topography, temperature and rainfall influence the increased risk of Schistosomiasis. The solutions proposed by the biomedical and geographic studies, as history shows, have underestimated the habits or customs that constitute the sociocultural and reproductive dimension of endemicity. Such socio cultural dimension observable through socio-behavioural indicators is the subject of this study. Unlike medical and geographical disciplines, this study is part of the anthropological perspective that has focused on human risk factors. It was therefore suggested considering how Schistosomiasis was seen among the diseases that are common locally, human factors underlying the increased risk of the disease and people's attitudes towards the treatment of this endemic disease.

Methodology of Work

Study area

The geographical area concerned is the region of TAABO where is located one of the six hydroelectric dams in Cote d'Ivoire (Ministry of Environment 1996). Observation sites include five locations that are: Ahondo, Bonikro, Léléblé, Taabo village and Tokohiri. These are rural communities located around the large dam of TAABO in central Cote d'Ivoire.

Nature of the study

The study is qualitative in nature. It is guided by the assumption that the perceptions and attitudes of members of the community are factors of increased risk of the endemic Schistosomiasis despite the proven effectiveness of parasitological treatment. These social and cultural considerations underpin the use of social science disciplines including the socio-anthropology. The contribution of the latter is to explain and understand the fundamentals of the reluctance observed. In the context of this social discipline, method of work is determined by two factors: the quality of the respondents and the specificity of observation units.

Survey population

Given the qualitative nature of the study, it was not necessary to determine a statistically-representative sample. It is thus that within each community visited, key informants were identified. They were likely to provide reliable information expected. They included the following:

- The chief and/or some very important people
- Primary school teachers present during our visit
- Community health workers
- A nurse or midwife
- Youth representatives
- Managers of health management committee (COGES)
- Representatives of students' parents
- Women's representatives

Data collection techniques

Regarding data collection, we used three types of techniques. These are: documentary research method, direct observation of the physical environment, and the group interview to collect the official version of facts according to the community.

Observation units

The facts observed involved the following:

- Ecological, socio-economic and cultural characteristics of the community;
- Epidemiological pattern in the community;
- Existing water points in the area;
- Experience of the community as regards Schistosomiasis.

From these focal points, a series of exchanges brought results

Results

Characteristics of the study area

The area is determined by quite a peculiar ecological environment, a composite socio-cultural environment and a variety of water points.

Ecological and climatic characteristics: TAABO is an area in the southern part of central Côte d'Ivoire, a hinge zone located between the forest in the south and the savannah in central Côte d'Ivoire. It is a landscape characterized by the presence of a chain of hills, lots of areas of shallow water, a tropical climate with a dry season and a rainy season. Local temperature varies between 28°C and 30°C.

Ethno-cultural environment: The ethno-cultural environment remains very mixed. It consists of native peoples, Akan (Baoule, Swamlin, Ngban), Kru (Dida) and many non-native communities, then aliens (Burkinabes, Malians, Nigeriens and Mauritanians) hailing from the West African sub-region.

The large dam and water points in terms of hydrology, the area are mainly characterized by the presence of the large dam on the Bandaman river, several lakes and seasonal streams.

These specific ecological, ethno-cultural and hydrological characteristics result in unique implications relating to health.

How is Schistosomiasis seen among the common diseases in the community: In the areas visited, the pathologies regarded as common, appear to be numerous. Among these, the most feared were identified. This socio-sanitary environment is described in (Table 1)

Urinary Schistosomiasis is endemic in the five locations visited. Yet, the group interviews resulted in two significant facts:

- Schistosomiasis is not recognised as a pathological fact in the Baoulé community;
- Schistosomiasis is not considered a serious morbid state because, of course, it is not a disease. Thus, it is not feared in this Baoulé community

Human risk factors of Schistosomiasis in the region: Factors observed in the community's concern water points, human activities and conditions of public health. Items of analysis are shown in (Table 2). SODECI: Company of Water Distribution in Côte d'Ivoire.

Table 2 noted three major items

- There are a multitude of surface water sources in the physical space of the study area

Localities	Common diseases mentioned	Feared diseases among those listed	Reason for fearing the diseases	Comments
Ahondo	Malaria Schistosomiasis Onchocerciasis	Onchocerciasis	Onchocerciasis causes sight loss	Schistosomiasis has been recognised as an endemic disease by all participants in the interview
Bonikro	Malaria Diarrhoea Buruli ulcer	No disease mentioned is feared except when there are complications at an advanced stage	Complications immobilise the patient or lead to death	Schistosomiasis has been reported among common diseases only by teachers present at the meeting
Leleble	Malaria Typhoid fever Buruli ulcer Measles	Typhoid fever	The symptoms of typhoid fever are difficult to distinguish from malaria; besides, treatment takes longer and is expensive	Schistosomiasis is endemic but not listed among the common diseases
Taabo-village	Malaria Buruli ulcer Typhoid fever Schistosomiasis	Typhoid fever	The treatment of typhoid fever is long because of its symptoms that are similar to malaria	Schistosomiasis has been mentioned among the common diseases only by teachers
Tokohiri	Malaria Buruli ulcer Onchocerciasis Rheumatism	Onchocerciasis	Onchocerciasis is feared because it causes sight loss	Schistosomiasis is endemic but it was not listed among the common diseases

Source: 2008 survey

Table 1: Epidemiological pattern of according to the community.

Localities	Drinking water sources	Water points in natural environment	Human activities in natural water points	Health facilities	Latrines
Ahondo	A water tower in a neighbourhood	dam fahasso koukouba	Drink, laundry, dishwashing, swimming, fishing	Presence of a health centre	Presence of some latrines
Bonikro	Two water pumps	Bandama several seasonal water points	Drinking, washing, bathing watering vegetable gardening	Presence of a health centre	No latrines
Leleble	SODECI water supply	dam behifon labâbrouha Doho 1 Doho 2	Drinking, washing, washing dishes, watering crops, swimming and fishing	Presence of a dispensary	No latrines
Taabo-Village	SODECI Water supply	dam Lake backwater	Drinking, washing, washing dishes, swimming fishing, recreation	No health centre	No latrines
Tokohiri	Two water pumps	kimbahongo kpadjagna dogo-n'zuhé	Drinking, washing, washing dishes, watering, bathing	No health centre	No latrines

SODECI: Company of water distribution in Côte d'Ivoire

Table 2: Risk factors relating to exposure to schistosomiasis in the localities.

- A large number of human activities associated with water are carried out in these water sources.
- Absence of latrines in communities is an increased risk factor for contamination of Schistosomiasis in the study area.

Social aetiology according to the community and its attitudes towards treatment: The social experience of the communities as regards this endemic disease is observed through their perception and attitudes.

The cultural communities' perception of Schistosomiasis: This perception is about describing the name, the symptoms and causes. In terms of nosology and symptomatology

Schistosomiasis has two different names in the Baoule Swamlin group that is the dominant group. The terms used for Schistosomiasis are:

- "*Bié-modja/*bjemodzæ/", meaning "pee from blood"
- "*Ako-liè* /ækɔliɛ/", which is equated with "*rooster's venereal disease*".

Reference to these images is due to the presence of blood in the urine. Urine colour remains the major symptom for the group.

The intestinal form of the disease remains unknown. Also, in the imagination of this cultural complex, Schistosomiasis is not considered a serious disease. In this community, any morbidity implying physical disability or any morbidity of a chronic nature is defined as a serious illness- Social aetiology

According to the groups visited, three cases are distinguished due to Schistosomiasis:

- Consumption of contaminated water;
- Pees on the traces of urine of a subject having the disease
- Sexual transmission.

These items indicate explicitly that the real causes of contamination due to Schistosomiasis remain ignored in the communities.

Attitudes vis-à-vis the treatment of Schistosomiasisare observed at TAABO through three social contexts:

- Treatment in the community through traditional African medicine; this treatment is performed by traditional healers. This is by and large the starting point of a series of types of therapy. The use of medicinal plants in the form of decoction is involved. Plant leaves, bark, roots or fruit are used. Both men and women are subject to this type of African medicine; adults, young people as well as children are all subject to the same treatment.

- Parasitological treatment at school; target population regarding praziquantel-based treatment at school is meant for all six to thirteen year-old primary school children. This population segment is the most affected by Schistosomiasis in the aforesaid areas. Tablets are sold CFAF100.00 (about 0.20 USD) each to school children by school teachers officially assigned thereto. Some difficulties are observed, albeit this ridiculous price. As a matter of fact, some parents appear to be reluctant to give their offspring the one hundred francs for their treatment. To them, the drug should be absolutely free of charge.

- The parasitological treatment in the community: target social groups in this context are mainly young people and adults living in the community. This is actually a community-based distribution where a Community Health Officer (ASC) is the key interface. For contaminated subjects, access to praziquantel-based treatment is subject to payment of a paltry amount of two hundred (200.00) CFAF. Again, reluctance appears clearly visible through arithmetical demonstrations of household heads. They clearly indicate that the larger the household, the higher the cost of treatment. This fact becomes for a considerable number of households a deterrent to parasitological treatment. Moreover, according to this same population, parasitological treatment does not seem to be quite effective to the extent that many cases of recurrence are experienced in the group.

After all, as one can see, disruption of the disease transmission chain is not obvious at the present stage. To be honest, only the biomedical sciences through epidemiology, parasitology and pharmacology cannot put an end to this public health issue caused by Schistosomiasis. The nature of this issue is not only of biological dimension. Through water-related lifestyle, social perceptions of the disease and attitudes towards treatment methods, a socio-cultural dimension is to be taken into account. How can one justify this reflection perspective?

Discussion

At this stage of the process, it is all about showing how and why it appears necessary for social sciences to be instrumental in controlling, together with biomedical sciences, Schistosomiasis defined as an endemic disease. Such multidisciplinary approach is determined by three major findings that are: tradition involving rapport with water, social perception concerning Schistosomiasis and perception of treatment.

Tradition involving rapport with water

The tradition concerning the rapport with water is the starting point. Indeed, the cultural community in question in this context is the Baoule subgroup called "Swamlin". Geographically settled around the large dam, this group has historically developed a tradition in its rapport with Bandama river. The existence of small surface water points in any season of the year in the area has, of course, strengthened this tradition of rapport with water. This is accounted for in Table 2.

- The presence of all kinds of human activities in various natural water points, including washing, washing dishes, bathing, watering crops, fishing and recreation;

- Access to various water points by all social strata, men and

women, adults, youth and children at any time and without conditions.

This data set cause's increased risk factors that help spread Schistosomiasis, especially as hygiene conditions are insecure because of the lack of latrines in the communities. For the *Swamlin* community, the river and its immediate environment are a sociological framework that defines itself as a continuation of the village site, regardless of the distance separating the two areas. This same finding is seen in the works of [5] that argue that the distance to permanent water courses was one of the most significant variables for predicting the increased risk of the disease. Water in nature is an area with many social and cultural functions. It is seen as:

- An area for relations and trade (taking community baths in the evening by adults);

- An area for gender education (young girls learning how to do washing and washing up under the supervision of their mothers);

- An area for learning and assertiveness (swims and swimming competitions for young people);

- An area for leisure and eroticism (place for seduction among adolescents);

- An access route to workplace for farmers (crossing for farm work)

In this way, the water points involved, depending on days and seasons, a relatively large proportion, time for various members of the community (men, women, adults, young people and children) in their various activities (farming, recreation , sexuality, education, etc.).

Consequently, these sources being recognized as the bases for the spread of the disease, the logical question that arises is how to minimize contact with the waters from the natural environment, while reducing the risk of contamination. This is the first issue which falls within the competence of social sciences.

The illness representation system

Schistosomiasis known as "bié-modja" is represented in the Swamlin community through a belief system completely separate from classical epidemiology [6]. This belief system has a causal diagram but unrelated to the epidemiological sense. This finding is revealed by the data in Table 1.

- Of the five communities visited, only that of AHONDO recognised as Schistosomiasis is a common disease in the population. Only teachers, having different cultural origin, and present in different interview groups drew attention to the endemic nature of this disease.

- In none of the five communities surveyed, Schistosomiasis was listed as critical illness, even at AHONDO where it was regarded by the population as a significant endemic disease.

These observations lead us to highlight another reason for involvement of anthropology in the control of the endemic Schistosomiasis. Indeed, the system of representation in these Baoule communities is wrong. In fact, Schistosomiasis is certainly identified as a disease. But it is not recognised as a serious disease. This perception stems from the fact that this condition does not lead to apparent disability on a short-term basis in the eyes of the members of these communities. This finding is the same made by WARDA (1999) stating that Schistosomiasis is simply not perceived as a threat to life or even a debilitating disease. This is because many infected people do not suffer unduly. Yet, the serious medical consequences of Schistosomiasis are real. "In case of repeated reinfection causing intense parasitism, one sees a hepato-intestinal syndrome. It is a chronic and severe form where diarrhoea is coupled with a large liver (hepatomegaly), ascites, splenomegaly (enlarged spleen), severe anaemia and weight loss" [7]. These physiological implications remain simply ignored by the cultural groups visited.

Treatment perception

The field survey revealed that the *"Swamlin"* community is aware of the limitations of parasitological treatment of Schistosomiasis as an endemic disease. The treatment is based on Praziquantel. However, this concept of limits needs to be explained.

- To these communities, the concept of limits appears to amount to "inefficiency", and in this respect, Praziquantel is comparable to placebo [8]. Its effect would only be that of a psychological nature since the same patient may have several episodes of the disease during the same year.

- According to the medical model, the concept of limits would mean "necessary but not sufficient".

This leads us to understand that besides Praziquantel, it is important to adopt good health behaviour regarding human wastes (urine and faeces). Such wastes ought to be dumped in protected areas (latrines) but not in surface waters available to the public.

Indeed, one needs to state that a recurrent symptom of Schistosomiasis in some patients despite treatment with praziquantel does not amount to the drug being ineffective [9]. It is rather due to the risk behaviour (contact with contaminated water points) that exposes these subjects permanently. 'Schistosomiasis would be extinct if a contaminated subject took the habit of urinating and going to toilet away from water points" [10]. One must say that healing the body appears necessary but not enough, since human behaviour ought to be healed at the same time. Only social sciences concerned with this behavioural dimension, will be able to achieve this goal. This is the only way the overall community health project can be effective. In other words, the scope of this community health is defined as a multidisciplinary framework. Skills sought in this area include biomedical sciences, socio-anthropology and communication sciences.

Conclusion

It appears from the analysis of the facts that not only is Schistosomiasis endemicity due to epidemiological and geographical factors, but also to a human factor that appears decisive. The experience of the Taabo area has shown that the Baoule *swamlin* cultural communities do not consider Schistosomiasis a disease. No fear in this respect. Indeed, the risk of contamination is further compounded by the fact that most agricultural, domestic and recreational activities are related to surface water, while at the same time, latrines are almost non-existent in the localities. To this is added the parasitological treatment considered ineffective by the people. This set of human factors related to lifestyle, perceptions and social behaviour leads us to think that anthropology appears as an essential discipline in the control of the endemic Schistosomiasis in Taabo region.

References

1. Bourardi C, Roussiau N, Larrue J (1998) Social cognitive approach to representational dynamics and its determinants. International books Social Psychology.

2. N'guessan NA, Acka CA, Utzinger J, N'Goran KE (2007) Identification of high risk areas of schistosomiasis in Côte d'Ivoire. Bull Soc Pathol Exot 100: 119-123.

3. Adoubryn KD, Ouhon J, Yapo CG, Assoumou EY, Ago KM, et al. (2006) [Epidemiological profile of the schistosomiasis in school children in the Agneby Region (south-east of Côte-d'Ivoire)]. Bull Soc Pathol Exot 99- 28-31.

4. Evi JB, Yavo W, Barro-Kiki PC, Menan EH, Kone M (2007) Intestinal helminthiasis in school background in six towns of southwestern Côte d'Ivoire. Bull Soc Pathol Exot 100: 176-177.

5. Raso G, N'Goran EK, Toty A, Luginbuhl A, Adjoua C, et al. (2004) Efficacy and side effects of praziquantel against Schistosoma mansoni in a community of western Côte d'Ivoire. Trans R Soc trop Med Hyg 98: 18-27.

6. WHO-Workshop on the role of human water contact in schistosomiasis transmission and control (1979) Geneva, Switzerland 277.

7. WHO-Manual of the health team (1979) Ed Saint-paul, Issy les Moulineaux, Geneva, Switzerland 282.

8. N'Goran EK, Utzinger J, Gnaka HN, Yapi A, N'Guessan NA, et al. (2003) Randomized, double-blind, placebo-controlled trial of oral artémether for the prevention of patent Schistosoma haematobium infections. Am J Trop Med Hyg 68: 24-32.

9. N'Goran EK, Utzinger J, N'Guessan AN, Muller I, Zamble K, et al. (2001) Réinfection with Schistosoma haematobium following school-based chemotherapy with praziquantel in four higly endemic villages in côte'ivoire. TopMed Int Health 6: 817-825.

10. Prevention and control of Schistosomiasis and soil transmitted Helminthiasis: Report of a WHO expert committe (2001) WHO technical report series 912, Geneva, Switzerland.

27

Evaluation of Combined Efficacy of Greeva Basti, Patra Pottali Sweda and Nasya in the Management of Cervical Spondylosis

Shettar RV[1] and Bhavya BK[2]*

[1]Assistant Professor, P. G. Department of Kayachikitsa, D. G. M. A. M. C. & H, Gadag, India
[2]P. G. Scholar, II year Kayachikitsa, D. G. M. A. M. C. & H, Gadag, India

Abstract

Cervical Spondylosis is one among the degenerative disc ailments. A recent study showed, the middle aged population shows increased incidence of degenerative disc changes. This may be because of faulty regimen and lifestyle. The study conducted here is a combined therapy of Nasya (Nasal therapy), Griva Basti (Neck care), and Patra Pottali Sweda (Specialized massage therapy using boluses of herbs) consecutively to get maximum relief in a minimal period of time. More attentiveness is on the Bahi Parimarjana Chikitsa (External purification therapy) on the affected part that being Griva (neck) and Manya pradesha (cerviacal spine region). At the initial stage because of Kapha Avarana (Kapha obstruction) there will be stiffness and later when it becomes chronic due to improper usage of cervical spine, Vata alone will lead to Dhatukshaya (tissue degeneration) because Dhatukshaya is an integral character of Vatadosha and Asti is always a victim.

Keywords: Cervical spondylosis; Paraesthesia; Nasya karma; Spine; Degenerative changes

Introduction

Degeneration is a natural process with aging. Elderly people are most affected with degenerative disorders. Today is an era of sophisticated and fast life; everybody is busy and leading a stressful life. So to meet each and every requirements of life there is a vigorous competition and consequently there is change in life style leading to several disharmonies in the biological system of humans.

Advancement of busy professional and social life, improper sitting postures in work places, continuous work in only one posture and over exertion, jerky movements during travelling and sports; all these factors create undue pressure and stress injury to the spine (cervical) and play a major role in producing diseases like Cervical Spondylosis.

Cervical Spondylosis is the most common disorder of the cervical spine. It is caused by degenerative changes in the vertebrae and intervertebral discs that occur as a result of constant improper stress on the cervical spine, injury, ageing, rheumatoid disease etc.

A number of factors are responsible for the development of signs and symptoms of Cervical Spondylosis:

- Osteophyte (bony growth).
- A narrowed spinal canal present since birth.
- Degeneration of the intervertebral discs.
- Changes in the spinal cord and nerves due to insufficient blood supply.

There is no exact clinical entity mentioned in Ayurvedic Classics as Cervical Spondylosis, however it can be considered as Greeva Hundana or Astigata Vata because of its pathogenesis:

- Shoshana (withering) of Asthi Dhatu (in Cervical Region).
- Dushana of Vata.
- Rooksha (drying) guna of Vata increases.
- Avarana of Shleshmaka Kapha and its Shoshana by Pravruddha Vata.

Thus the clinical aspects of Astigata Vata can be implemented in the disease, Cervical Spondylosis. It leads to pain and stiffness in neck, radiating pain into arm, headache, vertigo, giddiness, paraesthesia, numbness, etc. It disturbs the daily routine and overall life of the patient. Though it is not immediately fatal, it causes severe complications in later stage. It cripples the patient to an extent there is dependency on others. The individual cannot perform day to day work properly because of the severity of pain leading to a decreased quality of life [1].

Modern medical science provides both conservative and surgical treatment for Cervical Spondylosis but nothing has been satisfactory to date. Alternative medical sciences, like Ayurveda aims to present a better remedy for this condition, which is the purpose of this paper.

Materials and Methods

Study design

An open, randomized, preliminary clinical study.

Source of data

Patients were selected from O.P.D & I.P.D of D.G.M.A.M.C. & H. having classical signs & symptoms of Cervical spondylosis as well as fulfilling inclusion & exclusion criteria.

Sample size

Total 8 patients were registered, among them 1 dropped out, and 7 patients completed treatment schedule.

Inclusion criteria

Patients diagnosed as suffering from Cervical Spondylosis based on classical signs and symptoms were included in the study.

Exclusion criteria

Patients below age 20 or more than 60 years and patients who had history of fracture, surgical emergencies and systemic diseases were

***Corresponding author:** Dr. Bhavya BK, P. G. Scholar, II year Kayachikitsa, D. G. M. A. M. C. & H, Gadag, India, E-mail: drbhavyabk86@gmail.com

excluded from the study. Patients who are not fit for the Nasya Karma were also excluded from the study.

Assessment criteria

A special research Performa was prepared for the study incorporating all the relevant points from both Ayurvedic and modern views. Subjective parameters like Manya Shoola (cervical vertebrae pain), Manya Stambha (cervical spine stiffness), Bahu Shoola (relating or other pain), Griva Shoola (neck pain) and objective parameters like Flexion, Extension, Lateral (Right & Left) Flexion, Rotation, and Passive Neck Flexion were assessed. Each parameter was graded [2].

Hematological analysis, which was done on patients include-Hb%, T.C., D.C., E.S.R. and bio-chemical tests. Random Blood Sugar was carried out to exclude the possibility of any other disease as well as to know the present condition and diagnosis of patients. X-ray of cervical spine Anterio-posterior and Lateral view was taken to rule out fracture, joint obliteration and other possibilities of exclusion (Tables 1 and 2).

Intervention

Step 1 - Griva Basti with Prabhanjana Khuzumbu and Sahacharadi Taila

Step 2 – Patra Pottali Sweda

Step 3 - Nasya with Dhanvantara 101

Abhyantara

Dashamoola Kashaya: 15 ml twice daily with warm water, before food.

Method

Step 1-Griva Basti with Prabhanjana Khuzumbu and Sahacharadi Taila: All patients were first subjected for Greeva vasti. For this Prabhanjana Khuzambu and Sahacharadi Taila were taken in equal quantity and mixed together. Patients were asked to lie on their chest in a comfortable position or sit on a chair flexing their neck resting on a platform with extended arms to expand the cervical spine area. In this position the para-spinal muscles are completely relaxed. A brim made of Masha kalka (black gram paste) was prepared around the cervical spine area with due care to expose the affected part of the spine. Warm oil was poured into the masha brim and constant temperature was maintained by replacing oil periodically at the prescribed time [3].

Griva basti was carried in Arohana (ascending) and Avarohana (descending) pattern. Procedure was carried out for 30 minutes on 1st day and then increased by 5 minutes till 5th day and then 6th day onwards decreased by 5 minutes daily till 10th day (Table 3).

After the Greeva vasti, Sthanika abhyanga was done with same taila. Abhyanga was followed by Patra Pottali Sweda.

Step 2-Patra Pottali Sweda: Small sized chopped Patras (leaves) of Eranda, Nirgundi, Arka, Karanja, shigru, nimba, chincha, along with small pieces of Lemon, Coconut gratings and Saindava Lavana are fried in a pan using little quantity of the Sahacharadi Taila until golden brown. Then pottali is prepared for Sthanika Sweda that is done until Samyak Swinna Lakshanas (signs of proper sudation e.g. sweating) appears [4].

Step 3 - Nasya with Dhanvantara 101 Times Oil: After patra pottali sweda, 5 minutes rest is given to the patient and then Nasya procedure carried out. A poorvakarma mukha abhyanga is done with

Parameter	Grading	Observation
Manya Shoola	0	No Pain
	1	Mild Pain
	2	Moderate Pain But Tolerable
	3	Moderate Pain But Not Tolerable
	4	Severe Intolerable, Perhaps Suicidal Pain
Manya Stambha	0	No Movement
	1	Up to 25% Of Total Movement
	2	Up to 50% Of Total Movement
	3	Up to 75% Of Total Movement
	4	Full Range Of Total Movement
Bahu Shoola	0	No Pain
	1	Mild Pain Radiating From Neck On Movement
	2	Moderate Pain Radiating From Neck On Movement
	3	Severe Continues Pain Affecting Routine Work
	4	Severe Continues Pain Reducing Arm Strength
Griva Shoola	0	No Pain
	1	Mild Pain
	2	Moderate Pain But Tolerable
	3	Moderate Pain But Not Tolerable
	4	Severe Intolerable, Perhaps Suicidal Pain

Table 1: Shows gradation of subjective parameter.

Parameters of Cervical Joint	Grading	Observation
Flexion & Extension	0	Full Range
	1	Restricted Movements
	2	No Movements
Lateral Flexion & Rotation	0	Full Range
	1	Restricted Movements
	2	No Movements
Passive Neck Flexion	0	Without any difficulty
	1	With some difficulty
	2	With much difficulty
	3	Unable to do

Table 2: Shows gradation of objective parameter.

Days	Duration	Days	Duration
1	30 minutes	6	50 minutes
2	35 minutes	7	45 minutes
3	40 minutes	8	40 minutes
4	45 minutes	9	35 minutes
5	50 minutes	10	30 minutes

Table 3: Shows duration of Greeva vasti.

same oil and mrudu (mild) sweda given with a cloth dipped in hot water.

Patient was asked to lie in supine position with neck slightly extended. Dhanwantara 101 times Avartita Taila was taken in Nasya yantra and 8 drops of oil was poured in both nostrils in an uninterrupted stream i.e., *avicchinna dhara* and the patient asked to slowly inhale the medicine but not to swallow. Patient is required to remain in the same position for 5 minutes and then spit the descended medicine from the throat.

Luke warm water with little saindhava lavana was given for gargling. Dhoomapanartha Haridra dhooma was prepared for the process. All procedures were done for 10 days [5].

Results

Observation

Among the 8 patients registered for trial, 7 completed the treatment schedule successfully, all the patients were suffering from neck pain radiating to arm with neck stiffness (Tables 4-7).

Table 4 shows there are 2 males (28.571%) and 5 females (71.428%). The age group between 25-35yrs is 4 (57.142%), 36-45yrs is 2 (28.571%) & 46 – 55yrs is 1 (14.285%). Vegetarians are 2 (28.571%) & Non-Vegetarians are 5 (71.428%). Hindus are 3 (42.851%), Muslims are 2 (28.571%), Christian is 1 (14.285%) & Jain is 1 (14.285%). Based on occupation working people are 4 (57.142), sedentary is 1 (14.285%) & heavy labor worker is 2 (28.571%) in number.

Table 5 shows that most symptoms are present in all patients i.e. manya shoola, manya sthambha, bahu shoola, griva shoola and amsa (shoulder) shoola are present in all patients (100%). Shira shola (nerve), nidra nasha (insomnia), anga marda (body pain), klama (fatigue) are a second major clinical symptoms present in 85.714% of patients. Aruchi (loss of appetite), gourava (heaviness in body) and suptata (numbness) was observed in 5 patients (71.428%), and adhmana (bloating) was observed in 4 patients (57.142).

Table 6 shows that among 7 patients 5 patients were of vata kapha prakriti (71.428%) & 2 were of vata pitta prakriti (28.571%).

Table 7 shows that among 7 patients 6 patients were of non-traumatic and 1 had history of injury.

Results

Results were analyzed on the basis of gradations of subjective and objective parameters before and after the treatment using a statistical test. The observed grading in the patients on subjective and objective parameters is as follows (Table 8 and 9).

SL NO	SEX		AGE	FOOD		RELIGION				OCCUPATION		
	M	F		Veg	Mixed	H	M	C	Other	Active	Sedentary	Labor
1.		+	28		+	+				+		
2.	+		32	+		+					+	
3.		+	35		+	+				+		
4.		+	34	+				+		+		
5.	+		46		+		+					+
6.		+	40		+		+					+
7.		+	45		+			+		+		

Table 4: Shows general observation in patients.

Symptoms	No of Patients	%
Manya Shoola	7	100%
Manya Stambha	7	100%
Bahu Shoola	7	100%
Griva Shoola	7	100%
Aruchi	5	71.428%
Shira Shoola	6	85.714%
Admana	4	57.142%
Amsa Shoola	7	100%
Nidranasha	6	85.714%
Anga Marda	6	85.714%
Gourava	5	71.428%
Klama	6	85.714%
Suptata	5	71.428%

Table 5: Shows clinical presentation of patients.

Deha Prakriti	No of Patients	%
Vata Pitta	2	28.571%
Vata Kapha	5	71.428%
Pitta Kapha	0	0

Table 6: Shows Deha Prakriti.

Abhigata / Trauma	No Of Patients	%
Trauma	1	14.285%
Non Trauma	6	85.714%

Table 7: Shows Abhigataja Karana.

Effect of therapy in subjective parameter: In the present study the therapy has shown highly significant results in all the subjective parameters. The mean of Manya shoola before treatment (BT) was 2.714 and after treatment (AT) showed 0.285 with 89.4% relief, statistically highly significant with $P<0.001$ and $t=8.0645$. The mean of Manya stambha BT was 2.714 and AT showed 1.142 with 57.92% relief, statistically highly significant with $P<0.001$ and $t=7.779$. The mean of Griva shoola BT was 2.714 and AT showed 0.142 with 94.8% of relief, statistically highly significant with $P<0.001$ and $t=8.619$. The mean of Bahu shoola BT was 2.571 and AT showed 0.857 with 66.6% of relief, statistically highly significant with $P<0.001$ and $t=4.774$ (Table 10).

Effect of therapy in objective parameter: In the present study the effect of therapy in all the objective parameters statistically showed significant results. The mean of Flexion BT was 1 and AT showed 0 with 100% relief, shows statistically high significance with $P<0.001$ and $t=0$. The mean of Extension BT was 1 and AT showed 0.142 with 85.7% relief shows statistically high significance with $P<0.001$ and $t=6.0173$. The mean of Lateral flexion BT was 1 and AT showed 0.142 with 85.7% relief shows statistically high significance with $P<0.001$ and $t=6.0173$. The mean of Rotation BT was 1 and AT showed 0 with 100% relief, shows statistically high significance with $P<0.001$ and $t=0$. The mean of Passive neck flexion BT was 2 and AT showed 0.428 with 78.6% relief, shows statistically high significance with $P<0.001$ and $t=7.820$ (Table 11).

Radiological study does not reveal any significant changes in post treatment images. This conclusion was drawn after evaluating the results by Sing's index.

Overall effect: Pre and post test result was analyzed statistically for 'p' value using paired 't' test. The test is significant at 81.26% with $p<0.01$.

Overall results show that among 7 patients 5 patients produced good results. Moderate response and mild response were seen in 1 patient each (Table 12 and Figure 1).

Discussion

Cervical Spondylosis is one of the degenerative disorders of the spine and is an affliction in the middle aged due to provocation factors such as improper stress on spine, irregular postures in working places, and bad food habits. Degeneration of the cervical disc demands Brihmana and Rasayana Therapy. Inter vertebral disc is a cushion like structure that provides protection to vertebral bodies from friction. Degeneration in the disc leads to undue pressure over the nerve roots. Cervical Spondylosis is characterized by degeneration, disc protrusion, calcification and consequent pressure on the nerve roots of the cervical and brachial plexus.

Kshaya roga (wasting) is an integral character of Vata dosha with associated contribution of Kapha and Pitta dosha. Shoola is Vata

SL NO	Manya shoola		Manya stambha		Bahu shoola		Griva shoola	
	BT	AT	BT	AT	BT	AT	BT	AT
1.	3	0	3	1	3	0	3	0
2.	2	1	3	2	3	2	2	1
3.	3	0	2	1	3	0	3	0
4.	2	0	3	1	3	2	2	0
5.	3	0	3	1	1	0	3	0
6.	3	1	3	1	2	1	3	0
7.	3	0	2	1	3	0	3	0

Table 8: Subjective parameter data.

Sl no	Flexion		Extension		Lateral (right & left) flexion		Rotation	
	BT	AT	BT	AT	BT	AT	BT	AT
1.	1	0	1	0	1	0	1	0
2.	1	0	1	1	1	1	1	0
3.	1	0	1	0	1	0	1	0
4.	1	0	1	0	1	0	1	0
5.	1	0	1	0	1	0	1	0
6.	1	0	1	0	1	0	1	0
7.	1	0	1	0	1	0	1	0

Table 9: Objective parameter data.

Sl. No	Parameter	Mean Bt	Mean At	% of Improvement	SD	SE	t value	P value
1.	Manya shoola	2.714	0.285	89.4%	0.78	0.297	8.0645	P<0.001
2.	Manya stambha	2.714	1.142	57.92%	0.534	0.202	7.779	P<0.001
3.	Griva shoola	2.714	0.142	94.8%	0.786	0.297	8.619	P<0.001
4.	Bahu shoola	2.571	0.857	66.6%	0.951	0.359	4.774	P<0.01

Table 10: Subjective parameter statistical data.

Sl no	Parameter	Mean Bt	Mean At	% of Improvement	SD	SE	t value	P value
1.	Flexion	1	0	100%	0	0	0	P<0.001
2.	Extension	1	0.142	85.7%	0.377	0.1425	6.0173	P<0.001
3.	Lateral flexion	1	0.142	85.7%	0.377	0.1425	6.0173	P<0.001
4.	Rotation	1	0	100%	0	0	0	P<0.001
5.	Passive neck flexion	2	0.428	78.6%	0.533	0.201	7.820	P<0.001

Table 11: Objective parameter statistical data.

pradhana whereas sthambha, gourava are character of Kapha dosha. In cervical spondylosis, upasthambita vata dosha vikriti lakshanas are seen more however kaphanubandhi is associated some times. In the present study we find kevala vatajanya lakshanas more. General line of the treatment of vata vyadhi was adopted in the present study. Acharya Charaka mentioned Navanastarpanani susnigdam swedayetat means one should go for navana (nose oiling), tarpana (eye oiling), snehana (internal and external oleation) and swedana (steam therapy) for the basic line of treatment of any vatavyadhi. In the present study nasya was adopted using Dhanwantara taila 101 avartita, tarpana by means of Greeva vasti with Prabhanjana khuzambu and sahacharadi taila, and swedana by Patrapottali sweda. These upakramas (supporting therapies) help in the Samprapti vighatan (cure) [6-8].

Griva Basti and Abhyanga with Prabhanjana Khuzumbu and Sahacharadi taila are indicated in vata vyadis. Griva basti as procedure done as Sthanika Bahya snehana of affected area. It nourishes the Asthi in affected area and pacifies the vata dosha, thereby taila doesn't aggravate kapha thus counteracting the pathology. Abhyanga softens the skin, gives soothing effect, allows free movement, reduces

the spasticity and rigidity in joint as well as muscle, improves blood circulation to the muscles and relieves the pain. In the long term, muscle wasting may be prevented.

The Swedhana selected here is Patra Pottali which is of the Snigdha Rooksha type. The patras used were vatahara, kapha and pittahara. It does shaman of both vata and kapha. It clears the srotodusti or sanga. The area in contact gets more blood circulation, improves local metabolism, and relieves stiffness and variety of obstructions by widening of the pores which allows easy movement of the liquefied solid or semisolid materials. Patrapottali was a better option because it

- Relieves para-vertebral muscle spasm
- Strengthens Para-vertebral muscles
- Strengthens inter vertebral discs
- Helps repair damaged myelin sheath
- Has a local anti- inflammatory effect

Depending on vyadi lakshanas and sthana of vyadhi i.e., Urdhwajatru (Kapha Sthana), the dusti of vata, along with kapha was considered and treatment of Nasya was planned of Navana type with Dhanwantara 101 taila, having Snigdha and Rooksha affecting ingredients. So, here also the drugs and procedure counteract the underlying pathology. Patrapottali Sweda also helps in relieving Avarana by Kapha dosha [9,10].

Dashamula kwatha is vata kapha hara and indicated for all vata vyadhi. The ingredients of Dashamula kwatha pacifies the vata dosha and helps in counteracting the process of Kshaya (degeneration). Sushruthacharya has stated Dashamula kwatha as the best kapha pitta anila apaha, it does pachana of ama and sarva jwara vinasana as well as vatahara (to pacify vata). Bhavapraksha includes it in *Guduchyadi varga* which is Tridoshagna (alleviating all three doshas), Swasakasahara, Shirorujahara, Tandrahara (drowsiness), Shothahara (anti-inflammatory), Jwaragna (antipyretic), Parswapidahara and aruchihara (relieves anorexia) [11].

Conclusion

Cervical Spondylosis is emerging as one of the most common

SL NO	RESULTS	NO OF PATIENTS
1.	GOOD RESPONSE	05
2.	MODERATE RESPONSE	01
3.	MILD RESPONSE	01
4.	NOT RESPONDED	00

Table 12: Overall result.

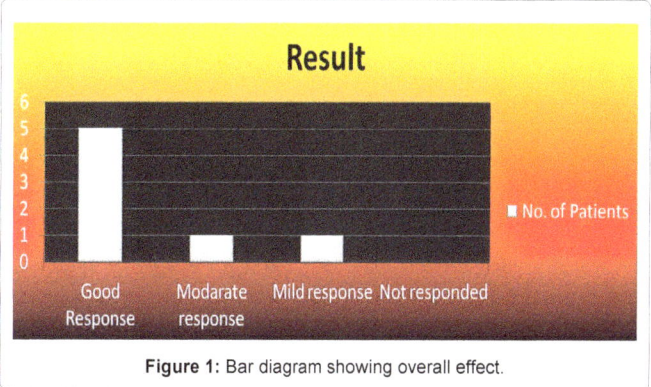

Figure 1: Bar diagram showing overall effect.

diseases especially in urban population. The prevalence of this disease has been expected to increase due to improper lifestyle, poor working, sleeping and sitting postures.

Conclusive results from the present study show a combined effect of griva basti, patra pottali sweda and nasya can offer benefits to reducing symptoms of cervical spondylosis.

Along with the above therapies, postural corrections during work, sleep, travel and avoiding elevated cushions below the neck, coupled with regular exercises go a long way in preventing Cervical Spondylosis.

References

1. Agnivesha, Charaka Samhita (4thedn), Chowkhambha Sanskrit Sansthan, Varanasi, India.

2. Michael Swash (2006) Hutchinson's Clinical Methods. (21stedn), Elsevier Health Sciences, London, United Kingdom.

3. Kaviraj Ambikadutt Shastri, Sushrutha Samhita (2009) (hindi commentary) Chowkhambha Sanskrit Series, Varanasi, India.

4. Kaviraj Atridev Gupta, Ashtanga Hridayam (hindi commentary), Chowkhambha Sanskrit Sansthan, Varanasi, India.

5. Srikanta Murthy KR, Madhava Nidanam (1987) Chowkhambha Sanskrit Series, Varanasi, India

6. Dr. Nirmala Saxena (1994) Vangasena samhita (4thedn), Chowkhambha Sanskrit Sansthan, Varanasi, India.

7. Sri Brahmashankara Mishra, Sri Rupalalaji Vaisya, Bhava Prakasha (5thedn), Chowkhambha Sanskrit Series, Varanasi, India.

8. Ram Nivas Sharma, Surendra Sharma (2004) Sahasrayogam, Chowkhambha Sanskrit Pratishtana, Delhi, India.

9. Dr. Siddharth Shah N (2003) API Textbook of Medicine. (7thedn), The Association of Physicians of India, Mumbai, India.

10. Mahajan BK (2005) Methods in Bio Statistics. (6thedn), Jaypee Brothers Medical Publishers (P) Ltd, New Delhi, India.

11. Gyanendra Pandey (2002) Dravyaguna Vijnana: Materia Medica Vegetable Drugs. (2ndedn), Krishnadas Academy, Varanasi, India.

28

Evidence-Base Unani Medicine: Need of Appropriate Research Methods

Malik Itrat* and Saba Khan

Department of Preventive and Social Medicine, National Institute of Unani Medicine, Bangalore, Karnataka, India

Abstract

Every health care system must be evidence based and Unani system of medicine ought to be no exception. An evidence base is needed at every level of health-care, right from diagnostics to the therapeutic decision making. Unani medicine requires thorough work to bring out evidence basis not only to support its interventions but also to its fundamental concepts to create scientific and logical basis on which therapeutic decisions are made. However, when pleading for evidence, problems associated with the nature of evidence and their relevance to Unani system of medicine ought to be thoroughly debated. Though Unani system and biomedicine share the same spirit of open and sincere scientific enquiry, their fundamentals, epistemology, logic and theories are distinct. Unani medicine is basically holistic, whereas biomedicine is reductionist. These epistemic variations call for the use of appropriate and acceptable research methods by involving experts from Unani system and biomedicine. The classical approach of this system should not be compromised for the convenience of prevailing research strategies. Various research strategies like reverse pharmacology to unravel the mechanism of action of drugs, pharmaco-epidemiology to study the toxicity of herbo-mineral preparations, retrospective treatment outcome surveys as a starting line to study the efficacy of drugs and whole system research to evaluate the efficacy of packaged interventions have been proposed by scientists to generate evidence in traditional medicine, that are also applicable to Unani system of medicine. In this paper research methods, which are appropriate to generate scientific evidence in Unani medicine are discussed.

Keywords: Unani medicine; Evidence-based medicine; Research methods

Introduction

The practice of Unani system of medicine stretches all the way back in to the misty dawn of time. The Asia-Pacific database on Intangible Cultural Heritage (ICH) by Asia-Pacific Cultural Centre for UNESCO (ACCU) has deemed Unani System of Medicine as one of the oldest and most acceptable systems of medicine. It is practiced in India and all over the world particularly in Egypt, Syria, Iraq, Iran and most parts of South East Asia [1]. The Unani system of medicine as its name suggests has its origin in Greece. The core philosophy of this system was conceptualized by Hippocrates. After him, Arab and Persian scholars made great contributions and hold a large share in what constitutes the Unani literature today. It was introduced in India by the Mughals and since then has enjoyed popularity amongst the masses and now forms an integral part of the healthcare delivery system of the country.

The strength of the system is in its holistic and individualistic approach to health promotion, disease prevention and treatment. It offers an effective treatment for various gastrointestinal, respiratory, genitor-urinary, musculoskeletal, neurological, cardiovascular, lifestyle and metabolic disorders [2]. Although the government has given great importance to the multi-faceted development of this system of medicine to make full use of its potential in the Indian healthcare delivery, the Unani system of medicine has not gained much recognition within the times.

A number of issues have been at the back drop of this lag, primary of which has been the lack of quality data on safety and efficacy of Unani drugs required to put the system's practices at par with contemporary medical systems. The main reason behind this inadequacy of research data is the lack of appropriate and accepted research methods that can be used for evaluating the system's practice. However the question, whether an evidence base is required for a system which has been in widespread practice for ages, has puzzled many a mind. This question needs to be analyzed in terms of extended benefits of putting an evidence basis for practice of Unani medicine, primarily for providing a prospectively better and dependable health care and secondarily for growth of Unani medicine as a contemporary science. Unani System of medicine indeed needs intensive work to bring out an evidence basis to its nosology, primarily to support its concepts and to make a sound scientific basis for its therapeutic interventions. Additionally, it also needs evidences to support its interventions in varied clinical conditions to the extent that their application in a given condition is justified.

The seemingly obvious task of deciphering and devising methods of furnishing this evidence leads us to a new set of questions. How can Unani drugs be standardized using parameters of another health system? Should all formulations used in the system be re-evaluated using biomedical parameters and would this process be affordable? While it is important to substantiate an evidence base for Unani medicine, it is equally important to ensure that the epistemological differences between the two systems are taken into account when developing research protocols.

The guiding dictum should be to identify such tools and methods for research in Unani medicine which are sensitive enough to respect the desired rigor of science as well as the original holistic nature of Unani medicine equally.

Unani Medicine: The Amendments Needed

In the context of recognition and resurgence of Unani system of medicine globally, there are certain issues that need to be critically understood and examined. In our opinion, Unani medicine requires extensive research in the following areas:

*Corresponding author: Malik Itrat, Department of Preventive and Social Medicine, National Institute of Unani Medicine, Bangalore, Karnataka, India, E-mail: malik.itrat@gmail.com

- Revalidation of Unani fundamentals so that they can be inexplicably stated and understood.

- To find out better treatment modalities for existing diseases and for newer diseases.

- To standardize the treatment procedures scientifically.

- To establish dose, duration, indication and side-effect profile of drugs.

- Unani and modern drugs interactions (Figure 1).

Applying Evidence Base to Unani medicine: What are the tools?

Evidence-Based Medicine (EBM) is defined as the systemic approach for finding and analyzing published data for the basis of clinical decision making [3]. It is also defined as the integration of the best research evidence with clinical expertise and patient values to make clinical decisions [4]. EBM bridges the gap between modern day research and physician, as current research findings and data are often required to diagnose and treat patients. EBM focuses on research dealing with day to day practice of patient care. The evidence may prove or disprove previously accepted methods or demonstrate new ways of care that are more accurate and effective and less harmful. In biomedicine, the golden standards of EBM are formulated from "Randomised Controlled Trials".

Although RCT usually considered to be amongst the top in the hierarchy of study designs, it is not the only tool that can be used unequivocally to provide evidence in traditional systems also. The RCT design made for testing a single entity cannot be used for testifying Unani medicine in which the hall mark of treatment itself is packaged intervention. Indeed, an RCT may be inappropriate or inadequate in answering determined questions and/or in certain contexts [5]. What reckons a clinical study to be better evidence is neither its logistics nor the sample size; rather it is the connexion of the research question with its design, the rigor of data collection and analysis along with explicit reportage of the observed effects [6].

Various scholars have explored different models of testing the validity and standardization techniques in traditional medicine. Verhoef and Van der Greef have considered observational studies to be better tools for evaluating the efficacy and safety of traditional medicine as they are cheaper, have higher external validity and accommodate better to the medical epistemology of the Unani system of medicine [7,8].

There are a number of research designs that can substantiate evidence base to the Unani system of medicine. They are: the retrospective treatment – outcome study, the prognosis – outcome study, the dose–escalating prospective study for detecting a dose-response phenomenon in humans, pharmaco-epidemiology - to document the safety of Unani medicines, especially herbo-mineral preparations and reverse pharmacology - to unravel the biological mechanisms behind the drug action.

Retrospective Treatment-Outcome (RTO) survey: The collection of clinical data, such as patient status and progress after the use of Unani medicines, can help in the study of the effectiveness and safety of Unani practices and products. These surveys can analyze records of patient's progress (outcome) along with the different treatments used for a given disease or syndrome. It will make possible to perform correlation tests between treatment and outcome, providing indices of effectiveness and safety. It will also provide data about precautions and contra-

indications. RTO surveys are usually conducted with a questionnaire applied to a representative sample of a population. Inclusion criteria are "having suffered from the disease of interest since weeks/months/year". For a benign health problem, the recall period is kept short (e.g., two weeks) for accuracy and for a severe problem, it can be longer (e.g., 1 year). Patient's progress under various treatments is recorded, and then analyzed with adjustment for confounding factors. If we find a good association between a given treatment for a health problem and patient cure with no significant side effects, this could mean that the treatment is effective and should be validated further with other methods. Precise data about drug collection, preparation and dosage that are of great importance, in order to facilitate future replication of the study, can also be gathered during the survey (Figure 2 and Table 1). These types of studies can also provide baseline information about known side effects, incompatibilities and limitations (including experience with small children and pregnant women), which can be the precious signs for further research on its toxicity [6,9].

- Last time you used this treatment for which health problem.
- What was the patient progress? (Cured/better/same/worse).
- After how many days?
- Have you experience any allergy or side effects during this treatment?
- Have you used this drug during pregnancy?
- Have you taken any precautions during this treatment?
- Is there anything that you have not eaten or done at the same time?

Table 1: Questions to be asked during field work to get basic information on effectiveness and safety of a traditional treatment [10].

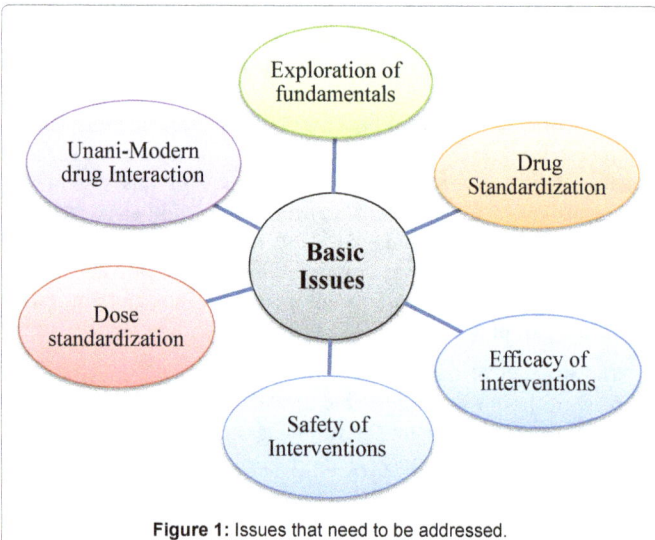

Figure 1: Issues that need to be addressed.

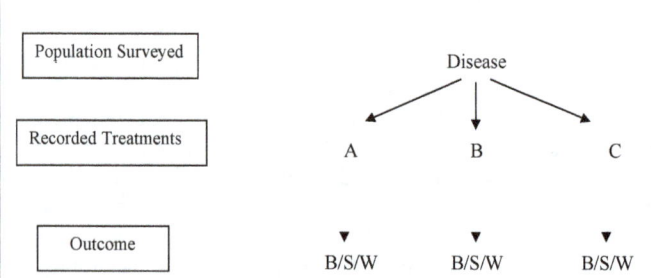

Figure 2: Design of a clinical study eliciting the best clinical outcome among numerous alternative treatments for the same ailment: the Retrospective Treatment-Outcome study. B: Best Outcome; S: Same Outcome; W: Worst Outcome [6].

Comparison of Prognosis and Outcome (CPO) study: It is also an observational study which can be useful to assess the overall results of therapeutic interventions of Unani medicine. It explores whether health care dispensed by Unani practitioners is as good as – or better than – what could be expected with allopathic medicine in the area. What could be expected with conventional medicine is an allopathic practitioner's prognosis which is compared with actual patient progress (clinical outcome) with Unani treatment.

A four-point relative scale allows comparisons between expected and observed patient progress. Analysis of results will show that, whether the outcome with Unani treatment is same, worse or better than standard modern medicine. Those cases, in whom outcome is better than expected, will suggest that Unani medicine has better results than standard modern medicine for those ailments, and it would be advisable to focus further research on such treatments in those diseases (Figure 3) [10,11].

Dose–escalating prospective study: When any drug is given in extremely variable doses and the preliminary observations indicate that the therapeutic range is large and the probability of toxicity at the doses used is very low, a Prospective Dose Escalating (PDE) trial can be organized on a small sample. In this study, patients are allocated into different groups and practitioner gives to one group, what he/she considers the lowest dose, to another group, the middle range dose and upper range dose to a third group. There should be no difference in inclusion criteria between the groups, and patients should be randomly allocated to a particular dosage group. If statistically significant difference appears in outcome between various doses groups, the presence of a dose–response phenomenon can be estimated, indicating specific activity at different doses. In the next step, if all pre-requisites are met, then a prospective randomized controlled trial can be conducted, with some adaptations [6] (Figure 4).

Reverse pharmacology: This research technique offers an effective answer in understanding how Unani drugs work. Reverse pharmacology is defined as the science of integrating documented clinical experiences and experimental observations into leads by interdisciplinary exploratory studies and further developing these into drug candidate or formulations through robust preclinical and clinical research [12]. This approach is especially applicable to traditional treatments, where the safety and efficacy are already known but need validation to support their usage. Such studies helps in revealing underlying mechanisms of drug action and give a better picture of their efficacy, safety thus hugely aiding their acceptability [13].

Reverse pharmacology approach helps in reducing three major bottlenecks: costs, time and toxicity. It comprises of three stages—experiential, exploratory and experimental. In Experiential phase, a number of clinical drug candidates can be shortlisted for going through the next two stages. It includes robust documentation of clinical effects of standardized drugs by meticulous record keeping. The exploratory studies will cover dose-activity in ambulant patients and selected *in-vitro* and *in-vivo* models to evaluate the key target. The experimental stage then employs relevant basic and clinical science to study the plant or a molecule at different levels of biological organization especially at the molecular level (Figure 5). This would define the safety, efficacy, preventive or therapeutic dimensions of the new or natural drug [14].

Pharmaco-epidemiology: As there are questions about efficacy of Unani drugs, there are also questions about the toxicity of its formulations especially herbo-mineral preparations. In this scenario, pharmaco-epidemiological studies can provide valuable information concerning the relationship between therapeutic agents and adverse and beneficial health outcomes. Although Unani formulations are in use since centuries which itself is a proof to their safety but such studies can be used to further hone their usage and acceptability. Pharmaco-epidemiology is the study of drug efficacy, toxicity and patterns of use in large populations. With the help of these studies, we can salvage safety data from pool of patients, who have already used Unani drugs. If Unani preparations are found to be safe, it can advance as major evidence in support of this system [15,16].

Conclusion

Validation gives credibility to practice. Structured validation is undoubtedly the key to furnish an evidence base to the Unani system of medicine. Current research in Unani Medicine uses modern scientific parameters as the exclusive yardstick. Unani treatment methodology is force fitted into conventional research designs and the knowledge so obtained is used within the framework of biomedicine. Packaged Unani interventions are broken down to their simpler components in an attempt to study the efficacy of these broken components in a

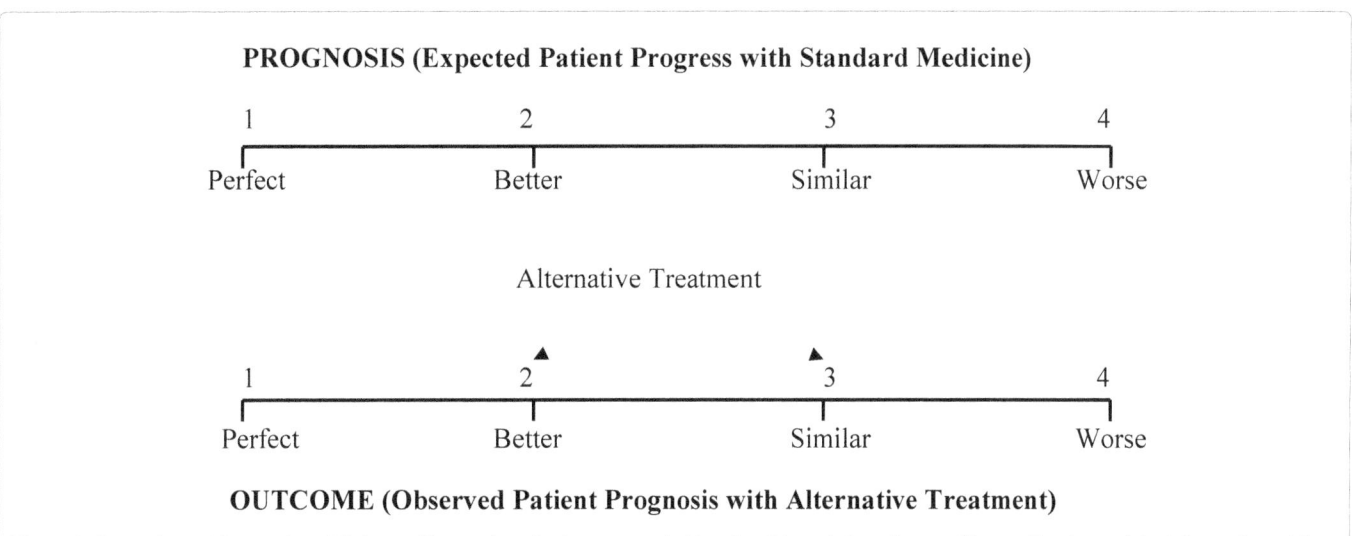

Figure 3: Comparison of Prognosis and Outcome, Prognosis and outcome are rated by allopathic and alternative practitioner with a four-point relative scale, and then compared.

specific disease. This leads to trimming and modification of Unani treatment to fit into the conventional research design. Consequently, the results of such ill designed studies are unlikely to add any value to this system. The focus of research has to shift from just the drugs and practices to the concepts that warrant their use. In Unani system of medicine it is not only desirable to re-validate the use of drugs but also the fundamentals on which therapeutic decisions are made. This may require appropriate methodological modifications. Research designs sensitive to the system need to be adapted and if necessary, reinvented. The three pronged strategy of leveraging the benefits of pharmaco-epidemiology, observational therapeutics and reverse pharmacology should be taken up as the primary step in this direction (Figure 6).

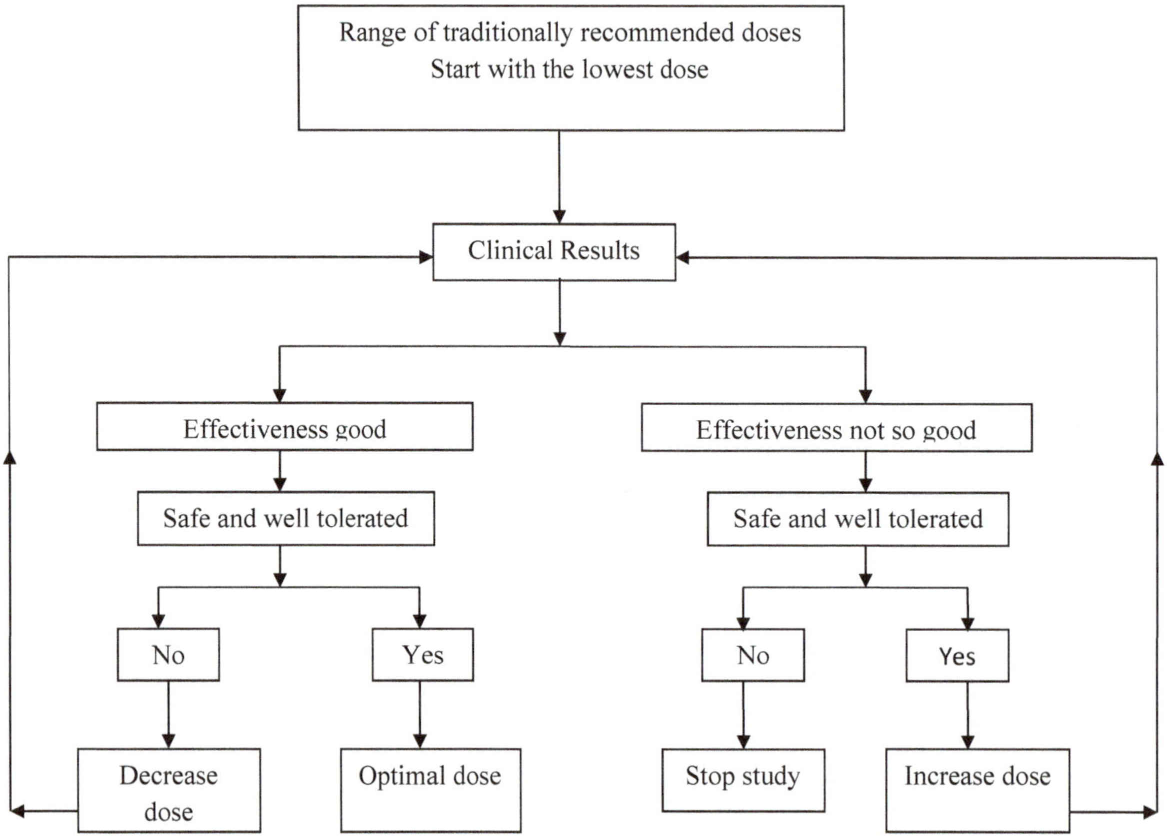

Range of traditionally recommended doses
Start with the lowest dose
Clinical Results
Effectiveness good
Effectiveness not so good
Safe and well tolerated
Safe and well tolerated
No
Yes
No
Yes
Decrease dose
Optimal dose
Stop study
Increase dose

Figure 4: Dose escalating study.

DRUG DEVELOPMENT PROCESS
Expensive, time consuming, numerous bottlenecks
TARGET IDENTIFICATION
LEAD IDENTIFICATION
LEAD OPTMIZATION
PRECLINICAL STUDIES
CLINICAL TRIALS
DRUG TO MARKET
8 to 10 yrs
Economical, time sparing, least bottlenecks
Reverse Pharmacology
LARGE SCALE TRIALS
RELEVANT SCIENCE
SAFETY STUDIES
PARACLINICAL STUDIES
CLINICAL TRIALS PHASE II & I
DRUG TO MARKET
4 to 5 yrs

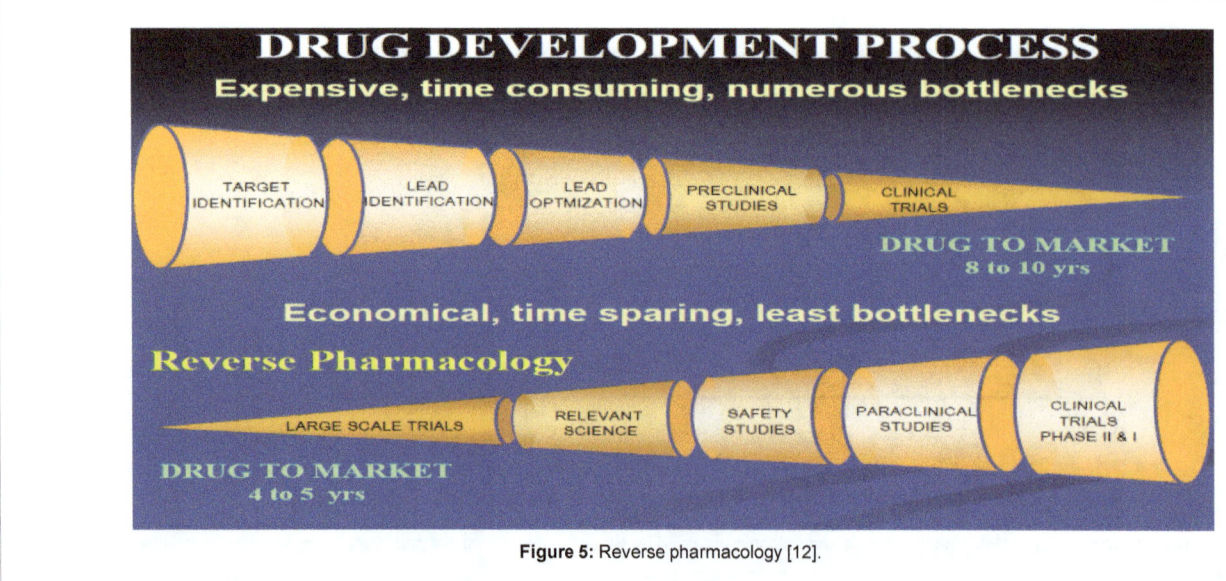

Figure 5: Reverse pharmacology [12].

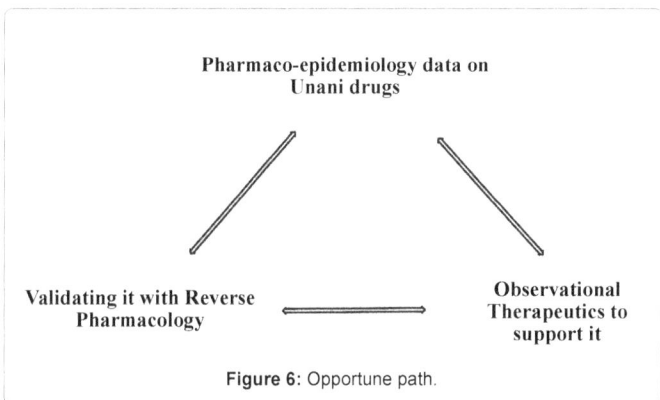

Figure 6: Opportune path.

References

1. Asia-Pacific Database on Intangible Cultural Heritage (ICH) by Asia-Pacific Cultural Centre for UNESCO (ACCU).

2. Husain A, Sofi G, Tajuddin, Dang R, Kumar N(2010) Unani System of Medicine-Introduction and Challenges. Med J Islamic World Acad Sci 18: 27-30.

3. Sacket DL, Rosenburg WM, Gray JA, Haynes RB, Richardson WS (1996) Evidence-based Medicine: What it is and it isn't. BMJ 312: 71-72.

4. Krishnan R (2013) Comprehending Evidence-Based Ayurveda. Int J Ayur Pharm Res 1: 1-3.

5. Black N (1996) why we need observational studies to evaluate the effectiveness of health care? BMJ 312: 1215-1218.

6. Graz B, Elisabetsky E, Falquet J (2007) Beyond the myth of expensive clinical study: Assessment of traditional medicines. J Ethnopharmacol 113: 382-386.

7. Verhoef MJ, Lewith G, Ritenbaugh C, Boon H, Fleishman S, et al. (2005) Complementary and alternative medicine whole systems research:Beyond Identification of Inadequacies of the RCT. Complement Ther Med 13: 206-212.

8. Van der Greef J (2007) Perspective: All Systems Go. Nature 480: S87.

9. Graz B, Diallo D, Falquet J, Willcox M, Giani S (2005) Screening of traditional herbal medicine: first, do a retrospective study, with correlation between diverse treatments used and reported patient outcome. J Ethnopharmacol 101: 338-339.

10. Graz B, Falquet J, Elisabetsky E (2010) Ethnopharmacology, sustainable development and cooperation: The importance of gathering clinical data during field surveys. J Ethnopharmacol 130: 635-638.

11. Graz B, Falquet J, Morency P (2003) Assessment of alternative medicine through a comparison of the expected and observed progress of patients: a feasibility study of the prognosis/follow-up method. J Altern Complement Med 9: 755-761.

12. Anju S, Sumit S, Sujata S (2015) Reverse pharmacology: A new approach to drug development. Inn original: Int J Sci Nat 2: 7-12.

13. Patwardhan B, Vaidya ADB (2010) Natural products drug discovery: accelerating the clinical candidate development using reverse pharmacology approaches. Indian J Exp Biol 48: 220-227.

14. Patwardhan B, Vaidya ADB, Chorghade M, P Joshi Swati (2008) Reverse Pharmacology and Systems Approaches for Drug Discovery and Development. Curr Bioact Compd 4: 1-12.

15. Brian L Storm (2000) Pharmacoepidemiology. (3rd ed.). Chicester: John Wiley and Sons Ltd. pp: 3-11.

16. Itrat M (2016) Research in Unani Medicine: Challenges and Way Forward. Altern Integr Med 5: 215.

29

Phytochemical Analysis of *Cynanchum callialatum* through GCMS and LCMS

Karthikeyan M[1]* and Balasubramanian T[2]

[1]*Research Scholar, Department of Pharmacy and Medical Sciences, Singhania University, Rajsathan, India*
[2]*Associate Professor, Department of Pharmacology, Alshifa College of Pharmacy, Kerala, India*

Abstract

Medicinal plants are still important source for drug discovery. Herbal medicines have gained importance in recent years because of their efficacy and cost effectiveness. The objective of the present study is to investigate the phytochemical present in the *Cynanchum callialatum*. The phytochemical analysis was done by preliminary phytochemical test for secondary metabolites, GCMS for volatile constituents and LCMS for nonvolatile constituents.

The phytochemical test confirms the presents of alkaloids, flavonoids, terpenoids, tanins etc. The GCMS analysis shows the presents of 52 compounds in which some have medicinal value. The LCMS analysis shows the presents of compounds in which most of them have the medicinal properties. The present study on *Cynanchum callialatum* reveals the presence of various phytochemical constituents like Betulinic acid, Lupeol, Germacrone and Longiverbenone. *Cynanchum callialatum* may be a potential source for anticancer, antiHIV, antiinflammatory, antimicrobial drug discovery.

Keywords: *Cynanchum callialatum*; Phytochemical analysis; GC-MS; LC/MS

Introduction

Plant still remains a major source for drug discovery in development of synthetic molecules. The use of traditional plant extract in the treatment of various diseases has been flourished. In the early 19th century, when chemical analysis first became available, scientists began to extract and modify the active ingredients from plants. The World Health Organization estimated that about 80% of the world population relays on herbal medicines.

Herbal medicines have gained importance in recent years because of their efficacy and cost effectiveness. These drugs are invariable single plant extracts or mixtures of extracts from different plants, which have been carefully standardized for their safety and efficacy. Substances derived from the plants remain the basis for a large proportion of the commercial medications used today for the treatment of heart disease, high blood pressure, pain, asthma and infectious diseases [1]. Nowadays medicinal plants receive more attention to researchers because of their safety and curative property which is due to the complex mixtures secondary metabolites.

Cynanchum is a genus of about 300 species including some swallowwort's, belongs to the milkweed family Asclepiadaceae. Most species are non-succulent, climbers or twiners. These plants are perennial herbs or sub shrubs, often growing from rhizomes. The leaves are usually oppositely arranged and sometimes are borne on petioles. The inflorescences and flowers come in a variety of shapes. These plants bear follicles, which are pod like dry fruits. These species are found worldwide in the tropics and subtropics. Several species also grow in temperate regions. *Cynanchum* varieties are prescribed in chinese medicine to treat fever, cough, pneumonia and asthma [2]. *Cynanchum callialatum* twiner to 4 m, latex milky, flowers white, widely distributed in India. *Cynanchum callialatum* has been used to treat wounds, headaches, infections and other skin related problems by tribes in Tamil Nadu, India.

Based on the literature review there is no scientific reports on phytochemical constituents of *Cynanchum callialatum*. The present study has made an attempt to identify the chemical constituents from the areal parts of *Cynanchum callialatum* through GCMS and LCMS.

Materials and Methods

Plant material

The plant *Cynanchum callialatum* was collected from Pollachi, Coimbatore District, Tamil Nadu, India and It has been identified and authenticated by Dr. Udyan P.S., Professor, Sreekrishna College, Guruvayur, Thrissur, Kerala, India.

The areal parts of the *Cynanchum callialatum* were collected during March-April month and washed with water. Then the plant material was shade dried for 10 days. The dried plant materials have been powdered using mechanical grinder to get uniform coarse particles. The powdered plant material was stored in polythene air tight containers at room temperature for further use.

Preparation of the crude plant extract

The shade dried coarse powdered bark of *Cynanchum callialatum* (250 g) was packed in the soxhlet extraction apparatus and extracted with 2 L of 95% ethanol at a temperature of 40-50°C for 72 hr. The extract was filtered and the filtered extract was then concentrated to dryness in a rotary evaporator under reduced pressure at temperature of 40°C. The resultant green color residue was stored in a desiccator for use in subsequent experiments and considered as the crude ethanol extract. The yield of the ethanolic extract was 14% w/w.

Phytochemical analysis

The preliminary phytochemical screening test was carried out in

*Corresponding author: Karthikeyan M, Research Scholar, Department of Pharmacy and Medical Sciences, School of Pharmacy and Medical Sciences, Singhania University, Pacheribari, Jhunjhunu, 333515-Rajsathan, India
E-mail: karthikeyanpgt@gmail.com

ethanolic extract of *Cynanchum callialatum* to find out the nature of chemical compounds as per the standard procedures [3-6] and the phytoconstituents were identified through GCMS and LCMS (Tables 1- 3).

GCMS specifications

Make: PerkinElmer Clarus 500

Software: Turbomass ver 5.2.0

Column Type: Capillary Column Elite-5MS (5%Phenyl 95% dimethylpolysiloxane)

Column length: 30 m

Column id: 250 μm

GC conditions

Oven Program: 50°C@6°C/min to 220°C (2 min)@6°C/min to 270°C (10min)

Injector temperature: 280°C

Carrier gas: Helium @ flow rate 1 ml/min

Split ratio: 1:20

MS conditions

Mass Range: 40-600 amu

Type of Ionization: Electron Ionization (EI)

Electron energy: 70 ev

Transfer line and source temperature: 200°C, 180°C

Library: NIST 2005

Sample injected: 1.0 microlitre

LCMS specifications

S.No	Test done for	Name of the test	Quantity present
1	Phenol	Lead acetate test	+
2	Flavonoids	Shinoda's test	+
3	Alkaloids	Dragondroff's test Wagners test Mayer's test Hager's test	+
4	Saponins	Foam test	-
5	Glycosides	Borntragers test	+
6	Proteins	Biuret test	-
7	Amino acids	Ninhydrin test	-
8	Carbohydrates	Anthrone test	+
9	Tannins	Ferric chloride test	+
10	Gums and Mucilage	Ruthenium red test	-
11	Flavones	NaoH test	+
12	Sterols	Liberman's test	+
13	Terpenoids	Tin and thionyl chloride test	+
14	Reducing sugars	Molishch's test	+
15	Terpenes	Plate derivatisation	+
16	Aromaticity	Organoleptic tests	+
17	Essential oil	Filter paper test	-

+ Presence   - Absence

Table 1: Preliminary Phytochemical carried out in ethanolic extract of *Cynanchum callialatum*.

S.No.	Peak Name	Retention time	% Peak Area	
1	Name: Hexanal Formula: $C_6H_{12}O$ MW: 100	4.32	0.2696	
2	Name: Octanal Formula: $C_8H_{16}O$ MW: 128	8.85	0.0067	
3	Name: Hexanoic acid Formula: $C_6H_{12}O_2$ MW: 116	8.97	0.0914	
4	Name: 1,3-Dioxane, 2-heptyl- Formula: $C_{11}H_{22}O_2$ MW: 186	9.48	0.8036	
5	Name: Bicyclo[2.2.1]heptan-2-ol, 1,7,7-trimethyl-, (1S-endo)- Formula: $C_{10}H_{18}O$ MW: 154	13.41	0.0347	
6	Name: Octanoic Acid Formula: $C_8H_{16}O_2$ MW: 144	13.65	0.6199	
7	Name: Myrcenylacetate Formula: $C_{12}H_{20}O_2$ MW: 196	13.90	0.0958	
8	Name: L-Glucose, 6-deoxy-3-O-methyl- Formula: $C_7H_{14}O_5$ MW: 178	14.31	0.7977	
9	Name: á-d-Allopyranoside, methyl 6-deoxy-2-O-methyl- Formula: $C_8H_{16}O_5$ MW: 192	15.19	2.1420	
10	Name: 2H-Pyran-2-one, tetrahydro-6-propyl- Formula: $C_8H_{14}O_2$ MW: 142	16.13	0.0819	
11	Name: Thymol Formula: $C_{10}H_{14}O$ MW: 150	16.50	0.5089	
12	Name: 2-Methoxy-4-vinylphenol Formula: $C_9H_{10}O_2$ MW: 150	16.88	0.3273	
13	Name: 3-Cyclohexene-1-methanol, à,à,4-trimethyl-, acetate Formula: $C_{12}H_{20}O_2$ MW: 196	17.27	0.5481	
14	Name: Cyclohexane, 1-ethenyl-1-methyl-2,4-bis(1-methylethenyl)-, [1S-(1à,2á,4á)]- Formula: $C_{15}H_{24}$ MW: 204	18.25	0.0448	
15	Name: à-Zingiberene Formula: $C_{15}H_{24}$ MW: 204	18.41	0.0600	
16	Name: Phenol, 4-(1,1-dimethylpropyl)- Formula: $C_{11}H_{16}O$ MW: 164	18.59	0.0377	
17	Name: (+)-2-Carene, 4-à-isopropenyl- Formula: $C_{13}H_{20}$ MW: 176	19.03	0.0704	
18	Name: 1,6,10-Dodecatriene, 7,11-dimethyl-3-methylene-, (E)- Formula: $C_{15}H_{24}$ MW: 204	19.45	0.1268	
19	Name: Phenol, 2-methoxy-4-(1-propenyl)-, (E)- Formula: $C_{10}H_{12}O_2$ MW: 164	19.91	0.0776	

20	Name: Curcumene Formula: $C_{15}H_{22}$ MW: 202	20.20	8.9064	
21	Name: à-Farnesene Formula: $C_{15}H_{24}$ MW: 204	20.56	0.2632	
22	Name: Di-epi-à-cedrene Formula: $C_{15}H_{24}$ MW: 204	20.76	6.6327	
23	Name: Cyclohexene, 3-(1,5-dimethyl-4-hexenyl)-6-methylene-, [S-(R*,S*)]- Formula: $C_{15}H_{24}$ MW: 204	21.08	0.5788	
24	Name: Nerolidol 2 Formula: $C_{15}H_{26}O$ MW: 222	21.83	0.1858	
25	Name: Dodecanoic acid Formula: $C_{12}H_{24}O_2$ MW: 200	22.13	0.0141	
26	Name: Benzenepropanoic acid, á,á-dimethyl-, methyl ester Formula: $C_{12}H_{16}O_2$ MW: 192	22.33	0.4125	
27	Name: Elemenone Formula: $C_{15}H_{22}O$ MW: 218	22.77	1.1606	
28	Name: Asarone Formula: $C_{12}H_{16}O_3$ MW: 208	22.96	0.3469	
29	Name: 6-(p-Tolyl)-2-methyl-2-heptenol Formula: $C_{15}H_{22}O$ MW: 218	23.92	3.2528	
30	Name: Bergamotol, Z-à-trans- Formula: $C_{15}H_{24}O$ MW: 220	24.40	0.1695	
31	Name: Germacrone Formula: $C_{15}H_{22}O$ MW: 218	24.74	1.3890	
32	Name: Longiverbenone Formula: $C_{15}H_{22}O$ MW: 218	25.12	0.3171	
33	Name: Phenol, 5-(1,5-dimethyl-4-hexenyl)-2-methyl-, (R)- Formula: $C_{15}H_{22}O$ MW: 218	25.80	13.7413	
34	Name:Tetradecanoic acid, ethyl ester Formula: $C_{16}H_{32}O_2$ MW: 256	26.13	1971073	0.2242
35	Name: 2-n-Propyladamantane Formula: $C_{13}H_{22}$ MW: 178	26.35	4544831	0.5170
36	Name: 3,7,11,15-Tetramethyl-2-hexadecen-1-ol Formula: $C_{20}H_{40}O$ MW: 296	27.03	27310200	3.1067
37	Name: 2-Pentadecanone, 6,10,14-trimethyl- Formula: $C_{18}H_{36}O$ MW: 268	27.26	12747370	1.4501
38	Name: Naphthalene, decahydro-1,1-dimethyl- Formula: $C_{12}H_{22}$ MW: 166	28.77	9831310	1.1184
39	Name: n-Hexadecanoic acid Formula: $C_{16}H_{32}O_2$ MW: 256	30.37	214922064	24.4485
40	Name: Hexadecanoic acid, ethyl ester Formula: $C_{18}H_{36}O_2$ MW: 284	30.45	7800140	0.8873
41	Name: Uridine, 2'-deoxy-3-methyl-3',5'-di-O-methyl- Formula: $C_{12}H_{18}N_2O_5$ MW: 270	31.28	4476319	0.5092
42	Name: Phytol Formula: $C_{20}H_{40}O$ MW: 296	32.75	6885792	0.7833
43	Name: (E)-9-Octadecenoic acid ethyl ester Formula: $C_{20}H_{38}O_2$ MW: 310	33.64	64711056	7.3612
44	Name: Octadecanoic acid Formula: $C_{18}H_{36}O_2$ MW: 284	33.95	37751912	4.2945
45	Name: Hexadecanoic acid, ethyl ester Formula: $C_{18}H_{36}O_2$ MW: 284	34.07	30412262	3.4595
46	Name: 3-Methoxytyrosine Formula: $C_{10}H_{13}NO_4$ MW: 211	34.99	5369919	0.6109
47	Name: 1H-Indene, 2,3,3a,4,7,7a-hexahydro-2,2,4,4,7,7-hexamethyl- Formula: $C_{15}H_{26}$ MW: 206	36.04	3164643	0.3600
48	Name: 2-(3,4-Methylenedioxyphenyl)cyclohexanone Formula: $C_{13}H_{14}O_3$ MW: 218	36.71	25409886	2.8905
49	Name: Ethyl 13-docosenoate(ethyl erucate) Formula: $C_{24}H_{46}O_2$ MW: 366	40.30	7670625	0.8726
50	Name: 4,4,6a,6b,8a,11,11,14b-Octamethyl-1,4,4a,5,6,6a,6b,7,8,8a,9,10,11,12,12a,14,14a,14b-octadecahydro-2H-picen-3-one Formula: $C_{30}H_{48}O$ MW: 424	40.84	11640140	1.3241
51	Name: Benzaldehyde, 4-methoxy-3-(3,7,11-trimethyldodeca-2,6,10-trienyl- (E,E)- Formula: $C_{23}H_{32}O_2$ MW: 340	45.03	12875374	1.4646
52	Name: Lupeol Formula: $C_{30}H_{50}O$ MW: 426	46.06	1775649	0.2020

Table 2: Shows the Peak name, peak area during GCMS analysis of ethanolic extract of *Cynanchum calilalatum*.

LC column: ReversePhaseC-18PUMP:SPD10AVP

Mobile Phase: water: Methanol (50:50)

Ionization Mode: Electronic Spray Ionization

Mode: Both Positive and negative

Injection Volume: 10 microlitre

Flow Rate: 2 ml/min

Column Temperature: 250°c

S.No	Compound name	Molecular mass
1	Betulinic acid	456.71
2	Benzoic acid	122.12
3	Palmitic acid	256.43
4	Sinapic acid	242.21
5	Pseudolaric acid A- glucopyranoside	550.60
6	Isoeugenol	164.20
7	Succinic acid	118.09
8	Conduritol	146.14
9	Daocosterol	576.85
10	Lupeol acetate	468.77
11	Taraxasterol	426.73
12	Amino Benzoic acid	137.14
13	Coumarin	146.15
14	Umbelliferone	162.15
15	Syringic acid	198.18
16	Diferulic acid	386.36
17	Beta amyrin	426.73
18	Palmitoyl acetate	660.85
19	Vanillic acid	168.15
20	Glucuronic acid	193.21
21	Abscisic acid	264.33
22	Erucic acid	338.58

Table 3: LCMS Analysis Library Search Results.

Column: PhenomenexRP18

Column Dimension: 25 cmx2.5 mm

LC Detection: 254 nm

M/Z Range: 50-1000

Software: classvp integrated.

Library: Metwin2.0

Results and Discussion

Cynanchum callialatum twiner to 4 m, latex milky, flowers white widely distributed in India. *Cynanchum callialatum* has been used to treat wounds, headaches, infections and other skin related problems by tribes in Tamil Nadu, India. As per our knowledge the chemicals constituents of *Cynanchum callialatum* was not yet scientifically reported. Moreover, identification of chemical constituents in the crude drugs is the basic goal to prove its pharmacological effects behind the folklore uses and ultimate discovery of novel therapeutics. In the present study phytochemical investigation on *Cynanchum callialatum* ethanolic extract has been done by preliminary phytochemical screening, GCMS and LCMS analysis (Figures 1-3). Our study reveals the presence of various natural bioactive compounds shown in table 1 and 2 and these chemical compounds also been found in other species of *Cynanchum* [7].

Expected pharmacological properties of *Cynanchum callialatum*

The photochemical investigations on *Cynanchum callialatum* ethanolic extract have revealed the presence of several natural compounds (Tables 1 and 2) and most of them have various biological activities.

Betulinic acid: Betulinic acid, is a naturally occurring pentacycliclupane- type triterpenoid which exhibits a variety of biological and medicinal properties such as inhibition of human immunodeficiency virus (HIV), anti-bacterial, anti-malarial, antiinflammatory, anthelmintic, antinociceptive, anti-HSV-1, anti-HSV-1 , and anti- cancer activities [8].

Lupeol: Lupeol, a phytosterol and triterpene, is widely found in edible fruits, and vegetables. In various in vitro and preclinical animal studies suggest that lupeol has a potential to act as an anti-inflammatory, anti-microbial, anti-protozoal, anti-proliferative, anti-invasive, anti-angiogenic and cholesterol lowering agent. Employing various *in vitro* and *in vivo* models, lupeol has also been tested for its therapeutic efficiency against conditions including wound healing, diabetes, cardiovascular disease, kidney disease, and arthritis. Lupeol has been found to be pharmacologically effective in treating various diseases under preclinical settings (in animal models) irrespective of varying routes of administration viz; topical, oral, intra-peritoneal and intravenous. It is note worthy that lupeol has been reported to selectively target diseased and unhealthy human cells, while sparing normal and healthy cells. Lupeol modulates the expression or activity of several molecules such as cytokines IL-2, IL4, IL5, ILβ, proteases,

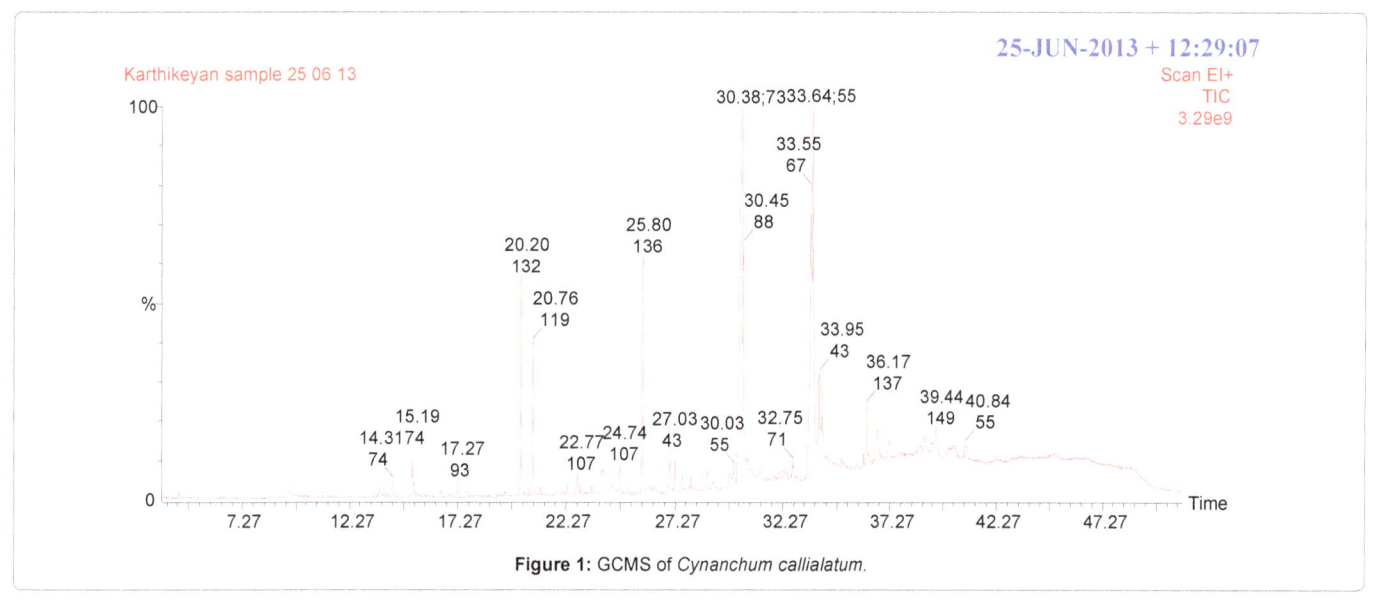

Figure 1: GCMS of *Cynanchum callialatum*.

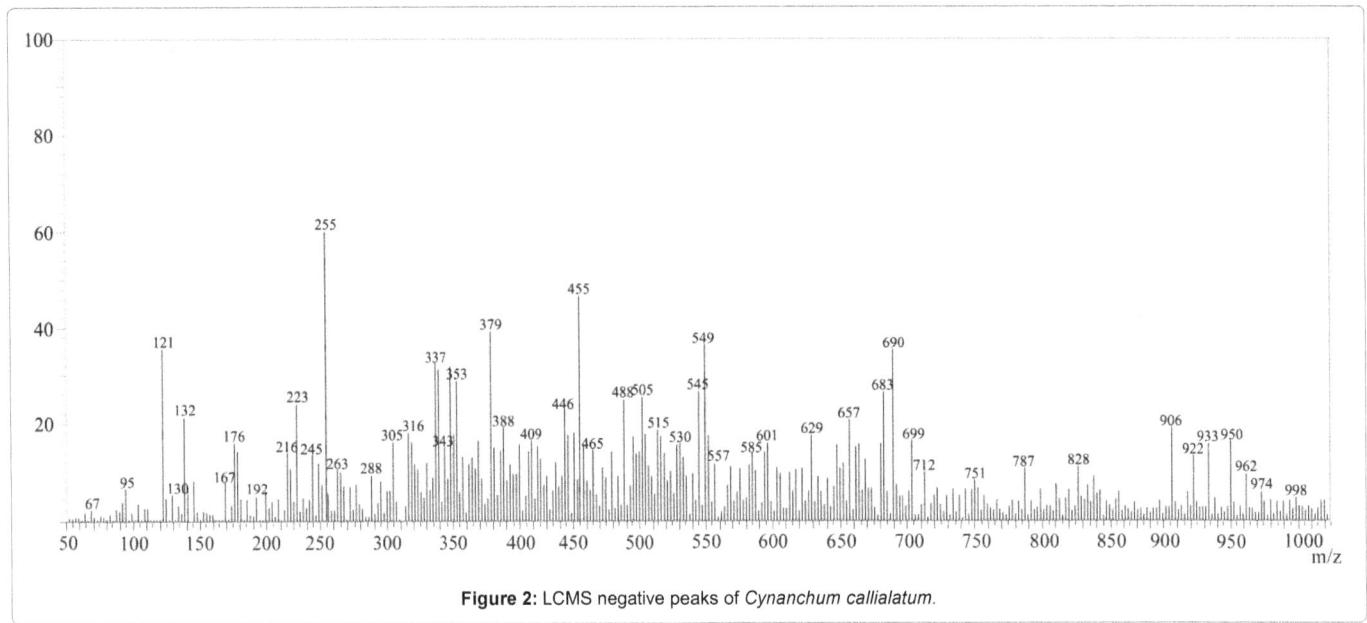

Figure 2: LCMS negative peaks of *Cynanchum callialatum*.

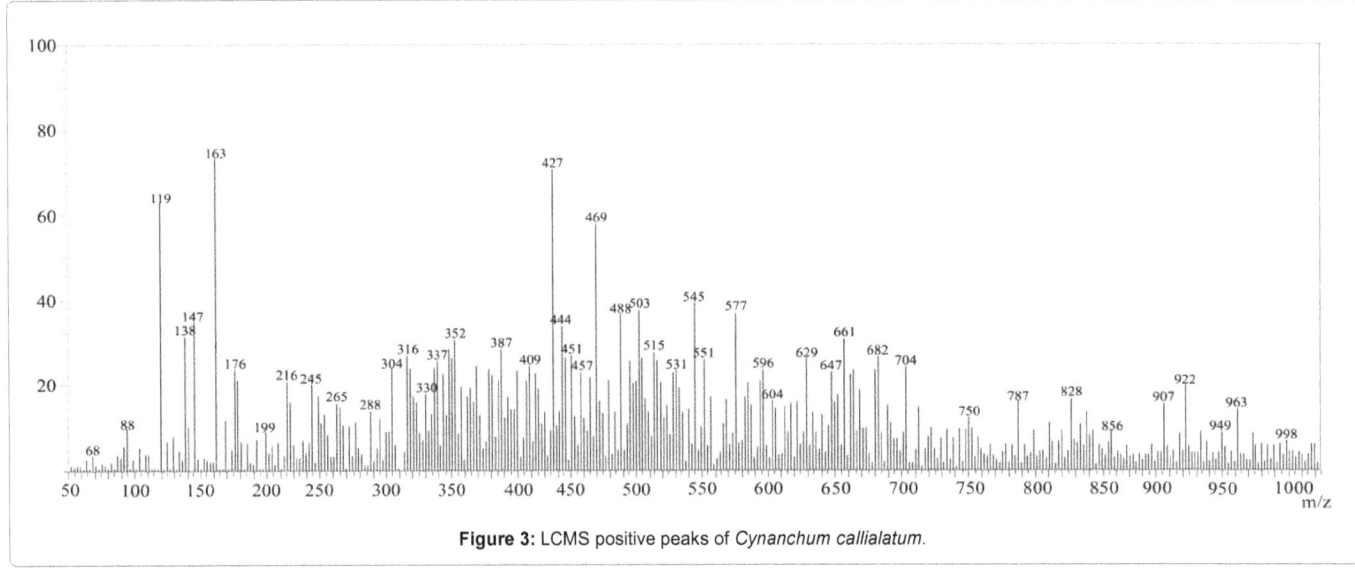

Figure 3: LCMS positive peaks of *Cynanchum callialatum*.

α-glucosidase, cFLIP, Bcl-2 and NFκB [9].

Germacrone: Germacrone possessed antiviral activity against the H1N1 and H3N2 influenza A viruses and the influenza B virus in a dose-dependent manner. The viral protein expression, RNA synthesis and the production of infectious progeny viruses were decreased both in MDCK and A549 cells treated with germacrone. In a time-of-addition study, germacrone was found to exhibit an inhibitory effect on both the attachment/entry step and the early stages of the viral replication cycle. Germacrone also exhibited an effective protection of mice from lethal infection and reduced the virus titres in the lung [10]. The germacrone possessed anti-proliferative effect of on the human hepatoma cell lines. Treatment of human hepatoma cell lines HepG2 and Bel7402 with germacrone resulted in cell cycle arrest and apoptosis in a dose-dependent manner as measured by MTT assay, flow cytometric and fluorescent microscopy analysis, while much lower effect on normal human liver cell L02 was observed. Germacrone might be a new potent chemo preventive drug candidate for liver cancer via regulating the expression of proteins related to G2/M cell cycle and apoptosis, and p53 and oxidative damage may play important roles in the inhibition of human hepatoma cells growth [11].

Longiverbenone: Is a sesquiterpene isolated which possess antibacterial and cytotoxic activity. The cytotoxic activity (LC50) of the compound longiverbenone new born brine shrimp (Artemiasalina) is presented in (Table 3). The LC50 of the compound against the brine shrimp was found to be 14.38 μg/ml. The cytotoxic bioassay result of longiverbenone may lead to the exploration of its potential and practical application as a novel less toxic and antimicrobial compound from this plant. Similar cytotoxic activities of plant constituents have been reported previously [12].

Sinapic acid (SA): shows cerebral protective and cognition-improving medicine.SA has anti-oxidative and anti-inflammatory activities, and may be an efficacious treatment for Alzheimer's disease [13].

Daucosterol: The treatment with DS-given mice with anti-mouse IFNγ, the protection was also abolished. These show that DS protects mice against disseminated candidiasis by the CD4[+] Th1 immune response [14]. Daucosterol improved blood circulation by inhibiting ether platelet aggregation and/or blood coagulation [15].

Taraxasterol: Have been shown experimentally to inhibit colon and breast cancer development. They act at various stages of tumor development, including inhibition of tumorigenesis, inhibition of tumor promotion, and induction of cell differentiation. Effectively inhibit invasion of tumor cells and metastasis [16]. Taraxasterol dramatically decreased the total inflammatory cell and reduced the production of Th2 cytokine IL-4, IL-5, IL-13 in BALF and OVA-specific IgE in sera, and suppressed AHR in a dose-dependent manner. Histological studies evidenced that the taraxasterol substantially suppressed OVA-induced inflammatory cells infiltration into lung tissues and goblet cell hyperplasia in airways [17].

Conclusion

The present study on phytochemical investigation of *Cynanchum callialatum* reveals the presence of various phytochemical constituents which support its use in folk medicine. This study also helps us to carry out researches based on the bioactive compounds, and to confirm scientifically the anticancer, antiretroviral, antimalarial, anti-inflammatory activities of *Cynanchum callialatum*. Our study suggests that *Cynanchum callialatum* may be a potential source for anticancer, antiHI, anti-inflammatory, antimicrobial drug discovery.

Acknowledgements

The Authors are thankful to Dr Udayan PS, Assistant Professor, P.G, Department of Botany and Research Centre, Sree Krishna College, Ariyannur P.O., Guruvayur,Thrissur District, Kerala, for the identification and Authentication of the plant material and to Dr. P.Brindha, SASTRA University, for providing full support to utilize their facilities. Authors also thank to Mrs.Sudha Palanivel ,SASTRA University for technical support and Dr.TNK SuriyaPrakash, Principal, Al Shifa college of Pharmacy,Kerala for his valuable support to complete this research work.

References

1. Balasubramanian T (2010) Phytochemical and pharmacological evaluation of indigenous medicinal plant *Stereospermum suaveolens* (Roxb.)DC, Jadavpur University, India: 1-20.

2. Navarra T (2004) The encyclopedia of vitamins, minerals and supplements. (2ndedn), Facts on File, New Jersey, USA.

3. Kokate CK, Purohit AP, Gokhale SB (1998) Pharmacognosy. (3rdedn), Nirali Prakashan, Pune, India.

4. Singh SP (1995) Practical manual of biochemistry, (3rdedn). CBS Publishers and distributors, Delhi, India.

5. Trease GE, Evans WC (1972) Pharmacognosy, (10thedn). Balliere Tindal, London, UK.

6. Tyler VE, Brady LR, Robbers JE (1998) Pharmacognosy, (9thedn), Lea and Febiger, Philadelphia

7. Mehdi D, Zoh R, Fereshteh J, Jasem E, Abbas H (2012) Antimicrobial activity of ethanolic and aqeous extract of *Cynanchumacutum*. British J Pharmacol Toxicol 3: 177-180.

8. Mansour GM, Faujan Bin HA, Alireza SK (2012) Biological Activity of Betulinic Acid: A Review. Pharmacology & Pharmacy 3: 119-123.

9. Hifzur RS, Mohammad S (2011) Beneficial health effects of lupeol triterpene: a review of preclinical studies. Life Sciences 88: 285–293.

10. Qingjiao L, Zhengxu Q, Rui L, Liwei A, Xulin C (2013) Germacrone inhibits early stages of influenza virus infection. Antiviral Research 100: 578–588.

11. Yunyi L, Wei W, Bin F, Fengyun M, Qian Z, et al. (2013) Anti-tumor effect of germacrone on human hepatoma cell lines through inducing G2/M cell cycle arrest and promoting apoptosis. European Journal of Pharmacology 698: 95–102.

12. Shafiqur RM, Nural AM (2008) Antibacterial and Cytotoxic activity of Longiverbenone isolated from the rhizome of *Cyperus scariosu*. Bangladesh J Microbiol 25: 82-84.

13. Lee HE, Kim DH, Park SJ, Kim JM, Lee YW, et al. (2012) Neuroprotective effect of sinapic acid in a mouse model of amyloid β(1-42) protein-induced Alzheimer's disease. Pharmacol Biochem Behav 103: 260-266.

14. Lee JH, Lee JY, Park JH, Jung HS, Kim JS, et al. (2007) Immunoregulatory activity by daucosterol, a beta-sitosterol glycoside, induces protective Th1 immune response against disseminated Candidiasis in mice. Vaccine 25: 3834-3840.

15. Koo YK, Kim JM, Koo JY, Kang SS, Bae K, et al. (2010) Platelet anti-aggregatory and blood anti-coagulant effects of compounds isolated from Paeonia lactiflora and Paeonia suffruticosa. Pharmazie 65: 624-628.

16. Ovesná Z, Vachálková A, Horváthová K (2004) Taraxasterol and beta-sitosterol: new naturally compounds with chemoprotective/chemopreventive effects. Neoplasma 51: 407-414.

17. Liu J, Xiong H, Cheng Y, Cui C, Zhang X, et al. (2013) Effects of taraxasterol on ovalbumin-induced allergic asthma in mice. J Ethnopharmacol 148: 787-793.

30

Ayurveda a Boon for Epileptics

Avinash Shankar[1]*, Amresh Shankar[2] and Anuradha Shankar[2]

[1]National Institute of Health & Research, Bihar, India
[2]Centre for Indigenous Medicine & Research, Bihar, India

Abstract

Apsmar denotes epilepsy, that usually persists in majority of patients with mental debility and disability, in spite of multidrug therapy with advanced anti-epileptics. But by supplementing Sodium valproate with indigenous composite of some Indian herbs as an adjuvant at 8 hourly dosing, tends to modulate the therapeutic outcome positively due to bioregulation of altered GABA bio kinetics and neurogenic action. Thus this adjunction seems a boon in epilepsy management.

Keywords: Epilepsy; Convulsions; Apsmar; Seizure; Neuronal disorder

Introduction

Apsmar, an Indian equivalent of Epilepsy, duly documented in vedic and post vedic literature of Charak and Sushrut 1000 BC is a non specific manifestation of hyper (synchronous discharge of cortical neurons and its prevalence in developing country is 57 in thousand, while in developed country like America and South Africa it is very high. Even in India also, incidences are increasing in geometric progression [1].

It is a complex brain disorder associated with both mental and physical debility, occurrence of recurrent convulsions causes neural hypoxia resulting in neuronal disorder or degeneration [2].

Improper drug scheduling among epileptics promote resistance to the receptor site causing recurrence even with wide range of available antiepileptic drugs such as; Phenobarbitone, Phenytoin, Sodiumvalproate, Carbamazepine, Ethosuccimide, Folvamate, Gabapentine, Labotegu, Oxycarbamazepine, Toperonoid, Tiagevin, Zenisonide, Tectal, Lamotrigine, Lavetiraceton, Pregabalin etc. But, non ensure complete cure of the disease except transient control of the seizure.

Almost one third of the people with epilepsy continue to have seizure (s) despite appropriate therapy with above mentioned drugs and possess considerable risk of cognitive and psychosocial dysfunction and increased health risk among the resistant epileptics. Mono therapy facilitates drug compliance, associated with lower risk of toxicity, affordability and regularity with minimized drug untoward effects.

Considering the IHO study of status of epilepsy patient taking treatment through an NGO Sanchar Kolkata and London epilepsy forum, majority cases presented with physical and mental debility in 90% cases while physical and mental handicap in 46%.

Hence a study was conducted to evaluate an indigenous composite as an adjuvant with conventional antiepileptic mono therapy in proper schedule to assess the therapeutic efficacy and safety profile [3].

Material and Methods

To evaluate the clinical efficacy of an indigenous composite as an adjuvant with widely prescribed antiepileptic monotherapy and study the status of old epileptic cases, a mass propaganda to create awareness for epilepsy patient in a multi centre epilepsy treatment camp was organized and 4568 cases of grand mal epilepsy were selected, duly interrogated (both patient and their parent), evaluated, investigated ,treated and follow-up observation was given by Centre For Indigenous Medicine & Research, RA. Hospital & Research Centre and Indian epilepsy forum.

Patients of convulsive disorder with associated other systemic diseases, patients of status epileptics and patients unable to follow the therapeutic and follow up schedule were excluded from the study.

Patient's non responsive to major therapeutics are termed resistant epileptics.

All the selected patients were investigated for CT scan, EEG, Hematological index and biochemical parameters to evaluate safety profile of the prescribed drug.

Irrespective of the disease duration, age of the patient, status of illness and previous therapeutics, all patients were given:

• Sodium valproate in recommended dose at 8 hourly schedule, strictly. (We practiced/administered doses at 6 AM, 2 PM and 10 PM)

• Indigenous composite containing (equal portions of)

- Acorus calamus (rhizome)

- Nardostachys jatamanshi (root)

- Convolvulus pluricaulis

- Herpestis monneiri (leaf)

- Crotalaria verrucosa (seed)

Dose: For adult: 1 cap of 500mg daily, while in children a 1/8th decoction 5 ml in >5 yrs; <5 yrs 2.5 ml; <1 year 1.25 ml every 12 hours.

Patients were examined and data were recorded in a follow up card.

Initially, weekly for 1st month, every 15th day for next 6 months and monthly for rest of the period during the therapy and every 3 month for 2 yrs post therapy follow up during the follow up, patients were evaluated for-

• incidence of attack of seizure

---

*Corresponding author: Dr. AvinashShankar, Chairman, National Institute of Health & Research, (RA. Hospital & Research Centre), Warisaliganj (Nawada), Bihar, 805130 India, E-mail: dravinashshankar@gmail.com

- frequency of seizure

- duration of seizure

- severity of seizure

- any untoward effect

- physical and mental status

To ensure 100% follow up with an instruction to the parent of the patient to enter the requisite information and observation in the follow up card.

To assess safety profile, patients were re-examined for hemato, hepato and renal status.

Therapeutic response was adjudged, analyzed and graded as per following index (Table 1).

Observations

- 4658 Patients of age range 5-40 years were selected for the present study. Among them 58% (2680) were male and rest female; 40.57% of all patients were of age group 10-20 years (Figure 1 and Table 2).

- Whereas disease status wise, 55.38% were recently detected, 38% were old cases of epilepsy without treatment, among them 21.9% patients were suffering from the past 1 year and others were 1-5 years old. Remaining 6.62% of patients were suffering from recurrent episodes of epilepsy in spite of a therapeutic regime (Figure 2 and Tables 3 and 4).

- As per clinical presentation 13% patients were presenting with convulsion, unconsciousness, frothing and autonomic dysfunction while old resistant cases (21%) were presenting with associated physical and mental debility (Table 5).

Grade	Characteristics
I	Complete absence of seizure, improved mental status and physical capacity without any untoward effect and Recurrence.
II	Complete absence of seizure without any untoward effect. Improved physical capabilities but unchanged mental state
III	No response

Table 1: Therapeutic response comparison as per index.

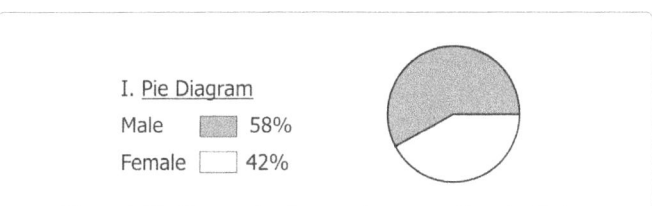

I. Pie Diagram

Male ▨ 58%

Female ☐ 42%

Figure 1: Pie diagram showing sex wise composition of patients.

Age Group	Number of patient			
	Male	Female	Total	%
<5 yr	72	48	120	2.6
5-10 yr	414	330	744	15.97
10-15 yr	480	320	800	17.17
15-20 yr	610	480	1090	23.4
20-25 yr	320	186	506	10.86
25-30 yr	318	236	554	11.89
30-35 yr	276	164	440	9.44
35-40 yr	190	114	304	6.52

Table 2: Distribution of patients as per age and sex.

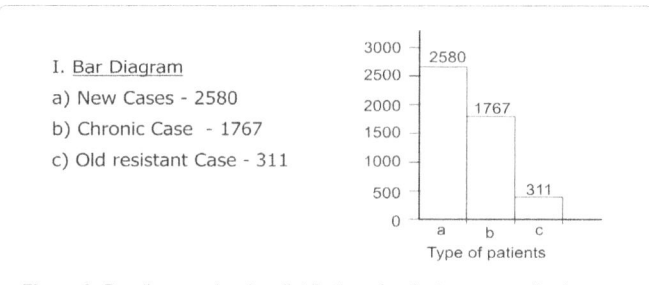

I. Bar Diagram
a) New Cases - 2580
b) Chronic Case - 1767
c) Old resistant Case - 311

Type of patients

Figure 2: Bar diagram showing distribution of patients as per epileptic state.

Duration of illness	Number of patients	Percentage
<12 month	1013	21.7
1-2 yrs	1662	35.7
2-3 yrs	804	17.2
3-4 yrs	672	14.4
4-5 yrs	120	2.7
>5 yrs	381	8.3

Table 3: Distribution of patients as per duration of illness.

Therapeutic regime	Number of patients	Percentage
Phenobarbitone+Carbamezipine	49	15.75
Phenytoin sodium+phenobarbitone	52	16.72
Sodium valproate+Phenobatbitone	57	18.32
Sodium valproate+Phenytoin sodium	73	23.47
Sodium valproate+Carbamezipine	43	13.82
Phenobarbitone+Phenytoin sodium & Carbamezipine	37	11.9
	311	

Table 4: Distribution of old resistant patients as per their therapeutic regime.

Presenting feature	Number of patients	Percentage
Convulsion with unconsciousness frothing from mouth and autonomic dysfunction	607	13.05
Convulsion with unconsciousness and Frothing from mouth	2002	42.97
Convulsion with transient unconsciousness	1394	29.93
Mental debility	970	20.82
Physical debility	970	20.82

Table 5: Distribution of patients as per clinical presentation.

- Among selected patients 42.01% were with hemoglobin less or equal to 10gm%, 1.05% with altered hepatic and 1.24% with altered renal functions (Table 6).

- All newly detected cases, 96.2% of old cases and 67% of chronic resistant cases had complete cessation of epileptic attack from beginning of therapy while 23% of old cases failed to respond within 48 hours but slowly severity, frequency and duration of convulsion regressed markedly. No patient exhibited autonomic dysfunction.

- Overall 99.76% patients revealed improved mental status in terms of psychosocial behavior and intelligence (mental ability) while 0.23% (11 cases) or 3.53% of resistant cases showed no change in their mental status but all had improved physical status.

- No post therapy recurrence of seizure was reported during 2 years follow-up observation

- All newly detected cases, 96.20% of old patients and 67.52% of resistant cases had grade I clinical response while 3.8% of old and 21.8%

Particulars	Number of patients	Percentage
Hematological:		
Hemoglobin-(%)		
8-10 gm	1957	42.01
10-12 gm	2423	52.01
12-14 gm	279	5.98
Hepatic parameters:		
Serum bilirubin-		
> 1 mg%	49	1.05
<1 mg%	4609	98.95
Renal parameters:		
Blood urea-		
>30 mg%	58	1.24
<30 mg%	4600	98.76
Serum creatinine		
>1.5 mg%	54	1.16
<1.5 mg%	4604	98.84

Table 6: Distribution of patients as per their base hemato, hepatic and renal parameters.

Particulars	Number of patients		
	New cases	Old cases	
		Chronic	resistant
	(2580)	(1767)	(311)
Convulsive attack-			
Absent	2580	1700	210
Declined	-	67	88
Non response	-	-	13
Mental status-			
Improved	2580	1767	300
Unchanged	-	-	11
Physical state-			
Improved	2580	1767	300
Unchanged	-	-	11
Safety profile-			
Recurrence of attack	None	None	109
Hepatic function-			
Altered	None	None	49
Unchanged	2580	1767	262
Renal function-			
Altered	None	None	54
Unchanged	2580	1767	257
Hematological-			
Improved	2580	1767	300
Unchanged	-	-	11
Post therapy convulsion-			
Absent	2580	1767	300
Grade of clinical response-			
Grade I	2580	1700	230
Grade II	-	67	68
Grade III	-	-	13

Table 7: Results of herbal adjunction therapy.

of resistant cases had grade II response and 4.18% of resistant cases failed to respond.

• The abnormal hemato, hepato and renal parameters of some old patients with refractory epilepsy were sustained or improved but not worsened (Table 7).

Discussion

Medical literature and study shows that available antiepileptic fails to ensure cure and prevent recurrent intense and repeated attack of seizure associated with physical and mental debility due to hypoxia, loss of GABA mediated inhibition of dentate granule and death of GABAergic inhibitory neuron results in attenuation of inhibitory control which in turn results in hyper excitation of the remaining neuron of the hippocampus. In spite of the fact that GABA neurons are more resistant to seizure induced neuronal death than other hippocampus neurons. Mossy cells (located in dentate hilus, a part of hippocampus) are extremely sensitive to seizure induced neuronal death and damage following intense synaptic activator i.e., excite-tonic mechanism of activator of NMDA (N methyl D aspartate) a sub type of glutamate receptor which results in excessive intracellular calcium.

Release of cellular zinc attenuate GABA response and induce hyper-excitability of neurons.

GABA binds to GABA-A (coupled to calcium/chloride channel and a main target of currently prescribed drugs) as excitatory post synaptic potential are the main form of communication between neurons and is mediated by release of excitatory amino acid-Glutamate from pre-synaptic elements which is mediated by

- NMDA (N methyl D aspartic acid/aspartate)

- AMPA(Alpha-amino-3 hydroxy 5 methyl isoxazole propionic acid) kinate

- Metabotropic

GABA-B (Couples to potassium channel, a cause of latency and long duration of action) located in pre-synaptic element of an excitatory pre-neuron and inhibits pre-synaptic neuron by

- direct induction of IPSP

- inhibition of release of excitatory neuro transmitters [4,5]

Hence clinical supremacy of the adjunct indigenous composite with Sodium valproate mono drug therapy can be attributed to bioregulative action of indigenous composites active ingredients for GABA neurodynamics i.e., Nardostachys jatamansi (Jatamansin, Jatamanose, Nardostachine) Herpestis monnieri(Monnerein) bio regulate GABA biokinetics and act in synergism with Sodium valproate and prompt control of the seizure, while Acorus calamus (Acorin, Beta asarone and calaminidine) and Crotolaria verrucosa (crotallidine and verrucosin) acts as a neurogenic and helps in regeneration and repair of damaged neuron due to epileptic attacks thus improve and check neural debility and alleviate physical disability .

In addition Convolvulus pluricaulis (Covolvulin) and Herpestis monnieri (Bacoside A & B) both promote neural growth due to activation of nerve growth factor-Tyrosine kinase A receptor, preserve m RNA level of muscarnic receptors and check accumulation of lipid and protein damage ,thus improve both mental ability and capability [6].

Hence bioregulation of altered GABA neuro kinetics prompt non recurrence of seizure even after drug withdrawal and neurogenic action improve mental capability and physical capability.

References

1. Shankar A, Shubham (2010) Epidemiological study of epilepsy among children in Jharkhand. The Holistic pediatrics 4: 230-236.

2. Shankar A (2013) Ayurveda for neurological disorder. J Homeop Ayurv Med 2: 130-131.

3. Shankar AC, Shankar AA, Shankar SA (2008) Epileptics debility a clinician idiosyncrasy. IJM Today 4: 143-145.

4. Shankar A (2009) Analysis of clinicopathology of grand mal epilepsy and present trend of its management. India epilepsy forum bulletin 4: 212-216.

5. Andrews DT, Sconfeld WH (1992) Predictive facts for controlling seizure using a behavioural approach. Seizure 1:111-116.

6. Shankar A (2013) Chemical constituents and pharmacodynamics of herbal constituents: The Pharmacological basis of Indigenous therapeutics. Bhalani Publication, Mumbai, India.

31

Acupuncture Prevents the Atrial Fibrillation through Improving Remodeling of Atrial Appendage in Rats

Zhu P[1], Zhang M[1], Yang M[1], Puji D[2], Ying Guo[1], Ao P[3] and Sun Y[1]*

[1]*The 2nd affiliated hospital of Heilongjiang TCM University, China*
[2]*TCM hospital of Daqing City, China*
[3]*The expriment center test cabinet of heilongjiang TCM University, China*

Abstract

The evidence from clinical experiments of acupuncture given at Neiguan (PC 6) spot has been proven effective in cardiovascular pathologies including cardiac arrhythmia. To understand how acupuncture prevents the atrial fibrillation (AF), the most common cardiac arrhythmia, an *in vivo* model of AF in rat was induced with continuous tail injection with $CaCl_2$ and ACH for 7 days. Meanwhile, bilateral acupuncture at PC6 was treated for 30 min just before the injection, and amiodarone worked as a positive control in this study. We found that both acupuncture (PC 6) and amiodarone treatments could effectively prevent the onset of arrhythmia and restore the sinus rhythm in AF rats. The analysis of ECG showed the AF maximal durations ($p<0.05$) and P-wave dispersion ($p<0.05$) in acupuncture (PC 6) were reduced. H & E-stained sections of the right atrial appendage from model group showed interrupted cardiomyocytes, myolysis, interstitial edema and increased extracellular space, which could be significantly improved by acupuncture at PC 6 group. Ultrastructure changes also were observed with electron microscope. Compared with the rats from model group, the sarcomeres were organized normally, and the number of swollen mitochondrial was reduced in the group of acupuncture at PC 6. Moreover, there were no major ultrastructure differences with the amiodarone group. These results suggest that the anti-arrhythmia effect of acupuncture may be mediated through the restoration and modification of remodeling of right atrial appendage.

Keywords: Acupuncture; Atrial fibrillation; Remodeling of atrial appendage

Introduction

Atrial fibrillation (AF) as the most common clinical cardiac dysrhythmia is a major cause of morbidity and mortality [1-2]. The number of patients with AF is constantly increasing as a result of aging, hypertension, cardiac infarction and congestive heart failure (CHF) [3-4]. Moreover, the lifetime risk of AF are high (1 in 6), even in the absence of CHF or cardiac infarction [5]. Patients with AF suffer a wide range of symptoms, such as palpitations, dyspnea, fatigue, dizziness, angina, and decompensated heart failure. In addition, Symptomatic AF can be combined with hemodynamic impairment, tachycardia-induced heart failure, and systemic thromboembolic events [6]. AF is emerging as a major public health concern and represents a major social and economic problem.

Cumulating evidences prove that AF is much more complicated than a simple electrophysiological disorder. The underlying mechanisms of AF susceptibility are not well characterized. Many triggers have the potential for initiation and maintenance of AF, which may therefore explain the difficulties in managing AF patients [4,7]. The present therapeutic strategies for atrial fibrillation generally are dependent on the antiarrhythmic and anticoagulant drugs in the sinus rhythm maintain, rate controlling and coagulation resisting [8]. There are many major limitations, including limited efficacy, risks of proarrhythmic events, a relatively high recurrence rate and hemorrhagic tendency [8-9]. These issues have inspired efforts to develop safer and more effective antiarrhythmic drugs and improved therapeutic approaches. More recent approaches for rate control, such as non-pharmacological ablation and atrioventricular node ablation, are improving, but safety and effectiveness are imperfect and remain uncertain. [10-11]. In China, acupuncture as one of tranditional treatment modalities is the most familiar to Western medicine [12]. Acupuncture given at Neiguan (PC 6) spot has been found effective for treatment of cardiovascular pathologies with regard to paroxysmal supraventricular tachycardia [13]. Recently, several clinical trials

demonstrate the efficacy of acupuncture in antiarrhythmias and preventing arrhythmic recurrences after cardioversion in patients with persistent AF [14,15]. To date, unfortunately, the evidence of acupuncture in the treatment of arrhythmias has not been well accepted because of the limited methodologic quality of the clinical trials and the lack of diverse patient populations.

Given the limitation and controversial in those clinical datum [14,16,17], we utilized drug-induced AF Sprague Dawley (SD) rats model by acupuncture at Neiguan (PC 6) spot, supposed to have a calming and sedative effect on cardiac excitability in patients [18,19] to confirm the efficacy of acupuncture in AF. The right atrial was harvested to evaluate the right atrial remodeling, which is closely related with the onset of AF [7,20]. The aim of our study was therefore to evaluate the antiarrhythmic effects of acupunctural therapy and make patients benefit from this ancient medical modality.

Methods

Animals

Male Sprague-Dawley rats (initial body weights ~250 g) were provided by the Department of Experimental Animal Sciences Center, Heilongjiang University of Chinese Medicine. The animals were kept on a 12-h/12-h light/dark cycle in a temperature-controlled (22°C) room and were given standard rat chow and water ad libitum throughout

*****Corresponding author:** Sun Y, The 2nd affiliated hospital of Heilongjiang TCM University, China, E-mail: 13069870666@163.com

the experiment. All animal procedures were strictly conducted in accordance with the international ethical guidelines and National Institutes of Health guide concerning the Care and Use of Laboratory Animals and were approved by the Animal Care and Use Committee of Heilongjiang University of Chinese Medicine.

Method for inducing AF and mortality

We followed the methods described by Tang et al. for induction of AF model [21]. SD rats were injected intraperitoneally with sodium pentobarbital (30 mg/kg) in a concentration of 10 mg/mL, followed by intravenous injection with $CaCl_2$ (10 mg/mL) and ACH (acetylcholine, 66 μg/mL) through the tail vein once a day for 7 days. A typical AF electrocardiogram (disappearance of the P wave and the appearance of the f wave) appeared immediately and recovered to sinus rhythm (disappearance of the f wave and the appearance of the regular P wave) in the following tens of seconds. The electrocardiogram (ECG) recording was maintained from rat anesthetized to administration finishing, approximately 30 minutes each rat each day for 7 days. Some rats died during the period of the induction of AF. The death rates were reported for this period based on the number of dead rats and the total number of the rats allocated to the given group.

Acupuncture methods and grouping

As illustrated in Figure 1B, the acupoints "Nei-Guan" (PC6) is located 3 mm lateral and distal to the wrist joint and between the radius and ulna in the fore limb. For acupuncture stimulation, stainless steel needles (0.25 mm in diameter) were vertically inserted into the selected acupoints (PC6) and applied for 30 min before the intravenous administration of $CaCl_2$ and ACH. Acupuncture treatment was given every day for 7 sessions in total.

A flowchart of the study protocol is shown in the schematic diagram in Figure 1A. Male rats were randomized into the following groups with 14 rats per group: Control group (injection of saline from day1 to day 7), Model group (injection of $CaCl_2$ and ACh mixture from day1 to day 7), Acupuncture group (Acupuncture treatment at PC 6 once a day for 30 min once a day, followed with injection of $CaCl_2$ and ACh mixture from day1 to day 7), Amiodarone group (oral treatment of 4.5 mg/kg Amiodarone once a day from day1 to day 7, followed with injection of $CaCl_2$ and ACh mixture 30 min later).

Electrocardiogram

ECG (lead II) recordings were performed to quantify ECG parameters (Heart rate, AF duration, P-wave width and P-wave dispersion). As shown in Figure 1C, Electrodes were placed under the skin for recording the conventional bipolar limb leads (II). In order to avoid errors in the position of the leads, the electrodes were always placed by the same person. The ECG was recorded using a three-channel digital ECG recorder with a paper speed of 50 mm/s and sensitivity of 0.5 mV/cm.

Histology

For Hematoxylin and eosin (H & E) staining, dissected right atrial appendages were immediately fixed with 10% formalin overnight at room temperature, dehydrated in an ethanol series, and paraffin embedded. Coronally sectioned tissues (5 μm) were deparaffinized in in a xylene-ethanol series and also dehydrated in an ethanol-xylene series. The sections were used to stain with hematoxylin/eosin (HE). Following washes in deionized water, dehydrated via ethanol, cleared in Xylene and slides were mounted. Each slide was examined by light microscopy.

Ultrastructure analysis

Right atrial appendages were fixed in cold 2,5-glutaraldehyde in 0.1

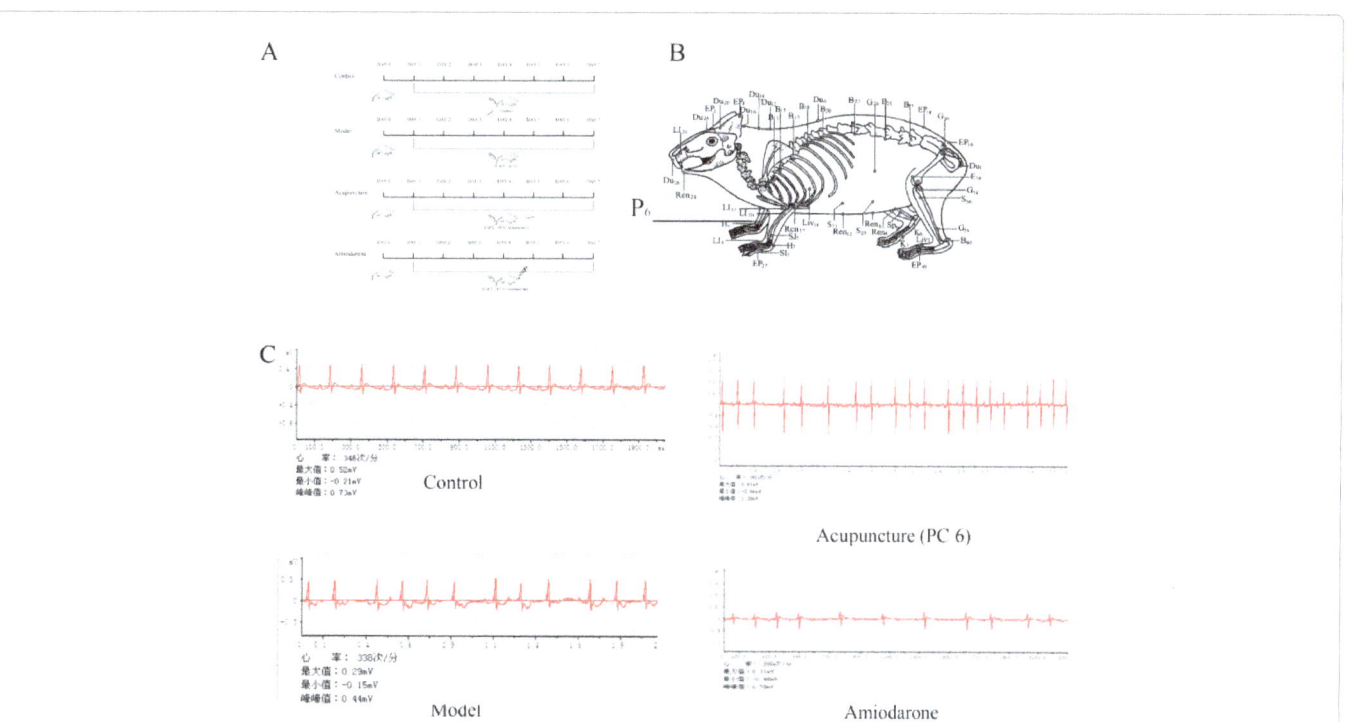

Figure 1: Experimental protocol, the location of Neiguan (PC 6) spot, and the ECG. **A)** 64 rats were used with 14 rats each in 4 groups, named with Control (treated with non-acupoint acupuncture); Model (without treatment); Acupuncture (treated with acupuncture at PC 6); Amiodarone (treated with amiodarone); **B)** The location of PC 6 in rat; **C)** Acupuncture at PC 6 could prevent the onset of atrial arrhythmia induced with $CaCl_2$ and ACh, and restore the sinus rhythm to some extent.

mol/L cacodylate buffer (pH 7.3), postfixed in 1%OsO4, dehydrated, and embedded in Epon. Thick sections (about 1 μm) were stained with toluidine blue and observed by light microscopy in order to select fields. Ultrathin sections were mounted on copper grids, stained with uranyl acetate and lead citrate, and examined under an electron microscope (4200 ×).

Statistical analysis

Normal data were expressed as mean±SD, whereas non-normal data were expressed as medians (interquartile range). Analysis of variance (ANOVA) and pairwise comparisons were used for normal data. Yates' chi-square test ($\chi 2$) was used for intergroup comparisons of mortality rates.

Results

Acupuncture at P6 showed no significant difference in survival data

Data from 56 SD rats were analyzed in this study (14 in each of the 4 groups). Survival after induction of AF differed among the four groups Figure 1D. In the model group, 6 rats died in model group within the first 7 days; 0, 4 and 3 rats died in the control, amiodarone and acupuncture group, respectively. The mortality rates on 7 d showed no marked difference among the four experimental groups ($p > 0.05$).

Effects of acupuncture on arrhythmic rats induced with AF

When the induction of AF was stable in the model group on the 7th day, the ECG data was selected for further analysis on the AF duration, P-wave width, and heart rate. Figure 1C shows the representative tracings of ECG recorded from the AF rat. The P wave was disappeared, the f wave was appeared and the duration of the R-R interval was prolonged, suggesting that a stable paroxysmal AF could be induced by intravenous injection of CaCl2 and ACh. Figures 2 and 3 is the statistical graphics among the groups. Compared with model group, both acupuncture and amiodarone could reduce the AF durations ($p<0.05$, n=8) and P-wave dispersion ($p<0.05$, n=8) by approximately 50%, except for P-wave width, within 30 min after the injection of CaCl2 and ACh.

Acupuncture improved morphological changes in right atrial appendage of AF rat

As shown in H&E-stained sections of the right atrial appendage, the injection of CaCl2 and ACh resulted in pronounced morphological responses. The characteristics were focal interrupted cardiomyocytes, myolysis, interstitial edema and increased extracellular space, which also could be observed in patients with chronic AF [22]. Compared with model group, the treatment of acupuncture or amiodarone could improve these morphologic changes.

Effects of acupuncture on the ultrastructure of right atrial appendage of AF rat

The right atrial cardiomyocytes in control group showed a tightly organized sarcomeric structure and Z-lines were clearly visible at higher magnification (arrows). As expected on basis of light microscopic observations, ultrastructure changes could be observed in the right atrial cardiomyocytes of AF model controls at day 7 (Figures 4 and 5). A significantly higher number of cardiomyocytes with disassembled sarcomeres, and an increased number of swollen mitochondria with fusion of mitochondrial were identified. The intercalated discs also appeared to be interrupted. In the Acupuncture groups, the

sarcomeres were organized normally and although some lightly swollen mitochondrial was observed, there were no major signs of ultrastructure compared with the amiodarone controls.

Discussion

As an important alternative therapy in China, acupuncture may be used to treat a variety of cardiovascular dysfunctions including reduction of arrhythmic events and recurrence [23]. However, the various antiarrhythmic effects of acupuncture were not based on formal clinical trials conducted in a rigorous scientific manner, and the weaknesses of standardized regimen and mechanic study have been considered the shortness in the field of evidence-base medicine [24,25]. In the present study, we established an *in vivo* AF model in rats and evaluated the Antiarrhythmic effects of repeated acupuncture stimulation at Neiguan point (P6). Our data suggested that the antiarrhythmic effects of acupuncture appeared to be similar to that of the amiodarone, inducing the restoration of morphometric and ultrastructural changes.

The development of numerous animal models of AF with clinically relevant disease paradigms has been a major advance over the last

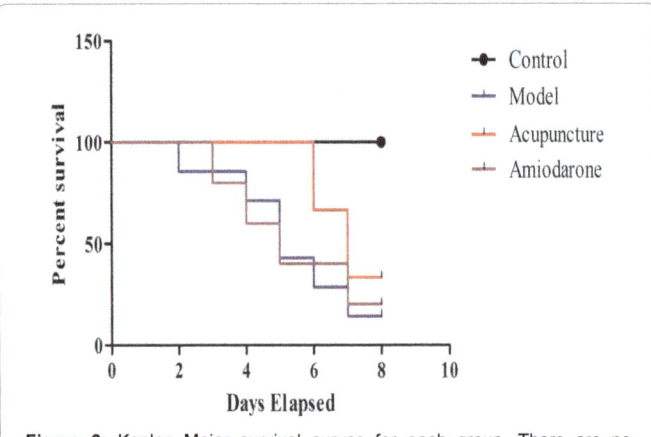

Figure 2: Kaplan–Meier survival curves for each group. There are no significantly different among model, Acupuncture and amiodarone groups.

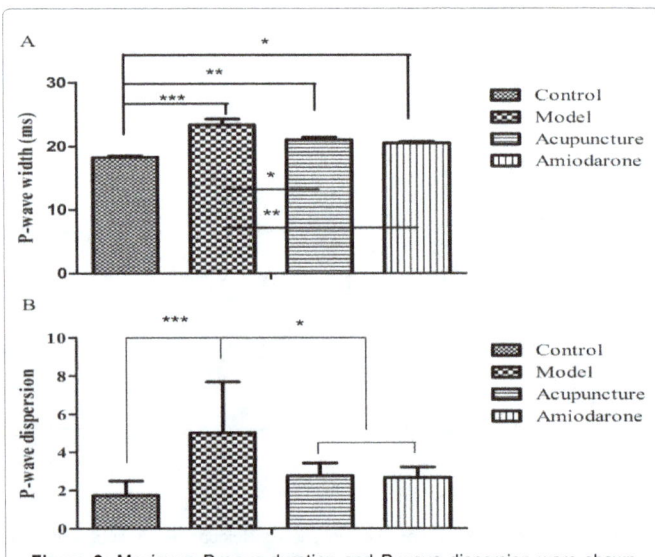

Figure 3: Maximum P-wave duration and P-wave dispersion were shown with Mean ± SEM for each group, (*=p<0.05, ***;=p<0.001).

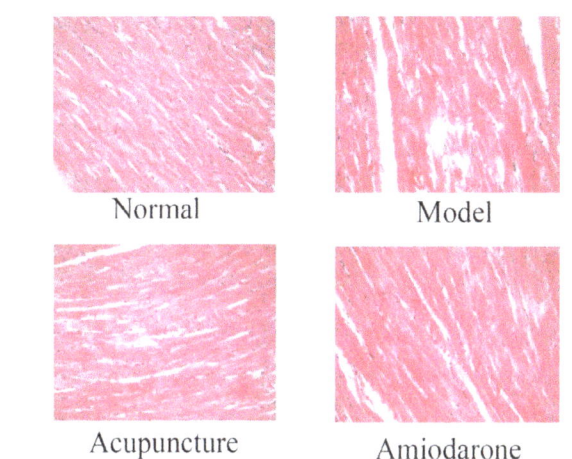

Figure 4: Morphological changes from each group. H&E staining showed there are interrupted cardiomyocytes, myolysis, interstitial edema and increased extracellular space in Model group. In acupuncture or amiodarone group, there are no significant morphological changes.

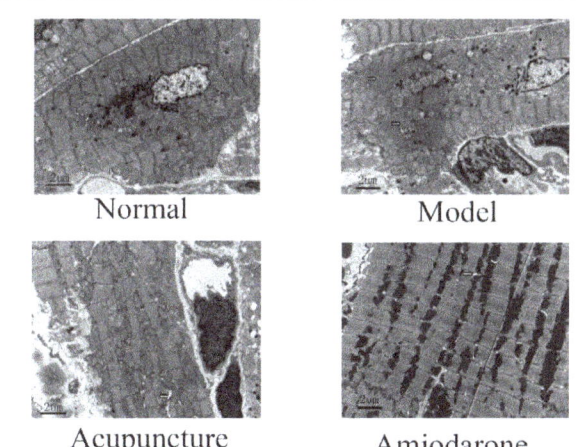

Figure 5: Figure 4: Electron microscopy of right atrial appendage from each group. Electron micrographs illustrated disassembled sarcomeres, swollen mitochondria and interrupted intercalated discs in Model group. In the Acupuncture groups, the sarcomeres were organized normally with lightly swollen mitochondrial. There were no major signs of ultrastructure compared with the amiodarone controls.

decades, which provided the practitioners a new insight to change the skepticism that acupuncture was based heavily on clinical subjective judgment, and lack of rigorous experimental evidence. With the going deep of the anti-arrhythmic mechanism of acupuncture, a plausible hypothesis on its antiarrhythmic effect could be through an action on the autonomic nervous system. Indeed, an increase in vagal or sympathetic neural activity directed to the heart might favor the initiation and maintenance of AF episodes in patients, and vagal nerve stimulation or acetylcholine infusion often was used to sustain AF in animals [26,27]. In this case, we utilized an infusion with acetylcholine and CaCl2 to induce the AF in animal with normal heart [21], which could be applicable to the impact of acupuncture on improving cardiac arrhythmias.

The Neiguan spot is located in the portion of the Meridian of the Heart Minister situated in the forearm, along the course between the two tendons, which controls blood-flow as well as pulse rate in

traditional Chinese medicine. In the early studies, Neiguan spot, as the point most commonly used for treating cardiac disorders, has been well known and proven effective in patients with symptomatic coronary artery disease [28-30], and the results have also been confirmed in experimental myocardial infarcted animals by stimulating the Neiguan point [31-33]. Whether the acupuncture on the Neiguan spot could be an effective non-invasive and safe antiarrhythmic tool in patients [34], further studies with rigorous controlled experiments should be made. The main finding of this study was that Naiguan acupuncture continued for 0.5 h was as effective as amiodarone in reducing duration of symptomatic AF episodes and P-wave dispersion by approximately 50%, without the suppression of heart rates compared with amiodarone treatment in conscious rats. More pertinent to our results was the experimental evidence that acupuncture of the Neiguan spot exerted an antiarrhythmic effect similar to that of amiodarone in patients with persistent AF [34], and Neiguan stimulation could augment sympathetic tone and improve the inhibited cardiovascular function under anesthetic dogs [35]. Moreover, Acupuncture pretreatment also exerted a modulatory function on the autonomic nervous system by regulating the firing rate of the amygdala nucleus [36], and attenuated the increase of [Ca2+]i in the myocytes isolated from the rat hearts subjected to ischemia-reperfusion by regulating L-type Ca2+ channel [25]. We could speculate anti-arrhythmic effects of acupuncture would primarily be due to the sympathetic tone activated, counterbalancing a reduction of action potential duration (APD) and reentry circuits [27].

In addition to electrophysiological dysfunctions, recent studies indicated that cardiomyocytes underwent dramatic structural alterations during AF, in which calcium overload and stretch appeared to be important regulating mechanisms [20,22]. In our *in vivo* rat model of AF, the structural remodeling, such as myolysis, focal interrupted cardiomyocytes and edema was also observed in AF rats induced with. However, the fibrosis was not obvious in our procedure. We speculated that short-term irritation with ACh and calcium could not induce the chronic structural remodeling. The electron microscope analysis of ultrastructure showed changes that were comparable to those histological changes seen in H&E staining heart of AF rats. Myolysis was illustrated accompanied with the presence of disassembled sarcomeres. Within the myolytic areas, the mitochondria displayed remarkable swollen, but their cristae appeared normal. The present results showed that acupuncture pretreatment restored the morphological and ultrastructural changes to some extent, even though the improvements of amiodarone pretreatment looked better. Given that interconnection between the structural remodeling and recurrence of AF [37,38]. We could speculate that acupuncture repeatedly over a period of days not only restored sinus rhythm but also reduced the recurrence rate of AF.

Our study was not designed to elucidate further details of anti-arrhythmic effects of acupuncture in cellular and subcellular levels, but we provided experimental evidence for participants willing to try this traditional non-pharmacologic therapy. Considering that acupuncture was safe, effective, without any pro-arrhythmic effect compared with the classical pharmacological therapy, this traditional Chinese medicine had a potential to become a more mainstream complementary intervention in the treatment of atrial fibrillation.

Reference

1. Benjamin EJ, Wolf PA, D'Agostino RB, Silbershatz H, Kannel WB, et al. (1998) Impact of atrial fibrillation on the risk of death: the Framingham Heart Study. Circulation. 98: 946-952.

2. Wolf PA, Mitchell JB, Baker CS, Kannel WB, D'Agostino RB (1998) Impact of atrial fibrillation on mortality, stroke, and medical costs. Arch Intern Med 158: 229-234.

3. Psaty BM, Manolio TA, LH Kuller, Kronmal RA, Cushman M, et al. (1997) Incidence of and risk factors for atrial fibrillation in older adults. Circulation 96: 2455-2461.

4. Allessie MA, Boyden PA, Camm AJ, Kleber AG, Lab MJ, et al. (2001) Pathophysiology and prevention of atrial fibrillation. Circulation 103: 769-777.

5. Lloyd-Jones DM, Wang TJ, Leip EP, Larson MG, Levy D, et al. (2004) Lifetime risk for development of atrial fibrillation: The Framingham Heart Study. Circulation 110: 1042-1046.

6. Go AS, Hylek EM, Phillips KA, Chang Y, Henault LE, et al. (2001) Prevalence of diagnosed atrial fibrillation in adults: national implications for rhythm management and stroke prevention: the AnTicoagulation and Risk Factors in Atrial Fibrillation (ATRIA) Study. JAMA 285: 2370-2375.

7. Nattel S (2002) New ideas about atrial fibrillation 50 years on. Nature 415: 219-226.

8. Wyse DG, Waldo AL, DiMarco JP, Domanski MJ, Rosenberg Y, et al. (2002) A comparison of rate control and rhythm control in patients with atrial fibrillation. N Engl J Med 347: 1825-1833.

9. Dobrev D, Nattel S (2010) New antiarrhythmic drugs for treatment of atrial fibrillation. Lancet. 375: 1212-1223.

10. Nattel S, Carlsson L (2006) Innovative approaches to anti-arrhythmic drug therapy. Nat Rev Drug Discov 5: 1034-1049.

11. Riley MJ, NF Marrouche (2006) Ablation of atrial fibrillation. Curr Probl Cardiol 31: 361-90.

12. Run-Ming Y (1985) The origin and development of chinese acupuncture and moxibustion. Anc Sci Life 4: 224-228.

13. Wu RD, Lin LF (2006) Clinical observation on wrist-ankle acupuncture for treatment of paroxysmal supraventricular tachycardia. Zhongguo Zhen Jiu 26: 854-856.

14. Lomuscio A, Belletti S, Battezzati PM, Lombardi F (2011) Efficacy of Acupuncture in Preventing Atrial Fibrillation Recurrences After Electrical Cardioversion. Journal of Cardiovascular Electrophysiology 22: 241-247.

15. VanWormer AM, Lindquist R, Sendelbach SE (2008) The effects of acupuncture on cardiac arrhythmias: A literature review. Heart & Lung 37: 425-431.

16. Celentano A, Palmieri V, Zulati P, Di Minno G (2003) Isolated episodes of atrial fibrillation and acupuncture. Nutrition Metabolism and Cardiovascular Diseases 13: 183-184.

17. Jonkman FAM, Jonkman-Buidin ML (2013) Integrated approach to treatment-resistant atrial fibrillation: additional value of acupuncture. Acupuncture in Medicine 31: 327-330.

18. Wu JH, Chen HY, Chang YJ, Wu HC, Chang WD, et al. (2009) Study of Autonomic Nervous Activity of Night Shift Workers Treated with Laser Acupuncture. Photomedicine and Laser Surgery. 27: 273-279.

19. Jang IS, Cho KH, Moon SK, Ko CN, Lee BH, et al. (2003) A study on the central neural pathway of the heart, Nei-Kuan (EH-6) and Shen-Men (He-7) with neural tracer in rats. American Journal of Chinese Medicine. 31: 591-609.

20. Dobrev D, Nattel S (2011) New insights into the molecular basis of atrial fibrillation: mechanistic and therapeutic implications. Cardiovasc Res 89: 689-691.

21. Tang YQ, Guo X, Chen CL, Yin YM, Wang MH, et al. (2010) Effects of Berberine Derivate CPU 86017 on IKur Currents and Experimental Atrial Fibrillation. Chinese Journal of Natural Medicines 8: 212-217.

22. Thijssen VL, Ausma J, Borgers M (2001) Structural remodelling during chronic atrial fibrillation: act of programmed cell survival. Cardiovasc Res 52: 14-24.

23. Longhurst J (2013) Acupuncture's Cardiovascular Actions: A Mechanistic Perspective. Medical Acupuncture 25: 101-113.

24. Dow J, Painovich J, Hale SL, Tjen-A-Looi S, Longhurst JC, et al. (2012) Absence of Actions of Commonly Used Chinese Herbal Medicines and Electroacupuncture on Myocardial Infarct Size. Journal of Cardiovascular Pharmacology and Therapeutics. 17: 403-411.

25. Gao JH, Zhang L, Wang YM, Lu B, Cui HF, et al. (2008) Antiarrhythmic Effect of Acupuncture Pretreatment in Rats Subjected to Simulative Global Ischemia and Reperfusion - Involvement of Adenylate Cyclase, Protein Kinase A, and L-Type Ca2+ Channel. Journal of Physiological Sciences 58: 389-396.

26. Nattel S, Shiroshita-Takeshita A, Brundel BJJM, Rivard L (2005), Mechanisms of Atrial Fibrillation: Lessons From Animal Models. Progress in Cardiovascular Diseases 48: 9-28.

27. Vigmond EJ, Tsoi V, Kuo S, Arevalo H, Kneller J, et al. (2004) The effect of vagally induced dispersion of action potential duration on atrial arrhythmogenesis. Heart Rhythm 1: 334-444.

28. Richter A, Herlitz J, Hjalmarson A (1991) Effect of Acupuncture in Patients with Angina-Pectoris. European Heart Journal 12: 175-178.

29. Ballegaard S, Pedersen F, Pietersen A, Nissen VH, Olsen NV (1990) Effects of Acupuncture in Moderate, Stable Angina-Pectoris - a Controlled-Study. Journal of Internal Medicine 227: 25-30.

30. Ballegaard S, Jensen G, Pedersen F, Nissen VH (1986) Acupuncture in Severe, Stable Angina-Pectoris - a Randomized Trial. Acta Medica Scandinavica 220: 307-313.

31. Redington KL, Disenhouse T, Li J, Wei C, Dai XJ, et al. (2013) Electroacupuncture reduces myocardial infarct size and improves post-ischemic recovery by invoking release of humoral, dialyzable, cardioprotective factors. Journal of Physiological Sciences 63: 219-223.

32. Zhou W, Ko Y, Benharash P, Yamakawa K, Patel S, et al. (2012) Cardioprotection of electroacupuncture against myocardial ischemia-reperfusion injury by modulation of cardiac norepinephrine release. American Journal of Physiology-Heart and Circulatory Physiology 302: 1818-1825.

33. Ho FM, Huang PJ, Lo HM, Lee FK, Chern TH, et al. (1999) Effect of acupuncture at Nei-Kuan on left ventricular function in patients with coronary artery disease. American Journal of Chinese Medicine. 27: 149-156.

34. Lombardi F, Belletti S, Battezzati PM, Lomuscio A (2012) Acupuncture for paroxysmal and persistent atrial fibrillation: An effective non-pharmacological tool? World J Cardiol 4: 60-65.

35. Syuu Y, Matsubara H, Kiyooka T, Hosogi S, Mohri S, et al. (2001) Cardiovascular beneficial effects of electroacupuncture at Neiguan (PC-6) acupoint in anesthetized open-chest dog. Japanese Journal of Physiology 51: 231-238.

36. Lai Z, Cao Q, Chen S, Han Z (1991) Role of amygdaloid nucleus in the correlation between the heart and the acupoint neiguan in rabbits. J Tradit Chin Med 11: 128-138.

37. Cosio FG, Aliot E, Botto GL, Heidbuchel H, Geller CJ, et al. (2008) Delayed rhythm control of atrial fibrillation may be a cause of failure to prevent recurrences: reasons for change to active antiarrhythmic treatment at the time of the first detected episode. Europace. 10: 21-27.

38. Lombardi F, Belletti S,.Battezzati PM, Pacciolla R, Biondi ML (2011) MMP-1 and MMP-3 polymorphism and arrhythmia recurrence after electrical cardioversion in patients with persistent atrial fibrillation. J Cardiovasc Med (Hagerstown) 12: 37-42.

32

Medicinal Herbs can Play Significant Role in Attenuation of Ischemia and Reperfusion Injury

Ipseeta Ray Mohanty[1]*, Suresh Kumar Gupta[2], Dharmavir Singh Arya[4], Nimain Mohanty[3] and Yeshwant Deshmukh[3]

[1]*Department of Pharmacology, MGM Medical College, Navi Mumbai, India*
[2]*Department of Clinical Research and Pharmacology, Delhi Institute of Pharmaceutical Sciences & Research, New Delhi, India*
[3]*Department of Pediatrics, MGM Medical College, Navi Mumbai, India*
[4]*Department of Pharmacology, AIIMS, New Delhi, India*

Abstract

Nature has been a source of medicinal treatments for thousands of years and plant-derived products continue to play an essential role in the primary health care of about 80-85% of the world's population. Medicinal herbs are widely used in Ayurveda, the Indian System of Medicine and have been observed to possess numerous activities with regard to cardiovascular system viz. antiplatelet, hypolipidemic, anti-inflammatory, hypoglycemic and hypotensive actions. Hence, these herbal extracts traditionally used have been evaluated scientifically in the present study with an aim to define the role of these agents in limiting the deleterious effects of myocardial ischemia and reperfusion (IR) injury by providing scientific data to validate their use as prophylactic approaches or as an adjunct to standard treatment (synthetic compounds employed in conventional treatment protocols) of ischemic heart disease. The efficacy of *Withania somnifera (Ws), Curcuma longa (Cl)* and *Ocimum sanctum (Os)*, and herbal combination (HCB) including {*Ws* (50 mg/kg) + *Cl* (100 mg/kg) + *Os* (75 mg/kg)} to limit injury in the setting of myocardial ischemia and reperfusion was explored in the present study. An open chest left anterior descending coronary artery (LAD) occlusion and reperfusion induced myocardial injury was used as the experimental model. Wistar albino rats were divided into ten groups and orally fed saline once daily (sham, control IR) or medicinal herbs (Ws/Cl/Os/HCB; Ws-IR, Cl-IR/Os-IR/HCB-IR) respectively for 1 month. On the 31st day in the rats of the Control IR and Ws-IR, Cl-IR/Os-IR/HCB-IR groups, LAD was occluded for 45 min, and reperfused for 1 h. Hemodynamic parameters were recorded at preset points and subsequently sacrificed for biochemical, immunohistochemical and pathological studies. In the control IR group, significant ventricular dysfunction, cardiac necrosis, apoptosis; decline in antioxidant status and elevation in lipid peroxidation was observed. Chronic oral treatment with HCB *per se* for 1 month resulted in significant enhancement of the myocardial endogenous antioxidant enzymes. Pretreatment with *Ws, Cl* and the herbal combination exerted significant cardioprotective effects in the experimental model of myocardial injury. The most remarkable observation of the present study was that cardioprotective effect exerted by HCB treatment was found to be superior to that shown by singular treatment with individual herbal extracts. The combination of herbal extracts was found to significantly ameliorate the ischemia and reperfusion cardiomyocyte apoptosis, cardiac dysfunction, compromised antioxidant status and histopathologic alterations as compared to control IR group. Cardioprotection by HCB treatment may be attributed to its favorable hemodynamic effects, myocardial adaptogenic properties, and significant antioxidant and antiapoptotic properties. Furthermore, HCB decreased the severity of pathological changes and significantly preserved the myocardial creatinine phosphokinase confirming its myocardial salvaging effects. Results clearly demonstrated the therapeutic potential of the herbal drugs in the treatment of myocardial ischemia and reperfusion injury. If the beneficial effects can be established in-patients, these findings may represent a novel adjunctive therapy of ischemic heart disease and Myocardial Infarction.

Keywords: Herbs; Ischemia; Reperfusion; Apoptosis; *Withania somnifera*; *Curcuma longa*; *Ocimum sactum*

Introduction

Myocardial ischemia initiated by occlusion or blockade of a major coronary artery leads to myocardial cell death. Thrombolytic therapy (i.e streptokinase, tissue plasminogen activator) by producing prompt reperfusion of ischemic myocardium relieves or reduces ischemia and the morbidity and mortality associated with an acute myocardialinfarction [1]. It has been well documented that early reperfusion of viable but ischemic jeopardized myocardium is essential to prevent cardiac damage. However, reperfusion itself has been shown to enhance myocardial injury and leads to further complications such as diminished cardiac contractile function and metabolic derangements. Myocardial injury associated with restoration of blood flow into previously ischemic tissue has been termed '**reperfusion injury**'. Reperfusion injury is defined as 'those metabolic, functional and structural consequences of restoring coronary artery flow that can be avoided or reversed by modification of the condition of reperfusion' [2].

The deleterious consequences of myocardial reperfusion include the hastening of the necrotic process of irreversibly injured myocytes, cell swelling, the no-reflow phenomenon, hemorrhagic myocardial infarction, the calcium and oxygen paradox, the production of oxygen derived free radicals which may further damage the ischemic myocytes, depletion of the antioxidant network of the myocardium and the prolonged post ischemic depression of ventricular function or the so called 'stunning' of the myocardium. Reperfusion of the ischemic tissue may also induce a number of important cardiac electrophysiological

changes, which in turn can cause a variety of arrhythmias, some benign, others potentially lethal [3,4].

Thus, myocardial reperfusion may be viewed as a 'double-edged sword', although it clearly exerts deleterious effects on the severely ischemic cells, when reperfusion is carried out relatively early in the course of ischemia its net effects are usually beneficial [5]. Thus, given the enormous potential clinical importance of early reperfusion in limiting infarct size, preserving antioxidant status, left ventricular function, and thus ensuring a significant decrease in patient morbidity and mortality, the development and identification of safe and effective interventions to reduce myocardial ischemia and reperfusion induced injury and/or optimize the benefit/risk ratio remain fertile areas for clinical and experimental investigation.

In the present investigation, modification of the condition of

*Corresponding author: Dr. Ipseeta Ray Mohanty, Department of Pharmacology, MGM Medical College, Navi Mumbai, India
E-mail: ipseetamohanty@yahoo.co.in

reperfusion has been achieved with the use of plant derived agents giving new insight to advanced therapeutic targets and strategies for the treatment of myocardial ischemic and reperfusion injury. The review summarizes the work undertaken in the laboratory to evaluate the cardioprotective potential of certain herbs {*Withania somnifera* (Ashwagandha), *Curcuma longa* (Turmeric), *Ocimum sactum* (Tulsi), the herbal combination including *Withania somnifera* (50 mg/kg) + *Curcuma longa* (100 mg/kg) + *Ocimum sanctum* (75 mg/kg)} and to elucidate their possible mechanisms of action on the basis of hemodynamic, biochemical and histopathological studies. The cardioprotective effects were evaluated in the in-vivo (coronary artery occlusion and reperfusion) and in the isoproterenol model of myocardial necrosis. In addition, the anti-apoptotic properties of the herbal extracts were studied using a combination of techniques of TUNEL positivity and immunohistochemical localization of Bax and Bcl-2 proteins.

The present study reveals that severe myocardial ischemia and reperfusion results in the biochemical derangements, deterioration of myocardial function and leads to the development of infarction. Although reperfusion is essential for the salvage of myocardium, it may enhance myocardial injury. Results clearly demonstrated the therapeutic potential of the herbal drugs in the treatment of acute Myocardial Infarction (MI). If the beneficial effects can be established in-patients, these findings may represent a novel therapy of ischemic heart disease and MI.

Materials and Methods

Experimental animals

Adult male Wistar rats, 10 to 12 weeks old, weighing 150 to 200 g were used in the study. The study protocol was reviewed and approved by the Institutional Animal Ethics Committee and conforms to the Indian National Science Academy Guidelines for the Use and Care of Experimental Animals in Research. Animals were obtained from the Central Animal Facility of All India Institute of Medical Sciences, New Delhi, India and were maintained under standard laboratory conditions in the department animal house. Rats were housed in polyacrylic cages (38×23×10 cm) with not more than four animals per cage. They were housed in an air-conditioned room and were kept in standard laboratory conditions under natural light and dark cycles (approximately 14 h light/10 h dark) and maintained at humidity 60 ± 5% and an ambient temperature of 25 ± 2°C. All experiments were performed between 9.0 and 16.0 h. The animals were allowed free excess to standard diet (Ashirwad; Chandigarh) and tap water *ad libitum* and allowed to acclimatize for one week before the experiments. Commercial pellet diet contained 24% protein, 5% fat, 4% fiber, 55% carbohydrates, 0.6% calcium, 0.3% phosphorous, 10% moisture and 9% ash w/w.

Chemicals

All Chemicals were of analytical grade, purchased from Sigma Chemical Co., St Louis, USA. The ABC staining kit and primary (Bax mouse monoclonal IgG_{2b} and Bcl-2 mouse monoclonal IgGI) & secondary antibodies (Anti mouse IgG) were procured from Santa Cruz Biotechnology, USA. TUNEL assay kit was purchased from Roche Diagnostics, USA. Double distilled water was used in all biochemical assays.

Test drugs

Hydro-alcoholic lyophilized extracts of *Withania somnifera and Ocimum sanctum* was procured from Dabur Research Foundation,

India. Aqueous extract of *Curcuma longa* was purchased from Sanat Research Laboratories, India. Standard Drugs: Vitamin E was procured from Sigma Chemical, Co., USA and Lisinopril from Cadila Pharmaceuticals, India.

Experimental Models of Myocardial Infarction

Dose selection studies (Isoproterenol model of myocardial necrosis)

The ISP (85 mg/kg) model of myocardial necrosis was used for the evaluation of therapeutic intervention of herbal extracts on the extent of jeopardized myocardium and evolution of infarction in ISP administered rats and select the optimum cardioprotective dose of the herbal extracts for further studies in the ischemia and reperfusion model of myocardial injury.

Experimental myocardial ischemia and reperfusion (IR) model: coronary artery occlusion and reperfusion

An open chest left anterior descending coronary artery (LAD) occlusion and reperfusion induced myocardial injury was used in the present study. In anesthetized rats, LAD occlusion was undertaken for 45 min, thereafter, the occlusion was released and reperfusion of the ischemic myocardium was allowed for a period of 1h. Baseline readings of all the hemodynamic variables were monitored and recorded after 15 min stabilization period, immediately before LAD ligation (time 0 min); thereafter, continuously throughout the experimental period (1 h 45 min) at preset time points. The hemodynamic variables were recorded at 5, 15, 25, 35, 45 min after ligation and at 5, 15, 30, 45, 60 min following reperfusion. At the end of the reperfusion period, animals were sacrificed by an overdose of anesthesia. Myocardial tissue was fixed in accordance to the specific methodology for biochemical, immunohistochemical and histopathological studies.

Experimental parameters evaluated

Cardiac function: The time-course of changes in {mean arterial pressure (MAP), heart rate (HR), left ventricular end diastolic pressure (LVEDP), left ventricular (LV) peak positive (+) dP/dt (rate of pressure development) and negative (-) dP/dt (rate of pressure decline)} were monitored and recorded during coronary artery ligation and reperfusion in different experimental groups.

Cardiac oxidant-antioxidant balance: In the present study, the biochemical indicators of myocardial oxidative damage, lipid peroxidation product; TBARS (thiobarbituric acid reactive substances), endogenous antioxidant: glutathione (GSH), antioxidant enzymes {superoxide dismutase (SOD), catalase (CAT), glutathione peroxidase (GSHPx)} and the myocardial enzyme creatine phosphokinase (CPK) were determined in the different experimental groups of the study.

Histopathologic evaluation: The Hematoxylin and eosin stained sections of the left ventricle were used to study the light microscopic architecture of the myocardial tissue and the degree of necrosis, edema and inflammation was quantified in the hearts of animals from the different experimental groups.

Apoptotic parameters: TUNEL positivity and the immunohistochemical localization of Bax and Bcl-2 proteins were studied to delineate the involvement of apoptosis in ischemia and reperfusion induced myocardial injury in the different experimental groups

Results

Pilot study (Isoproterenol model of myocardial necrosis)

In the present study 25, 50 &100 mg/kg doses of Ws; 25, 50, 100 & 200 mg/kg doses of Cl and 25, 75 & 150 mg/kg of Os were screened in the ISP model of myocardial necrosis in rats. Ws (50 mg/kg), Cl (100 mg/kg) and Os (75 mg/kg) were found to be most effective for functional recovery of the myocardium and the favorable restoration of biochemical and histopathological alterations. Hence, these doses were selected for further evaluation in the ischemia and reperfusion model of myocardial injury in rats.

Experimental myocardial Ischemia and Reperfusion (IR) model

Post-ischemic reperfusion injury resulted in significant cardiac necrosis, apoptosis; depression of left ventricular dynamics, peripheral hemodynamics (mean blood pressure) and heart rate; and decline in antioxidant status and elevation in lipid peroxidation. In addition, consistent with the increase in TUNEL staining in the control IR group, ischemia and reperfusion slightly reduced Bcl-2 expression and significantly increased Bax expression ($p<0.01$) compared with that observed in the sham group, demonstrating the phenomenon of ischemia and reperfusion induced enhanced myocardial apoptotic cell death.

Withania Somnifera: Augmentation of myocardial endogenous antioxidant reserve {SOD, CAT, GSHPx ($p<0.01$)} following chronic oral administration of Ws to healthy controls (study group of animals without any experimental challenge to the myocardium; via ISP administration or inducing ischemia and reperfusion injury) significantly improved defense against oxidative stress as compared to the sham group (oral administration of saline for one month to healthy experimental animals). Further, Ws treatment favorably reestablished the ischemia-reperfusion-induced abnormality of left ventricular functions {(+)LVdP/dt, (-)LVdP/dt and LVEDP}, restored the myocardial oxidant-antioxidant balance, corrected the metabolic derangements (reduced levels of TBARS and enhanced SOD, CAT, GSHPx and CPK activity); exerted marked antiapoptotic effects {(upregulated Bcl-2 ($p<0.001$) protein, decreased Bax ($p<0.01$) protein, and attenuated TUNEL positivity ($p<0.01$)}; and reduced myocardial damage as evidenced by histopathologic evaluation in the ischemia and reperfusion model of myocardial injury; emphasizing its beneficial action as a cardioprotective agent. Thus, favorable modulation of cardiac function by Ws and its myocardial adaptogenic, antioxidant and anti-apoptotic properties may contribute to the cardioprotective effects observed in the present study.

Curcuma longa: Chronic oral administration of Cl to healthy controls for one month significantly enhanced the myocardial activity of CAT ($p<0.05$) as compared to the sham group. The present investigation demonstrates that Cl has significant cardioprotective activity as shown by its mitigating effects on several myocardial injury induced hemodynamic {(+) LVdP/dt, (-) LVdP/dt & LVEDP}, biochemical {GSH ($p<0.001$), TBARS ($p<0.01$), CPK ($p<0.05$)} and histopathological perturbations. In addition, Cl administration significantly reduced the percent of TUNEL positive cells ($p<0.05$) as compared to the control IR group; demonstrating its significant anti-apoptotic activity. Treatment with Cl was associated with significantly increased expression of Bcl-2 ($p<0.001$) and attenuated Bax expression ($p<0.01$) in comparison to the control IR group.

Ocimum sanctum: In the present study, chronic oral administration

of Os *per se* to healthy experimental animals for 30 days resulted in significantly enhanced myocardial antioxidant status of basal SOD ($p<0.05$), CAT ($p<0.05$) as compared to the healthy sham control groups. Chronic administration of Os resulted in significant correction of oxidant-antioxidant balance {GSH ($p<0.001$), TBARS ($p<0.05$)} and modulation of the hemodynamic alterations (MAP, LVEDP) as compared to control IR group. However, this drug failed to significantly prevent leakage of myocardial CPK and prevent the histopathological alterations as compared to control IR group. Moreover, Os treatment did not demonstrate any significant anti-apoptotic activity as determined by TUNEL staining and immunohistochemical results. No significant change in the expression of Bax and Bcl-2 proteins was observed with Os treatment as compared to control IR group.

Herbal combination: To investigate whether a combination of the herbal extracts under investigation would offer any added advantage over treatment with individual herbal agents *per se*; the effects of chronic oral administration (30 days) of an herbal combination of (HCB) of Ws (50 mg/kg) + Cl (100 mg/kg) + Os (75 mg/kg) were evaluated. The effects of HCB were investigated in healthy experimental rats and compared with normal healthy sham control group and those of the HCB treated group submitted to myocardial ischemia-reperfusion protocol were compared to the control IR group. Furthermore, the efficacy of HCB was compared to that of both vitamin E and lisinopril used as standard reference drugs.

The results of the present study provide substantial evidence that HCB has significant cardioprotective potential. Although, the precise underlying mechanism of its cardioprotective effects is presently not fully understood; some explanations and likely mechanism(s) are being proposed based on the obtained data: Chronic oral treatment with HCB *per se* resulted in significant enhancement of the myocardial endogenous antioxidants; SOD, CAT, GSHPx ($p<0.01$) and reduction in myocardial TBARS level ($p<0.05$) as compared to the sham control group. Furthermore, HCB was effective enough to beneficially modify the ischemia-reperfusion-induced hemodynamic alterations. It significantly reduced the surrogate preload marker LVEDP as compared to control IR. It has been shown that interventions that decrease LVEDP improve myocardial blood flow in the deeper (endocardium) regions. Furthermore, HCB treatment significantly improved both inotropic and lusitropic function of the heart as evidenced by increased (+) and (-) LVdP/dt. HCB significantly restored the myocardial antioxidant network, as assessed by the increased levels of GSH content and SOD, CAT, GSHPx ($p<0.001$) activity, decreased level of TBARS ($p<0.01$)} as compared to control IR group. Most importantly, HCB demonstrated significant anti-apoptotic effects i.e. decreased Bax ($p<0.01$), upregulated Bcl-2 ($p<0.001$) expression and attenuated TUNEL positivity ($p<0.001$). Loss of contractile cells in the heart poses an additional workload on the remaining viable myocytes that may be unbearable, resulting in pathological stimuli and death signals. Hence, it is likely that chronic treatment with HCB might salvage these viable myocytes, which are at risk of irreversible injury and prevent cell loss induced by apoptosis and necrosis. Preserved myocardial CPK activity ($p<0.01$) and histopathologic evaluation further confirm its myocardial salvaging effects.

Discussion

Myocardial consequences of Ischemia and Reperfusion

Hemodynamic changes: Myocardial ischemia occurs when myocardial oxygen supply is insufficient to meet the demand. Hence, the evaluation of hemodynamic variables associated with myocardial oxygen demand and supply was done in the present study to assess this critical balance and the functional status of the heart specifically the left ventricular dynamics. Furthermore, the extent of myocardial injury couples with the degree of left ventricular dysfunction. Therefore, hemodynamic monitoring is essential to assess response to therapy. Because no single hemodynamic variable can reliably predict the outcome of myocardial ischemia and the effectiveness of a therapeutic approach, a combination of hemodynamic indices has been used to improve the value of hemodynamic monitoring. Alterations in MAP, HR, LVEDP, (+) LVdP/dt and negative (-) LVdP/dt during coronary artery ligation and reperfusion have been studied in different experimental groups.

In the present study, on occlusion of the LAD coronary artery there was a significant fall in MAP in conjunction with a non- significant change in HR. However fall in both these parameters progressed with the duration of ischemia and reached statistical significance at 45 min of ischemia. Coronary artery occlusion for 45 min and subsequent reperfusion for 60 min, resulted in a marked depression in myocardial contractility and diastolic function as evidenced by a fall in (+) and (-) LVdP/dt in concert with a significant elevation of LVEDP. Similar observations have been reported by other workers [6].

Following reperfusion, a further fall in MAP and HR was observed, which was sustained till the end of the reperfusion period. Fall in MAP ideally elicits reflex sympathetic activation, which should have increased HR. However, the significant fall in HR observed in the present study may be due to:

ı)   Anesthesia induced blunting of the reflex neural activity

ıı) Fall in MAP might not be biologically adequate for a reflex neural activation

ııı) Impairment of conduction (A-V block) of the heart following ischemia and reperfusion induced injury

Reperfusion of the ischemic myocardium also caused a further significant decrease in both (+) and (-) LVdP/dt, which failed to recover over the entire period of reperfusion. Such deterioration in the hemodynamic functions during reperfusion as observed in the present study is suggestive of an injury occurring following reinstitution of blood flow into the regionally ischemic myocardium. Similar observations (popularly known as ischemia and reperfusion injury) have also been made by several investigators in different experimental models [7]. Hasan and McDonough [6], have reported that reperfusion of the ischemic myocardium resulted in a significant and prolonged depression of contractile function in a rat model. Depression of (+) LVdP/dt has also been reported in a rat model subjected to ischemia and reperfusion. Reperfusion of the ischemic myocardium was effective in lowering LVEDP, which was ultimately corrected to near baseline levels after 1 hr. of reperfusion. These observations suggest that though the impaired contractility in reperfused myocardium is dependent on the preceding ischemic insult, yet reperfusion carriers with itself an injurious component. This is in accordance with the theory of post-ischemic dysfunction or stunned myocardium.

Biochemical changes: Several recent studies have demonstrated that altered oxygen utilization and/or increased formation of reactive oxygen species (ROS) contribute to myocardial infarction and its progression. While direct evidence of ROS-induced cardiac injury during hypoxia or ischemia and reperfusion in humans is lacking (due to inadequate methodology), many studies have shown increase in biomarkers of oxidant production and/or decrease in antioxidant

capacity during myocardial infarction [8]. In the present study biochemical indicators of oxidative damage, via the lipid peroxidation product, TBARS [9], endogenous antioxidant: GSH [10], antioxidant enzymes: SOD [11], CAT [12], GSHPx [13] and myocardial enzymes: CPK [14] and LDH [14] have been evaluated.

Lipid peroxidation marker: The level of TBARS, a biological marker of oxidative stress was elevated in the myocardium following ischemia and reperfusion. It is well established that a burst of oxygen free radicals (OFR) generation occurs immediately after reinstitution of blood flow to the previously ischemic myocardium. Due to reactions involving OFR and lipid component of cells, more stable lipid peroxidation components like malondialdehyde (MDA) are formed. MDA is measured in biological fluids by forming an adduct with thiobartituric acid, known as TBARS. Increase in TBARS as a marker of lipid peroxidation in conditions of myocardial ischemia and reperfusion is well documented both in clinical and experimental studies [15]. The results of the present study concur with earlier findings.

Myocardial antioxidants: In the present study, along with significant myocardial lipid peroxidation, myocardial GSH content, SOD and CAT activities were also depleted significantly following ischemia and reperfusion induced injury. However, the activity of the antioxidant enzyme, GSHPx was not significantly reduced. Superoxides are the major and the first formed OFRs and SOD is the enzyme, which dismutates superoxides to form H_2O_2 and O_2. The function of SOD has often been termed as primary defense against OFR, because this enzyme prevents further generation of free radicals. Catalase is also a major primary antioxidant enzyme that catalyses this function through the GSH system. Furthermore, cellular defense mechanisms rely on autolysis as well as inactivation of H_2O_2 by CAT to produce water and oxygen. It appears that, in the present study the major burden of neutralizing the ischemia and reperfusion induced oxidative stress, was borne out of GSH, SOD and CAT and to a lesser extent by GSHPx. This is reflected by the extent of depletion of the respective antioxidants. There are several studies, which have documented the evidence of depletion of different antioxidant compounds along with the increase of TBARS in different *in vitro* and *in vivo* models [16]. Thus, the increased TBARS production and the reduced levels of endogenous antioxidants provide strong evidence for the occurrence of oxidative stress during ischemia and reperfusion injury.

Histopathological changes: Morphologically, reperfusion after a certain period of ischemia can accelerate necrosis in irreversibly injured myocytes because of an increase in cell swelling, disruption of cell ultrastructure, formation of contraction bands, and deposition of intra-mitochondrial calcium phosphate granules. Sarcolemmal damage may also occur, leading to impairment of fluid regulation and ion flux balance [1]. The hematoxylin and eosin staining was used to study the light microscopic architecture of the myocardium and the degree of necrosis, edema and inflammation was quantified. On histopathological examination, control IR rat heart subjected to ischemia and reperfusion showed marked edema, confluent areas of myonecrosis, loss of myofiber and mild inflammation as compared to those in the sham group. Histopathological findings confirmed that ischemia and reperfusion resulted in significant myocardial damage.

Apoptotic changes: The recognition of a different cell death phenomenon, 'apoptosis', has recently become a major clinical interest. It accounts for a great proportion of cell death associated with myocardial infarction and/or myocardial ischemia and reperfusion. Cell loss through apoptosis contributes to the impairment of cardiac performance, and also plays an important role in myocardial and vascular remodeling processes. Induction of apoptosis is implicated in cardiac dysfunction. Not only ROS *per se*, but also their oxidative products and their secondary messenger molecules generated by ROS can trigger the programmed cell death. TUNEL positivity and the immunohistochemical localization of Bax, an inducer of apoptosis and Bcl-2 proteins, inhibitors of apoptosis were studied to delineate the involvement of apoptosis in ischemia and reperfusion induced injury. The TUNEL assay identifies single strand DNA breaks with free 3'-OH terminals. Several studies have raised doubts about the specificity of TUNEL staining. Collective evidence suggests that the TUNEL assay is useful in identifying apoptosis but should be complemented by additional evidence of apoptosis, such as the up-regulation of pro- or anti-apoptotic gene products or structural criterion [17].

TUNEL positive cells were expressed as percentage of total normal nuclei. In the sham myocardium, few cells stained TUNEL positive. In contrast, TUNEL positive nuclei were significantly increased in the control IR group as compared to non-ischemic sham group demonstrating the presence of enhanced apoptotic cell death. The process of apoptosis is regulated by the Bcl-2 family of proteins, which suppress (e.g. Bcl-2, Bcl-X_L) or promote (eg. Bax, Bad) apoptosis. The ratio of the anti-apoptotic proteins and pro-apoptotic proteins is critical in determining whether the cell survives or dies. Consistent with increase in TUNEL staining in the control IR group, ischemia and reperfusion slightly reduced Bcl-2 expression and significantly increased Bax expression as compared with sham group, suggesting a role of apoptosis in contribution of myocardial injury after ischemia and reperfusion. This observation receives support from earlier studies [18].

Pilot study (Isoproterenol model) for dose selection of herbal extracts: Isoproterenol (ISP), a synthetic β-adrenergic agent, causes ischemic necrosis in rats, which closely resembles human myocardial infarction. Rona et al. first described the production of myocardial necrosis and hypertrophy in the rat heart by intermittent subcutaneous administration of ISP. The pathological features observed in ISP treated rat concurs with earlier reports and consisted of myofiber degeneration, interstitial edema, subcutaneous congestion associated with infiltration of both neutrophils and lymphocytes [19].

A number of patho-physiogenic mechanisms have been outlined to explain the experimental lesions produced by ISP via altered membrane permeability, increased turnover of nor-adrenaline, generation of cytotoxic free radicals and marked inotropic and chronotropic actions resulting in greater oxygen demand. In addition to these, the reduction of blood pressure that is observed on administration of ISP, by means of peripheral vasodilatation is also suggested to cause myocardial necrosis [19].

Various studies have shown that oxidative stress results in the reduction of the efficacy of the beta-adrenoceptor agonists probably due to reduction in cAMP formation, caused by an impaired coupling between the receptor and adenylate cyclase. The reduction in maximal beta-adrenoceptor-mediated response might be the result of cytotoxic aldehydes that are produced during the oxidative stress. This beta-adrenoceptor hyperstimulation leads to cardiotoxicity. Oxidative stress may also impair the sarcolemmal Ca^{2+} transport and result in the development of intracellular Ca^{2+} overload and ventricular dysfunction. Hence, therapeutic interventions having antioxidant activity may be useful in preventing these deleterious changes [20].

In the present investigation, the biochemical and histopathological confirmation of the cardiotoxic effect produced by ISP (85 mg/kg), has

established the suitability of this model for studying the cardioprotective effect of the herbal extracts. This experimental protocol was used for the evaluation of the prophylactic and/or therapeutic intervention with the herbal extracts on the extent of the jeopardized myocardium and evolution of the irreversible tissue injury in ISP administered rats and select the optimum dose of the herbal extracts exhibiting maximum cardioprotective effects for further studies in the ischemia and reperfusion model of myocardial injury. In addition, hemodynamic, biochemical and histopathological parameters were incorporated in the study design to investigate the underlying mechanisms of their myocardial salvaging effects.

Withania somnifera

i) **Dose selection studies with *Withania somnifera*:** *Withania somnifera* (Ws) most commonly known as Ashwagandha, belongs to the natural order Solanaceae. The roots of Ws have been extensively employed as a valuable drug in Ayurveda, the ancient Indian system of medicine. Although its therapeutic potential on account of its immunomodulatory, adaptogenic, antioxidant, hypoglycemic and anticancer activities are reported [21], very few studies assessing its cardioprotective potential are presently available [22]. In the present study 25, 50 & 100 mg/kg doses of Ws were screened in the murine model of ISP-induced myocardial necrosis and the optimum dose exhibiting maximum cardioprotective effect was evaluated.

Myocardial injury was evident by leakage of myocardial CPK and a significant rise in TBARS. Superoxide radical generation and hydrogen peroxide formation after ISP administration may be the reason for lipid peroxidation in cell membrane. The metabolism of ISP produces quinones, which react with oxygen to produce superoxide anions and hydrogen peroxide leading to oxidative stress and depletion of the antioxidant system. The present data are in concurrence with the concept that the generation of highly cytotoxic free radicals through the auto-oxidation of catecholamines is one of the important causative factors for ISP induced myocardial necrosis. In the present study, ISP injection resulted in reduced GSH content as well as lowered activities of antioxidant enzymes; SOD, CAT and GSHPx in the cardiac tissue. These findings corroborate earlier reports [23]. In the present study, the fall in the activity of GSHPx in the ISP group might be correlated to the decreased availability of its substrate; that is, reduced GSH. Moreover, due to impairment in both enzymatic and non-enzymatic antioxidant defense mechanism, it is quite likely that the free radicals are not effectively neutralized and hence myocardium shows enhanced susceptibility to lipid peroxidation. The observation that Vitamin E (100 mg/kg) and Ws (50 & 100 mg/kg) treatment significantly restored LDH and CPK activity compared to ISP control group evidences their cardioprotective effect. Furthermore, both these drugs treatment restored the myocardial antioxidant status and maintained membrane integrity as evidenced by a decline in TBARS levels. Furthermore, histopathological examination confirmed the cardioprotective effects of Ws (50 & 100 mg/kg) and Vit E.

Various studies have shown that Ws possesses characteristic ginseng-like adaptogenic properties, which enhance myocardial tolerance subsequent to stress, a phenomenon known as 'adaptation' [24]. Although the exact mechanism of such an adaptation is not fully understood, but it may work through the induction of antioxidant enzymes such as SOD, CAT, GSHPx and antioxidants such as GSH and proteins like heat shock protein (HSP). In the present study, there was a concomitant increase in CAT and GSHPx along with SOD activity in the Ws (50 & 100 mg/kg) per se treated control groups. Vit E, however did not exhibit any such adaptogenic property as no significant increase in the levels of the endogenous antioxidants was observed in the Vit E treat group.

Measurement of the hemodynamic variables was also incorporated into the experimental design for better understanding and more precise information of the co-relation between biochemical and functional changes in the myocardium subjected to ISP induced damage. Previous studies have reported that exposure of the hearts to an oxidative stress depresses the ventricular functions and these changes are significantly prevented by antioxidants [24,25]. The results of the present study are consistent with these observations. In the ISP control group, myocardial dysfunction was clearly evident by a significant fall in MAP, HR, (+) & (-) LVdP/dt and a rise in LVEDP, which might be due to ISP induced myocardial necrosis. The (-) LVdP/dt was more markedly depressed indicating an increased diastolic dysfunction *per se* which may result in the persistence of the increase in LVEDP. Although Ws (25, 50 & 100 mg/kg) and Vit E (100 mg/kg) treatment did not significantly increase MAP, an increase in heart rate was observed as compared to ISP control group. Moreover, both the drugs appeared to preserve left ventricular function as evidenced by significant restoration of (+) and (-) LVdP/dt and correction of elevated LVEDP. Hence, it is suggested that preservation of cardiac reflexes resulting in improved ventricular dynamics may be on account of the myocardial protection exerted by Ws (50 & 100 mg/kg) and Vit E.

In summary, the present study strongly suggests that multiple mechanisms may be responsible for the cardioprotective effect of Ws. It produced myocardial adaptive changes (augmentation of endogenous antioxidants) on chronic administration to healthy experimental animals (that is animals without any myocardial pathologic challenge). In addition, it restored the antioxidant status of the myocardium, subsequent to ISP induced oxidative stress. These beneficial effects also translated into functional recovery of the myocardium as evidenced by favorable modulation of hemodynamic variables. Histopathological assessment further confirmed the protective effect of Ws on the myocardium. Taken together, the results of the present study demonstrate that although Ws (100 mg/kg) displayed modest protective effects, maximum cardioprotective effects were observed by pre- and co-treatment with Ws at the dose of 50 mg/kg. Ws (50 mg/kg) dose was found to be the most effective in functional recovery of the heart and favorable restoration of biochemical and histopathological alterations. Hence, Ws (50 mg/kg) dose was selected for further evaluation in the ischemia and reperfusion model of MI [26].

ii) Myocardial Consequences of Intervention with *Withania somnifera* during ischemia and reperfusion: It is well established that myocardial injury leads to loss of structural integrity and increased permeability. As described earlier, a good correlation between the histopathological evidence of myocardial necrosis and the enzymatic activity of enzyme CPK elucidates that the degree of CPK leakage from myocardium corresponds well with the myocardial injury [27]. In the present study, Ws (50 mg/kg) treatment significantly prevented leakage of myocardial enzyme CPK and preserved the myofiber architecture as compared to the IR control group.

As discussed earlier, a concept is now emerging of 'adaptogenic drugs', first time reported by Brekhman and associates in *Eleuthrococcus* and *Panax ginseng*, these are agents that increase non-specific resistance of the users to a variety of stresses. The definition of an adaptogen according to Brekhman (1969) is based on the following

ι.   Safety of the adaptogen's action on the organism

ιι.   A wide range of regulatory activity, but manifesting its action only against the actual challenge to the system.

ιιι. Act through a nonspecific mechanism to increase the non-specific resistance (NSR) to harmful influences of an extremely wide spectrum of physical, chemical and biological factors causing stress and has a normalizing action irrespective of the direction of forgoing pathological changes [28].

Adaptogenic property of various herbs like *Ocimum sanctum*, *Bacopa monniera* and *Withania somnifera* has already been reported in various experimental studies (Bhattacharya et al., Rege et al., Gupta et al.). These herbs allow one to adapt to a variety of heightened stressful circumstances. Although the exact mechanism of such adaptation is presently not known, it has been proposed that these drugs may act by inducing a number of antioxidant enzymes such as SOD, CAT, GSHPx and antioxidants such as GSH, proteins like heat shock protein (HSP) in the heart [25]. The present study demonstrated the adaptogenic property of Ws. Chronic oral administration of Ws per se to experimental animals; resulted in a significant increase in myocardial GSHPx, CAT along with SOD activity as compared to sham control group. Increase in antioxidant levels following chronic Ws treatment might considerably improve the myocardium's defense against oxidative stress and account for the cardioprotective effect of Ws. Any increase in SOD activity is beneficial in the event of increased free radical generation. However, it has been reported that an augmented SOD activity, without a concomitant rise in the activity of CAT and/or GSHPx might be detrimental, since S8D activity, generated hydrogen peroxide as a metabolite, which is more cytotoxic than oxygen radicals and must be scavenged by CAT or GSHPx. A simultaneous increase in CAT and/or GSHPx activity is essential for an overall beneficial effect of an increased SOD activity [16]. Thus, simultaneous increase in myocardial SOD, GSHPx and CAT activities observed in the present study with chronic administration of Ws underscores the distinct importance of enhanced beneficial effects of this herbal extract.

In addition, subsequent to ischemia and reperfusion induced myocardial injury, Ws treatment demonstrated significant antioxidant activity. It decreased the level of TBARS compared to control IR group, which could be imparted due to reduced formation of TBARS from fatty acids. Furthermore, protection against ischemia reperfusion induced oxidative stress in Ws treated rat hearts was evidenced by preservation of endogenous antioxidants enzyme SOD and GSHPx.

Monitoring of key hemodynamic variables was incorporated into the experimental design to demonstrate the close relationship between functional and biochemical changes in the myocardium subjected to ischemia and reperfusion induced injury. Exposure of the heart to an oxidative stress has been shown to depress left ventricular function and lower blood pressure and the use of antioxidants has been shown to reverse these hemodynamic alterations [19].

However, in the present study, Ws treatment appeared to preserve left ventricular function as evidenced by significant improvement of the inotropic and lusitropic state viz, (+) LVdP/dt and (-) LVdP/dt and correction of elevated LVEDP at various time points during the entire experimental period. However, these drugs at the doses used did not have significant effect on MAP and HR during the ischemic period. Cardioprotection afforded by Ws cannot be attributed to a reduction of myocardial oxygen demand as this drug did not significantly influence HR and MAP [29].

In addition, in the present study, Ws demonstrated significant anti-apoptotic property. In association with a reduction in the percentage

TUNEL positive cells in the ischemic myocardium, Ws treatment upregulated the expression of anti-apoptotic protein, Bcl-2 and down regulated the expression of pro-apoptotic protein, Bax. These effects may significantly reduce the marked apoptotic cell death in the myocardium of the control IR group. The anti-apoptotic property of Ws has been reported earlier in a rat model of stroke [30].

On the basis of the obtained hemodynamic, biochemical and histopathological data, it was concluded that Ws is a highly effective cardioprotective agent. The favorable modulation of ventricular function, significant antioxidant and anti-apoptotic properties may contribute to the beneficial effects of Ws [31]. The study provides scientific rationale for the use of Ws in Ayurveda, the ancient Indian system of medicine known as Maharasayana [24].

Curcuma longa

i) **Dose selection studies with** *Curcuma longa*: The cardioprotective effects of 25, 50, 100 and 200 mg/kg *Curcuma longa* (Cl), a perennial herb used in Ayurveda, the Indian System of Medicine, as a general health tonic and healing agent, were studied in the ISP model of MI. Cl (Turmeric), common Indian dietary pigment and spice has been shown to possess a wide range of therapeutic utilities in the traditional Indian medicine. It's role in wound healing, urinary tract infections, liver ailments are well-documented [32]. The active component of turmeric identified as curcumin exhibits a variety of pharmacological effects including antioxidant, adaptogenic, anti-inflammatory and anti-infectious activities [33]. However, only few studies are presently available that documents its cardioprotective potential.

In the present study, chronic oral administration of Cl *per se* to healthy experimental animals resulted in a significant increase in CAT activity with Cl-50, 100 and 200 mg/kg doses and inhibition of lipid peroxidation with Cl (50 & 100 mg/kg) doses. This adaptogenic property may contribute to its cardioprotective effect and strengthen the antioxidant defense mechanisms of the heart. However, none of the doses of Cl evaluated in this study resulted in significant augmentation of myocardial GSH content and SOD and GSHPx activity. Furthermore, the depressed myocardial antioxidant enzyme levels subsequent to ISP induced myocardial necrosis, were significantly restored by Cl treatment. However Cl failed to significantly prevent the loss of GSH subsequent to ISP challenge. In the present study, enhanced lipid peroxidation, as indicated by elevated myocardial levels of TBARS was observed in the ISP control group. However, Cl treatment significantly decreased the myocardial level of TBARS; this may be due to inhibitory action on the formation of lipid peroxides from fatty acids. It has been reported that curcumin, the active constituent of Cl inhibits the metabolism of arachidonic acid via the cyclo-oxygenase and lipo-oxygenase pathways that generates reactive oxygen species; resulting in a decrease in the levels of lipid peroxides [34]. Further, Cl (50, 100 & 200 mg/kg) treatment restored the activity of the marker enzyme CPK, demonstrating the biochemical basis of protective action of Cl against ISP induced myocardial injury.

Among the different doses of Cl studied, only 100 mg/kg dose of Cl appeared to preserve left ventricular function as evidenced by significant restoration of (+) LVdP/dt and (-) LVdP/dt and correction of elevated LVEDP subsequent to ISP challenge. Increase in (+) LVdP/dt and (-) LVdP/dt reflects an overall enhancement of myocardial contractility and relaxation respectively. Another consequence of reduced LVEDP is the increase in blood flow through the sub-endocardial region of the ventricular muscle that bears the maximum brunt of the ischemic insult. Under ischemic conditions, there is a disproportionate reduction

in blood flow to the subendocardial regions of the heart, which is subjected to the greatest extra-vascular compression during systole [35]. Cl (100 & 200 mg/kg) may indirectly tend to restore blood flow in these regions towards normal by correcting the elevated LVEDP. Correction of the altered hemodynamic variables observed with Cl treatment may be due to myocardial salvage exerted by the agent.

Thus, the present study demonstrates a significant protective effect of Cl in the ISP model of myocardial necrosis. It may be concluded that the cardioprotective effect of Cl is the result of the combination of its antioxidant and adaptogenic properties as well as its favorable modulation of the hemodynamic variables. Histopathologic evaluation further confirmed the protective effects of Cl on the myocardium.

Cl (100 & 200 mg/kg) doses significantly reversed myonecrosis via augmentation of endogenous antioxidants, maintenance of the myocardial antioxidant status and significant correction of the altered hemodynamic variables. Among the various doses evaluated in the present study, Cl at 100 mg/kg exhibited maximum cardioprotective activity [37].

ii) **Myocardial consequences of intervention with** *Curcuma longa* **during ischemia and reperfusion:** Augmentation of endogenous antioxidants is an adaptive mechanism against oxidative stress. As oxidative stress plays a significant etiopathological role in ischemic heart disease, such adaptive changes are supposed to be beneficial in combating ischemia-induced oxidative stress and its consequences. In the present study, chronic administration of Cl per se to healthy experimental animals (i.e without any experimentally induced ischemic insult), resulted in a significant increase in myocardial CAT activity along with a significant reduction in TBARS levels. It is proposed that this adaptogenic property may contribute to its antioxidant effect and its ability to protect the myocardium against the severity of ischemic damage.

Cl treatment significantly prevented the rise in TBARS as compared to control IR group suggesting that the antioxidant effect of Cl is responsible for lower TBARS generation in this group. However, Cl treatment showed modest corrective effects on the myocardial endogenous antioxidants enzyme: SOD, CAT and GSHPx. Nonetheless, myocardial GSH levels were significantly preserved by Cl, which might be responsible for lower TBARS generation in this group. This suggests that the direct antioxidant effect of Cl rather than a better antioxidant milieu was responsible for its cardioprotective effects.

The observation that Cl (100 mg/kg) treatment significantly restores the activity of the marker enzyme CPK as compared to control IR group evidences the protective effect of Cl on the myocardium. Histopathological evaluation confirmed its myocardial salvaging effects.

There are several reports supporting or refuting a direct antioxidant property of Cl [34]. However, till date there are no in vivo studies, which have explored the relationship between the putative antioxidant effects of Cl on the functional recovery of ischemic-reperfused myocardium. In the present study chronic (30 days) oral administration of Cl prevented the ischemia and reperfusion associated deterioration in the hemodynamic functions. Cl treatment resulted in preserved left ventricular function as reflected by a significant increase in the indices of contractility (+) LVdP/dt, relaxation (-) LVdP/dt and decrease in preload (LVEDP). It is speculated that, Cl treatment may have indirectly restored blood flow in the ischemic regions towards normal as assessed by its efficacy in improving cardiac performance, especially correcting the ischemia and reperfusion-induced increase in LVEDP. However, Cl did not significantly affect MAP and HR.

The present investigation indicates that Cl has significant cardioprotective activity as shown by its mitigating effects on several myocardial injury induced biochemical, hemodynamic and histopathologic perturbations. In addition, Cl administration significantly reduced the percent of TUNEL positive cells vs. the control IR group; demonstrating its significant anti-apoptotic activity. Treatment with Cl was associated with greater Bcl-2 and attenuated Bax expression as compared to the control IR group. Curcumin, the active ingredient of the rhizome of the turmeric plant (*Curcuma longa*), a commonly used spice, has been reported to prevent cancer in animal tumor models possibly by its apoptosis-inducing and [37] antiproliferative influences. However, in the present study, in contrast to earlier reports, marked anti-apoptotic activity of Cl was observed [38].

The anti-apoptotic effect of Cl, improved ventricular functions, restored endogenous antioxidant network along with improved histologic features suggests that treatment with this agent may exert cardioprotective effects following coronary ligation and reperfusion.

The data from the present study confirm the observations of earlier reports with respect to the antioxidant effects of Cl. The antioxidant activity of Cl is probably mediated through a mixture of curcuminoids such as curcumin, demothoxycurcumin, bis-demothoxycurcumin, and the active ingredients of the Cl rhizome. Curcumin is reported to inhibit nitrite radical induced oxidation of hemoglobin, prostaglandin biosynthesis, scavenge free radicals, inhibit lipid peroxidation, protect SH group of GSH and activate glutathione-s-transferase [34].

Ocimum sanctum

i) **Dose selection studies on *Ocimum sanctum*:** *Ocimum sanctum* (Os), commonly known, as Tulsi in India is a local herb containing potent antioxidants flavanoids (orientin, vicenin) and phenolic compounds (eugenol, cirsilineol, apigenin). The ancient systems of medicine including Ayurveda, Greek, Roman, Siddha and Unani, have mentioned its therapeutic applications in cardiovascular disorders, diabetes and asthma [39-41]. However, its potential as a cardioprotective agent has not been extensively studied. The cardioprotective potentials of Os at the doses of 25, 75 and 150 mg/kg were studied in the present investigation.

Augmentation of endogenous antioxidants may enhance the myocardial antioxidant reserve and strengthen the defense mechanisms operating in the myocardium. In the present study, chronic oral treatment with Os per se to healthy experimental animals resulted in a significant increase in the activities of GSHPx and SOD as compared to sham control group. This myocardial adaptation seems to be one of the likely mechanisms contributing to its cardioprotective effects. Furthermore, chronic oral treatment with Os significantly preserved the activity of the antioxidant enzymes SOD and CAT and exerted modest preservation of myocardial GSH content and GSHPx activity in the ISP-challenged group. Enhanced lipid peroxidation, as indicated by elevated TBARS level was observed in the ISP control group and Os treatment significantly decreased its levels by preventing the formation of lipid peroxides from fatty acids.

Administration of Os (75 and 150 mg/kg) significantly increased HR as compared to ISP control. Os at all the doses studied, significantly reduced the surrogate preload marker LVEDP as compared to ISP

control. However, it failed to significantly improve both inotropic and lusitropic functions of the heart.

In summary, the present study demonstrated that Os (75 mg/kg) significantly reduced ISP induced myocardial injury. Histopathologic examination further confirmed its cardioprotective effects. Most importantly, the study demonstrated that chronic oral treatment with Os augments the endogenous antioxidant status of the heart (myocardial adaptation), decreased myocardial necrosis, edema and inflammation and improved cardiac function. Decreased myocardial necrosis as evidenced by reduced CPK release, improved histologic picture, favorable hemodynamic and antioxidant effects; all contribute to its cardioprotective potential. In this context, it is critical to mention that Os at 25 and 150 mg/kg doses failed to demonstrate any significant myocardial salvaging effects [42].

ii) **Myocardial consequences of intervention with *Ocimum sanctum* in ischemia and reperfusion:** In the present study, oral administration of Os per se extract for a month resulted in a significant increase in the activities of CAT and SOD as compared to the baseline values of these biochemical parameters in the sham operated group. This is suggestive of the cardiac adaptogenic property of Os.

Chronic oral treatment with Os for one month significantly prevented lipid peroxidation and the loss of GSH content during myocardial ischemia and reperfusion; however, it exerted modest effects on myocardial antioxidant enzyme activity, which was comparable to that observed in the control IR group. Furthermore, it appears that the major burden of neutralizing the ischemia and reperfusion induced oxidative stress was borne by GSH and not by the antioxidant enzymes. Os treatment significantly prevented formation of lipid peroxides from fatty acids evidenced by reduced level of myocardial TBARS as compared to the control IR group.

Os markedly increased MAP, HR and significantly reduced the surrogate preload marker LVEDP as compared to control IR. However, it failed to significantly improve the left ventricular contractility and relaxation.

Although Os treatment demonstrated modest antioxidant effects and modified some of the hemodynamic changes, it failed to significantly prevent leakage of myocardial CPK and modulate the histopathologic alterations compared to control IR group. Moreover Os treatment did not demonstrate any significant anti-apoptotic activity as determined by TUNEL staining and immunohistochemical results. No significant change in the expression of Bax and Bcl-2 proteins was observed with Os treatment as compared to control IR in the present study [38].

In conclusion, Os treatment exerted modest cardioprotective effects; viz decreased preload and enhanced antioxidant status. Nonetheless, it failed to preserve the myocardial cellular integrity as evidenced by histopathologic evaluation and decreased myocardial CPK activity.

iii) **The science of herb combining and processing:** Although single Ayurvedic herbs and spices such as Brahmi, Turmeric and Ashwagandha are popular, one of the most significant contributions offered by Ayurveda is the science of herbal combination -- formulations that personify 'sanyoga', the fortuitous blending of a variety of herbs that results in a formulation offering the dual benefits of synergy and balance. An Ayurvedic formulation can often contain one or more herbs and spices -- primary herbs that target the area of imbalance, supporting herbs to enhance the benefits of the primary herbs, balancing herbs to counter any possible side-effects from the actions of the main herbs, and bio-availability enhancers to expedite the transfer of the benefits of the formulation to the parts of the physiology. The most complex of the traditional Ayurvedic herbal combinations are an elite group called rasayanas, extolled at length in the Ayurvedic texts for their positive impact on the physiology [43].

The second principle, 'sanskar', refers to the way the herbs are harvested, used and processed. Ayurvedic formulations traditionally use the whole herb instead of extracting the active ingredient from the plant. Nature's healing wisdom is perceived to reside best in the plant in its entirety. Using the whole herb rather than the isolated ingredient also contributes to a balanced formula less likely to have side-effects, because according to Ayurveda, each medicinal plant has both the primary effect and the antidote present in it in its natural state.

iv) Cumulative benefits: The Ayurvedic approach to health is gentle and comprehensive. The concepts of instant cures and pill-popping for immediate relief are foreign to Ayurveda. Because the endeavor is to seek and correct the source of problems -- imbalances in the physiology -- the best results from Ayurveda come to those who are patient and persistent, who diligently adopt the associated dietary and lifestyle changes needed, and take a degree of responsibility for their own well-being. For those who do make this commitment, Ayurveda offers rich, cumulative health benefits that can help you enjoy a long, healthy and blissful life [44].

Myocardial consequences of intervention with the herbal combination (HCB): *Withania somnifera* (50 mg/kg) + *Curcuma longa* (100 mg/kg) + *Ocimum sanctum* (75 mg/kg) vs. lisinopril and Vitamin E during ischemia and reperfusion : The HCB was effective enough to significantly ameliorate myocardial ischemic injury following LAD coronary occlusion and reperfusion when compared to control IR group. A significant finding of the present study is that the cardioprotection extended by the herbal combination was superior compared to that extended by the herbal extracts administered alone.

HCB did not significantly affect MAP and HR during the ischemic period; however during the latter half of the reperfusion period, HCB and Lsp, significantly restored MAP and HR. However, the modest beneficial hemodynamic effects on HR and MAP exerted by HCB do not explain the marked cardioprotection observed during ischemic and reperfusion injury. In contrast, Vit E did not exhibit any significant effect on these parameters.

In the present study, HCB exerted beneficial effects on left ventricular dynamics as evidenced by (a) the correction of the ischemia-reperfusion induced enhanced level of LVEDP and (b) by significant improvement in myocardial contractility and relaxation. It appears that the herbal extracts are more effective when administered together in preventing the hemodynamic deteriorations observed in the control IR group. However, Lsp treatment demonstrated superior recovery in left ventricular function as compared to HCB and Vit E. In the Vit E treated group, measurement of left ventricular diastolic function and systolic function revealed correction of LVEDP and partial prevention of the diastolic dysfunction; that is an increased (-) LVdP/dt. However, a parallel protective effect on the contractile status of the heart (+) LVdP/dt was not observed.

It is well known that one of the major causes of myocardial infarction is an imbalance between oxidants and antioxidant defenses. Hence, it is possible to prevent or ameliorate disease progression by favoring the balance towards lower oxidative stress. Potential antioxidant therapy should, therefore, include exogenous supplementation of natural antioxidants that affect augmentation of endogenous antioxidants [45].

In the present study, chronic treatment with HCB augmented basal endogenous antioxidants and inhibited the increase in TBARS levels i.e enhanced the antioxidant reserve, favorably modulating the antioxidant defense mechanisms of the myocardium in the healthy experimental animals. However, chronic treatment (30 days) with Lsp and Vit E *per se* did not show any marked effect on the baseline oxidant-antioxidant parameters. However, a key question, which remains unanswered in the present study, is the mechanism by which HCB augments basal endogenous antioxidants. Although the precise mechanisms of such an effect are not clear from the present protocol, several factors might be playing contributing roles. In this regard it has been reported earlier that both Ws and Os possess adaptogenic properties; hence, it is speculated that they may contribute to the myocardial adaptogenic activity observed in the HCB control group. Subsequent to ischemia and reperfusion induced oxidative stress it was observed that the HCB, Lsp and Vit E group demonstrated significant antioxidant property, which might contribute to the observed cardioprotective effect of these interventions.

In addition, in the present study, HCB and Lsp demonstrated significant anti-apoptotic potential as it upregulated the expression of anti-apoptotic protein, Bcl-2 and downregulated the expression of pro-apoptotic protein, Bax; in association with a reduction in the percentage of TUNEL positive cells in the ischemic -reperfused myocardium. The exact mechanism by which the herbal combination may reduce myocardial ischemia and reperfusion induced myocardial apoptosis is far from clear presently; and may not be answered fully by the present study. However it can be speculated that it may attenuate apoptosis via a number of mechanisms: Upregulation of Bcl-2 may result in formation of heterodimers with Bax, resulting in no/fewer free Bax protein available for homodimerization. If Bax homodimers predominate cell death will occur, but when Bcl-2 and Bax heterodimererization prevails cells can survive. Substantial evidence indicates that the mitochondria play a critical regulatory role in the signal transduction pathway leading to apoptosis. HCB may attenuate mitochondrial injury resulting from ischemia and reperfusion and preserve mitochondrial function. By this mechanism, it may prevent the formation of the permeability transition pore in the mitochondrial membrane, inhibit the release of pro-apoptotic molecules such as apaf-1 and apaf-2 (cytochrome c) from the mitochondria, and reduce myocardial apoptosis. HCB may also attenuate myocardial apoptosis through prevention of the dephosphorylation of Bad, a pro-apoptotic protein of Bcl-2 family, by calceneurin (a calcium/calmodulin dependent protein serine/thereonine phosphate). Preventing the activation of calcineurin keeps Bad in its phosphorlylated state and inhibits its translocation to the mitochondrial surface, preventing subsequent cytochrome c release. Moreover, free radicals have been demonstrated to directly activate calcium and magnesium dependent endonuclease (DNase I), thus resulting in DNA fragmentation and cell apoptosis [46]. The herbal combination treatment through its antioxidant mechanism may prevent this DNAase activation and reduce myocardial apoptosis. In contrast, Vit E did not exhibit any significant anti-apoptotic effect.

The protective effects of the HCB, Lsp and Vit E were supported by histopathologic examination and in concert with preserved myocardial CPK content. However, the cardioprotection afforded by Lsp was found to be superior as compared to that exerted by HCB treatment.

Finally, the potential of HCB as a novel therapeutic strategy for cardioprotection during ischemia and reperfusion injury has been well elucidated by the dosing protocol of the present study. The data of the current study evidence that the beneficial effects of chronic administration of the combination of the herbs under investigation were superior to those exerted by the respective agents administered singularly. Although the precise mechanism of the cardioprotective effects of HCB in this model of ischemia and reperfusion induced myocardial injury is not fully understood, however some of the likely mechanisms of its myocardial salvaging effects are being proposed on the basis of the obtained data: To summarize, administration of the HCB significantly augmented the levels of endogenous antioxidants in the healthy HCB control group (treated with HCB per se without any pathological challenge). Furthermore, HCB reduced the surrogate preload marker LVEDP as compared to control IR. The major consequence of the reduction in LVEDP is to increase blood flow through the sub-endocardial region of the left ventricular muscle that bears the maximum brunt of the ischemic insult. Under ischemic conditions, there is a disproportionate reduction in microcirculation and blood flow to the subendocardial regions of the heart, which is subjected to the greatest extra-vascular compression during systole. In addition, HCB significantly improved both inotropic and lusitropic function of the heart and significantly restored the antioxidant defense capacity of the myocardium subjected to ischemic and reperfusion injury. This effect maybe due to the free radical scavenging properties of the herbs under investigation. Most importantly, treatment with HCB demonstrated significant anti-apoptotic effects. Loss of contractile cells in the heart poses an additional workload on the remaining viable myocytes that may be unbearable, resulting in pathologic stimuli and death signals. In the present study, HCB treatment may have salvaged these myocytes and prevented cell loss induced by apoptosis. Preserved myocardial CPK activity and histopathologic evaluation further confirm the cardioprotective potential of such a combination [47].

Conclusions

Chronic oral pretreatment with *Withania somnifera*, *Curcuma longa* and the herbal combination (HCB) including *Withania somnifera* (50 mg/kg) + *Curcuma longa* (100 mg/kg) + *Ocimum sanctum* (75 mg/kg) exerted significant cardioprotective effects in the experimental models of myocardial injury. The most remarkable observation of the present study is that cardioprotective effect exerted by HCB treatment was found to be superior to that shown by singular treatment with individual herbal extracts. The combination of herbal extracts was found to significantly ameliorate the ischemia and reperfusion cardiomyocyte apoptosis, cardiac dysfunction, compromised antioxidant status and histopathologic alterations as compared to control IR group. Cardioprotection by HCB treatment may be attributed to its favorable hemodynamic effects, myocardial adaptogenic properties, and significant antioxidant and antiapoptotic properties. Furthermore, HCB decreased the severity of pathological changes and significantly preserved the myocardial CPK confirming its myocardial salvaging effects.

The present study provides scientific rationale of the employment of herbs/herbal extracts for cardioprotection, as described in Ayurveda, the ancient Indian system of medicine. These herbal extracts have the potential for the management of patients at risk of myocardial infarction. In view of the safety, efficacy and traditional acceptability of these agents, well-controlled prospective clinical trials should be contemplated to establish their efficacy in the treatment of ischemic heart disease.

References

1. Hearse DJ, Humphrey SM, Nayler WG, Slade A, Border D (1975) Ultrastructural damage associated with reoxygenation of the anoxic myocardium. J Mol Cell Cardiol 7: 315-324.

2. Opie LH (1989) Reperfusion injury and its pharmacologic modification. Circulation 80: 1049-1062.

3. Braunwald E, Kloner RA (1985) Myocardial reperfusion: a double-edged sword? J Clin Invest 76: 1713-1719.

4. Flitter WD (1993) Free radicals and myocardial reperfusion injury. Br Med Bull 49: 545-555.

5. Reimer KA, Lowe JE, Rasmussen MM, Jennings RB (1977) The wavefront phenomenon of ischemic cell death. 1. Myocardial infarct size vs duration of coronary occlusion in dogs. Circulation 56: 786-794.

6. Hasan A, McDonough KH (1995) Effects of short term ischemia and reperfusion on coronary vascular reactivity and myocardial function. Life Sci 57: 2171-2185.

7. Brunvand H, Rynning SE, Hexeberg E, Westby J, Grong K (1955) Non-uniform recovery of segment shortening during reperfusion following regional myocardial ischaemia despite uniform recovery of ATP. Cardiovasc Res 30: 138-146.

8. Marczin N, El-Habashi N, Hoare GS, Bundy RE, Yacoub M (2003) Antioxidants in myocardial ischemia-reperfusion injury: therapeutic potential and basic mechanisms. Arch Biochem Biophys 420: 222-236.

9. Ohkawa H, Ohishi N, Yagi K (1979) Assay for lipid peroxides in animal tissues by thiobarbituric acid reaction. Anal Biochem 95: 351-358.

10. Moron MS, Depierre JW, Mannervik B (1979) Levels of glutathione, glutathione reductase and glutathione S-transferase activities in rat lung and liver. Biochim Biophys Acta 582: 67-78.

11. Aebi H (1974) Catalase in: Methods of Enzymatic Analysis. Ed. Hans Elrich Bergmayer. Edit 2: 213-215.

12. Paglia DE, Valentine WN (1967) Studies on the quantitative and qualitative characterization of erythrocyte glutathione peroxidase. J Lab Clin Med 70: 158-169.

13. Lamprecht W, Stan F, Weisser H, Heinz F (1974) Determination of creatine phosphate and adenosine triphosphate with creatine kinase. In Bergmeyer HU. Ed. Methods of Enzymatic Analysis, Academic Press, New York, USA.

14. CABAUD PG, WROBLEWSKI F (1958) Colorimetric measurement of lactic dehydrogenase activity of body fluids. Am J Clin Pathol 30: 234-236.

15. Ferrari R, Ceconi C, Curello S, Cargnoni A, De Giuli F, et al. (1992) Occurrence of oxidative stress during myocardial reperfusion. Mol Cell Biochem 111: 61-69.

16. Yim TK, Ko KM (1999) Schisandrin B protects against myocardial ischemia-reperfusion injury by enhancing myocardial glutathione antioxidant status. Mol Cell Biochem 196: 151-156.

17. Kumar D, Jugdutt BI (2003) Apoptosis and oxidants in the heart. J Lab Clin Med 142: 288-297.

18. Maulik N, Yoshida T, Das DK (1998) Oxidative stress developed during the reperfusion of ischemic myocardium induces apoptosis. Free Radic Biol Med 24: 869-875.

19. RONA G, KAHN DS, CHAPPEL CI (1963) STUDIES ON INFARCT-LIKE MYOCARDIAL NECROSIS PRODUCED BY ISOPROTERENOL: A REVIEW. Rev Can Biol 22: 241-255.

20. Arya DS, Bansal P, Ojha SK, Nandave M, Mohanty I, et al. (2006) Pyruvate provides cardioprotection in the experimental model of myocardial ischemic reperfusion injury. Life Sci 79: 38-44.

21. Bhattacharya SK, Muruganandam AV (2003) Adaptogenic activity of Withania somnifera: an experimental study using a rat model of chronic stress. Pharmacol Biochem Behav 75: 547-555.

22. Dhuley JN (2000) Adaptogenic and cardioprotective action of ashwagandha in rats and frogs. J Ethnopharmacol 70: 57-63.

23. Csapó Z, Dusek J, Rona G (1972) Early alterations of the cardiac muscle cells in isoproterenol-induced necrosis. Arch Pathol 93: 356-365.

24. Rege NN, Thatte UM, Dahanukar SA (1999) Adaptogenic properties of six rasayana herbs used in Ayurvedic medicine. Phytother Res 13: 275-291.

25. Das DK, Engelman RM, Kimura Y (1993) Molecular adaptation of cellular defences following preconditioning of the heart by repeated ischaemia. Cardiovasc Res 27: 578-584.

26. Mohanty I, Arya DS, Dinda A, Talwar KK, Joshi S, et al. (2004) Mechanisms of cardioprotective effect of Withania somnifera in experimentally induced myocardial infarction. Basic Clin Pharmacol Toxicol 94: 184-190.

27. Boehm E, Ventura-Clapier R, Mateo P, Lechène P, Veksler V (2000) Glycolysis supports calcium uptake by the sarcoplasmic reticulum in skinned ventricular fibres of mice deficient in mitochondrial and cytosolic creatine kinase. J Mol Cell Cardiol 32: 891-902.

28. Brekhman II, Dardymov IV (1969) New substances of plant origin which increase nonspecific resistance. Annu Rev Pharmacol 9: 419-430.

29. Gupta SK, Mohanty I, Talwar KK, Dinda A, Joshi S, et al. (2004) Cardioprotection from ischemia and reperfusion injury by Withania somnifera: a hemodynamic, biochemical and histopathological assessment. Mol Cell Biochem 260: 39-47.

30. Adams JD Jr, Yang J, Mishra LC, Singh BB (2002) Effects of ashwagandha in a rat model of stroke. Altern Ther Health Med 8: 18-19.

31. Mohanty IR, Arya DS, Gupta SK (2008) Withania somnifera provides cardioprotection and attenuates ischemia-reperfusion induced apoptosis. Clin Nutr 27: 635-642.

32. Scartezzini P, Speroni E (2000) Review on some plants of Indian traditional medicine with antioxidant activity. J Ethnopharmacol 71: 23-43.

33. Dixit VP, Jain P, Joshi SC (1988) Hypolipidaemic effects of Curcuma longa L and Nardostachys jatamansi, DC in triton-induced hyperlipidaemic rats. Indian J Physiol Pharmacol 32: 299-304.

34. Balasubramanyam M, Koteswari AA, Kumar RS, Monickaraj SF, Maheswari JU, et al. (2003) Curcumin-induced inhibition of cellular reactive oxygen species generation: novel therapeutic implications. J Biosci 28: 715-721.

35. Grossman W, McLaurin LP (1976) Diastolic properties of the left ventricle. Ann Intern Med 84: 316-326.

36. Mohanty IR, Arya DS, Gupta SK (2009) Dietary Curcuma longa protects myocardium against isoproterenol induced hemodynamic, biochemical and histopathological alternations in rats. International Journal of Applied Research in Natural Products 1:19-28.

37. Kirana C, McIntosh GH, Record IR, Jones GP (2003) Antitumor activity of extract of Zingiber aromaticum and its bioactive sesquiterpenoid zerumbone. Nutr Cancer 45: 218-225.

38. Mohanty I, Arya DS, Gupta SK (2006) Effect of Curcuma longa and Ocimum sanctum on myocardial apoptosis in experimentally induced myocardial ischemic-reperfusion injury. BMC Complement Altern Med 6: 3.

39. Gupta SK, Prakash J, Srivastava S (2002) Validation of traditional claim of Tulsi, Ocimum sanctum Linn. as a medicinal plant. Indian J Exp Biol 40: 765-773.

40. Devi PU, Bisht KS, Vinitha M (1998) A comparative study of radioprotection by Ocimum flavonoids and synthetic aminothiol protectors in the mouse. Br J Radiol 71: 782-784.

41. Devi PU, Ganasoundari A (1999) Modulation of glutathione and antioxidant enzymes by Ocimum sanctum and its role in protection against radiation injury. Indian J Exp Biol 37: 262-268.

42. Arya DS, Nandave M, Ojha SK, Joshi S, Mohanty I (2006) Myocardial salvaging effects of Ocimum sanctum in experimental model of myocardial necrosis: a haemodynamic, biochemical and histoarchitectural assessment. Current Science 91: 667-672.

43. Muruganandam AV, Kumar V, Bhattacharya SK (2002) Effect of poly herbal formulation, EuMil, on chronic stress-induced homeostatic perturbations in rats. Indian J Exp Biol 40: 1151-1160.

44. Shao ZH, Vanden Hoek TL, Li CQ, Schumacker PT, Becker LB, et al. (2004) Synergistic effect of Scutellaria baicalensis and grape seed proanthocyanidins on scavenging reactive oxygen species in vitro. Am J Chin Med 32: 89-95.

45. Rajak S, Banerjee SK, Sood S, Dinda AK, Gupta YK, et al. (2004) Emblica officinalis causes myocardial adaptation and protects against oxidative stress in ischemic-reperfusion injury in rats. Phytother Res 18: 54-60.

46. Singal PK, Dhalla AK, Hill M, Thomas TP (1993) Endogenous antioxidant changes in the myocardium in response to acute and chronic stress conditions. Mol Cell Biochem 129: 179-186.

47. Mohanty I, Gupta SK, Arya DS (2007) Antiapoptotic and cardioprotective effects of a herbal combination in rats with experimental myocardial infarction. International J Integrative Bio 3: 178-188.

33

Effects of *Cleome gynandra* Linn: Leaf Extract on Ovarian Folliculogenesis of Albino Mice

Jupitara Deka* and J C Kalita

Department of Zoology, Gauhati University, Guwahati-781014, Assam, India

Abstract

It is well known that the plant kingdom contains numerous bioactive substances affecting the regulation of reproduction. *Cleome gynandra* plant extracts contain phytoestrogenic compounds. These compounds act as agonist or antagonist estrogen receptors, thus affecting the steroid hormones level. In traditional medicine, *Ceome gynandra* is used by lactating females for enhancement of milk and as a housing drug. The aim of this study was to investigate the effects of methanolic extract of *C. gynandra* leaves on the folliculogenesis of female albino mice. The effect of *C. gynandra* methanolic leaf extracts on folliculogenesis was studied in sixteen (N=16) sexually matured female albino mice with regular oestrus cycle. Mice were randomly divided into four (4) groups of four (n=4) mice per group. The experimental groups were treated as follows: Group I treated with 250 mg/kg, Group II with 500 mg/kg, Group III with 0.01 mg/kg 17β estradiol and Group IV with 1% Tween 80 (control). Follicular growth and changes were studied through standard histological protocols. For each ovary, every 12th and 20th section was examined for counting primordial, primary, secondary, graafian and atretic follicles, respectively to obtain an overall view of the follicular populations per ovary. In this experiment, the dose of 500 mg/kg BW/day showed a significant ($p<0.05$) decrease in primordial, primary, secondary and Graafian follicle compared to that of normal control mice. Significant increase in the number of atretic follicles was recorded in dose of 500 mg/kg BW/day compared to normal control mice. The dose of 250 mg/kg BW/day showed a similar decrease in primordial, primary, secondary and Graafian follicle compared to that of control mice ($p<0.05$). 17β Estradiol treated group showed a statistically significant ($p<0.05$) decrease in number of primordial, primary, secondary and Graafian follicle compared to that of normal control mice.

Keywords: *Cleome gynandra*, Folliculogenesis, Phytoestrogen, Nutraceuticals

Introduction

The relationship between female fertility and ovarian follicle development is well recognized [1]. Studies in mice [2] and rats [3,4] suggest that differential follicle counts may provide a sensitive means of estimating the extent of ovarian toxicity in females exposed to xenobiotics. As reported in a preliminary study [5] a three stage classification system based on follicle diameter and structure [6] as adapted by Mattison, et al. [7] appears to provide a quantifiable screening procedure for use in subchronic toxicity bioassays.

In 1989, DeFelice hypothesised the occurrence of biological interventions not related to pharmacological methods and wrote about "nutraceutical" products, i.e., "a food (or part of a food) that provides medical or health benefits, including the prevention and/or treatment of a disease" [8,9]. The original hypothesis was that these foods can protect the human body from adverse events because of the beneficial effects of some phytochemicals. Several studies have reported the validity of this idea in clinical practice [10-12]. Certain synthetic or natural compounds present in the environment mimic, enhance or inhibit endogenous hormones. These compounds are called as environmental estrogens [13]. These chemicals have been a source of concern because of their possible health threats to human being in particular. These are also called as xenoestrogens which cause change in cellular function of animals' body by binding with estrogen receptor sites [14,15]. These chemicals present in the environment interfere in the biosynthetic pathway of the endogenous hormones or modifying hormone metabolism thereby which an animal maintain a normal homeostatic system with which it responds to its surrounding environment.

Estrogens inhibit mouse oocyte nest breakdown and follicle assembly [16]. Estrogenic action reduces follicle assembly leading to fewer primary and subsequent developing follicles. Thus, the study of follicular populations provides important information about the function of the ovary, in particular the relationship between folliculogenesis and also environmental factors having estrogenic property that regulate it [17].

Plant kingdom contains numerous bioactive substances affecting the regulation of reproduction in animals and humans. *Cleome gynandra* plant extracts contain numerous bioactive compounds. There are reports that these compounds act as agonist or antagonist of estrogen receptors, thus affecting the steroid hormones level. In traditional medicine, *C. gynandra* was used by lactating females for enhancement of milk and as a housing drug. The aim of the present study was to investigate the effects of methanolic extract of *C. gynandra* leaves on the ovarian folliculogenesis in albino mice (Figure 1).

Materials and Methods

Collection of plant materials: Fresh leaves of *C. gynandra* were collected from different parts of Kamrup district. They in fresh condition were washed under running tap water and then again with distilled water. The plant material was air dried in the shade for 5 days and then homogenized to fine powder and stored in airtight bottles with proper labeling.

Preparation of extract: Powdered plant materials were collected and weighed carefully. A 50 g of the plant material was weighed and soaked in 300 mL of methanol. The mixture was kept in shaker for

*Corresponding author: Jupitara Deka Department of Zoology, Gauhati University, Guwahati-781014, Assam, India; E-mail: jdjupitara1@gmail.com

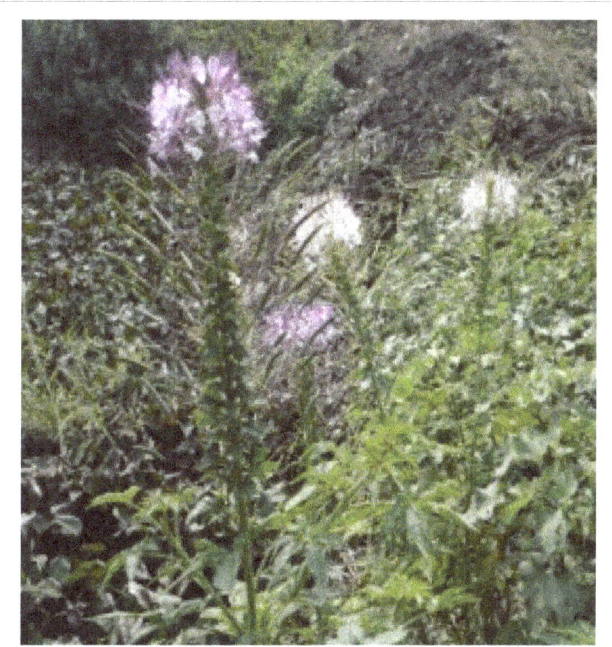

Figure 1: *Cleome gynandra* L. at natural habitat.

48 h and filtered. The filtrate was kept in a rotary evaporator in low temperature under reduced pressure till dryness. Extract thus obtained was examined chemically and screened for phytochemical screening. The extract was kept in a refrigerator when not in use.

Treatment procedure and route of administration: Two doses of 250 mg/kg BW and 500 mg/kg BW of plant extracts, respectively were used which corresponds to a 1/12th and 1/6th, respectively of the highest tested dose (3000 mg/kg BW). 1% v/v Tween-80 (P8074, CAS 9005-65-6) which is a polyethylene sorbitol ester was used to prepare the extract suspension of the test plant extract. To prepare the 17β-Estradiol stock solution, the same was dissolved in Ethanol (analytical grade) and it was diluted with normal saline to prepare the desired dose of working solution. Animals were exposed to the test compounds through standard gastric gavages feeding syringe (Feedy-I, FG-05). The doses were administered at 24 h of interval for a period of 21 days.

Morphological classification of follicles: Ovaries of five animals of each group were taken for the follicular studies. Ovaries were selected based on the stage and comparability of the weight with respective control ovaries. The ovaries were fixed in Bouin's fluid, embedded in paraffin and sectioned at 6 μm thickness. The sections were separated for every 10th section and stained with hematoxylin and eosin. Sections of the ovary were examined under a light microscope and the general histologic appearance of the ovary was assessed. All serial sections of the ovary were counted for various stages of development of follicles as described by Moawad, et al., [18,19]. Follicles and atretic follicles were classified according to the method described by Swartz and Mall and Bucci [20,21].

Quantification of follicles: To determine the total population of different types of follicles per ovary the method used by Pedersen and Peters and Butcher and Kirkpatric-Keller were followed [22]. At an average, about 200 serial sections were obtained and for each ovary, every 12th and 20th section was examined for counting smaller (primordial, primary and secondary) and larger (graafian and atretic) follicles, respectively to obtain an overall view of the follicular populations per ovary (Myers et al., [23].

Statistics: Statistical analyses for all the data of animal experimentations were performed using MS Office Excel 2007. The results were expressed as mean ± Standard Error (SE) of mean. The means in both negative as well as positive control versus treated animals were analyzed for significant by Student's independent t-test distribution. A value of $p < 0.05$ was considered statistically significant for all the tests.

Results

The results of the ovarian follicular counting on treatment with CGME were showed in the Table 1. In this experiment, the dose of 500 mg/kg BW/day showed a significant ($p < 0.0001$) decrease in primordial follicle (892.45 ± 5.97), primary follicle (252.34 ± 4.67), secondary follicle (152 ± 9.78) and Graffian follicle (11.89 ± 2.55) compared to that of normal control mice. Significant increase in the number of atretic follicles (48.12 ± 4.67) was also recorded in dose of 500 mg/kg BW/day compared to normal control mice (18.06 ± 3.27). The dose of 250 mg/kg body weight/day showed a similar decrease in primordial follicle (928.43 ± 4.11), primary follicle (268.51 ± 5.39), secondary follicle (159.72 ± 2.17) and Graffian follicle (16.44 ± 5.13) compared to that of olive oil control mice ($p < 0.0001$). 17β Estradiol treated group showed a statistically significant ($p < 0.0001$) decrease in number of primordial follicle (816.75 ± 44.47), primary follicle (179.42 ± 11.56), secondary follicle (142.51 ± 6.33) and Graffian follicle (12.34 ± 7.21) compared to that of normal control mice (Figure 2).

Discussion

In this experiment, the dose of 500 mg/kg BW/day showed a significant ($p < 0.05$) decrease in primordial follicle (892.45 ± 5.97), primary follicle (252.34 ± 4.67), secondary follicle (152 ± 9.78) and Graafian follicle (11.89 ± 2.55) compared to that of normal control mice. Significant increase in number of atretic follicle (48.12 ± 4.67) was also recorded in dose of 500 mg/kg BW/day compared to normal control mice (18.06 ± 3.27). The dose of 250 mg/kg body weight/ day showed a similar decrease in primordial follicle (928.4 ± 4.11), primary follicle (268.51 ± 5.39), secondary follicle (159.72 ± 2.17) and Graafian follicle (16.44 ± 5.13) compared to that of tween 80 control mice ($p < 0.05$). 17β Estradiol treated group showed a statistically significant ($p < 0.05$) decrease in number of primordial follicle (816.75 ± 44.4), primary follicle (179.42 ± 11.56), secondary follicle (142.51 ± 6.33) and Graafian follicle (12.34 ± 7.21) compared to that of normal control mice. The results showed a clear vision of the effect of CGME on the ovarian folliculogenesis of the albino mice. It is evident that the higher dose of CGME has much reductive activity on it than those of lower dose. The increasing number of atretic follicles due to the higher dose reveals that there are certain phyto-compounds in CGME which affect normal folliculogenesis. These compounds must have a definite estrogenic property which affects the steroid hormone level.

The experimental results of the present investigation showed a reducing effect upon the follicular development in all the experimental groups of female mice with respect to control upon treated with *C. gynandra* leaf extract (methanolic) for a period of consecutive 21 days. The number of primordial, primary, secondary and graafian follicles decreased significantly in both the CGME treated groups along with the Estradiol treated group, whereas degenerative nature was seen clearly resulting in the increase in the number of atretic follicles. Another study reported that methanolic extract of Rumex steudelii has potential to disrupt ovarian folliculogenesis when administered orally for 30 consecutive days by inhibiting further development of the recruited ovarian follicles (Solomon, [24]. Many other investigations

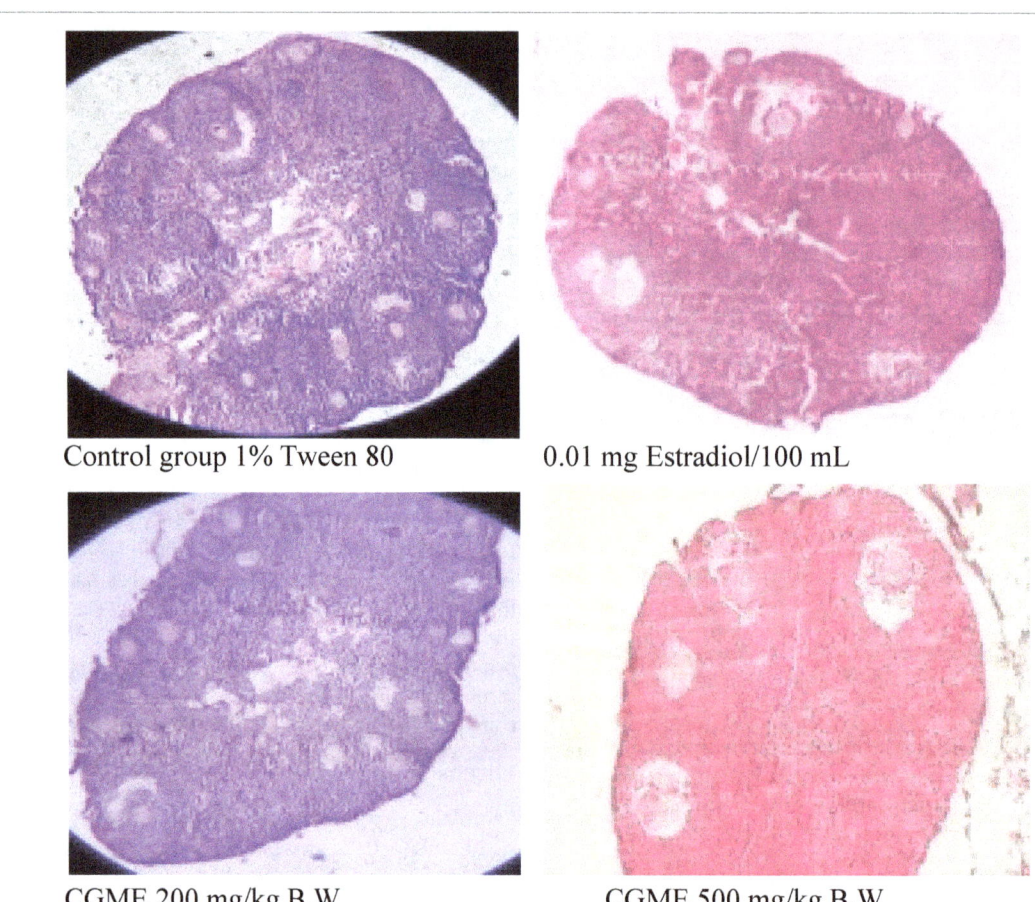

Control group 1% Tween 80   0.01 mg Estradiol/100 mL

CGME 200 mg/kg B.W   CGME 500 mg/kg B.W

PF: Primary Follicle; SF: Secondary Follicle; TF: Tertiary Follicle; AF: Atretic Follicle

Figure 2: Photomicrographs of hematoxylin and eosin stained representative section of the ovarian tissue illustrating the interstitial cell masses, follicular remnants and oocyte.

Treatment group	Primordial follicle	Primary follicle	Secondary follicle	Graffian follicle	Atretic follicle
Control, 1% Tween 80	983.62 ± 10.52	286.37 ± 6.48	169.26 ± 8.32	19.43 ± 4.86	18.06 ± 3.27
Estradiol treated, 0.01 mg/100 mL	816.75 ± 44.47'''	179.42 ± 11.56'''	142.51 ± 6.33''	12.34 ± 7.21''	52.81 ± 1.57'''
Low dose, 250 mg/kg BW	928.43 ± 4.11	268.51 ± 5.39	159.72 ± 2.17	16.44 ± 5.13	39.68 ± 2.41'''
High dose, 500 mg/kg BW	892.45 ± 5.97'''	252.34 ± 4.67''	152.53 ± 9.78	13.89 ± 2.55''	48.12 ± 4.6'''

Significance was estimated by student's t-test and compared with the untreated control group ('p<0.01, ''p<0.001, '''p<0.0001). Values are shown as mean ± SEM, (n=5)

Table1: Effect of CGME on the ovarian follicular population after 21 days of treatment.

reported the disrupting effect of various plant extracts on ovarian folliculogenesis. The number of primordial follicle reduced in the ovaries of gerbils when treated with Cannabis extract at 2.5 mg/day for 60 days [25]. There was a total loss of primordial follicles in the ovaries of rats treated with an aqueous extract of dried seed powder of Sapindus trifoliatus at dose level of 50, 100 and 150 mg/100kg BW for consecutive 30 days (Singh and Singh, [26] resembling the effect of hexane extract of *Ferula jaeschkeana* in guinea pigs (Pathak et al., [27]. Another study revealed the reducing effect of nicotine on the number of graafian follicles at a dose level of 0.3 mg/kg for 15 days (Patil et al., [28]. A study by Roop et al., [29], reported the significant reduction at 6 mg polar fraction of *Azadirachta* extract treatment. This significant reduction in the number of healthy follicles in all

the experimental groups leads to the assumption of disruption of the process of follicle selection due to atresia (Guraya), [30,36-39]. These changes in the oocyte growth and maturation have been influenced by gonadotrophins and steroids along with maturation promoting and growth factors (Guraya, Driancourt and Thuel), [31-35] suggesting the possible reason of the inhibitory effect of these plant extracts on the folliculogenesis in female [40-42].

Conclusion

Lots of researches are going on the phytochemicals of *C. gynandra* L. and its application in different aspects of human welfare. My aim was to investigate the estrogenic property of *C. gynandra* L. on ovarian folliculogenesis of the albino mice.

References

1. Takizawa K, Mattison DR (1983) Female reproduction. Am J Ind Med 4: 17-30.

2. Weitzman GA, Miller MM, London SN, Mattison DR (1992) Morphometric assessment of the murine ovarian toxicity of 7,12-dimethylbenz(a)anthracene. Reprod Toxicol 6: 137-141.

3. Toaff ME, Abramovici A, Sporn J, Liban E (1979) Selective oocyte degeneration and impaired fertility in rats treated with the aliphatic monoterpene, citral. J Reprod Fertil 55: 347-352.

4. Flaws JA, Doerr JK, Sipes IG, Hoyer PB (1994) Destruction of preantral follicles in adult rats by 4-vinyl-cyclohexene diepoxide. Reprod Toxicol 8: 509-514.

5. Anderson LD, Hirshfield AN (1992) An overview of follicular development in the ovary: from embryo to the fertilized ovum in vitro. Md Med J 41: 614-620.

6. Heindel JJ, Thomford PJ, Mattison DR (1989) Histological assessment of ovarian follicle number in mice as a screen for ovarian toxicity. In: Hirshfield AN (ed.) Growth Factors and the Ovary. Plenum, New York pp: 421-426.

7. Pedersen RA, Peters H (1968) Proposal for a classification of oocytes and follicles in the mouse ovary. J Reprod Fertil 83: 555-557.

8. Mattison DR, Nightingale MS (1982) Oocyte destruction by polycyclic aromatic hydrocarbons is not linked to the inducibility of ovarian aryl hydrocarbon (benzo(a)pyrene) hydroxylase activity in (DBA/2N X C57BL/6N) F1 X DBA/2N backcross mice. Pediatr Pharmacol 2: 11-21.

9. DeFelice SL (1995) The nutraceutical revolution: Its impact on food industry R&D. Trend Food Sci Technol 6: 59-61.

10. Kalra EK (2003) Nutraceutical–Definition and introduction. AAPS Pharm Sci 5: 27-28.

11. Estruch R., Ros E, Salas-Salvado J (2013) Primary prevention of cardiovascular disease with a Mediterranean diet. N Engl J Med 368: 1279-1290.

12. Massaro M, Scoditti E, Carluccio MA (2010) Nutraceuticals and prevention of atherosclerosis: Focus on omega-3 polyunsaturated fatty acids and Mediterranean diet polyphenols. Cardiovasc Ther 28: e13-e19.

13. Scicchitanoa P, Cameli M, Maiello M, Modesti PA, Muiesan ML, et al. (2014) Nutraceuticals and dyslipidaemia: Beyond the common therapeutics. J Funct Foods 6: 11-32.

14. Odum J, Ashby J, Sumpter JP (1998) Some alkyl hydroxy benzoate preservatives (parabens) are estrogenic. Toxicol Appl Pharmacol 153: 12-19.

15. Kummerer K (2001) Pharmaceuticals in the Environment: Sources, Fate, Effects and Risks (3rd edn.) Berlin: Springer publisher.

16. Fent K, Weston AA, Caminada D (2006) Ecotoxicology of human pharmaceuticals. Aquat Toxicol 76: 122-159.

17. Chen Y, Jefferson WN, Newbold RR, Padilla-Banks E, Pepling ME (2007) Estradiol, progesterone, and genistein inhibit oocyte nest breakdown and primordial follicle assembly in the neonatal mouse ovary in vitro and in vivo. Endocrinol 148: 3580-3590.

18. Raymond Whish S, Loretta PM, O Neal T, Martinez A, Sellers MA, et al. (2007) Drinking water with uranium below the U.S. EPA Water Standard causes estrogen receptor dependent responses in female mice. Env Health Perspect 115: 1711-1716.

19. Moawad AH, Rakoff AE, Kramer SA (1965) Histologic study of the effects of lowdosage irradiation of rabbit ovaries. Fertil Steril 16: 370-381.

20. Bolon B, Bucci IJ, Warbritlon AR, Chen JJ, Mattison DR, et al. (1997) Differential follicle counts as a screen for chemically-induced ovarian toxicity in mice: results from continuous breeding bioassays. Fundam Appl Toxicol 39: 1-10.

21. Swartz WJ, Mall GM (1989) Chloredecone induced follicular toxicity in mouse ovaries. Reprod Toxicol 3: 203-206.

22. Bucci TJ, Bolon B, Warbritton AR, Chen JJ. Heindel JJ (1997) Influence of sampling on the reproducibility of ovarian follicle counts in mouce toxicity studies. Reprod Toxicol 11: 689-696.

23. Butcher RL, Kirkpatri Keller D (1984) Pattern of follicular growth during the four-day oestrus cycle in the rat. Biol Reprod 31: 280-286.

24. Myers M, Britt KL, Wreford NGM, Ebling FJP, Kerr JB (2004) Methods for quantifying follicular numbers within the mouse ovary. Reprod 127: 569-580.

25. Solomon T, Largesse Z, Mekbeb A, Eyasu M, Asfaw (2010) Effect of Rumex steudelii methanolic root extract on ovarian folliculogenesis and uterine histology in female albino rats. Afr Health Sci 10: 353-361.

26. Dixit VP, Arya M, Lohiya NK (1976) Mechanism of action of chronically administered Cannabis extract on the female genital tract of gerbils Meriones hurrianae. Indian J Physiol Pharmacol 20: 38-41.

27. Singh SP, Singh K (1994) Effect of Sapindus trifoliatus seed on the fertility of female albino rats. Cell Signalling and Ova Implantation (Abstracts). The International Symposium on Cell Signalling and Ova-Implantation. All India Institute of Medical Science pp: 21-23.

28. Pathak S, Jonathan S, Prakash AO (1995) Timely administration of extract of Ferula jaeschkeana causes luteolysis in the ovary of cyclic guinea pig. Indian J Physiol Pharmacol 39: 395-399.

29. Patil SR, Ravindra Patil SR, Londonkar R, Patil SB (1998) Nicotine induced ovarian and uterine changes in albino mice. Indian J Physiol Pharmacol 42: 503-508.

30. Roop JK, Dhaliwal PK, Guraya SS (2005) Extracts of Azadirachta indica and Melia azedarach seeds inhibit folliculogenesis in albino rats. Braz J Med Biol Res 38: 943-947.

31. Guraya SS (1997) Ovarian Biology in Buffaloes and Cattle. Directorate of Information and Publications of Agriculture. Indian Council of Agricultural Research.

32. Guraya SS (2000) Comparative Cellular and Molecular Biology of Ovary in Mammals. Fundamental and Applied Aspects. Oxford & IBH Publishing Co. Pvt. Ltd.

33. Chen YT, Mattison DR, Feigenbaum L, Fukui H, Schulman JD (1981) Reduction in oocyte number following prenatal exposure to a diet high in galactose. Science 214: 1145-1147.

34. Halpin DM, Jones A, Fink G, Charlton HM (1986) Postnatal ovarian follicle development in hypogonadal (hpg) and normal mice and associated changes in the hypothalamic-pituitary-ovarian axis. J Reprod Fertility 77: 287-296.

35. Haque A, Kalita JC, Deka DD, Baruah BK (2010) Effect of effluent water downstream to the Nagaon Paper Mill, Assam on ovarian follicular population of immature female C3h mice. The Bioscan 2: 529-535.

36. Maheshwar A, Bhattacharya S (2007) Ovarian ageing and fertility-review. Current Women's Health Reviews 3: 63-67.

37. Mattison DR, Thomford PJ (1989) The mechanisms of action of reproductive toxicants. Toxicol Pathol 17: 364-376.

38. Mattison DR, Plowchalk DR, Meadows MJ, Miller MM, Malek A, et al. (1989) The effect of smoking on oogenesis, fertilization and implantation. Semin Reprod Endocrinol 7: 291-304.

39. Mattison DR, Shiromizu K, Nightingale MS (1983) Oocyte destruction by polycyclic aromatic hydrocarbons. Am J Ind Med 4: 191-202.

40. Osman P (1985) Rate and course of atresia during follicular development in the adult cyclic rat. J Reprod. Fertil 73: 261-270.

41. Tilly JL (2003) Ovarian follicle counts – not as simple as 1, 2, 3. Reprod Biol. Endocrinol 1: 11.

42. U.S. Environmental Protection Agency (1998) Health Effects Test Guidelines, OPPTS 870.3800, Reproduction and Fertility Effects. EPA 712-C-98-239. U.S. Environmental Protection Agency, Office of Prevention, Pesticides and Toxic Substances, Washington, DC.

43. U.S. Food and Drug Administration, Redbook (2000) Toxicologial Principles for the Safety Assessment of Food Ingredients. IV.C.9.a. Guidelines for Reproductive Studies. U.S. Food and Drug Administration, Center for Food Safety and Applied Nutrition, Washington, DC.

34

Mustard: the Great Gift of Danvantri for Vitiligo

Priya R*, ArunaV, Amruthavalli GV and Gayathri R

Dr.JRK's Siddha Research and Pharmaceuticals PVT Ltd, 18, 19, Perumal koil Street, Kundrathur, Chennai-600069, India

Abstract

The present study deals with mustard and its therapeutic potential for Vitiligo. We have created a Vitiligo like situation using mustard, *Pityrosporum ovale* and *Cryptococcus neoformans*. Our innovative experiment has not only opened door for the above simulation to be used for screening drugs for Vitiligo but also highlighted the enormous drug value of mustard.

Keywords: Vitiligo; Mustard; Cryptococcus; Pityrosporum

Introduction

Vitiligo is an autoimmune disorder of the skin occurs as a result of defective melanogenesis. The trigger for the disease is although unknown however the role of autoimmune factors responsible for the disease progression is well established. As on date no effective treatment is available for Vitiligo and use of steroids is often sought out medicament for Vitiligo.

Indian traditional system of medicine collectively called AYUSH (Ayurveda, Yoga, Unani Siddha and Homeopathy) has enormous claims on having effective treatment for Vitiligo. However such claims warrant scientific evidence. Several proprietary siddha products of Dr.JRK's Siddha Research and Pharmaceuticals are proven to be effective for the treatment of Vitiligo. Mustard (Brassica nigra) is highly venerated plant in Ayurveda and which is reported to have enormous medicinal values [1,2]. Shvitrahara kashaya is one of the famous Ayurveda drugs used for the treatment of Vitiligo [3]. Although several clinical evidences are available for mustard for increasing pigmentation of the skin still a credible scientific proof is lacking. A reliable scientific proof may help in the better exploitation of mustard for treating Vitiligo.

We have devised a novel tool in which we have mimicked melanocytes ex-situ as well as an auto-immune like trigger to evaluate the efficacy of the mustard.

For the above experiment we have used two different species of eukaryotic microbe viz., *Cryptococcus neoformans* and *Pityrosporum ovale*. *C. neoformans* is known to produce melanin like pigment in mustard medium [4,5]. Similarly *P. ovale* is known to produce Azelaic acid [6] that suppress tyrosinase and melanogenesis [7].

Finding of our research has shown a new dimension and promise for screening and developing novel drugs for the treatment of Vitiligo besides establishing the possible therapeutic benefits of mustard for Vitiligo.

Materials and Methods

Preparation of mustard medium

Mustard seeds were procured and subjected to quality check and then the seeds were powdered. Aqueous extract of mustard was prepared by adding 40 g of mustard powder to 200 ml of distilled water. It was boiled for 30 min. Then the mixture was filtered and the final filtrate was made up to 100 ml. To the mustard extract, 2 g of dextrose and 2 g of Agar agar were added and then autoclaved at 121°C for 15 minutes. The medium after autoclaving was then poured onto sterilized petriplates and was allowed to solidify. Similarly, Sabaurauds dextrose Agar (Hi media laboratories) medium plates were also prepared and used.

Details of the fungal culture used

The clinical isolates of *Cryptococcus neoformans* (procured from Dr.P. Balakrishnan, YRG care, Voluntary Health Service) and the human isolate of *Pityrosporum ovale* were used for the present experiment. In brief, 7 day old culture of *C. neoformans* and *P. ovale* were used. The organisms were inoculated separately onto SDA medium and mustard agar medium. Similarly, both the organisms were inoculated together onto both the media. All the above plates in quadruplicate were incubated at room temperature for 14 days with every alternative day observation. The presence or absence of melanoid pigmentation over the culture of *C. neoformans* with reference to the extent of pigmentation and the period of incubation were recorded. Similarly, the presence or absence of pigmentation over *C. neoformans* grown along with *P. ovale* was also noted.

Statistical Analysis

Simple average value was calculated and the data is presented accordingly.

Study Design

In the present study, we have grown the culture of pigment producing organism *C. neoformans* and *P. ovale* separately and together (mixed culture) in two media viz., mustard medium and Saboraud's dextrose Agar. Further both cultures were streaked adjacent to each other in the above media plates. The extent of pigment production/inhibition was read and scored.

Results

In mustard medium, *C. neoformans* produced intense melanoid pigment on day 14 and the pigment initiation was observed on day 10. On the contrary, no such pigmentation was observed in the above organism that was grown in SDA medium. *P. ovale* did not produce any pigment in either of the two media used. In co-culture environment i.e., *C. neoformans* grown along with the *P. ovale* in mustard medium, the

*Corresponding author: Priya R, Dr.JRK's Siddha Research and Pharmaceuticals PVT Ltd, 18, 19, Perumal koil Street, Kundrathur, Chennai-600069, India
E-mail: research@jrksiddha.com

melanoid pigmentation was observed over *C. neoformans* culture on day 5. The pigment initiation was observed on day 3 (Table 1 and Figure 1).

Discussion

Present study has opened vista of hope and promise for the treatment of Vitiligo from the Siddha system of medicine. The siddha system of medicine is very vibrant, brilliant, scientific and time tested. The medicines of Siddha system are holistic and all inclusive it means they could prevent the disease (preventive), promote health (promotive) and cure diseases (curative). Siddha drugs not just work at the symptom level but work at the root of the disease Tridosha i.e., Vata, Pita, Kapha.

This is the first study to the best of our knowledge, where we have simulated Vitiligo like situation by using the isolates of *C. neoformans*, *P. ovale* and mustard medium. It is known that *C. neoformans* produce melanin like pigment in mustard medium [4] and the duration of pigmentation may range from 3 to 14 days. The ecosystem of mustard medium and the property of *C. neoformans* producing melanin like pigment we have contemplated for a mammalian system. The *P. ovale* is known to produce azelaic acid that suppresses melanogenesis [7]. Therefore, we used *P. ovale* as constant trigger for suppressing the pigmentation in *C. neoformans* when grown in mustard medium. We have co-cultured both the organisms in SDA as well as mustard medium with the hypothesis that the pigmentation in *C. neoformans* will be suppressed by the azelaic acid produced by *P. ovale*.

Interestingly, we found an intense pigmentation over *C. neoformans* and was unaffected by *P. ovale*. We presume that the azelaic acid may be getting inactivated in mustard medium and therefore no suppression of pigmentation has occurred. Another possibility may be that *P. ovale* may not be producing azelaic acid in mustard medium.

Our earlier experiment on the role of azelaic acid prepared from *Pityrosporum ovale* in affecting the process of phenol oxidation has clearly shown that the phenol oxidase enzyme gets downregulated thus resulting in poor coloration [8].

The model used in the present experiment can be considered as a microcosm of Vitiligo wherein *C. neoformans* plays the role of melanocytes and Pityrosporum the likely spoilsport of melanogenesis (the likely auto-immune cause). When we mimicked the above situation in mustard medium we found that mustard extract could overpower the effect of azelaic acid of *P. ovale* on melanin pigmentation by *C. neoformans*.

The mustard has been used for the treatment of Vitiligo in Ayurveda [2,9]. Shvitrahara kashaya is one of the famous Ayurvedic products with mustard oil used for the treatment of Vitiligo [3]. In Siddha system of medicine also we can find several corollaries for mustard.

Finding of the present study has clearly shown that mustard has enormous therapeutic potential for Vitiligo which was already discovered and used by the great scholars of Ayurveda and Siddha. Further the present study also has revealed the unimaginable science and uncommon wisdom of our ancient Ayurveda and Siddha scholars. If the world passionately and prudently follows Siddha and Ayurveda they can not only live 'disease free life' but also can possibly attain eternity and salvation.

Details of media	Days	Organisms/Pigmentation		
		C. neoformans	*P. ovale*	*C. neoformans+P. ovale*
Saboraud's dextrose Agar	7	-	-	-
	14	-	-	-
Mustard agar medium	3	+	-	+
	5	+	-	++
	14	+++	-	+++

+	= pigment initiation
++	= moderate pigmentation
+++	= Intense pigmentation
–	= no pigmentation

Table 1: Pigmentation of *C. neoformans* in mustard medium.

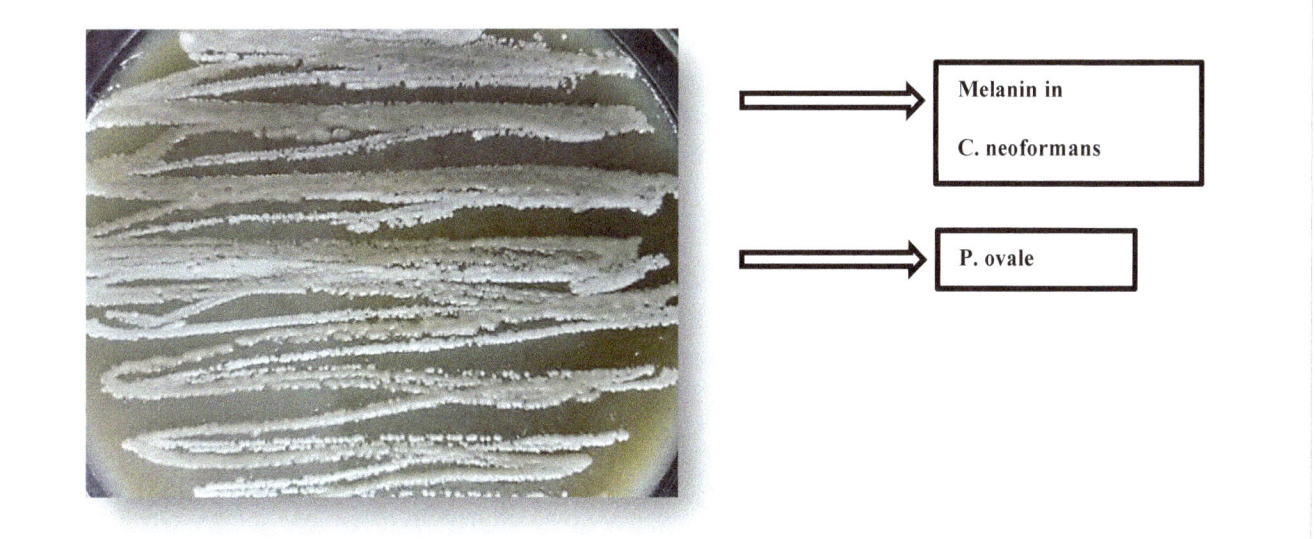

Figure 1: Production of melanin pigment by *C. neoformans* when grown with *P. ovale* in mustard medium.

Reference

1. Nauman SM, Mohammad I (2015) Role of Khardal (Brassica Nigra) in Non-Communicable Diseases: An Overview. Int j drug dev.

2. Manohar RP, Pushpan R, Rohini S (2009) Mustard and its uses in Ayurveda. International Journal of Traditional knowledge 8: 400-404.

3. Dhanik A, Sujatha N, Rai NP (2011) Clinical evaluation of the efficacy of Shvitrahara kashaya and lepa in vitiligo. Ayu 32: 66-69.

4. Nandhakumar B, Girishkumar CP, Prabu D (2006) Mustard Seed Agar, a New Medium for Differentiation of Cryptococcus neoformans. J Clin Microbiol 44: 674.

5. Xavier TF (2016) Comparison of Different Media for the Pigment Production of Pathogenic and Non Pathogenic Cryptococcus neoformans Isolates. Scholars Acad J Biosci 1: 263-266

6. Gaitanis G, Magiatis P, Hantschke M, Bassukas ID, Velegraki A et al. (2012) The Malassezia Genus in Skin and Systemic Diseases. Clin Microbiol Rev 25: 106 –141.

7. Yu JS, Kim AK (2010) Effect of combination of taurine and azelaic acid on antimelanogenesis in murine melanoma cells. J Biomed Sci 17: S45.

8. Priya R, Aruna V, Gayathri Rajagopal (2016) Novel Test for Developing Drugs-Hyper/Hypopigmentation. Int J Pharm Biol Sci 11: 70-72.

9. Lakhani DM, Deshpande AS (2014) Various Treatments for Vitiligo: Problems Associated and Solutions. Journal of Applied Pharmaceutical Science 4: 101-105.

35

Evaluation of Gutinous Rice Roots Decoction Sponge Bath Treatment for Sweating Syndrome in Children

Peiyi Chen[1], Yan He[2], Ziyu Zhao[3]*, Jiapeng Zhang[3], Jingyun Ye[3]

[1]*Professor, College of Nursing, Guangzhou University of Traditional Chinese Medicine, Guangzhou, China*
[2]*Lecture, Guangzhou Medical University, Guangzhou, China*
[3]*Master student, College of Nursing, Guangzhou University of Traditional Chinese Medicine, Guangzhou, China*

Abstract

Objective: Explore the effect of TCM external treatment of glutinous rice roots decoction sponge bath method treatment to the children with sweating.

Methods: To collect 70 sweating syndrome of children in the pediatric clinic of Guangdong Provincial Hospital of Traditional Chinese Medicine and the First Affiliated Hospital of Guangzhou University of Traditional Chinese Medicine, were randomly divided into 2 groups, the control group and the experimental group. Each group has 35 children. The control group is using traditional Chinese medicine Oral treatment, the experimental group is using traditional Chinese Herbs and sponging bath with the decoction of glutinous rice root.

Results: In this study, we had collected 70 cases of children suffering from sweating. Ultimately the effective number of cases: 29 cases in the control group and 31 cases in the experimental group. 7 days after the intervention, the related indicators of the experimental group of lung health is not solid and other evidence were improved. Sweating symptoms were improved, and have statistically significant in the efficacy difference compared with the control group (lung health is not solid of the two groups p=0.017, other syndromes of the two groups p=0.006). The effect was significantly of lung health is not solid of the two groups after the intervention in sodium food, urine, tongue (P<0.05). The effect was significantly of other syndromes of the two groups after the intervention in sodium food, urine (P<0.05).

Conclusion: The sponging bath with the decoction of glutinous rice root to the sweating syndrome of children, glutinous rice roots has been confirmed with the convergence of the antiperspirant effect, use it as raw material preparation to bath shall play its efficacy, low cost, the acceptability strong advantage; The research results will help to promote family self-treatment of the sweating syndrome of children, it is safe and will be treatment resides in daily life, with simple, convenient, effective, should be widely applied.

Keywords: Glutinous rice root; Sponge bath; Children; Sweating syndrome

Introduction

Sweating syndrome refers to some function can't operate normally, nutritional imbalance, the organ disability or couli unstable induced by the presence of various dominant or recessive factors inside and outside of the body, thereby causing a symptom of sweating, which is a common symptom in clinical miscellaneous disease [1]. Currently there widely exists the phenomenon of children with infectious diseases received antibiotics or glucocorticoid treatment, causing the increasing number of children suffering from sweating syndrome [2]. The internal treatment of Traditional Chinese Medicine (TCM) are commonly used in clinical treatment of sweating syndrome in children, but it is hard for children to take decoction and because of its bitter taste and long course of treatment, which results in failure to treatment [3]. Meanwhile, modern medicine often treat sweating syndrome through the regulation of autonomic nerve function, suppressing the secretion of sweat gland, etc. But these treatments are limited by the side effects of such drugs. Transdermal administration is the third generation of administration method recommended by WHO, which is a new treatment technology researched in recent years [4]. This research investigated the evaluation of glutinous rice roots decoction sponge bath treatment which belongs to external treatment of TCM for sweating syndrome in children, the results show that this method can offer good supporting effect in treating sweating syndrome of children compared with internal decoction treatment of TCM, which provide valuable reference for clinical treatment of sweating syndrome

in children and will actively outreached in hospitals and communities. The details of this research are reported as follows:

Methods

This study was a case-control study design and was approved by the medical ethics committee, and families have signed informed consent.

Sampling

Inclusion criteria were including patients with the diagnosis of sweating syndrome according to the standard of diagnosis and curative effect of traditional Chinese medicine, age ranging between 1-14 years, and sweating symptom lasted more than one month. Exclusion criteria were including that patients suffered from other diseases which can explain the symptoms of hyperhidrosis in children, patients resolutely refused to take TCM therapy or can't cooperate with intervention and investigations for other reasons, and patients may be allergic to

*Corresponding author: Peiyi Chen, College of Nursing, Guangzhou University of Traditional Chinese Medicine, Guangzhou, China
E-mail: hlcpy@gzucm.edu.cn

glutinous rice roots, yupingfen power or other traditional Chinese medicine.

Nursing intervention of experimental group

Patients receive sponge bath using glutinous rice roots decoction. 50 g glutinous rice roots were added into 2500 ml cold water and decocted together. According to the standard weight of 15 kg to children, 50 g glutinous rice roots and 500 ml of cold water should be added for each additional 2 kg in ascending order [5-7]. After the drug starting boiling for 20 min, the medicine juice is retained while the dregs are filtered. The glutinous rice roots decoction should be cooled to 32-34℃, and children get sponge bath for 15 min, the room temperature should be maintained at 25-27℃ during sponge bath. The appropriate time for sponge bath is 1 h after meal once a day and 7 days are a period of treatment. The curative effect was evaluated on the 8th day while parents are asked to fill out the questionnaire and follow-up evaluation (Appendix). Glutinous rice roots are provided by Guangdong Kong Mei Pharmaceutical Co., Ltd. and for the same batch. During sponge bath, first, the operator washes hands, prepare the substance ready and bring it to the bedside of patient. While patient gets comfortable supine position. Second, small towel is dipped into glutinous rice roots decoction, twisted to the semi-dry and wrapped in a glove-like shape around operator's hands to pat patient in centrifugal direction, each side should be patted for 3 min, finally dry patients with a large towel. The order of the sponge bath is upper limbs first: first lateral neck, lateral part of upper arm, arms, and then lateral breast, armpits, the inside part of upper arm, and finally the palm. The same method are used for the other side of the upper limbs; then the operator pat patient's back and waist for 3 min and the patient wear jacketing. Afterwards, the operator conduct sponge bath of lower limbs in sequence of iliac, outer side of thigh, dorsal, groin, inner thigh, ankle, and finally below the femur, the popliteal fossa, heel. And dry patients with a large towel 3 min later. The same method is used for the other side of the lower limbs, at last patient wears pants. During the whole process, the operator should pay close attention to the local and systemic reactions of patient.

Internal decoction treatment of TCM and nursing

According to different syndrome types and individual physique, patients receive dialectical medication (decoction), and 7 days are a period of treatment. Decoction should be taken after meal when it is warm, and the most appropriate choice is taken in the early morning or in the morning. The vital signs, hemoglobin and body weight of patients should be observed during treatment process. If patients suffer from exogenous cold, they should stop taking the tonic to prevent situation that "the invaders stay behind the closed doors" [5]. Patients' parents are told to conduct psychological counseling with patients well, and as for children are prone to produce negative emotions such as dysphoria, parents should give spiritual comfort and encourage them adhere to medication.

Routine care

The families of children are guide to arrange patients' daily life reasonably. The windows of patients' living room should be ventilated at regular time [6,7], maintaining proper temperature and humidity in order to keep children's personal hygiene and health.

Evaluation of curative effect on glutinous rice roots decoction sponge bath treatment

The parents conduct a total of twice evaluation on the first day and eighth day (namely, the seventh day after treatment), checking the shoulder, back and underwear of children and detecting their sweat loss status by hand.

Significantly effective: There are no sweating symptoms during evaluation on eighth day, and patients' food taking, urine and stool status, sleep status, mental state and index finger collaterals return to normal. Recurrence doesn't occur after one month's followed up.

Effective: The sweating symptoms alleviates during evaluation on eighth day, and patient's food taking, urine and stool status, sleep status, mental state and index finger collaterals improve.

Invalid: The phenomenon of spontaneous sweating or night sweating still exists 7 days later. And patients' food taking, urine and stool status, sleep status, mental state and index finger collaterals aren't changed or even worse

Evaluation of clinical symptoms

According to the clinical research guiding principles of new medicine on traditional Chinese medicine (2002 provisions) and other related reference materials, the 9 common accompanying situation of children with hyperhidrosis syndrome will be evaluated in accordance with the models of TCM, mainly for anorexia, loose stool, urine is scanty and dark, poor sleep at night, languid and fatigue, pale tongue, teeth marks on tongue, white and greasy tongue coating, pulse Shenxi and easy to catch a cold. The degrees of symptoms in patient is divided into cured, improved, incured and is referred to as 0, 1, 2, respectively. See appendix 3 (This table is made according to the clinical research guiding principles of new medicine on traditional Chinese medicine (2002 provisions), and complete the evaluation of reliability and validity) (Tables 1-3).

Adverse events

Adverse event refers to all conditions which go against to disease cure after a sort of treatment to patient who is under clinical receipts collection, however, there's no necessary connection exists between this condition and the use of drugs. The time and measures in adverse events of patients should be registered in this clinical observation.

Data collection and analysis

Data were collected from March 2012 and March 2013; all cases were recruited from pediatric outpatients in the First and Second

	Control	Experimental
Male	20	19
Female	9	12
Age	4.00 (3.38, 5.00)	3.50 (2.75, 5.00)
n	29	31
Lung health is not Solid type	18	21
Other syndrome types	11	10

Table 1: Comparison of basic conditions between control group and experimental group.

	Loss	Inclusion
Male	4	39
Female	6	21
Age	4.00 (3.00, 5.00)	5.00 (4.13, 5.00)
n	10	60
Lung health is not solid type	6	39
Other syndrome types	4	21

Table 2: Comparison of basic conditions between loss group and inclusion group.

Symptoms in TCM	Degree	Control (n=29)	Experimental (n=31)		Control (n=29)	Experimental (n=31)	
		Lung health is not solid type	Lung health is not solid type	P value	Other syndrome types	Other syndrome types	P value
Sweating	0	0	0	-	0	0	-
	1	14	17	-	6	7	-
	2	4	4	1.000	5	3	1.000
Food taking	0	3	5	-	3	4	-
	1	12	14	-	6	4	-
	2	3	2	0.712	2	2	0.514
Stool status	0	3	5	-	2	4	-
	1	11	15	-	6	5	-
	2	4	1	0.272	3	1	0.506
Urine status	0	2	7	-	1	3	-
	1	14	13	-	6	4	-
	2	2	1	0.373	4	3	0.315
Sleep status	0	6	10	-	3	4	-
	1	8	6	-	4	4	-
	2	4	5	0.602	4	2	0.647
Mental state	0	8	11	-	4	5	-
	1	7	5	-	4	3	-
	2	3	5	0.689	3	2	0.650
Tongue quality	0	2	4	-	2	3	-
	1	9	13	-	5	5	-
	2	7	4	0.442	4	2	0.727
Tongue coating	0	3	6	-	3	2	-
	1	9	10	-	4	6	-
	2	6	5	0.650	4	2	0.857
Pulse	0	5	6	-	3	4	-
	1	10	11	-	4	3	-
	2	3	4	1.000	4	3	0.857
Index finger collaterals	0	5	6	-	3	4	-
	1	8	11	-	3	4	-
	2	5	4	0.914	5	2	0.859

TCM: Traditional Chinese Medicine

Table 3: Comparison of clinical symptoms at pre-treatment in both groups.

Affiliated Hospital of Guangzhou University of Traditional Chinese Medicine. The Excel software is used to create the database and to input data of patient. SPSS17.0 software is used for statistical analysis of data obtained, and qualitative data is analyzed by chi-square test. With regard to the grid number whose theoretical value is less than 5, more than 20% of the sample is analyzed by Monte Carlo exact test. Meanwhile, the grade data is analyzed by non-parametric tests.

Results

The study included a total of 70 cases including 35 cases in the control group (comprising lung health is not solid type and other syndrome types) receive internal decoction treatment of TCM; 35 patients in the experimental group (comprising lung health is not solid type and other syndrome types) receive internal decoction treatment of TCM plus glutinous rice roots decoction sponge bath. During the study, 6 patients in the control group who refused to take medicine exited this study, and the remaining patients completed the measurement and assessment of relevant indicators. There are 4 patients in experimental group didn't take daily glutinous rice

roots decoction sponge bath in accordance with the requirements were excluded, and the rest patients completed glutinous rice roots decoction sponge bath intervention according to requirements. Finally there were 29 effective cases in the control group and 31 cases in the experimental group.

Comparison of basic conditions between two groups

The χ^2 value in gender is 0.659, P=0.417. The Z value in Age is -1.579, P=0.114. The χ^2 value in the comparison of syndromes is 0.66, P=0.4168 and the difference was not statistically significant (P>0.05).

Comparison of clinical symptoms before treatment in different syndrome types between two groups

The comparison of the degrees of different clinical symptoms before intervention between two groups including sweating, food taking, urine and stool status, sleep status, mental state, tongue quality, tongue coating, pulse, index finger collaterals, etc. There was no statistically significant difference (P>0.05) and the results are comparable (Table 4).

	Lung health is not solid type			Other syndrome types		
	Invalid	Effective	Significant effective	Invalid	Effective	Significant effective
Control group	4	11	3	5	5	1
Experimental group	2	6	13	1	2	7

Table 4: Comparison of curative effect on different syndrome types between two groups.

Symptoms in tcm	Degrees	Control group Lung health is not solid type	Experimental group Lung health is not solid type	P value	Control group Other syndrome types	Experimental group Other syndrome types	P value
Sweating	0	3	13	-	1	7	-
	1	11	6	-	5	2	-
	2	4	2	0.019	5	1	0.004
Food taking	0	5	15	-	2	7	-
	1	9	4	-	6	2	-
	2	4	2	0.029	3	1	0.019
Stool status	0	4	15	-	2	5	-
	1	10	5	-	7	4	-
	2	4	1	0.006	2	1	0.233
Urine ststus	0	7	17	-	2	6	-
	1	9	3	-	6	2	-
	2	2	1	0.025	3	2	0.040
Sleep status	0	13	18	-	6	7	-
	1	3	2	-	2	2	-
	2	2	1	0.603	3	1	0.566
Mental state	0	13	18	-	6	7	-
	1	3	2	-	2	2	-
	2	2	1	0.603	3	1	0.566
Tongue quality	0	3	12	-	5	6	-
	1	11	7	-	4	3	-
	2	4	2	0.040	2	1	0.597
Tongue coating	0	13	16	-	6	6	-
	1	4	3	-	3	3	-
	2	1	2	0.865	2	1	0.836
Pulse	0	14	17	-	6	7	-
	1	2	3	-	3	2	-
	2	2	1	0.859	2	1	0.553
Index finger collaterals	0	14	17	-	6	7	-
	1	2	3	-	3	2	-
	2	2	1	0.859	2	1	0.553
Recurrence after 1 month's follow-up	0	13	17	-	5	6	-
	1	2	3	-	4	2	-
	2	3	1	0.554	2	2	0.368
The cold after 1 month's follow-up	0	13	17	-	5	6	-
	1	2	3	-	4	2	-
	2	3	1	0.554	2	2	0.368

TCM: Traditional Chinese Medicine

Table 5: Comparison of the clinical symptoms at post-treatment.

Comparison of curative effect on different syndrome types between two groups

The comparison of lung health is not solid type between two groups are illustrated in Table 5, the sweating symptoms of patients in experimental group with glutinous rice roots decoction sponge bath significantly improved compared with the control group, and the Z value in non-parametric tests is -2.651, P=0.008, p<0.01, the difference was statistically significant. The comparison of other syndrome types index between two groups such as the degree of sweating was analyzed with non-parametric test, Z=-2.793, P=0.005, p<0.01, the difference was statistically significant.

In the comparison of curative effect on lung health is not solid type between two groups, the Z value in non-parametric tests is -2.651, P=0.008. In the comparison of curative effect on other syndrome types between two groups, Z=-2.793, P=0.005.

Comparison of the clinical symptoms after treatment of different syndrome types between two groups

Seven days after treatment, the related indexes of lung health is not solid type and other syndrome types in experimental group all improved, and the sweating symptom improved remarkable among these indexes. Analyzing the data from the associated symptoms and comparing data from clinical symptoms after intervention, we can conclude that the curative effect in experimental group was significantly effective. We also conducted variance analysis between two groups and found the difference in sweating, food taking, urine and stool status, tongue quality of the lung health is not solid type and in sweating, food taking, urine status of other syndrome types is statistically significant (P<0.05).

Discussion

The study conducted exploratory research of the clinical curative effect on glutinous rice roots decoction sponge bath adjuvant treatment for sweating syndrome in children, summarizing and discussing the preliminary results.

Influencing of glutinous rice roots on sweating symptoms in children with sweating syndrome

After receiving glutinous rice roots adjuvant therapy, the sweating symptoms in patients of experimental group improved significantly. And the comparison between two groups with lung health is not solid type showed that the sweating symptoms in patients of experimental group who received glutinous rice roots decoction sponge bath improved significantly compared with the control group. Compared with other syndrome types between two groups, there were also statistically significant in terms of the effects of glutinous rice roots such as nourishing Yin, removing antiperspirant fever, stopping sweating, etc. [8]. Glutinous rice roots decoction sponge bath treatment has good supporting effect on sweating syndrome in children [9]. Besides, glutinous rice roots decoction sponge bath has more significant effect on sweating syndrome in children of lung health is not solid type than other syndrome types. After using glutinous rice roots decoction sponge bath, there are 13 patients with sweating syndrome of lung health is not solid type improved markedly, whereas there are 7 patients of other syndrome types improved markedly. So our study showed that glutinous rice roots decoction sponge bath has more pronounced effect on children with sweating syndrome of lung health is not solid type.

Effects of glutinous rice roots on TCM symptoms of children with sweating syndrome

In recent years, the incidence of sweating syndrome in children has a rising trend [10]. Sweating syndrome refers to some function can't operate normally, nutritional imbalance, the organ disability or couli unstable induced by the presence of various dominant or recessive factors inside and outside of the body, thereby causing a symptom of sweating, which is a common symptom in clinical miscellaneous disease [11]. Since there widely exists the phenomenon of children with infectious diseases received antibiotics or glucocorticoid treatment currently, combined with weakness, deficiency of Qi and Yin, nutrition and health disorders, defence unstable, etc., the sweating syndrome occurs [12]. This study observed that two groups of patients all have varying degrees of anorexia, abnormal urine and stool, poor sleep, fatigue, undynamic, easy to catch colds and other accompanying TCM symptoms.

All symptoms of patients in both groups were improved 7 days after receiving treatment, while the curative effect of glutinous rice roots decoction sponge bath adjuvant therapy intervention in the experimental group is more significant, in which the sweating syndrome in children of lung health is not solid type improved more significantly than those only received internal decoction treatment of TCM, and the children's food taking, urine and stool habits, tongue quality and other clinical TCM symptoms also improved to a certain extent. Besides,

the difference of effect after treatment on two groups of patients with lung health is not solid type was statistically significant; but there was no statistically significant difference in sleep, mental state, tongue coating, pulse condition, follow-up of catching cold in two groups. In addition, the accompanying symptoms weren't improved significantly in other sweating syndrome types of patients using glutinous rice roots decoction sponge bath, only the difference in the symptoms of sweating, food taking and urine symptoms was statistically significant compared with the control group.

The mechanism of glutinous rice roots decoction sponge bath adjuvant treatment for sweating syndrome in children

The primary pathogenesis of sweating syndrome in children is absence of righteousness, defence unstable, deficiency of Qi and Yin and spleen health loss, which cause spleen deficiency and indigestion [13], so that the appetite loss, then wood flourishing and soil restrained as well as the Qi of spleen obstructed so that it is hard to stop sweating. When metabolism slows down, a large amounts of waste accumulates inside the body and results in poor mind, fatigue, small voice, poor appetite and loose stools, even result in diarrhea, urinate long or incontinence, abdominal cold combined with pain [14], easy to feel backache or leg pain, pale fat tongue, white greasy or tiny white greasy tongue coating, slow pulse or even the pulse is hard to feel, etc. These are all the physical manifestation of yang deficiency [15]. The glutinous rice roots have effects on nourishing Qi, reducing phlegm, benefitting stomach and producing saliva, calming Liver, dispelling rheumatism, nourishing Yin, removing antiperspirant fever and stopping sweating [16]. In this study, one week after intervention of patients in the experimental group, their symptoms improved significantly compared with the control group, and to a certain extent, glutinous rice roots decoction sponge bath help children recover their functions of spleen and stomach, production and conversion of Qi and blood, so that defense strengthens as well as cold symptoms improves.

The feasibility of applications in glutinous rice roots decoction sponge bath adjuvant treatment for sweating syndrome in children

Children usually refuse to take medicine because of the bitter taste of TCM, which affected the therapeutic effect to some extent. Using external treatment of TCM through transdermal administration has better curative effect and is simple to proceed as well as easy to be accepted by children and parents. All in all, the glutinous rice roots decoction sponge bath can improve the symptoms of sweating syndrome in children, which can resides in the way of daily life and is safe and effective. Besides, this treatment reduces drug use and is more in line with the actual situation of children. In addition, glutinous rice roots can either be edible or be medicinal, so using glutinous rice roots to treat sweating syndrome is quick to be operated and its effect is obvious.

Conclusions

The glutinous rice roots has characters such as sweet, flat and safe, it also has effects such as benefitting stomach and producing saliva, stopping sweating and removing fever. Besides, the glutinous rice roots are easy to obtain and inexpensive, according to this drug's efficacy, changing the way of using glutinous rice roots is very helpful to treat sweating syndrome in children. In addition, the use of glutinous rice roots decoction sponge bath has many advantages: convenient operation, reducing children's agony by changing the way of medication and easily to be accepted by parents and children.

Meanwhile, using glutinous rice roots decoction sponge bath can not only shorten the treatment time and improve the effect of traditional internal medication treatment; but also make for the rehabilitation of primary disease, providing valuable reference for clinical treatment of sweating syndrome in children. Finally, the glutinous rice roots decoction sponge bath treatment for sweating syndrome in children has superiorities such as effective, low-cost and easy operation over internal decoction treatment of traditional Chinese medicine. It is worthy to outreach applications this treatment in hospitals and communities.

References

1. Wangjian (2008) Yin-deficiency sweating, Yang-deficiency sweating clinical brief analysis. Bright Chinese Medicine 2 : 667-668.

2. Yunbi X (2000) Conferences about sweating of children. Hainan Medical College Academic Journal 6120.

3. Ma C, Wang R (2011) The heart enlightenment of sweating syndrome and treatment. Funct J Tradit China Med 27: 267-267.

4. Yuyua (2005) Gaoshen Research Progress on enhancement methods of drug percutaneous absorption. China J Pharmaceut.

5. Song J, Zeng C (2004) Overview of study on external therapy of traditional Chinese medicine fever in children. Practical Clinical Journal of Integrated Traditional Chinese and Western Medicine 5: 86-87.

6. Li X (2005) Pray for the dialectical treatment of children with hyperhidrosis 50 examples Liaoning. J Tradit Chinese Med 32: 439.

7. Peiyi C (2002) Evaluation of glutinous rice roots decoction sponge bath treatment for sweating syndrome in children 27 examples. Journal of New Chinese Medicine.

8. Tongji W (2004) Evaluation of glutinous rice roots decoction bath treatment for sweating syndrome in children. Journal of Traditional Chinese Medicine.

9. Ailian T, Guixing T, Chaohui L (2008) A preliminary study on the chemical constituents of roots of glutinous rice Lishizhen Medicine and Materia Medica Research.

10. Yuanling S (1998) Eight methods of treating childhood hidrosis. Journal of Shanxi College of Traditional Chinese Medicine 21: 12.

11. Yuxia Li, Fengzhen C (2009) Chinese medicine treatment of sweat. China Practical Medicine 4: 194.

12. Yanzhan C (2006) Children night sweats diet. J Educ Dev.

13. Ye L (2010) The local meridian of night sweats pathogenesis and treatment of spontaneous. Morden Traditional Chinese Medicine 30: 48-50.

14. Huo L, Zhu S (2006) The application of the liver and spleen in childhood hidrosis in Tongzhi Huan. J Tradit Chin.

15. Lu M (2002) Yang–heat and Y in-deficiency sweating brief analysis Shanxi Chinese correspondence.

16. Tang A, Luo C, Tang G, Liu X, Ou X (2008) Identification of Glutinous Rice Root Granule Preparation and free amino acid. Central South Pharmacy 6: 398-400.

Evaluation of Acaricidal Effect of Ethnoveteinary Medicinal Plant by *in vivo* and *in vitro* against *Sarcoptes scabiei* var. *caprae* of Infected Goats in North Shoa, Oromia Regional State, Ethiopia

Bedaso Kebede[1]* **and Tsegaye Negese**[2]

[1]Veterinary Drug and Animal Feed Administration and Control Authority, Ministry of Livestock and Fisheries, Addis Ababa, Ethiopia
[2]Hirna Regional Veterinary Laboratory Center, Hirna, Oromia region, Ethiopia

Abstract

This study was conducted to determine parasiticidal efficacy of seven ethnomedicinal plants against *Sarcoptes scabiei* var. *caprae* of goats using *in vivo* and *in vitro* techniques. *In vitro* techniques for evaluation of efficacy of medicinal plants essential oils and fixed oils of seven medicinal plant extracts diluted at different concentrations (essential oils from 2.5% to 0.15625% and fixed oils from 160 mg/ml to 5 mg/ml) were added to petridishes containing adult stage of *Sarcoptes scabiei* var. *caprae*. After 3 h of contact, all concentrations of essential oil of *Eucalyptus globulus* and *Cymbopogon citractus* showed a good *in vitro* acaricidal efficacy as compared with the non-treated controls (p<0.05). However, *Nicotiana tobacum* fixed oil had significant (P<0.05) effect at a concentration of 160 mg/ml and 80 mg/ml. *Pyrethrum cineraria folium* fixed oil showed lower acaricidal efficacy (P<0.05) in all the concentrations of the extract as compared to the reference drugs. *In vivo* techniques undertaken for evaluation of efficacy essential oil of *Eucalyptus globulus* and *Cymbopogon citractus* at a concentration of 0.625% in 2% Tween 80 on two groups of (six animals each) *Sarcoptes scabiei* var. *caprae* infested goats were topically treated two times at 14 days interval and its compared with non-treated and treated (diazinone and ivermectin) controls of six goats in each group. The infected goats treated with the essential oils were cured completely. Statistically insignificant (p>0.05) difference was never observed in mite count, Mean Recovery Response (MRR) and degree of Skin Lesion Quality (SLQ) between goats treated with plant extracts and those treated with diazinone and ivermectin. Therefore, *Eucalyptus globulus* and *Cymbopogon citractus* extracts should be licensed for the treatment of *Sarcoptes scabiei* var. *caprae*.

Keywords: *In vitro* test; *In vivo* test; Mange mites; Medicinal plants; Goat; *Sarcoptes scabiei* var. *caprae*

Introduction

Ethiopia's economy is based on agriculture that account for 85% of the total employment and 75% of exports [1]. Livestock is the second major source of foreign currency through export of live animals, skin and hides [2]. The leather industry is one of the fast growing economic sectors in the country. However, this sector of trade and the country as whole, lost revenue due to a decline in quality and fall in export prices [3]. The current utilization of hides and skins is estimated to be 77.3% for cattle hide, 58.4% for goats skin and 29.7% for sheep skin with expected off take rate of 33%, 35% and 7% for sheep, goats and cattle respectively [4]. Even though, small ruminants are important components of the farming system in Ethiopia, their contributions are far below the expected potential. This is because small ruminant production in Ethiopia is confronted by several factors like diseases, poor feeding and poor managements [5,6].

Ectoparasitic skin diseases of small ruminants caused by mange mites, lice, fleas, keds, ticks and fleas are among the major diseases causing enormous economic losses to smallholder farmers, the tanning industry and the country as a whole. Infestation with ectoparasites is responsible for blood loss, irritation which results in downgrading and rejection of skins, poor growth, decreased production and reproduction performances and mortality [5]. The major observed economic losses due to mites, lice and keds is associated with skin damage. In 1996/97 six tanneries in and around Addis Ababa have rejected 2,037,745 pieces of skins which caused loss of USD 6.3 million [7] and in 1998/99 three tanneries that are found in Amhara Regional State have reported 443,602 pieces of skin rejection per annum which worth USD 1.4 million loss. According to Kassa ectoparasitic skin diseases due to ticks, lice, sheep keds and mange mites cause 35% of sheep skin and 56% of goat skin rejections. The ectoparasitic mites of mammals and birds inhabit the skin, where they feed on blood lymph, skin debris or sebaceous secretions, which they ingest by puncturing the skin, scavenge from the skin surface or imbibe from epidermal lesions. Most ectoparasitic mites spend their entire lives in intimate contact with their host, so that transmission from host to host is primarily by physical contact. The generalized veterinary term for an infestation by mites in an animal is called acariasis and can result in severe dermatitis, known as mange or scabies, which may cause significant welfare problems, economic losses and outright deaths [8,9].

Mange is a widespread and most important ectoparasitic disease of animals. Mange infestation is spread mainly by direct contact between hosts and all the three stages: the larvae, the nymph and the adults are capable of migrating and inert materials such as bedding and grooming tools can act as a carrier. Adult mites do not usually survive more than two weeks away from the host, but in optimum conditions they may remain to three weeks [10,11]. Female mites produce relatively large eggs, from which a small, six-legged larva hatches. A few species are ovoviviparous, producing live offspring's. The larva moults to become an eight legged nymph. There may be between one and three nymphal stages, known respectively as the protonymph, deutonymph and tritonymph. At least one of these nymphal stages is usually inactive

*Corresponding author: Bedaso Kebede, Veterinary Drug and Animal Feed Administration and Control Authority, Ministry of Livestock and Fisheries, Addis Ababa, Ethiopia, E-mail: kebede.bedaso@yahoo.com

and development proceeds without feeding. The nymph then moults to become adult. The number of eggs produced per female is highly variable but lifetime reproductive outputs may be as low as 16 eggs per female. Nevertheless, the life cycle of many parasitic species may be completed in less than 4 weeks and in some species may be, as short as 8 days. Hence, the mites have the potential for explosive increases in their population size. High temperature, humidity and sunlight favor mange mite infestations [12]. The disease affects all age groups and runs a more chronic course in adults than younger animals. Animals in poor condition are most susceptible to manage [13]. Mange cases due to *Sarcoptes* and *Psoroptes* are often fatal. The mortality rate is higher in younger and poor condition animals [14]. Death may be due to dehydration, a direct result of the feeding of huge number of mites, inability to move and feed due to severe lesions on the face, muzzle and on the joints or to secondary causes such as pneumonia or bacterial septicemia introduced through self-inflicted bite and scratch wounds [13,15]. In infestations, which do not end fatally, a marked regression of lesions, with healing of the skin and re-growth of the wool or hair occurs during dry season. Exposure of lesion and mite to direct sunlight and desiccation may reduce the survival potential of mite populations.

The clinical signs of erythema, pruritus and scale or crust formation are due to the inflammatory response of the skin and resulting excoriation. This response is stimulated by feeding, burrowing or the production of antigenic material by the mite. Some observers suggest that infra-orbital, inguinal pouches, scrotum, under tail, ears, inter digital pouches, perineum, and skin folds are foci for mites and serve as potential dry season hiding places where the mites tend to migrate to the general body surface with the onset of cold season [16]. According to the study reports, mange was noticed throughout the year but the incidence was higher during the wet cold months where the moistness and temperature is optimum condition for mite development [17]. Mange in sheep and goats is caused by four genera of mites, namely Sarcoptes, Psoroptes, Chorioptes and Demodex [18].

Sarcoptic mange is burrowing mites. It occurs in all species of animals and is caused by mite *Sarcoptes scabiei* that has a number of subspecies that affect different hosts but this host specificity is not complete and transference from one host species to another can occur [9,13]. *Sarcoptes* may be transmitted to unusual host in which it might burrow in to the skin and set up a typical mange lesion [19]. *Sarcoptes mites* are economically the most important cause of mange in sheep and goats. Sarcoptic mange in sheep and goats is caused by *Sarcoptes scabiei* var. *ovis* and *Sarcoptes scabiei* var. *caprae* respectively [20]. *Sarcoptic scabiei* var. *caprae* of goats and *Sarcoptic scabiei* var. *ovis* of sheep are widely distributed in many goat and sheep raising arid and semi-arid areas of Ethiopia. Sarcoptic mange seems more common in goats than in sheep. Sarcoptic mites are highly specialized for life with in the skin. Female mites burrow in to the skin and lay eggs in tunnels they made. Mating takes place on the surface of the skin [21]. The life cycle from egg to egg lying female may take 10-14 days [19]. The feeding activity of Sarcoptes causes intense itching and scratching due to a marked irritation, which causes self-inflicted lesions that aggravates the conditions [22]. Sarcoptic mange usually start on relatively hairless part of the skin and may latter generalize [19]. The course of Sarcoptic mange is rather more acute than the other forms of mange and may involve the entire body surface in a short time. It is highly contagious and the spread of *Sarcoptes scabiei* is usually by close physical contact. As a result single cases are rarely seen in groups of animals kept together. Infestation may also occur by indirect transfer, since the mites have been shown to be capable of surviving off the host for short periods. The length of time that *Sarcoptes scabiei* can

survive off the host depends on environmental conditions but may be between 2 and 3 weeks [11]. The ideal approach for diagnosis of skin diseases in general is a logical progression from history to an overall clinical examination, to a detailed examination of the skin, and finally to confirmatory testing or diagnosis by response to treatment [22,23].

Ectoparasites of small ruminants can be controlled by using commercial acaricides, but their accessibility and affordability to the resource poor farmers, and safety towards the environment makes them less preferable compared to other alternatives such as medicinal plants. The majority of farmers and pastoralists in the developing countries rely on traditional health care practices to keep their livestock healthy. These indigenous practices include the use of medicinal plants or ethno-veterinary medicine. It provides a vital contribution to livestock health needs throughout Ethiopia and is especially important to the resource poor rural communities. Treatment of mange with various acaricides like diazinon, fenvalerate, deltamethrin and avermectin has been attempted with different grades of success. Rapid development of resistance [24,25], high cost and environmental contamination [26,27] and health hazards to humans during treatment of animals [28] are the major problems associated with the use of synthetic acaricides. Concern about toxicity of many acaricides limits their use and reduces the number of safe effective products available. These problems have lead to research efforts to discover new effective compounds. The identification of novel active plant derived natural compounds could increase the number of available chemotherapeutic agents, thereby reducing the frequency of development of resistance and providing alternative drugs with greater acceptance, especially in terms of environmental safety [29]. In view of all these problems, use of botanical acaricides against highly pathogenic and economically important ectoparasites like mange is extremely important. Different indigenous plants like *Cedrus deodara, Pongamia glabra, Diospyros scabra, Dobera glabra, Euphorbia abtyssinica*, and *Sterculia alexandri* have been tried against sheep mange mites [30]. Various parts of different plants are being used in Ethno Veterinary Medicine practices for the treatment of mange mites in animals in different part of the world. Therefore, the objective of this study is to evaluate the acaricidal ability of *Eucalyptus globulus, Cymbopogon citractus, Nicotiana tobacum, Jatropha curcas, Melia azadarachta, Ximenia caffra* and *Pyrethrum cinerariifolium* extracts by *in vitro* and *in vivo* techniques against *Sarcoptes scabiei* var. *caprae* on infected goats.

Materials and Methods

Study area

The study was conducted in Dera and Hidabu Abote districts of North Shoa, Oromia regional state from November 2011 to May 2012. These districts comprise different agro climates namely highlands (>2000 m), midlands (1500-2000) and lowlands (<1500 m). The production system of the area is mixed crop livestock.

Study animals

Indigenous goats managed under extensive management system in the different agro-climates were used for the present study. Mange mite infested goats from different parts of the study sites were brought to Ejere town for the experimental study. According to the guide line set by Vercruysse et al. [25], all animals were selected from the same parasitological background (exposure of parasite infestation) those acquired the disease naturally, having similar weight, age and breed. During the study, the animals were identified by uniquely numbered ear tags. Animals were managed similarly and with due regard to their wellbeing. All study groups were confined separately, offered food under similar conditions according to local practice. Fresh water was available *ad libitum* throughout the study period. The health of the animals was also observed regularly. Other acaricides were never given to the study animals during the study period.

Study design

This study was designed using parameters of plant collection and extraction, *in vivo* and *in vitro* efficacy test and questionnaire survey.

Plant collection and extraction

The plants to be evaluated in this study were collected from their natural habitat and identified by taxonomists using standard flora, and voucher specimens was deposited in the national herbarium, Addis Ababa University. Air dried and powdered plant material (300-550 g) was extracted exhaustively with hydrochloric solvent by percolation at room temperature. The menstruum was filtered and concentrated in rotary evaporator or lyophilizer to give the crude extracts. The concentrated extracts were kept in tightly closed bottle in refrigerator until used for efficacy study. Small portion of the extract/fraction was used for the identification of the constituents (secondary metabolites) of the extract by examining the developed Thin Layer Chromatography (TLC) with appropriate chromogenic reagents.

In vivo and in vitro **acaricidal efficacy test:** Goats with mange like lesion of natural infestation were selected for the *in vivo* study. Infestation was confirmed by skin scraping examination. Infested animals were randomly divided into 6 groups (n=6) and were assigned to different treatments randomly based on the result of *in vitro* test. Plant extracts with good *in vitro* efficacy were selected and tested *in vivo*. Animals in all the treatment groups were individually sprayed with approximately 1 liters of the extract (until sufficiently became wet by the fluid) at a concentration of 0.625% two times, at 14 days interval [31,32]. The positive controls were treated two times again with ivermectin (Chengdu Qiankum Pharmaceuticals Co. Ltd., China, Lot: 09YW0705, Mfg. Date 10/07/09, Exp. Date: 09/07/2012) at a dose rate of 0.2 mg/kg body weight subcutaneously and diazinon (Shandong Luxy Animal Medicine Share Co. Ltd. No.1, Zhquqiao Road, West Ofqihe County, 251100, Shandong PR China Bach No.:20080330, Mfg. Date: 03/30/ 2008, Exp. Date: 03/ 29/2011)topically in the form of spray 14 days apart. The negative control groups were left none treated. The animals in each group were housed in separate rooms (Table 1).

Clinical examination of animals was carried out on the day of the first treatment (D0), the day of the second treatment (14 days after D0) and subsequently 21, 28 and 56 days post treatment [31,33]. All animals were individually examined and response to the treatment was monitored on days 14, 21, and 28 and 56 days in terms of Mean Recovery Response (MRR) and % reduction in mite counts according to the method described by Vercruysse et al. After the start of the trial, degree of lesions on individual animals were ranked using grading codes from 1-4 indicating an increasing degree of skin reaction and mean Skin Lesion Quality (SLQ) of each group were determined. After treatment (from Day 0 till end of trial) recovery in individual animals were ranked with grade codes from 0 to 4 and MRR of each group were determined to compare the effect of treatments (Table 2).

For parasitological examination skin scrapings were taken from the part of the lesions bordering healthy tissue by scraping as the method described by Fthenakis et al. [26]. Samples were examined within 12 h of collection. Scrapings were collectively placed into a test tube with 5 ml of distilled water and 10% KOH and heated until hair and epidermal scales dissolved and centrifuged at 2000 rpm for 2 min. The sediment then suspended in distilled water and re-centrifuged. The sediment was examined under a microscope and mites were identified with the help of morphological characteristics described by Souls by, Das; Wall and Shearer [18,28,11].

The total numbers of mites present were counted and % efficacy of each treatment was calculated as given by Khan [30]:

$$\% \text{ efficacy} = \frac{\text{No. of mites before treatment - No. of mites after treatment}}{\text{No. of mites before treatment}} \times 100$$

Data Analysis

Collected raw data was carefully recorded and stored in Microsoft Excel database system used for data management. Statistical software package called SPSS for windows version 17.0 was used for data analysis. Statistical significance was set at $P<0.05$ and Analysis of variance (one-way ANOVA-Tukey test) was also used to compare the means of different treatments (concentrations) of the extracts and controls in different time used for *in vitro* and *in vivo* efficacy studies of medicinal plants.

Results

Questionnaire survey

The results of the questionnaire survey forwarded to small ruminant owners were summarized by agro-ecology.45/90 (50%) of the respondents indicated mange to be treated traditionally by local healers using herbal medicine 17/90 (18.9%), non-herbal treatment 14/90 (15.6%) and 17/90 (18.9%) both. Results of the questionnaire survey on the participation in the treatment campaign program launched by the government for sheep and goats against ectoparasites revealed that 88/90 (97.8%) of sheep and goat owners have participated and treated their animals. According to that program each animal should have been treated 4 times at 10-14 days interval annually for a maximum of three years, but only 65/90 (72%) of the respondents who have participated in the program have treated their animals more than 3 times. In addition the interval between treatments was not regularly performed.

Focus group discussion

They said that inhabitant of the districts use modern medical care for treatment of animal diseases in general and skin problems in particular. But due to inaccessibility and high costs of modern drugs, traditional medical care like drenching, branding, vein puncture and washing with crude plant extracts are highly practiced in the area. Most traditional healers use plant preparations to treat livestock skin diseases. The people usually seek assistance from knowledgeable community members. The knowledgeable community members (traditional healers) do not charge for their assistance. But the individual who need assistance offer materials in kind like coffee and sugar. They believe that the treatment

Animals	Control (non-treated)	Diazinone treated	*Eucalypus*	*Eucalyptus* 0.625%	*Cymbopogon* 0.625%	Total
	Group 1	Group 2	Group 3	Group 4	Group 5	
Goat	6	6	6	6	6	30

Table 1: Schematic design of the experimental study.

No.	Description of lesions	Grade codes
1	Reddening of skin	1
2	Bare, exposed, moist lesions with serious exudation	2
3	Dry lesions with scab formation and loss of hairs	3
4	Thick, wrinkled skin with hyper keratinization	4
	Description of recovery	
5	No response	0
6	Dryness of lesions and loss of itching	1
3	Start of shrinkage of lesions and hair growth	2
4	Marked hair growth with smooth skin surface	3
5	Complete recovery	4

Table 2: Degree of lesion and mean recovery response of experimental animals.

would be effective (curable) when they offer materials as a gift to the healers. But compared to the cost of modern drugs this contribution is too cheaper. The participants also indicated the presence of secrecy with the knowledge of traditional medicine to treat livestock diseases. The traditional healers believed that the treatment will remain curable if they keep it secret. They inform the name of the medicinal plants that are used for treatment of ectoparasites only to the respected family members especially their elder sons when they get mature. In addition to this there are some plants which are known by the public to treat mange mites. These plants include *Accacia tortilis* ('Dhadacha'), *Aloe scundiflora* ('Chakke'), 'Sensel' and Lemon. The interviewed persons forwarded suggestions for scientific investigation of medicinal plants so as to develop herbal based drugs. They also forwarded the idea that researchers should address traditional healers in the investigation and development process.

In vitro acaricidal efficacy evaluation

Mortalities for the mite treated with the different concentration of *Eucalyptus globulus* essential oil are shown in Figure 1. When compared to the reference drugs (diazinon and Ivermectin), the extract was found to have comparable effects (p>0.05) against *S. scabiei* var. *caprae* at all test concentrations of 0.15625-2.5%. The concentration of 2.5% of the extract had the highest acaricidal efficacy causing 100% mortality after 10 min of exposure. But the concentration of 1.25% and lower showed 100% mortality after 120' of exposure. 0.625% was the lowest concentration that caused 100% mortality of mites compared to others at this 120'. After 3 h of contact all the concentrations of *Eucalyptus globulus* essential oil showed statistical significant (p<0.01) difference in mortality of mites with respect to the solvents (negative controls) and untreated controls (distilled water).

Mortalities of the mite treated with the different concentration of *Cymbopogon citractus* are shown in Figure 2. When compared to the control, the extract was found to have significant effect against *Sarcoptes scabiei* var. *caprae* at all test times and concentrations of 1.25-2.5%. These concentrations of the extract had the highest acaricidal efficacy with 100% mortality after 10 min of exposure. There was no significant difference (P>0.05) at all concentration of 0.15625-2.5% after 3 h of exposure when compared to the positive control. This implies all concentrations had comparable effect with the reference drugs. But 0.625% was the lowest concentration that caused 100% mortality of mites compared the others after 2 h of exposure. After 3 h of contact all the concentrations of *Cymbopogon citractus* essential oil showed a high mortality (p<0.01) when compared to the solvent (negative control) and non-treated control (distilled water).

Mortalities for the mite treated with the different concentration of the extracts of *Nicotiana tobacum* fixed oil are shown in Figure 3. When compared to the positive control, the extract was found to have

significant (P<0.05) effects against *Sarcoptes scabiei* var. *caprae* at all test times at a concentration of 160 mg/ml. 80 mg/ml and 160 mg/ml concentrations of the extract had the highest acaricidal efficacy with 100% mortality after 3 h of exposure. There was no significant effect (P<0.05) at a concentration of 40 mg/ml and below even after 3 h of exposure compared to the positive control. *Nicotiana tobacum* fixed oil 160-40 mg/ml showed a high mortality (p<0.01) When compared to the solvent (negative control). But only 20 mg/ml and above of the extracts with respect to untreated control (distilled water) showed statistically significance difference (p<0.01) in causing mortality of mites.

Mortalities for the mite treated with the different concentration of *Jatropha curcas* fixed oil are shown in Figure 4. When compared to the positive control, the extract was found to have comparable effects against *Sarcoptes scabiei* var. *caprae* at 120 min and concentrations of 160 mg/ml and 80 mg/ml. But after this time their effect seems to remain constant at about 80% when the positive controls continue to cause death of mites up to 100%. After 3 h of contact the extract showed no acaricidal efficacy (P>0.05) except the concentration of 160 mg/ml as compared to the reference drugs (diazinon and ivermectin). But when compared to the untreated control (distilled water) all the concentrations of the extract showed statistically significance difference (p<0.05) in causing mortality of mites. Only the concentration of

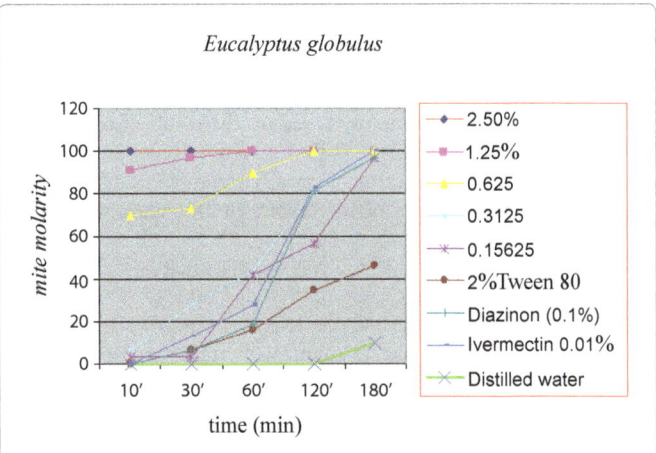

Figure 1: Mortalities of *Sarcoptes scabiei* var. *caprae* treated with the extracts of *Eucalyptus globules* essential oil *in vitro*.

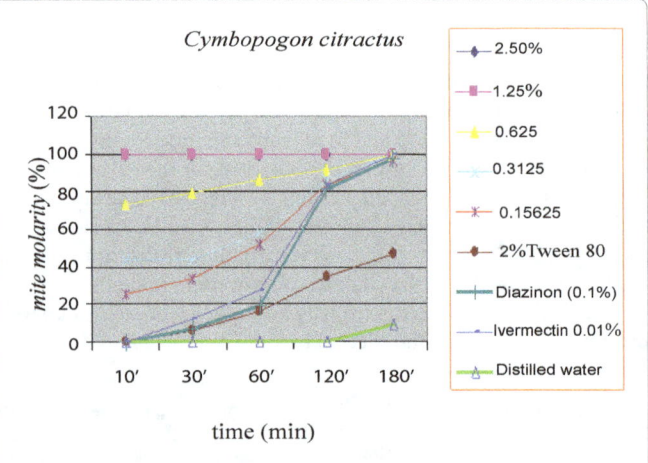

Figure 2: Mortalities of *Sarcoptes scabiei* var. *caprae* treated with the extracts of *Cymbopogon citractus* essential oil *in vitro*.

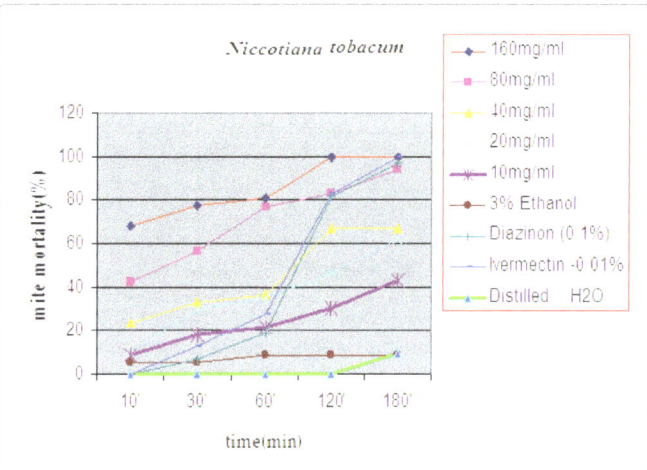

Figure 3: Mortalities of *Sarcoptes scabiei* var. *caprae* treated with the extracts of *Nicotiana tobacum* fixed oil *in vitro*.

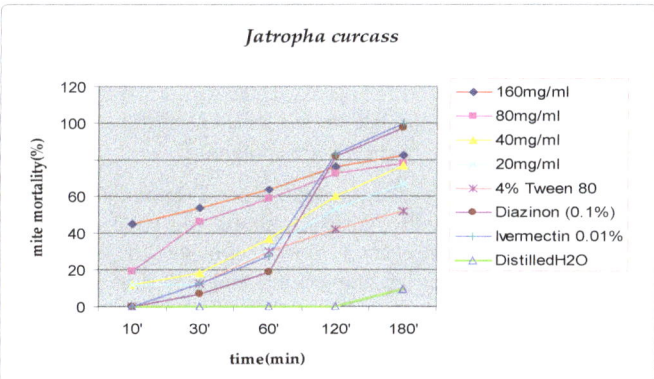

Figure 4: Mortalities of *Sarcoptes scabiei* var. *caprae* treated with the extracts of *Jatropha curcas* fixed oil *in vitro*.

80 mg/ml and 60 mg/ml showed statistically significance (p<0.05) difference on mite mortality to the solvent (negative control).

After 3 h of contact *Melia azadarachta* fixed oil showed comparable acaricidal efficacy (P>0.05) in causing mite mortality at concentrations of higher than 10 mg/ml of the extract when compared to the reference drugs (diazinon and ivermectin). But compared to non-treated control (distilled water) all the concentrations of the extract showed statistically significance difference (p<0.05) to cause mortality of mites (Figure 5).

After 3 h of contact the extract of *Ximenia caffra* (fixed oil) showed comparable acaricidal efficacy (P>0.05) in all the concentrations above 20 mg/ml of the extract as compared to the reference drugs (diazinon and ivermectin). But compared to untreated control (Distilled water) all the concentrations of the extract showed statistically significance (p<0.05) difference to cause mortality of mites (Figure 6).

After 3 h of contact *Pyrethrum cinerariifolium* fixed oil showed no acaricidal efficacy (P<0.05) in all the concentrations of the extract compared to the reference drugs (diazinon and ivermectin). The highest concentrations (160 mg/ml and 80 mg/ml) showed lower efficacy of mite mortality only 49% and 46.7% respectively (Figure 7). Even though there is statistically significant (p<0.05) difference compared to untreated control (distilled water) all the concentrations of the extract showed no significant (p<0.05) difference when compared with the solvent to cause mortality of mites.

In vivo acaricidal efficacy

For *in vivo* efficacy evaluation 0.625% concentration of both *Eucalyptus globulus* and *Cymbopogon citractus* was selected due to the promising efficacy of these plants after *in vitro* test. Table 3 shows the major results of the *in vivo* trial. At day 0 no difference was observed among all groups, both for the parasitological (presence of mites) and clinical score (presence of lesion). From day 21 after the beginning of the treatment, *Eucalyptus globulus* treated group, *Cymbopogon citractus* treated groups and treated control groups (ivermectin and diazinon treated groups) were negative for mites and/or eggs and significant differences (p<0.05) was recorded in their clinical lesion scores, Mean Recovery Responses (MRR) and percentage of mite count reduction

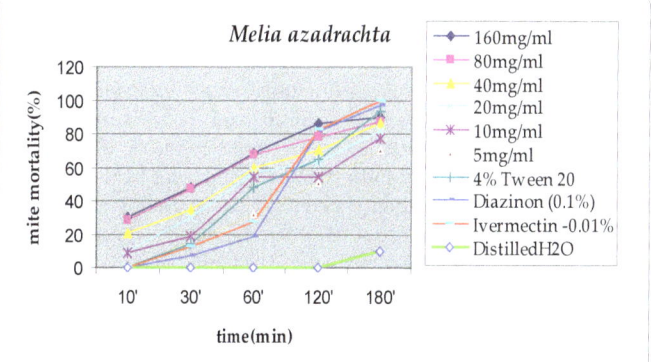

Figure 5: The mortalities of *Sarcoptes scabiei* var. *caprae* treated with the extracts of *Melia azadarachta* fixed oil *in vitro*.

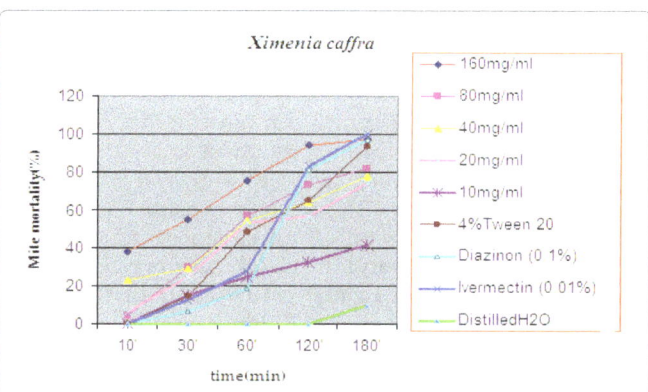

Figure 6: The mortalities of *Sarcoptes scabiei* var. *caprae* treated with the extracts of *Ximenia caffra* fixed oil *in vitro*.

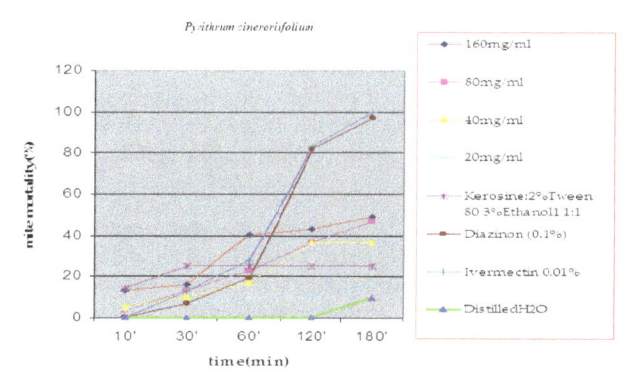

Figure 7: Mortalities of *Sarcoptes scabiei* var. *caprae* treated with the extracts of *Pyrethrum cinerariifolium* fixed oil *in vitro*.

Day	Eucalyptus globulus			Cymbopogon citractus			Ivermectin			Diazinon			Non-treated control		
	Mite count% efficacy	MRR	SLQ	Mite count %efficacy	MRR	SLQ	Mite count %efficacy	MRR	SLQ	Mite count %efficacy	MRR	SLQ	Mite count% efficacy	MRR	SLQ
0	0	0	3.2	0	0	3.2	0	0	2.7	0	0	2.8	0	0	3.3
14	45	2.0	1.8	83.3	3.1	1.17	80.7	2.67	1.33	80.3	2.67	1.5	-0.7	0	3.3
21	100	2.8	1.6	100	3.5	0.8	100	3.6	0.6	100	3.3	0.7	-0.7	0	3.3
28	100	3.0	1.0	100	3.8	0.33	100	4.0	0.00	100	4.0	0.00	-0.7	0	3.3
56	100	3.6	0.6	100	4.0	0.17	100	4.0	0.00	100	4.0	0.00	-0.7	0	3.3

Table 3: *In vivo* acaricidal efficacy of *Eucalyptus globulus* and *Cymbopogon citractus* against *Sarcoptes scabiei* var. *caprae*.

compared to non-treated group. Plant extracts of both of the essential oils and positive controls resulted in a clinical cure in all groups. The untreated control group remained positive for mite infestation until 14th day of the trial and the mite count increases progressively and the conditions of the lesions get worse and worse ending in death of the animals. On day 14, in this latter group the degree of infestation was significantly (p<0.01) higher when compared to *Eucalyptus globulus and Cymbopogon citractus* treated groups and treated control group in both the degree of skin lesion and mite count % efficacy. The Mean Recovery Responses in the treated groups and treated controls significantly increased without difference in these groups and the skin lesion reduced significantly (p<0.05) when compared to the non-treated groups and healing was observed after day 28 that was maintained to exist until day 56, the end of the *in vivo* experimental period.

Discussion

In the present study *Eucalyptus globulus* showed comparable acaricidal efficacy as compared to the reference drugs (diazinon and ivermectin) killing up to 100% of sarcoptic mites from goats. *Eucalyptus* essential oil has been previously reported to possess biocidal properties. *Eucalyptus globulus* essential oil has been tested for its acaricidal effect against other mites [34]. Oil from *Eucalyptus globulus* proved to be toxic to the mites in a separate study that tested the toxic effect of the essential oil from the same species of eucalyptus against *Dermanyssus gallinae* [35]. The present study confirmed *E. globulus* to be toxic to *Sarcoptes scabiei* var. *caprae*. In other studies, essential oils from other spp. of Eucalyptus proved to be effective in killing mites achieving more than 65% mortality. In contrary to the present study, essential oils from *Eucalyptus globulus* displayed a much reduced acaricidal effect, killing only 11% of mites after exposure [36,37]. This may be due to numerous factors which may affect the composition of essential oils. Geographic origin [38], seasonality [39], method of oil extraction [40], year of harvest [41] and even storage conditions are all factors that have been reported to influence essential oil chemistry and its efficacy against ectoparasites. The compound is commonly reported to have acaricidal [42,43] and pesticidal [44] properties. Essential oils with more complex chemical compositions may have an additional advantage over simpler oils if developed for use as acaricides. It has been observed the most important advantage of such products for pest management would be that the numerous active compounds in essential oils would make development of resistance to any essential oil based product extremely difficult [43].

All concentrations of *Cymbopogon citractus* essential oil had comparable efficacy with the reference drugs (diazinon and ivermectin). Even though there is very little study so far conducted on the acaricidal activity of this oil, several studies reported antimicrobial activities by *Cymbopogon citractus* essential oil [45-48]. Indeed, the oil exhibited a broad spectrum of fungi toxicity and its fungi toxic potency remained unaltered for 210 days of storage, with considerable interests in the application of the oil for the preservation of stored food crops [49].

Cymbopogon citractus essential oil inhibited microorganisms examined at ≤2% (v/v). The current study also showed mite mortality at ≤2.5% (v/v). Fungi colony growth and sporulation was completely retarded by this essential oil [50,51]. The initial idea of the current study was originated from these works on plant pest. Therefore the essential oil acts not only on crop pests but also animal pest particularly mange mites.

Nicotiana tobacum has a Jasmonic acid and its cyclic precursors and derivatives are members of a lipid-based signaling cascade originating from polyunsaturated fatty acids. It plays a role in development and defense including plant response to wounding and abiotic stress, and defenses against insects and pathogens [52]. This and other constituents of the plant may be responsible for the toxic effect of the mites that caused mortality of mites in the *in vitro* evaluation.

Jatropha curcas is used in the treatment of various disorders in man and animals, including goats and sheep, and are also ingested by grazing animals particularly at times of drought. The seed of this plant was used as purgatives, anthelmintic and molluscicides [53]. In the current study the extract was found to have goodacaricidal efficacy similar to conventional drugs *in vitro* against *Sarcoptes scabiei var. caprae* at concentrations of 160 mg/ml and 80 mg/ml even the effect seems to remain constant at about 80% when the positive controls continue to cause death of mites up to 100%. But in recent study by Abdel-Gadir et al. [52] the oral administration of *Jatropha curcas* seed to Nubian goat kids caused toxic manifestations and death of goats. But acaricides are applied topically; toxicity might not be as that of lethal as oral administration.

Some reports have confirmed that *Melia azadarachta* is an effective botanical acaricide for mange mites (*Sarcoptes scabies* var. *caniculi*) (*Sarcoptes scabies varovis*) [54,55] and ticks (*Boophilus microplus*) [56]. The pesticide activity of this fixed oil is generally thought to be due to azadirachtin, which is a well-known potent insecticide [57]. However, Walton et al., [58] reported that the product containing 0.3-0.5% azadirachtin had no effect on *Sarcoptes scabiei* var. *hominis* by *in vitro* test. Mortality of mites in the present study showed comparable efficacy with standard drugs even at lower concentrations.

Ximenia is a key part of native African medicine. Its principal use is as an emollient, hair oil, conditioner and skin softener, in soap manufacture, and as component of lipsticks and lubricants. The root, bark and leaves are used for medicinal purposes; the bark is used to treat toothache, mouth infections and stomach aches [59]. In the present study the extract of *Ximenia caffra* (fixed oil) showed comparable acaricidal efficacy with respect to the reference drugs (diazinon and ivermectin) *in vitro*.

The term *"Pyrethrum cinerariifolium"* refers to the plant, flower or flower extract, with the active insecticidal components known as "pyrethrins" [60]. *Pyrethrum cinerariifolium* is a plant widely used for insecticide production [61]. It also used as crop pest (grain weevil) [62].

It is a toxic agent for pest insects with a century-long history of safe use [63]. The great advantages of *Pyrethrum cinerariifolium* are its action against a wide variety of different insect species [64], a low mammalian toxicity and a rapid metabolism [63]. But in the current study *Pyrethrum cinerariifolium* fixed oil showed no acaricidal efficacy (P<0.05) in all the concentrations of the extract as compared to the reference drugs (diazinon and ivermectin). Even the higher concentrations (160 mg/ml and 80 mg/ml) showed lower acaricidal efficacy (only 49% and 46.7% respectively) against mites which is much lower to say effective. This may be due to physiological differences between acaris and insects.

Products prepared from both *Eucalyptus* and *Cymbopogon* extracts were found safe for goats in the *in vivo* application as they did not show the sign of irritation or restlessness at the time of application or afterwards. From the scanty previous information on the herbal acaricides *in vivo*, *Azadirachta indica* (50% oil) has been reported to cause 87.7% recovery [65,66], 100% recovery [32] in sheep with sarcoptic mange. Yand et al. [40], have also reported the efficacy of this ointment (neem) *in vivo* against ear canker of rabbits (caused by *Psoroptes cuniculi*). In the present study, 100% recovery was observed in goats treated with *Eucalyptus globulus* and *Cymbopogon citractus* at 0.625% concentration which were comparable with modern treatments. Other plant materials like linalool also showed acaricidal activity against Psoroptes mite *in vivo* on rabbits and goats [67]. In a recent study [45], linalool and cinnamyl acetate showed insecticidal activity against *Pediculus humanus capitis*.

In general along with the economic benefits, additional advantage of using plant pesticides is that, they have low environmental persistence [68] do not induce resistance readily in insects [69,70] and are relatively nontoxic to mammals. These results consolidate the belief that the use of herbal acaricides may provide a better way of combating a menace such as mange in domestic animals and they can be used more safely and effectively.

Conclusion and Recommendations

All medicinal plants showed acaricidal efficacy *in vitro* comparable to the reference drugs except *Pyrethrum cineraria folium* especially at higher concentrations. *In vivo* evaluation of both *Eucalyptus globulus* and *Cymbopogon citractus* resulted in complete elimination of mites. So results obtained in the *in vitro* and *in vivo* evaluation in the present study indicated that essential and fixed oils of the extracts tested could represent a possible alternative for the topical treatment of sarcoptic mange in goats.

Based on the above concluding remarks, the following recommendations are forwarded:

- The efficacy of the preparations, techniques and practices need to be further investigated in other areas to identify promising plants for use.

- Further studies should be conducted on the socio economic situation, drug formulation and licensing of the extracts so as to develop herbal based treatments.

References

1. Zewdu K (1995) Hides and skins in Ethiopia. In proceedings of the second Annual conference of the Ethiopian society of Animal production.

2. Ayele S, Assegid W, Jabbar MA, Ahmed MM (2003) Livestock Marketing in Ethiopia, A Review of Structure, Performance and Development Initiatives.

3. Pittards (1999) Ethiopian partnership review meeting.

4. MOARD (2005) Mange, Lice and Sheep Ked control project in Amhara, Tigray and Afar regions. MOARD Animal Health Department, Addis Ababa, Ethiopia.

5. Getachew T (1995) Parasites of small ruminants. In Gray GD and Vilenberg G (eds.) Parasitological Research in Africa 52: 198-232.

6. MOARD (2008) The effect of hide and skin quality on domestic and export markets and evaluation of the campaign against ectoparasites of sheep and goats in Amhara, Tigray and Afar regions. Official report to regions and other sectors, Addis Ababa, Ethiopia.

7. Kassa B (1998) Control of sheep and goat skin diseases. In Proceedings of Control of Sheep and Goat Skin Diseases for Improved Quality of Hides and Skins.

8. Sertse T, Wosene, A (2007) A Study on ectoparasites of sheep and goats in eastern part of Amhara Regional State, north east Ethiopia. Small Ruminant Res 69: 62-67.

9. Radostitis OM, Blood DC, Gay CC (2000) Veterinary Medicine, Text Book of Cattle, Sheep, Pigs, Goats and Horses, Ninth Edition, Bailliere Tindall, UK pp: 1280-1308.

10. Smith KE, Wall R, Berriatua E, French NP (1999) The effects of temperature and humidity on the off-host survival of Psoroptes ovis and Psoroptes cuniculi. Vet Parasitol 83: 265-275.

11. Pangui LJ (1994) Mange in domestic animals and methods of control. Rev Sci Tech 13: 1227-1247.

12. Olubunmi PA (1995) The prevalence of mange due to Sarcoptes scabiei Var Capri in Ile-Ife area of Nigeria, its control and management. Bulletin Animal Health and Production in Africa 43: 115-119.

13. Urquhart GM, Armour J, DuncanJL, Dunn AM, Jennings FW (1996) Veterinary Parasitology (2nd edn.) Blackwell Science Ltd, UK pp: 141-205.

14. Berriatua E, French NP, Wall R, Smit KE, Morgan KL (1999) Within- flock transmission of sheep scab in naive sheep housed with single infested sheep. Vet Parasitol 83: 277-289.

15. Okoh AE, Gadzama JN (1982) Sarcoptic mange of sheep in Plateau State, Nigeria. Bull Anim Health Prod Afr 30: 61-63.

16. Sewell MMH, Brockesby DW (1990) Hand Book on Animal Disease in the Tropics (4th edn.) Bailliere Tindall pp: 2-28.

17. Kaufmann J (1996) Parasitic Infections of Domestic Animals, Diagnostic Manual, Birkhauser, Germany pp: 188-201

18. Jackson P (1991) Skin Diseases in Goats. In Boden E (eds) Sheep and Goats Practice, Bailliere, Tindall pp: 34-67.

19. Bowman DD, Lynn CR, Eberhard LM, Alcaraz A (2003):Georgis' Parasitology for Veterinarians, Eighth Edition, USA pp: 1-78.

20. Smith MC, Sherman DM (1994) Goat Medicine, Williams and Wilkins, Maryland pp: 17-47.

21. Synge BA, Bates PG, Clark AM, Stephen FB (1995) Apparent resistance of P ovis to flumethrin. Vet Rec 137: 51.

22. O'Brien DJ (1999) Treatment of psoroptic mange with reference to epidemiology and history. Vet Parasitol 83: 177-185.

23. Alawa CBI, Adamu AM, Gefu JO, Ajanusi OJ, Abdu PA, et al. (2003) In vitro screening of two Nigeria medicinal plants (Vernonia amygdalina and Annona senegalensis) for anthelmintic activity. Vet Parasitol 113: 73-81.

24. Teshale S, Merga B, Girma A, Ensermu K (2004) Medicinal plants in the ethno veterinary practices of Borana pastoralists, Southern Ethiopia. J Appl Res Vet Med 2: 220-225.

25. Vercruysse J, Rehbein S, Holdsworth PA, Letonja T, Peter RJ (2006) World Association for the Advancement of Veterinary Parasitology guidelines for evaluating the efficacy of acaricides against (mange and itch) mites on ruminants. Vet Parasitol 136: 55-66.

26. Fthenakis GC, Karagiannidis A, Alexopoulos C, Brozos C, Papadopoulos E (2001) Effects of sarcoptic mange on the reproductive performance of ewes and transmission of Sarcoptes scabiei to newborn lambs. Vet Parasitol 95: 63-71.

27. Soulsby EJL (1982) Helminthes, Arthropods and Protozoa of Domesticated Animals (7th edn.) Lea and Febiger, Philadelphia pp: 375-502.

28. Das SS (1996) Effect of a herbal compound for treatment of sarcoptic mange infestations on dogs. Vet Parasitol 63: 303-306.

29. Wall R, Shearer D (1997) Veterinary Entomology (1st edn.) Chapman and Hall, UK pp: 1-438.

30. Khan MN, Hayat CS, Iqbal Z (1998) Evaluation of acaricidal efficacy of Ivermectin, Diazinon, Permethrin and Coumaphos in cattle and buffaloes. Pakistan Entomologist 19: 58-60.

31. Choi W, Lee S, Park H, Ahn Y (2004) Toxicity of plant essential oils to *Tetranychus urticae* (Acari Tetranychidae) and *Phytoseiulus persimilis* (Acari Phytoseiidae). J Economical Entomol 97: 553-558.

32. Kim S, Yi J, Tak J, An Y (2004) Acaricidal activity of plant essential oils against *Dermanyssus gallinae* (Acari Dermanyssidae).Vet parasitol 120: 297-304.

33. George DR, Callaghan K, Guy JH, Sparagano OA (2008) Lack of prolonged activity of lavender essential oils as acaricides against the poultry red mite (*Dermanyssus gallinae*) under laboratory conditions. Vet Sci 85: 540-542.

34. George DR, Olivier DM, Sparagano AE, Guy JH (2009) Variation in chemical composition and acaricidal activity against *Dermanyssus gallinae* of four eucalyptus essential oils. Experimental Appl Acarol 48: 43-50.

35. Raal A, Orav A, Arak E (2007) Composition of the essential oil of *Salvia officinalis* L. from various European countries. Nat Prod Res 21: 406-411.

36. Flamini G, Cioni PL (2007) Seasonal variation of the chemical constituents of the essential oil of *Santolina etrusca* from Italy. Chem Biodivers 4: 1008-1019.

37. Chiasson H, Belanger A, Bostanian N, Vincent C, Poliquin A (2001) Acaricidal properties of *Artemisia absinthium* and *Tanacetum vulgare* (Asteraceae) essential oils obtained by three methods of extraction. J Ecol Entomol 94: 167- 171.

38. Chalchat JC, Ozcan MM, Dagdelden A, Akgul A (2007) Variability of essential oil composition of *Echinophora tenuifolia* subsp sibthorpiana Tutin by harvest location and year and oil storage. Chem Nat Comp 43: 225-227.

39. Macchioni F, Cioni PL, Flamini G, Morelli I, Perrucci S, et al. (2002) Acaricidal activity of pine essential oils and their main components against *Tyrophagus putrescentiae*, a stored food mite. J Agric Food Chem 50: 4586-4588.

40. Yang YC, Lee HS, Clark JM, Ahn YJ (2004) Insecticidal activity of plant essential oils against *Pediculus humanus* capitis (Anoplura Pediculidae). J Med Entomol 41: 699-704.

41. Miresmailli S, Bradbury R, Isman MB (2006) Comparative toxicity of *Rosmarinus officinalis* essential oil and blends of its major constituents against *Tetranychus urticae* Koch (Acari Tetranychidae) on two different host plants. Pest Managem Sci 62: 366-371.

42. Appendini P, Hotchkiss JH (2002) Review of antimicrobial food packaging. Innov Food Sci Emerg Tech 3: 113-126.

43. Daferera DJ, Ziogas BN, Polissiou MG (2003) The effectiveness of plant essential oils on the growth of *Botrytis cinerea*, *Fusarium* spp. and *Clavibacter michiganensis* sub spp. Michiganensis. Crop Protect 2: 239-244.

44. Plotto A, Roberts D, Roberts RG (2003) Evaluation of plant essential oils as natural postharvest disease control of tomato (*Lycopersicon esculentum*). Acta Hortic 628: 737-745.

45. Martinez-Romero D, Serrano M, Castillo S, Guillen F, Valero D (2005) The use of the natural antifungal compounds improves the beneficial effect of MAP in sweet cherry storage. Innov Food Sci Emerg Tech 6: 115-123.

46. Adegoke GO, Odesola BA (1996) Storage of maize and cowpea and inhibition of microbial agents of biodeterioration using the powder and essential oil of lemon grass (*Cymbopogon citractus*). Int Biodeterior Biodegradation 6: 81-84.

47. Hammer KA, Carson CF, Riley TV (1999) Antimicrobial activity of essential oils and other plant extracts. J Appl Microbiol 86: 985-990.

48. Tzortzakis NG, Economakis CD (2007) Antifungal activity of lemongrass *Cymbopogon citractus*) (essential oil against key postharvest pathogens. Innov Food Sci EmergTech 8: 253-258.

49. Browse J, Howe GA (2008) New weapons and a rapid response against insect attack. Plant Physiol 146: 832-838.

50. Liu SY, Sporer F, Wink M, Jourdane J, Henning R, et al. (1997) Anthraquin ones in *Rheum palmantum* and *Rumex dentatus* and phorbol esters in Jatropha curcas with molluscicidal activity against the schistosome vector snails Oncomelania, Biornphalaria and Bulinus. Trop Med Int Health 2: 179-188.

51. Dafalla AA, Amin MA (1976) Laboratory and field evaluation of the molluscicidal properties of Habat Elmoluk (*Jatropha* spp). East Africa J Med Res 3: 185-195.

52. Abdel-Gadir WS, Onsa TO, Ali WE, El-Badwi SM, Adam SE (2003) Comparative toxicity of Croton macrostachys, *Jatropha curcas* and *Piper abyssinica* seeds in Nubian goats. Small Ruminant Res 48: 61-67.

53. Du Y, Jia R, Yin Z, Pu Z, Chen J, et al. (2008) Acaricidal activity of extracts of neem (*Azadirachta indica*) oil against the larvae *Sarcoptes scabiei* var cuniculi *in vitro*. Vet Parasitol 157: 144-148.

54. Srivastava R, Ghosh S, Mandal DB, Azhahianambi P, Singhal PS, et al. (2008) Efficacy of *Azadirachta indica* extracts against *Boophilus microplus*. Parasitol Res 104: 149-153.

55. Isman MB, Koul O, Luczynski A, Kaminskis J (1990) Insecticidal and anti feedant bioactivities of neem oils and their relationship to azadirachtin content. J Agric Food Chem 38: 1406-1411.

56. Walton SF, Currie BJ (2007) Problems in diagnosing scabies, a global disease in human and animal populations. Clin Microbiol Rev 20: 268-279.

57. Tomas R, Karel S (2007) Identification of very long chain in saturated fatty acids from Ximenia oil by atmospheric pressure chemical ionization liquid chromatography-mass spectroscopy. Photochemistry 68: 925-934.

58. Morris SE, Davies NW, Brown PH, Groomd T (2006) Effect of drying conditions on pyrethrins content. Industrial Crops Prod 23: 9-14.

59. Wainaina JMG (1995) Pyrethrum cinerariifolium flowers production in Africa. In Casida JE and Quistad GB (eds.) Pyrethrum cinerariifolium Flowers Production, Chemistry, Toxicology and Uses. Oxford University Press, New York pp: 49-54.

60. Biebel R, Rametzhofer E, Klapal H, Polheim D, Viernstein H (2003) Action of *Pyrethrum cinerariifolium*-based formulations against grain weevils. Int J Pharmaceutics 256: 175-181.

61. Katsuda Y (1999) Development and future prospects for pyrethroid chemistry. Pest Sci 55: 775-782.

62. Silcox CA, Roth ES (1994) Pyrethrum cinerariifolium for pest control. In Casida JE and Quistad GB (eds.) *Pyrethrum cinerariifolium* Flowers. Oxford University Press, Oxford pp: 285-301.

63. Satelle DB, Yamamoto D (1988) Molecular targets of pyrethroid insecticides. Insect Physiology 20: 147-213.

64. Hirudkar US, Deshpande PD, Narladkar BW, Vadlamudi VP (1997) Effect of herbal treatment with himax ointment and neem oil in sarcoptic mange in sheep. Indian Vet J 74: 506-508.

65. Tabassam SM, Iqbal Z, Jabbar A, Sindhu ZU, Chattha AI (2008) Efficacy of crude neem seed kernel extracts against natural infestation of *Sarcoptes scabiei* var. *ovis*. J Ethnopharmacol 115: 284-287.

66. Perrucci S, Cioni PL, Cascella A, Macchioni F (1997) Therapeutic efficacy of linalool for the topical treatment of parasitic otitis caused by *Psoroptes cuniculi* in the rabbit and in the goat. Med Vet Entomol 11: 300-302.

67. Sundaram KMS, Curry J (1994) Initial deposits and persistence of azadirachtin in fir and oak foliage after spray application of Margosan-O® formulation. Pestic Sci 41: 129-138.

68. Feng R, Isman MB (1995) Selection for resistance to azadirachtin in the green peach aphid, Myzus Persicae. Experientia 51: 831-833.

69. Jacobson M (1995) Toxicity of neem to vertebrates and side effects on beneficial and other ecologically important non-target organisms toxicity to vertebrates. In: Schmutterer H (ed.) The Neem Tree Source of Unique Products for Integrated Pest Management, Medicine, Industry, and other Purposes, Weinheim, New York pp: 484-495.

70. Larson RO (1989) The commercialization of neem. In: Jacobson M (ed.) Focus on Photochemical Pesticides. The Neem Tree, CRC Press, Boca Raton, FL pp: 155-168.

37

Health Seeking Pattern among Halakki Vokkalu Tribe of Karnataka

Praveen Hoogar[1]*, Ashwini Pujar[1] and Basavanagouda TT[2]

[1]Department of Studies in Anthropology, Karnatak University Dharwad, Karnataka State, India
[2]Karnataka State Tribal Research Institute, Mysore, Karnataka State, India

Abstract

The current article has produced as a part of Ph. D. thesis entitled "A study on Health Seeking Behaviour among Halakki Vokkalu Community of Uttara Kannada District, Karnataka." In this article the term tribe has been used invariably and instead of the term Community. Health is a prime priority in every tribe/community and every part of the globe. Every society has a patterns to deal with situations followed by many socio, religious and geoghical factors. Multiple medical streams are serving simultaneously through their own mode of methods. Every medical system is and should work as complementary to other. The availability, accessibility, and affordability of any treatment or medicine plays very important role in the selection of treatment and medicine from. The main objectives of this paper are: 1) Briefly making an academic account of the Halakki Vokkalu tribe of Karnataka; and 2) To briefly explain about Health Seeking Pattern of Halakki Vokkalu Tribe.

Keywords: Health seeking behaviour; Treatment pattern; Indigenous medicine; Halakki Vokkalu; Uttar Kannada; Medical anthropology

Introduction

The current article has produced as a part of Ph. D. thesis entitled "*A study on Health Seeking Behaviour among Halakki Vokkalu community of Uttara Kannada District, Karnataka.*" In this article the term *tribe* has used invariably and instead of the term *Community*.

Health is a common theme in most of the cultures; in fact, all communities have their own concepts of health and illness as part of their culture. Based on their earlier experiences with illness, various training on symptoms, different people of different societies has different conception of health. What is considering as being healthy in one society might not be consider so healthy in another. In the same ways the pattern of seeking health will also be change among different tribes or communities Illness perception on the one hand and treatment choice on the other are interdependent (Rake 1961:205). Health behaviours are a set of actions that the elderly perform to ensure they eat and keep well, and protect, promote and maintain health [1,2].

Halakki Vokkalu of Karnataka

'Halakki Vokkalu' is a small group in Karnataka and is settled down in four taluks of Uttara Kannada district namely Karwar, Ankola, Kumta and Honnavar. They are thickly populated in and around Ankola and Kumta taluks.

Halakki Vokkalu is mild, sober and economically poor people. In Karnataka they are considered as very backward community and placed in the category I group (Government Order No. SKE 225 BCA 2000, dated 30-03-2002) [3]. In the 2001 census Halakki Vokkalu are mixed with the other backward communities. Hence, it is very difficult to authentically about their total population.

Derivation of the Name

There are many versions regarding derivation of the name 'Halakki Vokkalu'. In Kannada, the term 'Halakki' denotes milk and rice (Halu=Milk and Akki=Rice). Halakki Vokkalu is white rice growers (Gazetteer of the Bombay Presidency 1883) [4].

According to Bhat, the name 'Halakki' probably because, these people are asked to sprinkle milk and rice at the marriage procession of Having Brahmin to prevent evil eye on the newlywed couple. According to the people, acquisition of the name may be due to their occupations like agriculture and dairy work. There is no unanimous opinion regarding the origin of the term [5].

Methodology

As mentioned in beginning itself this has produced as a part of Ph. D. research. That was a mixed research method study, but observations, interactions with respondents at the field and critical observation of data has used for this article. This is more of explanatory note of observed situations and mostly very general pattern found among the studied community.

Health seeking behaviour is preceded by a decision-making process that is further governed by individual and/or household behaviour, community norms and expectations. For this reason, the nature of care seeking is varied depending on cognitive and non-cognitive factors that call for a contextual analysis of care seeking action. This context may include factors such as cognition or awareness, as well as socio-cultural and economic factors.

The health seeking pattern directly dependent on health seeking behavior. In the present paper authors just wish to provide the pattern generally followed by the Halakki Vokkalu tribe. How they respond to an illness episode, how and what decision they take to address that illness, what is their preference of taking treatment for those are the concerns of this article. If there is an illness episode they directly don't go to the any Medical Specialist, they decide the treatment sources on the bases of illness, intensity of illness, severity of illness then they try to get cured from different modes [6-10]. If one is not effectively resulted gradually shift to another to resolve that particular illness. Observations and interactions with respondents were put together and tried to understand with anthropological perspectives, then the pattern which has presented below appears. It is a commonly existing pattern among Halakki Vokkalu. These are the some cues observed at field were motivated authors to write this article.

*Corresponding author: Praveen Hoogar, Research Scholar, Department of Studies in Anthropology, Karnatak University Dharwad, Karnataka State, India
E-mail: praveenhoogar@gmail.com

Discussion

The following diagram shows health seeking pattern of Halakki Vokkalu tribe. The diagram says that In case of any illness Halakkis do not directly go for any kind of treatments. They leave that to be cured by it. They wait for some time if they get result *Yes* just lead routine life then there is no question of taking further treatment. If the result is *No*, then they move to the step of *Mane maddu (Homemade) or Kai maddu (Handmade)* medicines.

In this stage try to medicate them at home by using some techniques of *Patthe* means avoid some food stuffs during illness episode or taking some foods and beverages. After this if result is *No*, they opt for medicine from counter.

Halakkis collect medicine from counters. The counters were *General Shops and Medical Shops (Chemist)*. The observation from field acknowledges the fact that availability of medical shops is comparatively less than any other general shops. If here also they do not cured, they will be going for *popular practitioner sector*. Popular practitioner means the lay, non-professional, non-specialist domain of the society which is treating for many illnesses since a long back. Halakkis go to these people because they live among and nearby, especially at rural areas where majority of the professional or trained doctors do not prefer to be there and serve in these places. It is purely an issue of availability, accessibility and affordability of a specialist of a treatment. Hence the preference for specialist treatment is at last they try to get out from the illness episode through their prior preferences of treatment gradually shift from one to other [11].

Halakkis sought treatment for their illness from one of the sector mentioned above then they lead routine life. Along this pattern of health seeking they follow one more practice that is magico-religious treatment or healing. Every treatment travel along with this parallel practice of healing. It means whichever treatment they opt till homemade medicine practice to treatment from professional doctors the magico-religious practices will be performed and it will be a fixed element (Figure 1).

Conclusion

This is the pattern found among the Halakki Vokkalu tribe's seeking health. This shows that they have their own style of identifying, diagnosing and treating an illness. The parallel system of seeking health is continuing with very strong beliefs and practices, according to a respondent because, it provides a moral and psychological strength and support to both patient and family. By this patient's belief in treatment and medicine get stronger and stronger. Once patient gets enough belief in treatment and medicine his mind starts reacting positively to the treatment and it results with cure. The respondent's statement denotes that the importance of psychological consideration for any treatment and medicine leads to proper responding from the patients. Wish to conclude this article with all sort of treatments have got their own set of pros and cons, they must work in complimenting to each other instead of any contradictions. Of course it is true that each type of sectors have very different style of diagnosing, treating and following-up the cases but the motto behind those is and must be one that is the betterment of mankind. We don't support any ill practices in the name traditional or indigenous medicine, but the concern is many of illnesses/disease are successfully treated by traditional or indigenous medicine. It has to be recognized and used in public health sector by which more numbers of people get benefited in terms of health and finance.

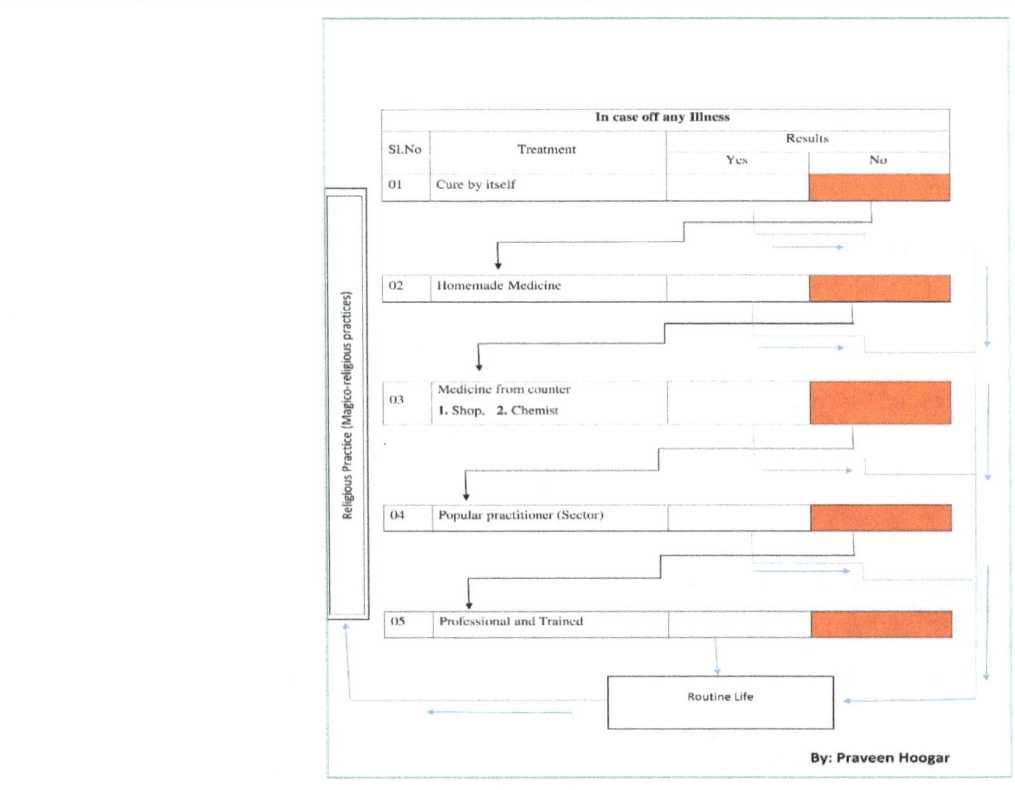

Figure 1: Religious practice (Magico religious practices).

Acknowledgement

Authors acknowledge the each and every member of the community Halakki Vokkalu for their cooperation and constant support during the research work.

References

1. Probart CK, Davis LG, Hibbard JH, Kime RE (1989) "Factors that influence the elderly to use traditional or nontraditional nutrition information sources". J Am Diet Assoc 89: 1758-1762.

2. Fajemilehin BR, Odebiyi AI (2011) "Predictors of elderly person quality of life and health practices in Nigeria". Int J Sociol Anthropol 3: 245-252.

3. http://backwardclasses.kar.nic.in/PDF/Caste/GB-Caste7.PDF

4. Gazetter of the Bombay Presidency (1883) Government of central press, Bombay.

5. Mazzilli C, Daris A (2009) "Health care seeking behavior in somalia: A literature view" UNICEF, Unite for Children.

6. Foster GM, Anderson BG (1978) Medical Anthropology. John Wiley and sons Inc. USA.

7. Majumdar DN (1961) Anthropology and Primitive Medicine, Majumdar DN (ed.) 'Races and Cultures of India (4th edn.). Asia Publishing House, Bombay, India pp: 452-456.

8. Nayak NR (2012) Halakki Vokkaligaru-A cultural study. In: Prakashana G (ed.). Bangalore, India.

9. Kumari P (2006) 'Etiology and healing practices: A study in primitive societies of jarkhand'. Serial Publications, New Delhi, India pp: 487-499.

10. Pujar A, Hoogar P, Basavanagouda TT (2016) An Assessment of Nutritional Status among Jenukuruba Tribe of Kodagu District. J Commun Med Health Educ 6: 468.

11. Pujar A, Hoogar P, Basavanagouda TT (2017) An Anthropometric Profile among the Koraga Tribe of Udupi District, Karnataka State. Int J Adv Res 5: 685-689.

38

Perceptions and Use of Medicinal Herbs among College Students at a Jordanian University in Amman-Jordan: Traditions Supersedes Education

Abdelmalek SMA*, Alkhawaja B and Darwish DA

Department of Pharmacology and Biomedical Sciences, University of Petra, Amman, Jordan

Abstract

Herbs serve as valuable remedies in many cultures. They offer an alternative to increasingly ineffective drugs. This study assesses the perceptions and determinants of medicinal herbs use among students at University of Petra, Amman, Jordan. A cross-sectional study involving randomly selected students from pharmacy and non-pharmacy specialties is conducted based on self-administered questionnaire. The sample involved 350 students (168 pharmacy and 182 non-pharmacy students). Medicinal herbs use as an alternative to medication is reported by 80% of pharmacy and 65% of non-pharmacy students. Sixty three percent of all students prefer using medicinal herbs over visiting a physician, as it is perceived easier and safer by 63% and 35% of pharmacy and 65% and 30% of non-pharmacy students, respectively. Lack of medical insurance significantly encouraged herbal use (p<0.001). Major sources of information on medicinal herbs use included family as reported by 71% of non-pharmacy and university education (53%) as reported by pharmacy students, however, 33% of pharmacy students reported family to be their major source of information of which 76% of them were second year students who were not yet exposed to education about herbs. Wrong choice and preparation of herbs are noted in 91% of non-pharmacy and 63% of pharmacy students. Abdominal pain is the primary reason for using medicinal herbs as reported by 98% and 87% of non-pharmacy and pharmacy students, respectively. Followed by upper respiratory tract infections (URTI), reported by 11% of pharmacy and 2% of non-pharmacy students. One per cent of pharmacy students who were in their fourth year mentioned diabetes and hypercholesterolemia as ailments that can be treated by herbs. None of the participants chose depression, insomnia, headache or migraine as an indication for which medicinal herbs can be used. The use of medicinal herbs among students is prevalent. It is primarily influenced by culture, however, further guidance to avoid faults in herbal choice and preparation is demanded.

Keywords: Medicinal herbs; College students; Traditions; Jordan

Introduction

Herbs are a valuable source of remedies in many cultures worldwide. Human beings used herbs for culinary as well as curative purposes for several thousand years [1]. Herbal medicine is a popular branch of alternative medicine. It offers an alternative to the increasingly ineffective drugs. According to the World Health Organization (WHO) more than three-quarters of the world's population rely on traditional medicine, mainly medicinal herbs [2]. Arabs are no exception to this; they used herbal medicine long time ago. In fact, the traditional Arabic and Islamic medicine is based on the use of a single plant or a mixture of plants to treat diseases [2]. Medicinal herbs fall under the category of traditional nutraceuticals that have been used in prevention and treatment of several non-infectious (e.g., diabetes [3], depression [4], insomnia [5] and dyslipidemia [6]) as well as infectious diseases [7]. Their action is fundamental when considering patients who are intolerant to certain medications [6].

In the international setting, use of herbs was investigated among various populations; young and elderly. In the Middle East, many studies discussed use of medicinal herbs among adult populations [1,8-11]. Nonetheless, little is known about herbs use among college students in this region of the world. Being a wide societal segment, it is important to understand college students' health patterns and practices. They are young, active and more approving of new approaches to health care [12,13]. Besides, students can play a significant role in the spread of health-related information to the society particularly if they will become members of the medical field.

In the Arab world, however, strong connections between family members prevail. Siblings are adherent to their families and show respect to their ancestors' experiences [14]. This led to the assumption that herbal use among Arab students would be influenced by their families. The current study is set to assess the awareness, perceptions and use of medicinal herbs among students at University of Petra, Amman, Jordan. It also aims at identifying factors that impact use of herbs, and examines the assumption that cultural beliefs and ancestors' advice have a greater influence over students' herbal use practices compared to education.

Materials and Methods

A cross-sectional self-administered questionnaire-based survey was conducted between October 2009 and January 2010. The study proposal was reviewed and approved by the Scientific Research Council at the University of Petra.

The sample involved university students from pharmacy and non-pharmacy faculties, namely; the faculties of Arts and Science and Information technology, at the University of Petra-Amman, Jordan. Pharmacy students were randomly enrolled from second, third and fourth year levels. This was intended in order to reflect the impact of education on herbs use, as the pharmacy program includes three academic courses on herbs introduced at the third year level. These courses are a pharmacognosy course, that introduces students to medicinal herbs, their constituents, methods of collection, drying, preparation, and preservation, as well as uses, and two phytochemistry courses (1&2), that focuses on the biosynthesis and the chemical and

*Corresponding author: Abdelmalek SMA, Department of Pharmacology and Biomedical Sciences, The Faculty of Pharmacy and Medical Sciences, University of Petra, Amman, Jordan, E-mail: sabdelmalek@uop.edu.jo

physiochemical properties of the principal classes of natural mixtures used in therapy.

The students were invited to participate in the study and verbal consent was sought before handing in the questionnaires, confidentiality and anonymity of the results were assured. To organize the process of questionnaire distribution and prevent overlap or repetition, questionnaires were given simultaneously to all students attending lectures from 9 to 10 am and collected at the end of the lecture.

The questionnaire was constructed upon reviewing relevant literature. It was field-tested to assure its applicability and comprehensiveness. The questionnaire was primarily written in English, and then translated into Arabic; the mother tongue spoken in Jordan. Translation was validated by a fluent speaker of both languages. The questionnaire comprised of 26 questions, which enquired about students' demography, specialty and year of study, medical insurance status and having a physician in the family. It also asked about relatives' use of herbs and whether herbs were used for culinary or medicinal purposes. Sources of information about medicinal herbs were investigated by giving students the choices of family, physicians, university education, or media (television, radio, newspaper) to choose from. Moreover, it explored the use of herbs as an alternative to drug therapy, as a prophylaxis versus treatment, and as self- directed therapy versus visiting a doctor. Also students' knowledge of the proper uses of certain herbs in the management of common diseases was explored. This was by providing a list of commonly used herbs in the local setting (e.g., chamomile, thyme, sage, mint, green tea, cinnamon, cardamom and senna) and diseases (e.g., upper respiratory tract infections, abdominal pain, constipation, weight loss, insomnia, headache, and diabetes) to match. The method of preparation of herbs (infusion versus decoction) and whether any education was received in this regard were also investigated.

Data handling and statistical analysis

Data were entered onto and analyzed for frequencies using Microsoft Office Excel 2013. Statistical significance calculated using χ^2 test on SPSS. Significance was defined as a p value ≤ 0.05. Missing data were omitted from the analysis, which were believed to be minimal.

Results

Sample demography

Three hundred and fifty students participated in this study. The sample consisted of two groups; pharmacy students (n=168) and non-pharmacy students (n=182). Pharmacy students were distributed as 53 (31.5%), 73 (43.5%), and 42 (25%) in second, third and fourth year levels, respectively. More than half of sample have no medical insurance. Both student groups were similar in terms of having a doctor in the family (Table 1).

Use of medicinal herbs among college students: A majority of all students (82% of both pharmacy and non-pharmacy students) kept herbs at home (Table 2), they did so for culinary purposes over remedy. Third year pharmacy students constituted the majority of pharmacy students who kept herbs at home whether for cooking (n=48,44) or for treatment purposes (n=25, 43%). They were followed by second year then fourth year students (Table 3).

Eighty percent of pharmacy and sixty five percent of non-pharmacy students stated that they used herbs as an alternative to medication. Sixty four percent of pharmacy and non-pharmacy students used herbs for treatment rather than prophylaxis purposes (Table 2). However,

variations existed among pharmacy students at different study years in terms of intention behind using herbs (Table 3). Moreover, self-medication with herbs is practiced by 63% of all students over visiting a doctor when feeling ill. This was similar between both pharmacy and non-pharmacy students (Table 2).

Determinants of using medicinal herbs: Insurance status was found to be inversely correlated with the use of medicinal herbs. Uninsured students reported a significantly higher level of herbal use (p<0.001) compared to insured ones (Figure 1). Insurance also significantly (p<0.001) determined the tendency of students to visit doctors for treatment. 28.4% have insurance and go to the doctor versus 13.7% don't have insurance and go to the doctor.

Other factors which rendered self-medicating with herbs preferred over visiting a doctor included primarily easiness of herbs use (63% of pharmacy and 65% of non-pharmacy), and a perceived safety of herbs compared to drugs by 35% of pharmacy and 30% of non-pharmacy students. The relatively low cost of medicinal herbs, on the other hand, did not impact choosing them over visiting a doctor in both groups (Table 2). A majority of pharmacy (71%) and non-pharmacy (77%) students had a family member that used medicinal herbs at some time. Almost 90% of pharmacy and non-pharmacy students had a doctor in their families (Table 1). Nonetheless, the presence of a doctor in the family did not have a significant impact on controlling use of herbs (P=1) instead of medicine, since 64.4% of these students used herbs. Oppositely, 25% of those who did not have a doctor in their families also used herbs (Figure 2).

Variable	Number of students [%]
Specialty	
Pharmacy	168 [48]
Non-pharmacy	182 [52]
Total	350 [100]
Insurance status	
Insured	150 [44]
Uninsured	192 [56]
Total	342 [98]
Number of students with a doctor in the family	
Pharmacy	149 [89]
Non-pharmacy	163 [90]
Total	312 [89]

Table 1: Demography of the study sample.

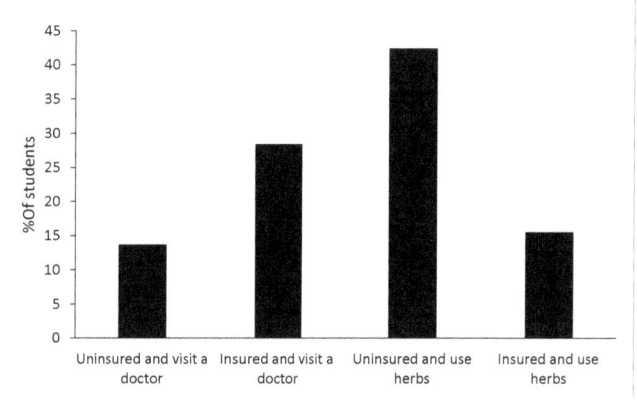

Figure 1: Effect of having medical insurance on the use of herbs. Correlation study performed between having medical insurance and tendency to use herbs. χ^2 Test applied. p≤0.05 is considered significant. P=0.001.

	Pharmacy students	Non-pharmacy students	Total %
Do you keep herbs at home?	**137 [81.5]**	**149 [81.9]**	**286 [81.7]**
Reason for keeping herbs at home			
Cooking	110 [65]	154 [85]	264 [75]
Remedy	58 [35]	28 [15]	68 [19]
Does any member of your family use herbs?	**120 [71]**	**141 [77.5]**	**261 [75]**
Did you ever use herbs as an alternative to medicine	**134 [80]**	**118 [65]**	**252 [72]**
Do you use herbs for:			
Prophylaxis	60 [36]	66 [36]	126 [36]
Treatment	108 [64]	116 [64]	224 [64]
If you exhibit symptoms of disease, you:			
Self-medicate with herbs	106 [63]	114 [63]	220 [63]
Visit a physician	62 [37]	68 [37]	130 [37]
Why do you prefer using herbs over going to the doctor when ill			
Safer	59 [35]	55 [30]	114 [33]
Easier	106 [63]	118 [65]	224 [64]
Lower cost	3 [2]	9 [5]	12 [3]

*Only yes answers are recorded.

Table 2: Perceptions* and use of medicinal herbs among the study sample.

	Pharmacy Students N [%]			
Study year	**2nd**	**3rd**	**4th**	**Total**
You keep herbs at home for:				
Cooking	34 [31]	48 [44]	28 [25]	110
Treatment	18 [31]	25 [43]	15 [26]	58
You use herbs for:				
Prophylaxis	19 [31]	26 [43]	15 [26]	60
Treatment	33 [31]	48 [44]	27 [25]	108
You prefer to use herbs over visiting a physician when you feel ill because it is:				
Safer	13 [22]	29 [49]	17 [29]	59
Easier	38 [36]	42 [40]	25 [24]	106
Less cost	1 [25]	2 [50]	1 [25]	4

Table 3: The use of Medicinal herbs by pharmacy students as classified by study year.

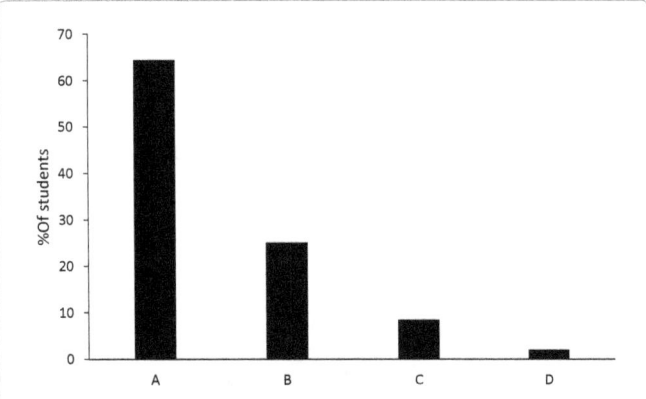

Figure 2: Does the presence of doctors in families influence the use of herbs. Correlation study performed between having a doctor in the family and the tendency to use herbs. χ² Test applied. p≤0.05 is considered significant. P value =1. (A): Have doctor in the family and use herbs. (B): Have doctor in the family and don't use herbs. (C): No doctor in the family and use herbs. (D): No doctor in the family and don't use herbs.

Sources of information on medicinal herbs: Eighty one percent of pharmacy students acknowledged receiving education about medicinal herbs whereas 75% of non-pharmacy students gave a negative answer.

Sources of information among both student groups differed, where university education on herbs was the major source of information for pharmacy students (53%), this was not applicable to non-pharmacy students who received no education about herbs at university (Table 4). A majority of pharmacy students who indicated university education as a source of information were in third year (63%) compared to 37% who were fourth year students (Table 4). Non-pharmacy students (71%) considered family the primary source of information about herbs, and 29% obtained their information from television. However, 33% of pharmacy students considered family as a source of information on this matter those were mainly second year students (76%) (Table 4).

Physicians were not considered as a source of information on medicinal herbs by any of the sample. Seventy percent of students who visited doctors stated that even when physicians asked about herbal use they did not provide relevant advice nor education.

Preparation of medicinal herbs: A majority of non-pharmacy and pharmacy students, 91% and 65%, respectively, prepared herbs by decoction (boiling) (Figure 3). Among pharmacy students third year students were the most to apply decoction (53%), whereas fourth year students were the least to use it (9%). On the other hand, infusion was applied by 39% of pharmacy students, most of which were fourth year students. This latter method was used by only 9% of non-pharmacy students (Figure 3).

	Pharmacy students %				Non-pharmacy students %			
Did you receive any education about herbs	**Yes**			**No**	**Yes**			**No**
	81			19	25			75
Sources of information on herbs*	**2ndt**	**3rdt**	**4tht**	**total**	**Non-pharmacy**			
University education	0	63	37	53	0			
Family	76	15	9	33	71			
TV	48	33	19	13	29			
Magazine	0	67	33	2	0			
Did Physicians ask about use of herbs	**Yes**			**No**	**Yes**			**No**
	74			26	66			34

'Participant could choose more than one of the listed sources of information.
†2nd, 3rd, 4th: Study year.

Table 4: Sources of student information on medicinal herbs.

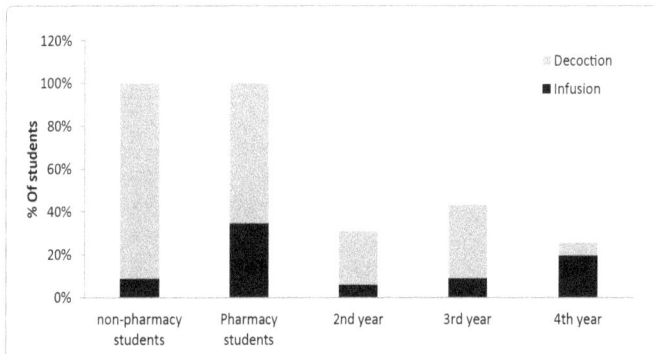

Figure 3: Are herbs consumed through decoction or infusion. Percentage of 2nd, 3rd, 4th year pharmacy students is calculated from total pharmacy students using a certain method.

Use of medicinal herbs to treat common illnesses: Abdominal pain is the major reason for which herbs were used as reported by 98% and 87% of non-pharmacy and pharmacy students, respectively. This is followed by upper respiratory tract infections (URTI), reported by 11% of pharmacy and 2% of non-pharmacy students (Figure 4). Most of the pharmacy students who used herbs to treat abdominal pain and URTI were in their third year level (Figure 4). In the management of URTI, 50% of non-pharmacy and 32% of pharmacy students preferred using medication over medicinal herbs (Figure 5A). The majority of pharmacy students who preferred using medication were in their second year level. The rest of pharmacy students who used herbs (68%), listed a variety of medicinal herbs, namely thyme, chamomile and sage (Figure 5A). Thyme was the herb chosen by most pharmacy and non-pharmacy students to manage URTI (Figure 5A). As for abdominal pain, 48% of non-pharmacy and 43% of pharmacy students preferred visiting a doctor over using medicinal herbs. Sage was the primary herb used for abdominal pain by both groups (Figure 5B). Constipation was managed in 42% of non-pharmacy and 51% of pharmacy students by drinking green tea, a minority used thyme (almost 10% of both groups), those were mainly either second year pharmacy or non-pharmacy students. Senna was used to a lesser extent, mainly by fourth year pharmacy students (Figure 5C). As for weight loss, green tea was the primary herb used by 86% of pharmacy students (46% in third year level) and 61% of non-pharmacy students (Figure 5D). One percent of pharmacy students who were in their year mentioned diabetes and hypercholesterolemia as ailments that can be treated by herbs. None of the participants chose depression, insomnia, headache or migraine as an indication for which medicinal herbs can be used.

Discussion

Use of medicinal herbs is prevalent between college students in this study, which complied with a previous Jordanian study [15]. Our assumption that students' use of medicinal herbs is positively affected by their families proved to be valid. Yet, a major determinant that affected herbal use, whenever provided, was education. A proof of this is the resemblance in responses between second year pharmacy and non-pharmacy students. Being not yet exposed to herbs-relevant academic courses at their second year of study rendered them depending on their families to obtain information about herbs. Whereas third year pharmacy students showed more awareness of the medicinal uses of herbs, their prophylactic and treatment effects compared to second and fourth year students. However, when it comes to the handling of herbs, education didn't seem to correct faulty cultural believes. It is known that herbs containing volatile oils decompose and/or lose activity if exposed to high temperatures for long periods [16]. Having the majority of students in this study boiling herbs before use revealed unawareness of proper preparation.

The indications for medicinal herbs reported herein were much fewer than those named in other studies [14,17]. While most participants in this study agreed that herbs are mainly used for abdominal pain and URTI, participants in a similar study carried in the USA indicated that the most frequent conditions for which herbs are used, musculoskeletal conditions, stomach or intestinal illnesses, anxiety/depression, insomnia, severe headache or migraine, menopause, cholesterol, and recurring pain [17]. This reflected the unawareness of the current study population of the potential uses of herbs. In fact, having a minority of pharmacy students acknowledging the role of herbs in the management of diabetes and dyslipidemia indicated substantial unawareness of medicinal herbs use. The choice of correct medicinal herb in treating some common illnesses constituted another challenge to non-pharmacy and pharmacy students. The use of sage for respiratory conditions is an incorrect practice. Sage is mainly indicated in cases of fever, digestive disorders and stomachache [18]. Similarly, the use of thyme to treat constipation is a suboptimal practice, as senna proved to be more effective [19].

It was interesting to note that the presence of a physician in a family did not affect the use of herbs. This could be explained by the lack of physician input into patients' education on the use of herbs as shown in the results. The literature showed how health care professionals, among which physicians, could play an important role in raising public's awareness on the proper use of herbs in treating diseases [20].

Also, of worth reporting is the tendency of pharmacy students in this study not to apply the information gained from the academic courses taught. This was clearly reflected by the responses of fourth year pharmacy students, which posed a question on how effective were the academic courses provided to them.

Despite the proven benefits from using medicinal herbs, the potential harm associated with their use should be emphasized [21], having a majority of students preferring the use of herbs, because they believed they were safe, is a prevalent misconception. In fact, there is an increasing concern about the safety of some medicinal herbs. Accidental herbal toxicity occurs not only as a result of lack of quality

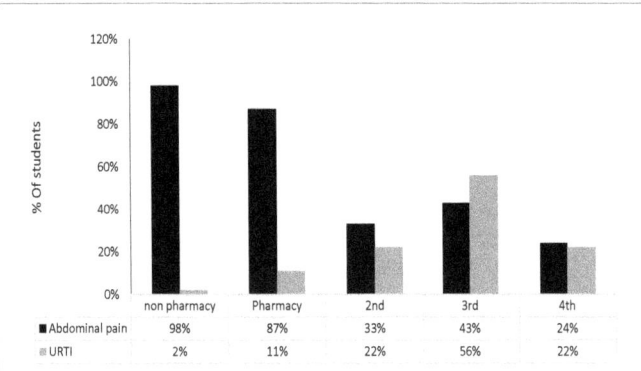

Figure 4: Common illnesses for which herbs are used. Students were questioned about illnesses they would use herbs for. Eight major disorders were included: abdominal pain, URTI, depression, insomnia, headache, diabetes, migraine, hypercholesterolemia. Answers came only for abdominal pain and URTI. And all other disorders were not chosen. Only two students from 4th year chose diabetes and hypercholesterinemia. Percentage of 2nd, 3rd, 4th year pharmacy students is calculated from total pharmacy students.

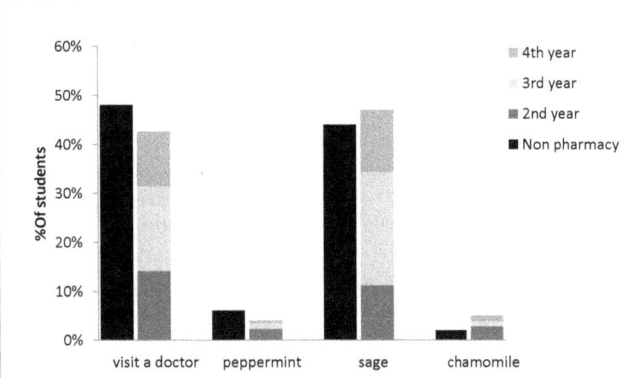

Figure 5A: Managing URTI infections. Students were questioned about how they would react at URTI infections, whether they would go to a specialist to seek medication or choose from a variety of herbs. Percentage of 2nd, 3rd, 4th year pharmacy students is calculated from total pharmacy students.

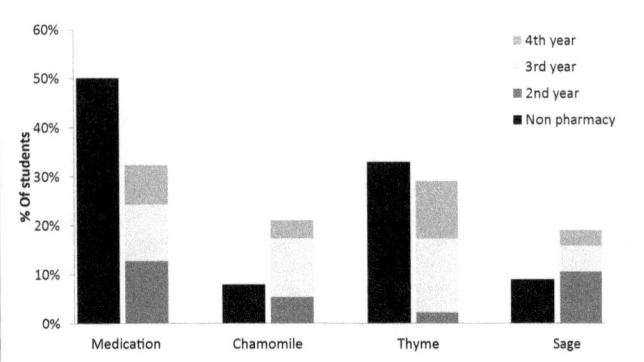

Figure 5B: Managing abdominal pain. Students were questioned about how they would react at abdominal pain, whether they would go to a specialist to seek medication or choose from a variety of herbs. Percentage of 2nd, 3rd, 4th year pharmacy students is calculated from total pharmacy students.

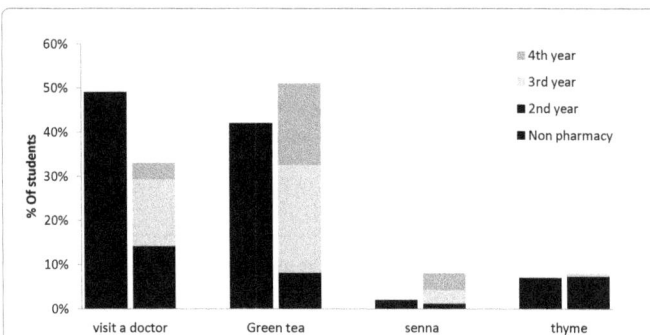

Figure 5C: Managing constipation. Students were questioned about how they would react at constipation, whether they would go to a specialist to seek medication or choose from a variety of herbs. Percentage of 2nd, 3rd, 4th year pharmacy students is calculated from total pharmacy students.

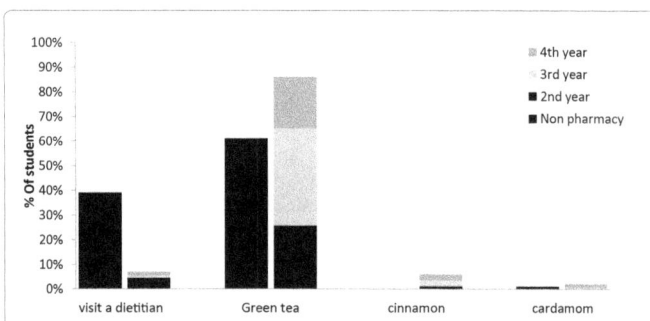

Figure 5D: Managing weight loss. Students were questioned about how they would react at weight loss, whether they would go to a specialist to seek medication or choose from a variety of herbs. Percentage of 2nd, 3rd, 4th year pharmacy students is calculated from total pharmacy students.

control over harvesting and preparing herbs, but also due to the false belief they are harmless [21].

Lack of insurance and the low income per capita evident in Jordan supported the use of herbs. This was further endorsed by the fact that those who had medical insurance reported using medicine over herbs to treat illnesses.

Study Limitations

Limitations to the study are those expected with self-administered surveys, first, where students might have over or under reported their use of herbs. Second, the fact that there are too many herbs sold in the market used for a wide array of indications and not all of them were listed in our study. However, we chose the most popular ones that are believed to be known by everyone regardless of their background and used for very common illnesses.

Conclusion

The use of medicinal herbs among students is prevalent. The influence of traditional beliefs on use of herbs is substantial. However, whenever education is provided it does shape practices relevant to herbs. Yet gaps in the awareness of the potential uses of herbs and their proper preparation are evident. More relevant education and hands-on practice are required to fill these gaps.

References

1. Abu Rabia A (2005) Herbs as a food and medicine source in Palestine. Asian Pacific J Cancer Prev 6: 404-407.

2. Azaizeh H, Saad B, Cooper E, Said O (2010) Traditional Arabic and Islamic medicine, a re-emerging health aid. Evid Based Complement Alternat Med 7: 419- 424.

3. Rizvi SI, Mishra N (2013) Traditional Indian medicines used for the management of Diabetes Mellitus. J Diabetes Res 2013.

4. Basti AA, Moshiri E, Noorbala AA, Jamshidi AH, Abbasi SH, et al. (2007) Comparison of petal of Crocus sativus L and fluoxetine in the treatment of depressed outpatients: a pilot double-blind randomized trial. Prog Neuropsychopharmacol Biol Psychiatry 31: 439-442.

5. Wing YK (2001) Herbal treatment of insomnia. Hong Kong Med J 7: 392-402.

6. Scicchitano P, Cameli M, Maiello M, Modesti PA, Muiesan ML, et al. (2014) Nutraceuticals and dyslipidaemia: Beyond the common therapeutics. J Funct Foods 6: 11-32.

7. Ewam UP (2014) Evidence based antibacterial potentials of medicinal plants and herbs countering bacterial pathogens especially in the era of emerging drug resistance: An integrated update. Int J Pharmacol 10: 1-43.

8. Afifi FU, Abu-Irmaileh B (2000) Herbal medicine in Jordan with special emphasis on less commonly used medicinal herbs. J Ethnopharmacol 72: 101-110.

9. Abu Irmaileh BE, Afifi FU (2003) Herbal medicine in Jordan with special emphasis on commonly used herbs. J Ethnopharmacol 89: 193-197.

10. Alzweiri M, Al Sarhan A, Mansi K, Hudaib M, Aburjai T (2011) Ethnopharmacological survey of medicinal herbs in Jordan, the Northern Badia region. J Ethnopharmacol 137: 27-35.

11. Wazaify M, Afifi FU, El-Khateeb M, Ajlouni K (2011) Complementary and alternative medicine use among Jordanian patients with diabetes. Complement Ther Clin Pract 17: 71-75.

12. Rogers EM (1995) Diffusion of Innovations (4th edn.) ACM The Free Press.

13. Dwairy M (2003) Validation of multigenerational interconnectedness scale among Arab adolescents. Psychol Rep 93: 697-704.

14. Johnson SK, Blanchard A (2006) Alternative medicine and herbal use among university students. J Am Coll Health Assoc 55: 163-168.

15. Khader Y, Sawair FA, Ayoub A, Ayoub N, Burgan SZ, et al. (2008) Knowledge and attitudes of lay public, pharmacists, and physicians toward the use of herbal products in North Jordan. J Altern Complement Med 14: 1186-1187.

16. Turek C, Stintzing FC (2013) Stability of essential oils: a review. Compr Rev Food Sci Food Saf 12: 40-53.

17. Gardiner P, Graham R, Legedza AT, Ahn AC (2007) Factors associated with herbal therapy use by adults in the United States. Altern Ther Health Med 13: 22-29.

18. Lima CF, Andrade PB, Seabra RM, Fernandes FM, Pereira WC (2005) The drinking of a Salvia officinalis infusion improves liver antioxidant status in mice and rats. J Ethnopharmacol 97: 383-389.

19. Kinnunen O, Winblad I, Koistinen P, Salokannel J (1993) Safety and efficacy of a bulk laxative containing senna versus lactulose in the treatment of chronic constipation in geriatric patients. Pharmacology 47: 253-255.

20. Bauer BA (2000) Herbal therapy: what a clinician needs to know to counsel patients effectively. Mayo Clinic Proceedings.

21. Saad B, Azaizeh H, Abu-Hijleh G, Said O (2006) Safety of traditional Arab herbal medicine. Evid Based Complement Alternat Med 3: 433-439.

39

Oral Hygiene – Knowledge, Attitude and Practice among the Health Worker (ANM/ASHA) of Kamrup (Metro) District in North East Region of India

Umakanta Prusty*

Regional Research Institute (H), Guwahati, Assam, India

Abstract

Background and aim: Oral health is an integral part of the general health and wellbeing of an individual to maintain the quality of life. As there is no valid and reliable instrument for identifying the Knowledge, Attitude and Practice (KAP) among the grass root level health workers (ANM/ASHA) in the field of oral hygiene. Therefore an instrument has been designed to identify their concerns i.e., KAP. So that their KAP on oral health awareness could be updated through different training programs and thereby we can achieve the aim to assess the oral hygiene awareness and practice among the ANM/ASHA to provide insight into educational programs.

Design and methods: A cross sectional survey was carried out to assess the KAP among the health workers (ANM/ASHA) through self-constructed, 28-items and a close-ended questionnaire. The questionnaire was pilot tested on 34-ANM to identify its internal consistency and the reliability for the different subscales (KAP). After the questionnaire is pilot tested on ANM, then it was again tested on 172-ASHA of the pre-selected zones.

Results: The entire questionnaire was developed and evaluated by using Cronbach's alpha (α) and found to be 0.719. This indicates a high level of internal consistency (α>0.71). Since the internal consistency of subscale items is<0.70, it needs to be further evaluation and development of questionnaire with respect to subscale. In this study it was found that there is a lack of knowledge on oral health awareness among the primary health care provider (ANM/ASHA). Hence there is a need to educate and spread knowledge of proper dental care and to prevent dental disease through motivation, training and education for the health workers to make a healthy individual and healthy society.

Keywords: Knowledge; Attitude; Practice; KAP; Oral hygiene; ANM and ASHA

Introduction

Oral diseases are a major public health concern owing to their high prevalence and their effects on the individual's quality of life [1]. Oral health attitude and beliefs are significant for oral health behavior [2]. One of the most important factors that decide the dental health of a population is the outlook of its people toward their dentition [3]. Oral health knowledge is considered to be an essential prerequisite for health related behavior [4,5]. Keeping a healthy oral profile requires joint efforts from the dentist as well as the patient himself.

The majority of the people in India from the low socioeconomic strata of society have never visited dentist or been for a dental check-up. This is primarily because of economic constraints, insufficient awareness and low literacy rates. Poor oral health can cause discomfort, pain, disability and diminish the quality of life. Sometimes it even contributes to systemic diseases like diabetes, cardiovascular and lung disease. Community based oral health and hygiene can be improved and various oral/dental diseases can be prevented by creating awareness among the public which can be carried out by grass root level health workers (ANM/ASHA). Such workers who are the connecting link between the public and health care delivery system should possess minimum knowledge regarding oral health and hygiene. While education should be promoted, especially in high-risk communities and population groups (low-income families and native population), it should be carried out by the trained grass root level health workers. Therefore a study is carried out to assess the training need through KAP study regarding oral hygiene. According to the literature, no study has been done to assess the oral hygiene awareness and practice in North East Region (NER) of India till now. Kamrup (Metro) District is being the largest city in the state of Assam with an area of 1,527.84 square km and population of 1,260,419 (census 2011) [6]. Keeping in this view, Central Council for Research in Homoeopathy (CCRH), autonomous bodies under Ministry of AYUSH, Govt. of India has planned to

conduct a pilot study on 'Health promotion during Dentition' under Capital and Dhirenpara zone of Kamrup (Metro) District of Assam in North East Region (NER) with a target age group (6 month–36 month) of 28885.

The program has been implemented through ANM/ASHA worker of the concerned zone for the age group (6 month–36 month) of children. Before implementing the program an instrument has been designed and tested to identify the Knowledge, Attitude and Practice (KAP) amongst the ANM/ASHA through a close-ended questionnaire.

Aims of the Survey

1. To develop an instrument for assessing the KAP for oral hygiene among the grass root level health worker.

2. To assess the need of training among the ANM/ASHA in Kamrup (Metro) District of Assam regarding the oral hygiene awareness and practice.

3. To evaluate the effectiveness of the training programs to be organized by CCRH professionals for grass root level health workers.

Materials and Methods

An institutional cross sectional survey was carried out to assess

***Corresponding author:** Umakanta Prusty, Regional Research Institute (H), Guwahati, Assam, India, E-mail: druprusty@gmail.com

the Knowledge, Attitude and Practice among the health workers (ANM/ASHA) of two adopted zones (Capital and Dhirenpara) of Kamrup (Metro) District of Assam in North East Region (NER). A self-constructed, 28-item, close-ended questionnaire having four options (A-D) was translated into regional Assamese version using a standardized forward-backward translation process which was conducted independently by two translators. Then the questionnaire was further pre-tested on a small group of study population which consists of 34-ANM, then it was further analyzed, interpreted and finally the questionnaire has been modified after pretesting. The reliability of the questionnaire has been tested by adopting the methods of Cronbach's Alpha test.

The duration of the study spanned over a period of one month from January 2014 to February 2014. A specially designed questionnaire consisting of three sections was used, these consisted of firstly questions based on the dental knowledge which included ten questions, secondly section based on the attitude of dental health, which included five questions and the last section was based on practice of oral hygiene which comprised of thirteen questions. All the 230- health workers (ANM/ASHA) were approached personally, 24-refused; finally 206 had given their written consent for participation. So final sample size was 206 (ANM-34 and ASHA-172) (n=206) who submitted their completed questionnaires in sealed envelope, hence the response rate was 89.56%.

Total 206-health workers (ANM-34 and ASHA-172) were explained the purpose of the study along with handing over of the questionnaire. The questionnaire took about 30 min. to complete. Instructions on the questionnaire promised anonymity. No identifiable information was required, thus protecting participant privacy. The completed questionnaires were concealed inside opaque envelopes, which were sealed at the survey site by participants themselves. It was also mentioned that responses would remain confidential. All survey forms were collected by the Research Associates and were sent for data analysis. All the subjects were interviewed in the premises of Regional Research Institute for Homoeopathy, Guwahati, Assam. The interviews were conducted in regional language Assamese, as it was the medium of instruction.

All demographic data and the quantitative data obtained via the questionnaires were analyzed by SPSS (Statistical package for social sciences) Windows version 20. Frequencies and cross-tabulations were performed. The reliability of the qualitative data analysis was enhanced by the independent investigation of the responses by a team approach. The team comprised of one Research Associates (H), two paramedical staff (Lab Technician), four field workers (MPHW) and two Data Entry Operator (DEO) took part of the evaluation. From this, level of agreement was assessed. Pearson's chi-square test was used to find the statistical significance among the health workers (ANM/ASHA) for their responses based on dental knowledge, attitude and practice on systemic conditions related to oral health.

Study Sample and Sampling Technique

The sampling method employed in this survey is convenient sampling. Health workers (ANM-34 and ASHA-172); (n=206) belonging to the two adopted zones (i.e., Capital and Dhirenpara) of Kamrup (Metro) District, Assam were selected.

Ethical clearance

This proposed study was reviewed by the Institutional ethical committee and informed consent was taken from each participant.

Pilot testing of questionnaire

The questionnaire was tested among 34-ANM and the reliability for the different subscales (such as knowledge, attitude and practice) for the questionnaire was evaluated by using Cronbach's alpha, and the results are shown (Tables 1 and 2). The criteria of Cronbach's alpha for establishing the internal consistency reliability: Excellent ($\alpha>0.9$), Good ($0.7<\alpha<0.9$), Acceptable ($0.6<\alpha<0.7$), Poor ($0.5<\alpha<0.6$), Unacceptable ($\alpha<0.5$) [7]. It considered that the Cronbach's alpha value for entire questionnaire was found to be 0.719. This indicates a high level of internal consistency for our scale with this specific sample [8]. Since the internal consistency of subscale items is<0.70, it is suggested that the scale is used in totality and individual subscales are not used until the scale is further developed and the internal consistency of subscale items increases [9]. The scale used in the study is in the process of development. This is the first survey study conducted using this questionnaire. More studies of similar nature are required to develop the scale fully.

As the questionnaire was found to be reliable after testing it upon 34-ANM for the entire questionnaire, the same was used for evaluating 172-ASHA of the preselected zones. The demographic data related to the above two professions are shown (Figure 1) and the evaluation of questionnaire was shown (Figure 2) [10].

All the 28 questions were individually stratified based on designation (ANM/ASHA). As per their response in terms of correct and incorrect answer the observed verses expected values were tested with K-way and higher-order effects using the Chi-Square test. There was a significant difference of response among the profession which is shown (Table 3).

Discussion

Oral health is an essential for one's overall wellness and it is an integral part of one's physical, social and mental wellbeing. Majority of the people are unaware about the relationship between oral hygiene and systemic diseases. Many diseases show their first appearance through oral signs and symptoms and they remain unchanged or untreated because of the lack of Knowledge, Attitude and Practice (KAP) on oral hygiene. Health workers could play a pivotal role in public health awareness. As a health worker, it is their responsibility to educate and

S. No.	Sub-scale	No. of items (N)	Cronbach's α	Cronbach's α based on Standardize d items	ICC	95%CI		F test with True value 0			
					Avg.	LB	UB	Value	df1	df2	p value
1	K	10	0.584	0.544	0.584	0.340	0.765	2.406	33	297	0.000
2	A	5	0.234	0.254	0.234	-0.265	0.576	1.306	33	132	0.148
3	P	13	0.285	0.098	0.285	-0.126	0.593	1.399	33	396	.075
4	KAP	28	0.719	0.673	0.719	0.563	0.839	3.556	33	891	0.000
K: Knowledge; A: Attitude; P: Practice; ICC: Intra Class Correlation; CI: Confidence interval											

Table 1: Reliability statistics for subscales (KAP).

motivate the peoples to visit a dentist to acquire basic dental knowledge [11-14]. In this context, an Institutional cross sectional survey was carried out to assess the knowledge, attitude and practice (KAP) among the health workers (ANM/ASHA) of two selected zones (Capital and Dhirenpara) of Kamrup (Metro) District, Assam through a self-constructed, 28-item, close-ended questionnaire. Out of ten nos. of

Cronbach's Alpha	Cronbach's Alpha Based on Standardized Items	N of Items
0.719	0.673	28

Table 2: Reliability statistics.

K		df	Likelihood Ratio		Pearson	
			Chi-Square	Sig.	Chi-Square	Sig.
	1	111	3891.912	0.000	4027.650	.000
K-way and Higher Order Effectsa	2	82	936.976	0.000	882.457	.000
	3	27	22.542	0.709	21.827	.746
	1	29	2954.936	0.000	3145.193	.000
K-way Effectsb	2	55	914.435	0.000	860.630	.000
	3	27	22.542	0.709	21.827	.746

Table 3: K-way and higher-order effects.

dental knowledge related questionnaire, 1049 (50.92%) responses were incorrect which shows that lack of knowledge on oral health awareness. Out of five questionnaires from attitude, 758 (73.59%) responses were wrong. Though 49.08% having some knowledge on oral hygiene but 73.59 % have no attitude for maintaining oral health and hygiene. It also showed that, out of rest thirteen questionnaires belong to practice, 1503 (56.12%) responses were negative. It shows that more than 50% of health workers were not even practicing good oral hygiene. In the present study, out of 206 of health workers (ANM/ASHA) 133 (64.6%) of them have no knowledge to visit a dentist at least once in six months. 156 (75.7%) of health workers did not know the use of dental floss/rinse in maintaining good oral health. 32 (15.5%) were only maintaining good oral health. It was also found that only 29 (14%) ANM/ASHA have visited dentist for their routine oral health checkup. 111 (53.8%) do not take their oral health problem so seriously. 22 (10.67%) have opined that tobacco or betel nut chewing benefits their oral health. 135 (65.5%) of ANM/ASHA didn't know how to do brushing.

The study suggests that there are some definite gaps in KAP among the health workers (ANM/ASHA) of the selected zone and which the clear indication of lack of awareness is. This is confirmed as the health workers could not describe oral health (84.5%), didn't visit dentist (85.9%) and used addictives (79.1%) in the present study [15-17].

This type of study was conducted for the first time in North East

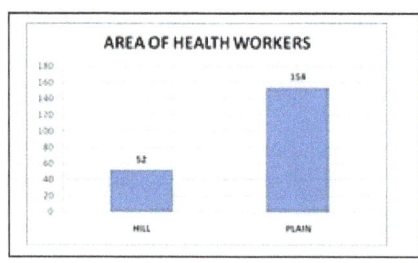
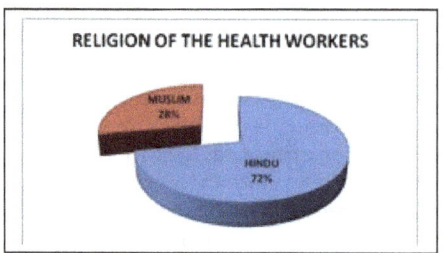
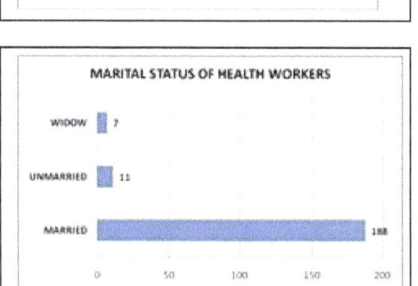
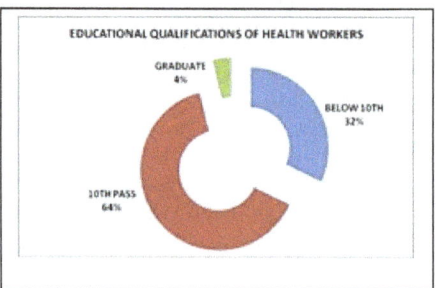

Figure 1: Demographic data of lath workers.

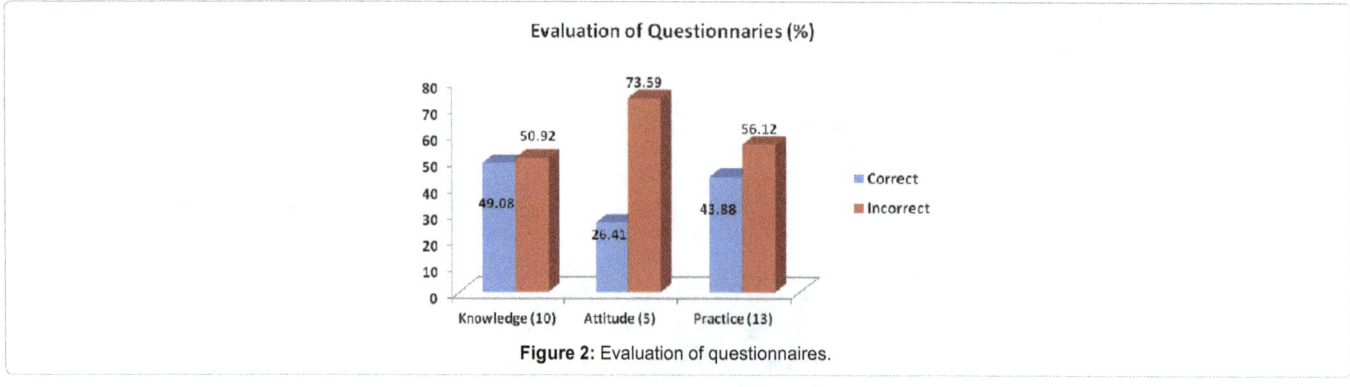

Figure 2: Evaluation of questionnaires.

Questions	KAP	A	B	C	D	Frequency of correct answer	%	Frequency of incorrect answer	%
Q1. What should be ideally used for cleaning teeth	K	11	153	40	2	153	74.3	53	25.7
Q2. How many times should you brush teeth in a day	K	5	154	45	2	154	74.8	52	25.2
Q3. When should you brush your teeth	K	21	4	176	5	176	85.4	30	14.6
Q4. What kind of brush should you Use	K	95	107	2	2	95	46.1	111	53.9
Q5. How often should one use dental floss/ rinse	K	50	80	19	57	50	24.3	156	75.7
Q6. How often one should go for dental scaling	K	58	87	22	39	87	40.2	119	57.8
Q13. How much do you think dental problem can affect your general health	K	119	57	8	22	119	57.8	87	42.2
Q14. How often should one visit a dentist	K	29	73	93	11	73	35.4	133	64.6
Q15. How would you describe your oral health	K	32	131	22	21	32	15.5	174	84.5
Q23. How often did you have teeth or gum problem in last one year	K	15	74	72	45	72	35	134	65
Knowledge(10)	-	-	-	-	-	1011	49.08	1049	50.92
Q21. Why did you last visited a dentist	A	29	57	6	114	29	14.1	177	85.9
Q22. What was the reason that you couldn't go for dental treatment that was needed	A	18	17	111	60	60	29.1	146	70.9
Q24. How often you had treatment for gum disease like dental scaling in last one year	A	15	28	136	27	28	13.6	178	86.4
Q26. Do you think Tobacco or betel nut chewing benefits your oral health	A	22	44	82	58	82	39.8	124	60.2
Q27. Did any oral health professional ever suggested you about benefit of giving up your addiction	A	58	73	36	39	73	35.4	133	64.6
Attitude(5)						272	26.41	758	73.59
Q7. How do you brush your teeth	P	61	71	71	3	71	34.5	135	65.5
Q8. How often do you clean your Teeth	P	19	161	25	1	161	78.2	45	21.8
Q9. Do your toothpaste contain Fluoride	P	118	4	18	66	118	57.3	88	42.7
Q10. How often do you change your Brush	P	45	116	9	36	116	56.3	90	43.7
Q11. How much toothpaste do you use for brushing	P	92	93	17	4	93	45.1	113	54.9
Q12. How often do you take addictive's like tobacco or betel nut	P	9	36	118	43	43	20.9	163	79.1
Q16. Do you have cavities in your Teeth	P	43	64	78	21	78	37.9	128	62.1
Q17. Do you have bleeding gums	P	19	73	102	12	102	49.5	104	50.5

Q18. Do you have bad breath in mouth	P	7	78	70	51	70	34	136	66
Q19. Do you have tartar deposits in Teeth	P	9	97	52	48	52	25.2	154	74.8
Q20. How often did you visit a dentist during last one year	P	60	12	126	8	60	29.1	146	70.9
Q25. How often in last one year dental problem hampered your job/work	P	9	63	26	108	108	52.4	98	47.6
Q28. How do you clean your tongue	P	42	103	56	5	103	50	103	50
Practice (13)	-	-	-	-	-	1175	43.88	1503	56.12

Table 4: The results of the response to the questionnaires after applying it to the 34-ANM and 172-ASHA are shown.

Region (NER) of India on this specific cohort but further studies on different cohorts, on larger samples, and in different geographic areas are needed to identify the gap of KAP. Conducting similar studies a few years later may also prove fruitful to assess the effectiveness of training/education programs. Preventive oral health education is in transitional stage in India. Population based oral health community programs are yet to be implemented for primary health care provider (ANM/ASHA).

Statistical Analysis

The data was first transferred to Microsoft Excel and then the results were analyzed by using IBM SPSS software (v. 20.0). Associations between discreet variables were tested by Chi-square test. In all the cases, $p<0.05$ was considered significant. The demographic details of the respondents were expressed in frequency and percentage (Figure 1). The evaluation of questionnaire was shown (Figure 2). Internal consistency was calculated using Cronbach's coefficient alpha (α) for the three domains (KAP) and total score (Table 4). Intra-class coefficients for each item and total score were estimated (Table 3).

Reliability

The Cronbach's alpha for three parameter (KAP) and their internal consistency along with reliability shown (Tables 1 and 2) respectively. According to the rule of thumb [7]. Cronbach's alpha (α=0.71, $p<0.001$) was acceptable for the questionnaire.

Conclusion and Recommendations

The present study shows that there is need for updating the knowledge of oral health awareness among primary health care provider (ANM/ASHA/AWC) through training/education programs. Moreover, majority of them were not aware of the fact that improper maintenance of oral health may contribute to systemic diseases.

Hence, there is a need to educate and spread knowledge of proper dental care and prevention of dental diseases through training and education for the health workers, outreach programs and relevant public health awareness measures to make a healthy individual and a healthy society.

Although dental health education is a relatively new discipline within dentistry, it is suggested that this education should start at an early stage in life, be delivered by trained personnel and be carefully integrated in general health through homoeopathy system of medicine. Further evaluation of such training program may be ascertained through testing and retesting.

Acknowledgments

The authors would like to acknowledge Dr. Tapan Nath, Research Associates, Regional Research Institute for Homeopathy, Guwahati, Assam for development of the questionnaire and collection of the data. Both Dr. Chintamani Nayak and Dr. Prashant Rath, Lecturer, National Institute of Homoeopathy (NIH) to assist in statistical analysis. Dr. Akshaya Kumar Prusty and Dr. Chittaranjan Kundu, Research Officer(H), R.R.I.(H), Puri, Odisha to assist in preparation of manuscript. The author is grateful to Mr. Sanjoy Das for their sincere efforts in data compilation. The author is also thankful to the entire team of Dentition program and all the ANM/ASHA of adapted two Zone of Kamrup (Metro) District for their participation in this study.

Author Contributions

The author is wholly developed the concept, design, literature search, data interpretation, statistical analysis, manuscript preparation and also edited and reviewed.

References

1. Butt AM, Ahmed B, Parveen N, Yazdanie N (2009) Oral Health related quality of life in complete dentures. Pak Oral Dent J 29: 397-402.

2. Tash RH, O'Shea MM, Cohen K (1969) Testing a Preventive- Symptomatic Theory of dental health behavior. Am J Public Health Nations Health 59: 514-521.

3. Chander Shekar BR, Reddy C, Manjunath BC, Suma S (2011) Dental health awareness, attitude, oral health- related habits, and behaviors in relation to socio-economic factors among the municipal employees of Mysore city. Ann Trop Med Public Health 4: 99-106.

4. Dagli RJ, Tadakamadla S, Dhanni C, Duraiswamy P, Kulkarni S (2008) Self-reported dental health attitude and behavior of dental students in India. J Oral Sci 50: 267-272.

5. Bhat PK, Kumar A, Aruna CN (2010) Preventive oral health knowledge, practice and behavior of patients attending dental institution in Banglore, India. J Int Oral Health 2: 1-6.

6. http://www.census2011.co.in/census/district/156-kamrup-metropolitan.html

7. George D, Mallery P (2003) SPSS for Windows Step by Step: A Simple Guide and Reference. 11.0 Update (4th edn.). Boston: Allyn and Bacon.

8. Mohsen T, Reg D (2011) Making sense of Cronbach's alpha. Int J Med Educ 2: 53-55.

9. Taneja D, Khurana A, Mathew G, Padmanabhan M, Sharma S (2015) Knowledge, attitude, practice, and beliefs about drug proving in students of Homoeopathy. Indian J Res Homoeopath 9: 230-238.

10. Kaliyaperumal K (2004) Guideline for Conducting a Knowledge, Attitude and Practice (KAP) Study. AECS Illuminat 4: 7-9.

11. Mehrotra V, Garg K, Sharma P, Sajid Z, Singh R (2015) A Study Based on Dental Awareness, Knowledge and Attitudes among the Medical Practitioners in and Around Kanpur City (India). J Inter Discipl Med Dent Sci 3: 183.

12. Ghosh S, Panja S, Ghosh T, Sharma P, Sarkar P (2014) Dental Practice Scenario in a Government Homeopathic Hospital in West Bengal, India, J Evid Based Complement Altern Med 19: 200-204.

13. Koley M, Saha S, Arya JS, Choubey G, Ghosh S (2016) Knowledge, Attitude, and Practice Related to Diabetes Mellitus Among Diabetics and Nondiabetics Visiting Homeopathic Hospitals in West Bengal, India J Evid Based Complement Altern Med 21: 39-47.

14. Kapoor D, Gill S, Singh A, Kaur I, Kapoor P (2014) Oral hygiene awareness and practice amongst patients visiting the Department of Periodontology at a Dental College and Hospital in North India. Indian J Dent 5: 64-68.

15. Jain N, Mitra D, Ashok KP, Dundappa J, Soni S (2012) Oral hygiene-awareness and practice among patients attending OPD at Vyas Dental College and Hospital, Jodhpur. J Indian Soc Periodontol 16: 524-528.

16. Mehta A, Pradhan S, Pradhan S, Pradhan S (2013) The Oral Hygiene Habits and General Oral Awareness in Public Schools in Mumbai. Int J Laser Dent 3: 60-67.

17. Bhatnagar R, Kim J, Joyce E (2014) Many, "Candidate Surveys on Program Evaluation: Examining Instrument Reliability, Validity and Program Effectiveness." Am Edu Res J 2: 683-690.

40

Ayurvedic Plants in Brain Disorders: The Herbal Hope

Balkrishna A and Misra LN*

Patanjali Research Foundation, Haridwar-249405, Uttarakhand, India

Abstract

Synthetic drugs for human brain disorders are expensive symptomatic long treatments, sometimes showing serious and unavoidable side effects with poor patient compliance. Therefore, the herbal and Ayurvedic treatments are preferred over synthetic drugs for a range of human brain disorders including, Alzheimer's disease, Parkinson's disease, depression, epilepsy, schizophrenia, anxiety, etc. Ayurvedic system of medicine has traditionally been used in several neurological conditions. The accessibility, negligible incidence of side effects and cost effectiveness of plant products offer considerable advantages. These days much attention is drawn towards the established traditional systems of herbal remedies for many brain disorders, generating positive hopes for the patients. It is estimated that more than 60 million Indian populations suffers from mental disorders while the country lags far behind the world for treatments and spending in the hospitals for mental cure. Nearly 1-2% Indians suffered from schizophrenia and bipolar disorder whereas 5% population showed common mental disorders like depression, anxiety, convulsion, etc. The term mental disease is not restricted to mean insanity and allied conditions of mental derangement but also includes, to a certain extent, the emotional disorders. When emotional factors cross the state of normalcy, one gets deranged to show the syndromes of mental disorder, very often. With the current alarming situation, it is high time to look back to the ancient Indian Ayurvedic system of medicine wherein a number of plants have been described for specific uses for a range of mental disorders, including migraine, epilepsy, convulsion, hysteria, paralysis, memory loss (Alzheimer's), insomnia, anxiety, Parkinson's disease, insanity, depression, etc. The Ayurvedic prescriptions which contain either a single identity of plant or a mixture of plant materials have been proven to be very useful against such disorders. The plant materials prescribed for these problems range from herbs to perennial trees with varied plant parts, ranging from whole plant, roots, stem, bark, leaves, flowers, fruits to seeds. The chemical structure of the major compounds from these plants range from straight chain fatty acids to terpenoids, steroids, flavonoids, alkaloids, peptides, etc. It has been attempted to review the current situation of mental disorder in the society vis-a-vis its effective solution described in the Ayurveda and problem of side effects in synthetic medicines.

Graphical Abstract

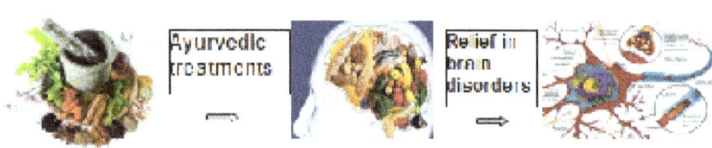

Keywords: Ayurvedic plants; Herbals; Medicinal plants; Brain disorder; Ayurvedic treatment; Ayurvedic uses; Chemical constituents

Introduction

It is rightly accepted that the nature has best answers to all the diseases affecting the human body from time to time. When the synthetic drugs fail to be effective or show serious side effects, it is the plant medicine which brings relief. Many of the plant species distributed throughout the world, have some pharmacological action on the body. Herbal treatment is the natural form of healing therapy to cure the diseases of mankind. Now-a-days, the herbal medicines are back into the prominence because the synthetic medicines, which once had universal acceptance, are now known to often cause side effects. Recently, it has been clinically proved that the treatment of high blood pressure using synthetic medicines is having a negative impact on their patient's mental health [1].

Right from the Vedic period, in India, the traditional knowledge on medicinal plants has been passed on through generations. Ayurveda, which was sourced from Atharvaveda, developed and grew into a well-established medical system due to the untiring efforts and great minds of the sages of "gurukulas". The impact of Ayurveda on the public mind in our country was so deep that even the influence of Middle East and Europe could not deter its popularity among the masses of India and neighboring countries. Herbal medicines in the form of Ayurvedic medicines are still popular and available for common masses due

to the untiring efforts of herbal industries of India, especially the Patanjali, Dabur, Zandu, Baidyanath, Himalaya, etc. These days, the drug discovery is based on the reverse pharmacology of Ayurveda in which the drug candidates are first identified based on their traditional medicinal knowledge, followed by the validations through clinical trials. Although the scattered or selective information on medicinal plants, useful in mental disorders, is available in previous reviews [2-4] but a comprehensive compilation, incorporating the Ayurvedic prescriptions, botanical and chemical aspects of the plants, is hardly traceable. Our continued interest on the chemistry and biology of medicinal and aromatic plants [5-9] prompted us to come up with this review article on some of the plants prescribed in Ayurvedic system of medicine for brain disorders.

***Corresponding author:** Misra LN, Patanjali Research Foundation, Near Patanjali Yog Peeth, NH 58, Haridwar-249405, Uttarakhand, India
E-mail: laxmisra@hotmail.com

Current Situation

Every year 10th October is the date when world mental health day is celebrated all over the world. The awareness regarding the balanced mental health is increasing and it is now recognized as a major cause of morbidity worldwide. As per WHO estimate, depression will be second only to cardiac diseases as the leading cause of morbidity and disability worldwide by 2020 [10]. India is, unfortunately, the leading country in adolescent and young age suicides. The condition is made worse by poor socio-economy, substance abuse, gender inequality and poor health infrastructure to deal with mental health issues. Unfortunately, India has got just 4000 psychiatrist for more than a billion populations. Further, in India, being a mentally ill patient carries huge stigma, this perhaps is the biggest of all barriers for mental treatment. Because of the stigma people don't prefer going to a mental health professional for an early evaluation [11-13].

In a global study, India has been ranked 143rd among 188 countries on a range of health indicators including its poor performance on hygiene. However, India scored well for its better performance in areas like neglected tropical diseases including communicable diseases, overweight and harmful alcohol consumption [14]. As India lags behind the world in medical professionals and spending on mental health issues, it is obvious that more than 60 million Indian populations suffers from mental disorder. Nearly 1-2% of its population suffers from severe mental disorders such as schizophrenia and bipolar disorder. About 5% of the population suffered from common mental disorders like depression and anxiety related problems as per the last report available in 2005. This data was recently quoted by Indian health and family welfare minister from national commission on macroeconomics and health forum. According to a more recent report by National Mental Health Survey (NMHS) commissioned by Government of India and implemented and coordinated by National Institute of Mental Health and Neuro Sciences (NIMHANS), Bangalore, about 150 million Indians aged 18 and above and 7.3% of those aged 13 to 17 years of the total population are suffering from various mental disputes and are in need of mental care service. India's health budget on mental health care is surprisingly 7.5 times lesser than Bangladesh. There is acute shortage of psychiatrists in India with 3 psychiatrists per million populations which is 18 times lesser than the commonwealth nations' norm of 56 psychiatrists per million people. Keeping these facts in mind, a new Bill was passed through Indian Parliament in August 2016 increasing the government funding a little more than before [10-13].

Common Brain Disorders

The term mental disease or brain disorder is not restricted to mean insanity and allied conditions of mental derangement but also includes, to certain extent, the emotional disorders. Often the emotional factors, when cross the state of normalcy, get deranged to become the syndromes of mental disorder. It is stated that the brain has 100 billion nerve cells (neurons) and each of them connect with many others to form communication networks. These nerve cells have special jobs like thinking, learning, remembering as well as to see, hear, and smell. To do their work brain cells, like tiny factories, receive supplies, generate energy, construct equipment, and get rid of the waste. Brain cells also process and store information to communicate with other cells. Keeping everything functional, it requires large amounts of fuel and oxygen for proper coordination [15]. Once the system is disturbed, a range of human brain disorders start appearing, for example, Alzheimer's disease, Parkinson's disease, Huntington's disease, depression, epilepsy, schizophrenia, anxiety, etc. These diseases have

very complex disturbance in the brain function and are beyond the scope of this review. However, a brief description is added here for primary information and understanding the most common brain illnesses.

Alzheimer's disease

Alzheimer's disease (AD) was originally defined as presenile dementia and means an acquired mental disorder with loss of intellectual abilities to interfere with social or occupational functioning. It is associated with localized loss of neurons and brain shrinkage, mainly in the basal fore brain and hippocampus. The beta-amyloid peptide (BAP) plays a significant role in the development of AD. Although there is no cure for AD by synthetic drugs, but, to certain extent, it can be managed with them. Several studies have revealed that natural antioxidants, such as vitamin E, vitamin C, and beta-carotene are useful in scavenging free radicals generated during the progression of this disease. The loss of memory is considered to be the result of shortage of a nerve transmitter, acetylcholine. By inhibiting the activity of the enzyme, acetyl cholinesterase, which splits or breaks down the transmitter substance, it is possible to increase the level of this transmitter in the brain. Synthetic drugs that inhibit the breakdown of the messenger or transmitter acetylcholine, may delay the development of the disease [16,17].

Anxiety

Anxiety is a psychological and physiological state characterized by cognitive, somatic, emotional, and behavioral factors. These factors combine to create an unpleasant feeling that is typically associated with fear, worry or uneasiness. Without an identifiable triggering stimulus, anxiety is a generalized mood state. In fact, it is distinguished from fear, which occurs in the presence of an external threat. As such, anxiety is the result of threats that are perceived to be uncontrollable or unavoidable whereas fear is related to the specific behaviors of avoidance and escape [18].

Depression

Depression is a common affective disorder of mood rather than disturbances of thought or cognition. It is the most common affective disorder which is accompanied by delusions and hallucination. In this disease condition, the neurotransmitters levels such as dopamine, acetylcholine, nor epinephrine etc., in the brain are increased. The symptoms of this disease are of two types (i) biological symptoms: retardation of thought, loss of libido, sleep disturbance and loss of appetite (ii) emotional symptoms: feelings of guilt, loss of motivation, ugliness etc. There are 2 types of depressive syndrome e.g., (i) unipolar depression: mood swinging always in the same direction; (ii) bipolar depression: depression alternates with mania [19].

Huntington's disease

This incurable, neurodegenerative disorder was named after the American physician George Huntington who could explain it in late 19th century. It is called as Huntington disease or simply HD, Huntington's chorea, chorea major, and is the genetic cause of chorea. In Western Europe, it affects up to 70 people per million populations, and can be much higher in localized regions. Onset of physical symptoms can begin at any age but it may start mostly from 35 to 44 years of age. In 1990s, genetic testing was made possible but as such the counseling for HD had to be developed and became a model for other dominant disorders also. The mechanism of the disease is not fully understood, but a number of factors have been identified. There is no cure for HD, although there are treatments to relieve some of its symptoms. The characteristic initial physical symptoms are jerky, random, and uncontrollable movements called chorea. As the disorder progresses, rigidity and dystonia become evident gradually leading to the dominant physical symptoms [20].

Epilepsy

A seizure is the characteristic event in epilepsy. In fact, epilepsy is associated with high frequency discharge of impulses by a group of neurons in the brain. It can be of two types: (i) Partial epilepsy: In this the localized areas of brain are damaged. Its symptoms depend on the brain regions involved and (ii) Generalized epilepsy: In this case total brain including reticular system is damaged. With the common synthetic medicines for epilepsy relief is possible on long term use but side effects have to be borne [21].

Parkinson's disease

It occurs mainly in the elderly and is a progressive disorder of movement showing continuous shivering. It is commonly associated with dementia and the symptoms include tremor at rest usually starting in the hands. The muscle rigidity can be detectable as an increased resistance in passive limb movement and hypokinesis suppression of voluntary muscles. In this condition the neurotransmitter levels, such as dopamine, 5- hydroxytryptamine, acetylcholine, nor-epinephrine, are decreased, mainly in the substantia nigra and carpus striatum of brain. With synthetic drugs short relief is possible but complete cure is, normally, unachievable [22].

Schizophrenia

The patients of this disease don't know what is happening at present and he does not cooperate with the society and physician for treatment. This disorder has 2 types of symptoms: (i) Positive symptoms: abnormal behavior, delusions, Hallucination, thought disorders. (ii) Negative symptoms: flattening of emotional responses and withdrawal from social contact. In this condition the level of neurotransmitter such as dopamine, 5-hydroxytryptamine, acetylcholine, nor-epinephrine level is increased in the brain. Synthetic drugs can reduce symptoms such as hallucinations, delusions and abnormal thinking. Some people have troubling side effects, including tremors and gaining weight and these drugs may also interfere with other medicines or supplements. It is needless to state that in most cases, medication is a must to treat schizophrenia [23].

Attention Deficit Hyperactivity Disorder (ADHD)

It is considered as a disorder of children but it is not limited to them. In fact, 30- 70% of kids with this disorder, continue showing symptoms of ADHD when they grow up. In addition, people who were never diagnosed ADHD in childhood may develop more obvious symptoms when grown up, causing trouble on the job or in relationships. In people with ADHD, the neurotransmitters are less active in areas of the brain that control attention. It is exactly not known what causes this chemical imbalance, but it is thought that genes may play a role as this disorder often runs in families. It has been found that adults given stimulants have fewer ADHD symptoms and some of them may feel better concentration, but complete cure is often not seen [24].

Natural Ways of Healing of Mind

With the passage of time, new techniques in the medical field are being re-introduced that include herbal healing, yoga, meditation, naturopathy, acupressure, etc. Several individuals as well as organizations are working

in this regard with the aim of fulfilling basic healing requirements of the body. As a matter of fact, there has been enormous change in the mind set of people who once depended on painkillers, are now looking for natural treatments, including Ayurvedic, traditional Chinese, Siddha, Unani, Homeopathy and a number of folklore medicines [25]. Yoga and meditation are also the major key for the fitness of body and mind by enhancing the blood flow in the whole body and calming down the worries and excitements of the mind [26,27]. Throughout the world the plant based systems of medicine have been doing wonders in treating various diseases. So is the case with the mental disorder problems. It is well proven that herbs have excellent properties for treating panic and anxiety affecting the central nervous system, in much the same way as some prescription drugs, without the negative side effects. Lemon balm is good for relieving stress and anxiety. Chamomile tea has been a highly touted herb for anxiety. The roots of kava are used for anxiety and are also well known in the treatment of sleep disorders such as insomnia. Passion flower is also used as herb for anxiety when given in tea or food. Chinese have used ginseng since long for anxiety and natural immune booster. *Cannabis sativa* is usually smoked and can be eaten for anxiety relief. People worldwide are aware of this relief but are sometimes abusing the remedy. Valerian is used throughout the world as a natural sedative and is used for insomnia and panic attacks. It is also a mild painkiller and is considered safe for short term use. *Ginkgo biloba* and *Hypericum perforatum* are very well known Chinese and European plants with neuroprotective properties and useful in improving memory and treating the learning dysfunction [16,28].

Ayurvedic plants mainly described for brain related disorders

Currently, the world is looking towards brain healing prescriptions of traditional medicines, including Ayurveda, for a reliable cure with no or minimal side effects for psychiatric disorders. Indian systems of medicine are very well developed for treating the brain related disorders. The most important among the Indian systems of medicine is Ayurveda which describes the use of hundreds of plants individually or in combination for treating brain related disorders. Description of each and every plant is beyond the scope of this review and has been taken up independently [29], however, the Ayurvedic prescriptions including these plants have been summarized in Table 1. In this Table, the list contains the majority of Indian plants which have been described in the treatment of mental disorders and are currently part of the regular Ayurvedic prescriptions. The plants belong to different plant Families and range from wild and cultivated herbs to shrubs and forest trees. Most of the prescriptions include more than one plant part which supports the synergistic approach of most of the Ayurvedic drugs. Except genetically rooted brain disorders, the Ayurvedic plants have potential to cure most of the mental diseases as given in Table 1.

Current trend on preference for Ayurvedic treatment over synthetic drugs

Most of the synthetic mental drugs act in the brain to produce their euphoric effects. However, sometimes they also cause damage due to seizures, stroke and direct toxic effects on brain cells. A brain disorder also occurs when repeated drug use leads to changes in the function of multiple brain circuits controlling the stress, decision-making, pleasures, impulse control, memory, learning and other functions. These changes make it harder for those with an addiction to experience pleasure in response to natural rewards, such as food, positive social interactions, sex, etc. Additionally, most of the synthetic drugs for brain disorders are prescribed for a long term use and have been showing some kind of side and after effects. There is a long list of synthetic drugs for brain disorders floating in the market, most of

S. No.	Botanical name	Family	Hindi name	English name	Major chemical constituents	Ayurvedic recommendations
1	*Achyranthes aspera*	Amaranthaceae	Chichdha, Chirchita, Latjira, Onga chichri Bach, Ghoda bach	Prickly chaff flower	Oleanolic acid glycosides, amino acids	When inhaled the powder of the seeds, it gives relief from stiffness and headache of migraine.
2	*Acorus calamus*	Araceae	Bach, Ghoda bach	Sweet flag root	β-Asarone, α-asarone	(i) Bark powder enhances memory and cures forgetfulness. (ii) It is beneficial in anxiety and epilepsy when its powder is taken with honey. (iii) Equal weights of its powder and "shunthi" powder (ginger) are recommended to cure facial paralysis.
3	*Adhatoda zeylanica*	Acanthaceae	Adusa, Adusi, Safed vasa, Vakas, Visotta	Malabar nut	Vasicine, vasicinone	Its powder with honey cures old epilepsy disorder.
4	*Albizzia lebbek*	Mimosaceae	Siris, Siras	Siris tree	Budmunchiamine alkaloids, saponins	(i) Its seeds and black pepper powder when applied near eyes, cures unconsciousness. (ii) Its seed powder is one of the constituents for treating psychosis, insanity, anxiety, hysteria.
5	*Allium cepa*	Liliaceae	Pyaz, Kanda	Onion	Dialkenyl sulfides	Tea from its seeds is beneficial in sleeplessness.
6	*Anacyclus pyrethrum*	Asteraceae	Akarkara, Karkara	Pellitory, pyrethrum	Pyrethrin	(i) When ground with vinegar and licked with honey, it controls the intensity of hysteria. (ii) When a decoction with "brahmi" is given, it controls the epilepsy. This mixture also improves in mental retardation. (iii) Massaging its root powder in mahua oil, heals paralysis. If the powder is mixed with honey and licked regularly morning and evening, effect of paralysis is checked.
7	*Bacopa monnieri*	Plantaginaceae	Brahmi, Jalneem	Thyme leaved gratiola, Indian pennywort	Bacosides A, B, C	Its juice is taken with "kuth" (Costus speciosus root) powder in honey to help in hysteria. It is also recommended by adding "kuth" and "shankhapushpi" to cure epilepsy and hysteria. It is very useful in the recovery of memory power.
8	*Benincasa hispida*	Cucurbitaceae	Kushmanda, Petha	Wintermelon, Wax gourd	Multiflorenol and its acetate	(i) Its juice is given with "kuth" powder and honey to cure hysteria. (ii) Its juice when given with "mulethi", helps in epilepsy.
9	*Brassica nigra*	Brassicaceae	Raee	Black mustard	Gallic acid, quercetin	(i) Its seeds and pigeon's droppings after grinding, are applied on forehead. It helps relieve migraine. (ii) Its fresh oil when massaged, reduces fatigue and laziness.
10	*Caesalpinia bonduc*	Caesalpiniaceae	Kat Karanj	Fever nut	Hematoxylol, stereochenol A	(i) Seeds in combinations when given as "nasya", cures headache. (ii) Juice of leaves is beneficial in epilepsy.
11	*Calotropis procera*	Asclepiadaceae	Madar, Aak, Akwan	Swallow wort, Madar	Ursane triterpenoids	(i) Flowers and its milk have been described to be useful in epilepsy. (ii) Yellowish dried leaves are used as "nasya" for migraine. When the mixture of its shade dried leaves with cardamom, peppermint and camphor is inhaled, it relieves migraine pain. (iii) Its roots, in a complex herbal combination, are recommended for relief in paralysis.
12	*Cannabis sativa Linn.*	Cannabinaceae	Bhang	Marijuana	Tetrahydro cannabinoids	Its leaves along with asafoetida have been used for epilepsy type problem in women. It is also useful in treating sleeplessness.

13	*Cassia occidentalis*	Caesalpiniaceae	Kasaundi	Negro coffee	Flavonoid glycosides	Decoction of whole plant or its roots, are useful in relieving the epilepsy and hysteria. Inhaling the flowers or their decoction is beneficial in hysteria.
14	*Cassia tora*	Caesalpiniaceae	Panvad, Chakravada	Foetid carria, Ringworm plant	Cassiside, toralactone	The seeds are ground in "kanji" (gruel of beans) and applied on forehead to get relief from migraine attack.
15	*Celastrus paniculatus*	Celastraceae	Malkangani, jyotishmati	Black oil plant, staff tree, intellect tree	Celapanin, celapanigin triglycerides	Its seed powder is used in combination of almond, pepper and cardamom powder to improve memory.
16	*Centella asiatica*	Apiaceae	Brahmi, Gotu Kola	Indian penny wort	Asiaticosides	(i) Dry plant when taken in preparations of combinations, improves memory power. (ii) Its powder when mixed with unboiled cow milk and taken, shows relief in insomnia. (iii) Its powder is mixed with honey or pepper or cow's "ghee" (purified butter) and taken to ease in anxiety.
17	*Citrullus colosynthis*	Brassicaceae	Indrayan	Colocynth, Bitter apple	Cucurbitacins colosynthosides	(i) Fruit juice or oil cooked root bark when applied on head, cures migraine and ear pain. (ii) "Nasya" of its root powder cures epilepsy.
18	*Citrus aurantifolia*	Rutaceae	Neembu, Kagaji nimbu	Lemon	Bergamottin, bergapten	(i) Seeds and juice are beneficial in insanity related disorder. (ii) Lemon juice is given to the patient of anxiety to regularize the heart beat.
19	*Clitorea ternatea*	Papilionaceae	Aparajita, Koel	Winged leaved clitoria, Butterfly pea	Inositol, hirsutene	The paste of seeds and roots when taken in equal amount and applied as "nasya", it relieves from the migraine pain.
20	*Convolvulus microphyllus*	Convolvulaceae	Shankhapushpi, Shankahuli	Shankhapushpi	Convoline, convolamine	(i) Its powder is mixed with milk or "bach" (Acorus calamus roots) or honey and "ghee" and taken to improve the memory power. (ii) Its juice with honey cures the epilepsy, psychosis and insanity. Shade dried powder alone or with "bach" or Indian pennywort strengthens the mind.
21	*Coriandrum sativum*	Apiaceae	Dhania	Corriander	Linalool, geranyl acetate	When its extract is regularly taken, the vertigo and headache is relieved.
22	*Cuscuta reflexa*	Cuscutaceae	Amarbail, Akashbail	Dodder plant	Cuscutoside A and B	Its juice is taken in water for improvement in brain disorders.
23	*Cynodon dactylon*	Poaceae	Doob, Doorba	Conch grass, Doob grass	Flavonoids, β-sitosterol	Extract of whole plant helps cure madness and epilepsy.
24	*Cyperus scariosus*	Cyperaceae	Nagarmotha	Nutgrass	Cyperene, Patchouli alcohol	It cures epilepsy when given with cow milk.
25	*Datura metel*	Solanaceae	Dhatura	Thorn apple	Hyoscine, hyocyamine	Its seeds are ground with black pepper and given for treating psychosis.
26	*Daucus carota*	Apiaceae	Gajar	Carrot	Carotenoids, α-Pinene, sabinene	Leaves are extracted with warm "ghee" and drops given in nose and ears to cure migraine through sneezing.
27	*Eclipta alba*	Asteraceae	Bhangra, Bhangraiya	Trailing eclipta	Widelolactone and glycoside	After mixing black pepper powder in its juice, it is applied on forehead for relief in migraine.
28	*Ficus benghalensis*	Moraceae	Bargad, Badha	Banyan tree	Bengalenosides, Leucopelargonidin glycoside	Its root bark powder when taken in sugar and cow's milk, improves memory power.
29	*Ficus religiosa*	Moraceae	Peepal	Peepal tree, Sacred	Pelargonidine glycosides, sterols	Extract of branches cures madness.
30	*Glycyrrhiza glabra*	Papilionaceae	Mulethi	Fig, Liquorice root	Phenolics, glabridin	Root powder in ghee brings improvements in epilepsy.
31	*Helianthus annuus*	Asteraceae	Hurhul	Sunflower	Diterpenoids, Kaurenoic acid	Its leaves' juice and seeds are grinded together and applied on forehead to get relief from migraine.

32	*Hibiscus rosasinensis*	Malvaceae	Gudahal	Shoe flower, China rose	Cyanidin, quercetin	Dried leaves and flowers are powdered together and given in sweet milk for improving memory power.
33	*Hyoscyamus niger*	Solanaceae	Khurasani ajawayan	Henbane	Hyoscine, coumarinolignans	Taking few drops of henbane oil in water at frequent intervals, controls hysteria in women.
34	*Juglans regia*	Juglandaceae	Akhrot	Walnut	Fatty acids, linoleic acid	Walnut seeds are ground in "nirgundi" (Vitex negundo) juice and given as nasal drop for hysteria.
35	*Lawsonia inermis*	Lythraceae	Mehendi	Henna	α- and β-ionones, lawsone	Seeds in honey or decoction of flowers are given to cure giddiness.
36	*Moringa oleifera*	Moringaceae	Sahijan, Munga	Drum stick plant	Moringine, Moringinine	(i) After grinding the bark, the liquid is squeezed and put into the nostrils or given orally as drink to cure meningitis. (ii) Decoction of its roots is given for epilepsy and hysteria in women.
37	*Mucuna pruriens*	Fabaceae	Kapikachhu, Kewanch	Velvet bean	L-DOPA, amines, alkaloids	In Ayurveda, it has been described for use in several illnesses and overall body strength. Scientifically it has also been found to be effective in Parkinson's disease.
38	*Nardostachys jatamansi*	Valerianaceae	Jatamansi, Balchhad	Spikenard	Jatamansone and terpenoids	It is useful in hysteria, epilepsy when taken with "ghee". "Jatamansi", "bach" and "brahmi" juice are mixed in honey and given in mental problem.
39	*Papaver somniferum*	Papaveraceae	Posta, Post, Afeem	Poppy, Opium	Morphine, codeine, thebaine, papaverine	Poppy is beneficial in delirium, sleeplessness, convulsion, etc.
40	*Piper longum*	Piperaceae	Peepal	Long pepper	Piperine, Piperlongumine	(i) Its roots in jaggery are given to overcome sleeplessness. (ii) Mixture of "peepal" and "bach" are given in milk to cure migraine pain.
41	*Piper nigrum*	Piperaceae	Kali mirch	Black pepper	Piperine and related alkaloids	On empty stomach, pepper powder and "bach" are given to treat hysteria.
42	*Psidium guajava*	Myrtaceae	Amrud, Safari	Guava	Oleanolic acid, ursolic acid	(i) Decoction of leaves is given to cure mental and physical deformities. (ii) Tincture of leaves is massaged on the backbone of children for convulsions.
43	*Punica granatum*	Punicaceae	Anar	Pomegranate	1-(2-propenyl)- piperidine in leaves, anthocyanins in fruit	(i) Leaves after boiling with water and concentrating, the extract is given in warm milk to cure fatigue, tiredness and insomnia. (ii) Leaves and rose flowers are cooked in water and concentrated. It is given in ghee to cure madness.
44	*Sapindus mukorossi*	Sapindaceae	Reetha	Soapnut tree	Triterpenoid, sesquiterpenoid, saponin, glycosides	(i) Its fruits are ground with black pepper and few drops are poured in the nostrils to get relief from migraine pain. (ii) Its seeds along with kernel and peel are ground and to be inhaled regularly to cure epilepsy, completely.
45	*Sesbania grandiflora*	Fabaceae	Agastiya, Agust	Sesbane	Leucocyanidin, cyanidin, triterpenoids	(i) Sesbane leaves and black pepper are ground in cow urine and made to inhale. It brings immediate relief from epilepsy. (ii) Few drops of leaf or flower extract are put in the opposite nostril of migraine pain giving immediate relief.

46	*Sida cordifolia*	Malvaceae	Jangli methi, Bariyar, Khrainti	Country mallow	Sidasterone A and B	(i) Its powder after cooking in milk, is given to the patient or massaged, giving relief in facial paralysis. (ii) To control the excessive anxiety, the plant and "apamarg" (Achyranthes aspera) are boiled in milk until concentration and given.
47	*Solanum surratense*	Solanaceae	Bhatkataiya, Kantakari, Laghukai	Yellow berried night shade	Solasodine, solasonine	Its roots and poppy seeds are grinded in child's urine and put in the nose to be relieved from epilepsy.
48	*Sphaeranthus indicus*	Asteraceae	Mundi, Gorakhmundi	East Indian globe thistle	Sterols, sesquiterpenoids	It and clove powder are given in honey to cure Parkinson's disease.
49	*Syzygium aromaticum*	Myrtaceae	Lavang, Laung	Clove	Carvacrol, thymol, eugenol	Cloves are grinded in water and the paste is applied on the earlobes to cure migraine.
50	*Terminalia chebula*	Combretaceae	Harad	The chebulic or black myrobalan	Ethyl gallate, luteolin	Seeds are grinded in warm water and applied on forehead for relief in migraine.
51	*Valeriana jatamansi*	Valerianaceae	Tagar	Valerian	Jatamansone, jatamansinol	Its juice is useful in epilepsy. When taken in honey, it helps in hysteria. "tagar" when taken in combination of other plants, helps controlling the delirium.
52	*Vitex negundo*	Verbenaceae	Samhalu, Meudi	Five leaved chaste	Negundoside	The powder of its fruits is given in mental disorder.
53	*Vitis vinifera*	Vitaceae	Munakka, Angur, Dakh	Grapesvine, Raisins	Glycosides of pelargonidin, cyanidin	(i) Grapes and "amla" (Phyllanthus emblica) are boiled together and crushed and Ginger powder is added. When given in unconsciousness due to fever, it helps. (ii) "Munakka", pomegranate bark, khus khus are grinded together and soaked in water overnight. Strained and given for faintness. (iii) "Munakka" is roasted and given for dizziness.
54	*Withania somnifera*	Solanaceae	Ashwagandha, Asagandha	Winter cherry, Poisonous gooseberry	Withaferin A, withanolide A	In Ayurveda, this plant has been described for use in several illnesses and overall body strength. Scientifically, it has also been found to be effective in ischemia.
55	*Xeromphis spinosa*	Rubiaceae	Main phal	Emetic nut	Oleanolic acid glycoside	Its fruits and sugar are grinded in cow milk and given as "nasya" to treat migraine headache.
56	*Zizyphus mauritiana*	Rhamnaceae	Ber	Jujube	Peptide and cyclopeptide alkaloids, sanjoinenine	Although not prescribed in Ayurveda, its fruit is used in mental healing as scientifically proved for epilepsy.

Table 1: List of commonly recommended Ayurvedic plants in brain disorders.

them with proven side effects on brain function or other organs of the body [30]. Therefore, discussing each of them individually, is beyond the scope of this paper, however, the basic difference in the ground of treatments between the two, have been discussed below and listed in Table 2.

Side and after effects of synthetic drugs for brain disorders

The effectiveness of allopathic medicines during an emergency is the main reason why it is adopted by most of the people all around the world. In allopathy, the doctors are restricted to concentrate on the symptoms of a disease and not on the causes of those symptoms. It appears that there is a pill for each symptom and then, a pill for all their side effects. It is known that allopathy offers only partial cure, as these drugs are made to mostly cure the symptoms, not the root cause. It is important to note that there is no place for individuality in allopathy

as the same pill is given to the patients suffering from different diseases of similar symptoms. The synthetic drugs for brain related disorders have been studied for harmful side effects and have been covered in a number of documents for psychostimulants, antidepressants, antipsychotics, antianxiety, etc. [30]. Therefore, the adverse effects for all drugs need not be covered in this paper but an example can be cited for the anticonvulsant drugs, as follows. They are used to control the convulsions by inhibiting the discharge and then producing hypnosis. These synthetic drugs, viz. phenytoin (PHT), diazepam, valproate (VPA), leviteracetam, etc., are being marketed for the treatment of the epilepsy. Although these agents have new spectrum of efficacy but show alarming adverse effects [31]. On the other hand, the treatment of epilepsy with Ayurvedic herbal drugs as adjuvant seems to be more beneficial and is gaining more popularity due to their negligible side effects (Table 1).

Ayurvedic drugs with negligible side and after effects

Ayurveda follows the fundamental principle of five great elements, which insists that the fault, issue and the impurity should be in perfect harmony with all the five elements used to form the human body, i.e., earth (prithvi), water (jal), fire (agni), air (vayu) and space (akash). According to this, there should be a balance in the three elemental energies, Vata (air+space=wind), Pitta (fire +water=bile) and Kapha (water+earth=phlegm). Ayurveda explains that, when these three energies are in a balanced state or exist in equal proportion, the body will remain healthy otherwise it becomes unhealthy in many ways [32]. Ayurveda is mainly connected with the cures accessible from nature and deals with the root cause of the disease and provides permanent cure in most of the cases. Normally, a patient treated with Ayurvedic medicines, not only gets cured but also achieves the permanent immunity. The main advantage that Ayurveda has over allopathy is that the former uses only the natural means to cure a disease and is the most eco-accommodating approach to get everlasting cure (Table 2).

It is therefore well accepted that the Ayurveda not only treats a patient with mental diseases, but also increases the overall mental capability by strengthening the immunity, thus keeping the mind and the body free from further damages. The consumption of the prescribed Ayurvedic medicines, improve the concentration and other mental capabilities. Popularly, the extracts of *Bacopa monnieri (brahmi), Acorus calamus (vach), Celastrus paniculatus (jyotismati)* are considered extremely beneficial in strengthening mental condition. Although a detailed list of Ayurvedic plants and their potential to treat brain related disorders are given in Table 1, some specific examples of Ayurvedic treatments for common mental diseases could be discussed. For example, the depression is a feeling of dejection affecting the natural functioning of our mind and body thus tend to become unhappy. It can be treated with herbal medicines rich in ingredients like, *Crataegus oxyacantha (hawthorn), Eschscholzia californica (California poppy), Ginkgo biloba, Lavandula angustifolia (lavender)*. Stress and anxiety tend to make us

hyper and unaware about mood swings. Following Ayurvedic plants are effective to counter stress and anxiety, mulungu bark, Rhodiola rosea, ashwagandha, lavender, etc. Similarly, ADHD reduces a mind's capability to pay concentration, to focus or pay attention to anything. Ayurvedic medicines for ADHD is made from natural herbs that cure mental disabilities, for example, *Centella asiatica (mandukparni), Bacopa monnieri (brahmi), Withania somnifera (ashwagandha), Celastrus paniculatus (jyotismati)*, etc. The bipolar disorder results in an unusual shift in mood, and activities affecting the mental ability of a person to carry out regular day to day activities. To cure this, brahmi, passion flower and several other Ayurvedic herbs are quite useful [33].

Since Ayurvedic system treats the cause of illness in the body by balancing the act of vata, pitta and kapha, therefore the treatment is long lasting and certainly irreversible. This is the reason that Ayurvedic medicine is almost free from side effects making it more acceptable in the society than the synthetic drugs which focus mainly on the symptoms in the patients leading to the temporary relief but with side effects in most of the cases [30,34]. Apart from this, most of the prescriptions in Ayurveda are in the form of Poly Herbal Formulations (PHF). It has gained its popularity owing to the fact that PHF possesses clear advantages, which is not available in allopathic drugs, by expressing high effectiveness in a vast number of diseases. The therapeutic effect of herbal medicines are exerted due to the presence of different bioactive phytoconstituents and the effects are further potentiated when compatible herbals are formulated together in PHFs. PHFs are usually found to have wide therapeutic range and most of them are effective even at a low dose and safe at high dose, thus exhibiting superior risk to benefit ratio [32].

Conclusion

The allopathic and Ayurvedic systems of medicine work through independent principles. Allopathic drugs are prescribed on symptomatic principle while Ayurvedic through the balance of three

S. No.	Condition	Allopathic treatment	Ayurvedic treatment
1.	Taking up the disease	Allopathy takes the body in pieces, is objective and incomplete in nature.	Ayurveda takes the body as a whole and the physician has knowledge of all the systems of body.
2.	System of treatment	Allopathy is a system of physical health and it believes in the replacing/changing of the systems or organs for treatment and not much worried about the cure.	Ayurveda focuses on the wellness as a complete package, be it physical, psychological, spiritual or social.
3.	Possibility of side effects	Allopathy is mostly a system of internal or external side effects.	Ayurveda is a natural cure in which scope of side effects is very less or mild.
4.	Focus of the treatment	Allopathy focuses on suppressing the signs and symptoms of a disease and never appreciates to remove the disease causing factors, completely.	Ayurveda considers that until a body devoids the disease causing factors, it will keep on relapsing. It considers the detoxification as a primary part of the treatment.
5.	Nature of effect	Allopathic medicines partially cleanse the body.	Ayurvedic medicines decontaminate the whole body by balancing the three energies (vata, pitta and kapha).

Table 2: Main differences between principles of allopathic and Ayurvedic treatments.

energies (vata, pita and kapha) required for maintaining good health. Therefore, direct comparative study on the efficacy of the drugs for brain related illnesses, has not been properly studied yet. However, it is well understood that in most of the cases, the synthetic drugs generally bring relief through a symptomatic treatment and hardly promise permanent cure. Since more than 60 million Indian population suffers from mental disorders and the country lags far behind the world for treatments and spending in the hospitals for mental cure, it is high time to look for the established alternative system of medicine. It was estimated that nearly 1-2% Indians suffer from schizophrenia and bipolar disorder whereas 5% population showed common mental disorders like depression, anxiety, convulsion, etc. The Ayurvedic prescriptions have been proven to be very useful against such disorders. Currently, the world is rightly looking towards brain healing properties of traditional medicines, including Ayurveda, for a reliable cure with no or minimal side effects. The present review clearly explains that the Ayurvedic system of medicine is very well developed for treating most of the brain related disorders. This review has right timely included some of the Ayurvedic treatments, which have been described for mental disorders and are currently part of the Ayurvedic prescriptions. Thus, it could be concluded that the Ayurvedic system of herbal medicine is certainly a treasury of plant drugs which brings back the much sought after hope for the complete and permanent treatment of mental disorders through natural means with minimum side effects as compared to the allopathic drugs.

References

1. http://health.economictimes.indiatimes.com/

2. Sandhya S, Vinod KR, Sravan K (2010) Herbs used for brain disorders. Hygeia J D Med 2: 38-45.

3. Rao RV, Olivier D, John V, Bredesen DE (2012) Ayurvedic medicinal plants for Alzheimer's disease: a review. Alzheimer's Res Ther 4: 22-30.

4. Younus M, Younus A, Shahbaz I (2015) Value of Ayurvedic medicinal plants as psychotherapeutic agents-A review. Intern J Innov Sci Engg Tech 2: 144-148.

5. Tewari R, Rout PK, Misra LN (2016) Simultaneous RP-HPLC-PDA-RI separation and quantification of pinitol content in Sesbania bispinosa vis-a-vis harvesting age. Plant Biosyst.

6. Gupta M, Rout PK, Misra LN, Gupta P, Singh N, et al. (2016) Chemical composition and bioactivity of Boswellia serrata Roxb, essential oil in relation to geographical variation. Plant Biosyst. 151: 623–629.

7. Ahmad F, Misra LN, Gupta VK, Darokar MP, Prakash O, et al. (2016) Synergistic effect of (+)-pinitol from Saraca asoca with β-lactam antibiotics and studies on the in-silico possible mechanism. J Asian Nat Prod Res 18: 172-183.

8. Ahmad F, Misra LN, Tewari R, Gupta P, Gupta VK, Darokar MP (2016) Isolation and HPLC profiling of chemical constituents of Saraca asoca bark. Indian J Chem B 55B: 353-361.

9. Ahmad F, Misra LN, Tewari R, Gupta P, Mishra P (2016) Anti-inflammatory flavanol glycosides from Saraca asoca bark. Nat Prod Res 30: 489-492.

10. http://www.who.int/mental_health/evidence/atlas/profiles/ind_mh_profile.pdf?ua=1

11. Anonymous (2016) Nearly 60 million Indians suffer from mental disorders.

12. Anonymous (2016) World Mental Health Day: Stigma continues to be the biggest barrier for mental health care in India.

13. http://health.economictimes.indiatimes.com/news/diagnostics/150-million-adult-indians-suffer-from-mental-disorder-nmhs/55043069

14. http://timesofindia.indiatimes.com/india/On-health-front-India-143rd-among-188-nations-Study/articleshow/54473135.cms

15. http://www.human-memory.net/brain_neurons.html

16. Hassan MAG, Balasubramanian R, Masoud AD, Burkan ZE, Sughir A (2014) Role of medicinal plants in neurodegenerative diseases with special emphasis to Alzheimer's disease. Int J Phytopharmacol 5: 454-462.

17. Perry E, Howes MR (2011) Medicinal plants and dementia therapy: Herbal hopes for brain aging? CNS Neurosci Therap 17: 683-698.

18. Martin EI, Ressler KJ, Binder E, Nemeroff CB (2009) The neurobiology of anxiety disorders: Brain imaging, genetics, and psychoneuroendocrinology. Psychiatr Clin North Am 32: 549-575.

19. Benedetti F, Bernasconi A, Pontiggia A (2006) Depression and neurological disorders. Curr Opin Psychiatry 19: 14-18.

20. Finkbeiner S (2011) Huntington's disease. Cold Spring Harbor Perspect Biol 3: 1-24.

21. Brodtkorb E, Torbergsen T, Nakken KO, Andersen K, Gimse R, et al. (1994) Epileptic seizures, arthrogryposis, and migrational brain disorders: a syndrome? Acta Neurol Scand 90: 232-240.

22. Ríos J, Onteniente M, Picazo D, Montesinos M (2016) Medicinal plants and natural products as potential sources for antiparkinson drugs. Planta Med 82: 942-951.

23. DeLisi LE, Szulc KU, Bertisch HC, Majcher M, Brown K (2006) Understanding structural brain changes in schizophrenia. Dialogues Clin Neurosci 8: 71-78.

24. Curatolo P, D'Agati E, Moavero R (2010) The neurobiological basis of ADHD. Ital J Pediatr 36: 79-85.

25. Misra LN (2013) Traditional phytomedicinal systems, scientific validations and current popularity as nutraceuticals. Int J Trad Nat Med 2: 27-75.

26. Balkrishna A (2008) Secrets of Indian herbs for good health. Divya Prakashan, Patanjali Yogpeeth, Haridwar, India pp: 1-420.

27. Balkrishna A (2014) Ayurved jadi-buti rahasya (Vol. 1-3). Divya Prakashan, Patanjali Yogpeeth, Haridwar, India pp: 1-1650.

28. Husain A, Virmani OP, Popli SP, Misra LN, Gupta MM, et al. (1992) Dictionary of Indian Medicinal Plants, CIMAP, Lucknow, India pp: 1-546.

29. Balkrishna A, Misra LN (2017) Brief chemo-botanical account of some Ayurvedic plants useful in mental health. Nat Prod J Commun.

30. Anonymous (2008) The side effects of common psychiatric drugs-A report by the citizens commission on human rights international.

31. Pandey SK, Jangra MK, Yadav AK (2014) Herbal and synthetic approaches for the treatment of epilepsy. Intern J Nutr Pharmacol Neurol Dis 4: 43-52.

32. Parasuraman S, Thing GS, Dhanaraj SA (2014) Polyherbal formulation: Concept of ayurveda. Pharmacogn Rev 8: 73-80.

33. http://www.dalmiahealth.com/ayurvedic-treatment-for-mental-health-problems/

34. Lavretsky H (2009) Complementary and alternative medicine use for treatment and prevention of late-life mood and cognitive disorders. Aging Health 5: 61-78.

41

Cordycepin from Hot Water Extract of *Cordyceps militaris* Induce Apoptosis in Human Non-Small Lung Carcinoma upon Activation of A3 Adenosine Receptors

Felix Shih-Hsiang Hsiao[1], Yu-Hsiang Yu[2], Pramod Shah[3], Witold Stanisław Proskura[4], Andrzej Dybus[4], Ching-Han Huang[2], Yi-Lin Chen[2] and Yeong-Hsiang Cheng[2]*

[1]*Department of Animal Science and Biotechnology, Tunghai University, Taichung 40704, Taiwan*
[2]*Department of Biotechnology and Animal Science, National I-Lan University, Yilan City, Yilan County, Taiwan*
[3]*Department of Biomedical Science and Engineering, National Central University, Taoyuan City 32001, Taiwan*
[4]*Laboratory of Molecular Cytogenetics, West Pomeranian University of Technology, 71-466 Szczecin, Poland*

Abstract

Cordyceps militaris hot water extract (CMHW) containing cordycepin (cordycepin-CMHW) was used to study the anti-cancer effects in human A549 non-small cell lung carcinoma cells. Our results showed cordycepin-CMHW can inhibit cell proliferations in A549 cells by activating A3 adenosine receptor (A_3AR) *via* the inactivation of Akt pathways. Cordycepin-CMHW can also induce apoptosis in the A549 cells by enhancing DNA fragmentation and chromatin condensation. We further observed that cordycepin-CMHW up-regulated caspase-9 and increased cleavage of caspase-3 and poly ADP ribose polymerase (PARP) in A549 cells. The results suggested cordycepin-CMHW is a highly selective treatment to de-regulation of the cell proliferation and apoptosis in non-small cell lung carcinoma *via* signaling pathways generated by A_3AR activation.

Keywords: *Cordyceps militaris*; Cordycepin; A_3AR; Apoptosis

Introduction

Adenosine receptor belongs to the superfamily of G-protein-coupled receptor, which plays a key role in the regulation of cell survival and cell death [1]. In humans, four distinct subtypes of adenosine receptors have been identified: A1, A2A, A2B and A3 [2]. Constitutive activation of A3 adenosine receptor (A_3AR) has been linked to the suppression of tumor growth [3]. For example, A_3AR has been reported to enhance transcription factors that inhibit transcription of tumor-related genes. These mechanisms guards against the cell proliferations and further instruct the lethal damage in developing tumors [4]. Different molecular pathways have been revealed to explain the anti-tumor activity of A_3AR. Signaling through the A_3AR involves suppression of downstream protein kinase, Akt, in diverse tumors [5]. Inhibition of Akt has been demonstrated to alter Wnt/*GSK-3β pathways* [6], and lead to the inactivation of Lef/Tcf and β-catenin-responsive cell cycle progresses factor c-myc and cyclin D1, which in turn suppress the cell survival [7]. Concurrently with the suppression of tumor growth, functional A_3AR inactivating Akt has also been described to enhance susceptibility of tumor cells toward apoptosis [8]. Indeed, down-regulated Akt has shown to prompted many agent-induced apoptosis through the caspase family of proteins [9,10]. Thus, it is tempting to speculate that Akt inhibitors promotes the apoptosis in cancer cells, and lowers their threshold for lethal effects by A_3AR activation [6].

Lung cancer is one of the major causes of death in the world. Two main types of lung cancer have been revealed: Non-small cell lung cancer and small cell lung cancer [11]. Non-small cell lung cancer is the major type of epithelial lung cancer which accounts for 85% of all lung cancer cases [12]. Although patients with non-small cell lung cancer can be treated by using surgery and/or in combination with chemotherapy, such disorders can be very difficult to be cured [13]; it develops resistance against chemotherapy agents render current treatments in non-small cell lung cancer remains elusive [14].

Cordycepin, also known as 3-deoxyadenosine, is the major bioactive component of *Cordyceps militaris* [15]. Cordycepin has been reported to exert many biological activities including anti-cancer, anti-oxidant and anti-inflammatory effects [16-18]. However, the molecular pathways of its anti-cancer effect in non-small cell lung cancer are not well understood. In this study, we have investigated whether cordycepin from *C. militaris* hot water extracts (cordycepin-CMHW) show anticancer activity towards an *in vitro* model of human non-small lung carcinoma.

Materials and Methods

Cell culture and reagents

Human A549 non-small cell lung carcinoma was purchased from the American Type Culture Collection (ATCC, Manassas, VA, USA). Cell was maintained in Ham's F-12k medium (Sigma-Aldrich, St. Louis, MO) supplemented with 10% fetal bovine serum (Sigma-Aldrich, St. Louis, MO), 100 units/ml penicillin, 100 mg/ml streptomycin (Gibco, Gaithersburg, MD) at 37°C in under 5% CO_2 and 95% humidity. The cells were split twice a week at a ratio of 1:3 to 1:8.

Cordycepin-CMHW isolation

Cordycepin was isolated from the mycelium of *C. militaris* (BCRC, Hsinchu, Taiwan) as previously descriptions [19]. In brief, the seed culture of *C. militaris* was first prepared using PDA (Nissui Pharmaceutical Co., Ltd., Japan) plate (seed plate). Inoculant from the seed plate was then transferred to 200 ml of PDB (Nissui

*Corresponding author: Cheng YH, Department of Biotechnology and Animal Science, National Ilan University, No. 1, Sec. 1, Shennong Road, Yilan City, Yilan County 260, Taiwan
E-mail: yhcheng@ems.niu.edu.tw

Pharmaceutical Co., Ltd., Japan) medium and inoculated at 22°C on a rotary shaker incubator at 150 rpm for 7 days. Mycelium of *C. militaris* was afterwards developed in a jar fermenter containing wheat-based medium consisting of 43.7% wheat, 5% yeast powder, 0.1% $CaCO_3$, 0.05% $MgSO_4$, 0.1% NaH_2PO_4, 0.05% KH_2PO_4 1% glucose and 50% H_2O and inoculated at 22°C for 28 days. The fermenters were dried at 50°C for 24 hrs, homogenized and dissolved in water at ratio of 1:5 (w/v); the fermenters/water mixtures were then incubated at 100°C oven for 24 hrs (*C. militaris* hot water extract, CMHW). Cordycepin amounts in CMHW were analyzed by high performance liquid chromatography (HPLC; Shimadzu, Japan) with a LiChrospher 100 RP-18 column (5 μm; Merck-Millipore, Watford UK). The mobile phase was a mixture of 15% methanol containing 0.02 MKH_2PO_4, with a flow-rate of 1 ml/min. The effluent was monitored by a UV detector at 254 nm. The concentrations of cordycepin in CMHW were 40 μg/mg dried material.

Cell proliferation assay

The 3-(4,5-dimethylthiazol-2-yl)-2,5-diphenyltetrazolium bromide (MTT) assay was used to determine the cell proliferation as previously descriptions [20]. In brief, cells were cultured in 96-well plate and treated with different concentrations of cordycepin for 24 hrs. MTT (500 μg/ml) was subsequently added to each well and incubated at for 3 hrs. The produced formazan was solubilized by dimethyl sulfoxide. Absorbance was measured at 570 nm with a reference wavelength of 690 nm.

Reverse Transcription PCR (RT-PCR)

Total cellular RNA was extracted using TRIzol reagent (Invitrogen) and then treated with RNase free DNase Set (Promega) according to manufacturer's instructions. The quantity of RNA was determined using a NanoDrop ND-1000 spectrophotometer (Thermo Scientific). Five μg of total RNA samples were reverse-transcribed for 120 min at 37°C with the Omniscript RT-PCR kit according to the manufacturer's instructions (QIAGEN). PCR was performed with 1 μL of the single-stranded cDNA sample. Annealing temperature was 55°C. Each assay was run in triplicate. The sequences of primers used were as follows: forward 5′-TGAAGGTCGGAGTCAACGGATTTGGT-3′, reverse 5′-CATGTGGGCCATGAGGTCCACCAC-3′ for *Glyceraldehyde-3-phosphate dehydrogenase* (*GAPDH*); forward 5′-TACCCTCTCAACGACAGCAG-3′, reverse 5′-TCTTGACATTCTCCTCGGTG-3′ for *c-myc*. *GAPDH* was used as a reference gene to normalize specific gene expression in each sample.

Western Blot Analysis

Total protein was extracted with 0.5 mL of ice-cold lysis buffer containing 10 m*M* Tris-HCl (pH 7.5), 150 m*M* NaCl, 1% Nonidet P-40 (Sigma-Aldrich), and 0.1% SDS for 15 min on ice. After being heated for 5 min at 95°C, 30 μg of protein lysate was analyzed on a 12% SDS-PAGE gel. Afterward, proteins were transferred to polyvinylidene fluoride membrane filters, probed with goat anti-GFP polyclonal antibody (Abcam, Cambridge, UK), and developed with enhanced chemiluminescent reagents (Amersham Bioscience).

Hoechst 33342 Fluorescent Staining

Cells grown on 6-well plate were fixed in 1.5% paraformaldehyde for 10 min. After washing, cells were permeabilized with 0.1% Triton X-100 in PBS for 5 min. Cells were then incubated with 10 uM Hoechst 3342 (BD Biosciences, San Jose, CA, USA) for 20 min in the dark, rinsed in PBS and fluorescence was observed microscopically.

Statistical Analysis

Data were expressed as mean ± standard error. Student's t-test was used to assess significance of the differences; *p*-values <0.05 were considered statistically significant.

Results

Cordycepin-CMHW inhibits lung cancer cell proliferations

It was revealed that cordycepin from *Cordyceps militaris* have anti-cancer activity [16]; therefore, we investigated the role of cordycepin-CMHW in lung tumor growth inhibitions. The non-small cell lung carcinoma A549 cells were used as tumor cell model. Different concentrations of cordycepin-CMHW (10-80 μg/ml) were incubated with A549 cells for 24 hrs; cell proliferation was determined using MTT test. The result showed that cordycepin-CMHW inhibited cell proliferations of A549 cell line in a dose dependent manner (Figure 1A). Microscopy examinations revealed most of the cells were detached from the plate surface after treating with cordycepin-CMHW. The attached cell did not form the well-spread morphology that was observed even the cells were cultured in a low concentration of cordycepin-CMHW (10 μg/ml; Figure 1B). This result indicated cordycepin-CMHW inhibits lung cancer cell proliferations.

Cordycepin-CMHW activate A_3AR signaling in lung cancer cells

Because of structural similarity of adenosine, cordycepin could activate adenosine subtype receptors to mediate tumor growth, especially the A_3AR [6,7]. Stimulation of A_3AR was reported to mediate suppression of tumor growth through the inactivation of downstream Akt. The inhibited Akt cause phosphorylation of GSK-3β and prevent division and proliferation of cancer cell by targeting the β-catenin-responsive cell cycle progresses factor c-Myc [21]. To reveal this

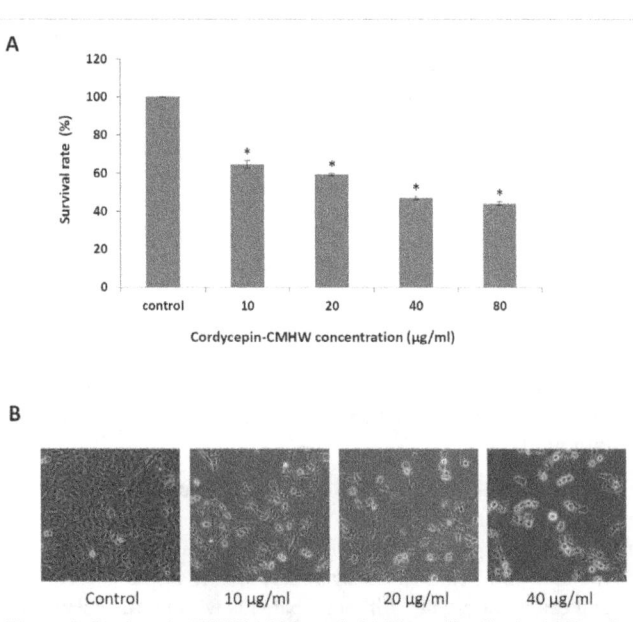

Figure 1: Cordycepin-CMHW inhibits cell viability proliferation in A549 cells. (A) A549 cells proliferation in respond to different concentration of cordycepin-CMHW (10, 20, 40 and 80 μg/mL). Controls were set to 100%. The asterisks represent the statistically significant difference in the survival rate of A549 cell treated with Cordycepin-CMHW compared with that of the non-treated control (p<0.05). (B) Image of A549 cells attach to plate surface at different concentration of cordycepin-CMHW (10, 20 and 40 μg/mL) after 24 hrs. Magnifications were 200X.

mechanism in non-small cell lung carcinoma, different concentrations of cordycepin-CMHW (10-80 μg/ml) were added to A549 cells and the expression of Akt, phosphate Akt (pAkt) and phosphate GSK-3β (pGSK-3β) were determined by Western blotting. As shown in Figure 2, the expression levels of total Akt and pAkt at A549 cells were dose dependently inhibited by cordycepin-CMHW. Inhibition of pGSK-3β was only observed at the higher dose of cordycepin-CMHW (40 and 80 μg/ml). These results indicated cordycepin-CMHW was able to suppress the downstream signaling through A_3AR. We further examined the time course effects of cordycepin-CMHW on these proteins. Cordycepin-CMHW (40 μg/ml) was added to the A549 cell cultures at 15, 30, 60, 120 and 240 min and the expression levels of A_3AR, Akt and pGSK-3β were observed (Figure 3A). Our result showed that cordycepin-CMHW is able to enhance the expression levels of A_3AR on A549 cells in a time dependent manner. Specifically, the expression levels of Akt were found to be down-regulated after the treatment of A549 cells with cordycepin-CMHW for 60 min. The inhibitory effects of cordycepin-CMHW were also shown in downstream GSK-3β at 120 min in culture. Moreover, RT-PCR analysis revealed the down-regulated expressions of c-Myc in A549 cells at 60 min after cordycepin-CMHW treatments. This result suggests cordycepin-CMHW can activate the signaling pathways through the activation of A_3AR in A549 lung carcinoma.

Cordycepin-CMHW induce apoptosis in lung cancer cells

A_3AR stimulation is integrally to signaling pathways governing apoptosis [22]. Since cordycepin-CMHW was able to enhance the expression levels of A_3AR (Figure 3B). We next examined the apoptotic effects of cordycepin-CMHW in A549 cells. Cytological observations by an inverted phase contrast microscope and Hoechst 33342 staining assay showed nuclear condensation in A549 cells upon treatment of cordycepin-CMHW (40 μg/ml) for 12 hrs (Figure 4A). Also, the formation of nuclear condensation was increased after incubation with cordycepin-CMHW for 24 hrs. We then used terminal deoxynucleotidyl transferase (TdT) dUTP Nick-End Labeling (TUNEL) assay to measure apoptotic cells, which undergo extensive DNA degradation during apoptosis. Upon treatment of cordycepin-CMHW (40 μg/ml) for 6 hrs, a nuclear mediated apoptosis was observed with the direct TUNEL labeling (Figure 4B). This result indicated cordycepin-CMHW induces apoptosis in A549 lung carcinoma.

Cordycepin-CMHW induce A549 cells apoptosis through caspase signaling

Activation of apoptosis is tightly regulated at several levels. Caspases are a family of cystine proteases which serve critical roles

in apoptotic signaling driven by A_3AR [23]. We next investigated the role of caspase proteins in cordycepin-CMHW-induced apoptosis. A549 cells were incubated with cordycepin-CMHW (40 μg/ml) for 3, 6, 12, 24 or 48 hrs, and levels of initiator caspase, caspase-9, were firstly assessed using RT-PCR (Figure 5A). Cordycepin-CMHW induced expressions of caspase-9 were observed after 3 hrs treatment, with maximal expressions at 6 hrs. The caspase-9 expressions decline to normal after 12 hrs as compared to non-treating control. Then, we examined the expression proteins that involved in the execution-phase of cell apoptosis included caspase-3 and its substrate Poly (ADP-ribose) polymerase (PARP). Western blot analysis revealed cordycepin-CMHW enhanced the activation of caspases-3 (cleaved-caspase-3) in A549 cell at 6 hrs. Furthermore, the elevated cleaved-caspase-3 was associated with their down-regulating at substrate PARP

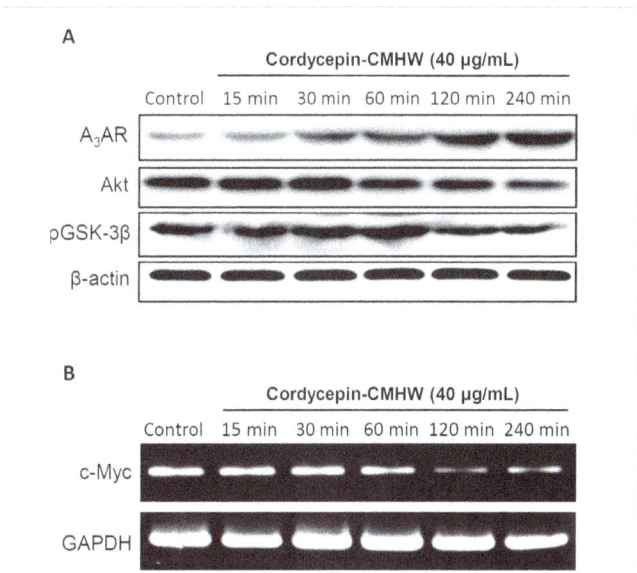

Figure 3: Effect of Cordycepin-CMHW on different proteins: (A) A549 cells were treated with cordycepin-CMHW (40 μg/mL) for 0 to 240 min and the proteins levels of A3AR, AKT and phosphate GSK-3β (pGSK-3β) were determined by Western blotting. β-actin was used as loading control. (B) Expression of c-Myc treated with cordycepin-CMHW (40 μg/mL) for 0 to 240 min by RT-PCR analysis. The house keeping gene *GAPDH* was used as internal control.

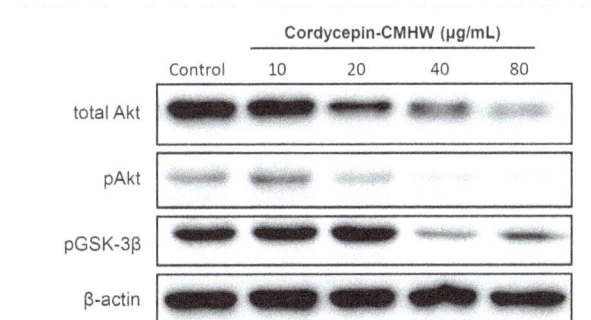

Figure 2: Expression of A3AR downstream signaling proteins in A549 cells in response to different concentration of Cordycepin-CMHWC-CMHW. Expression levels of total AKT, phosphate AKT (pAKT) and phosphate GSK-3β (pGSK-3β) were identified using Western blotting. β-actin was used as loading control.

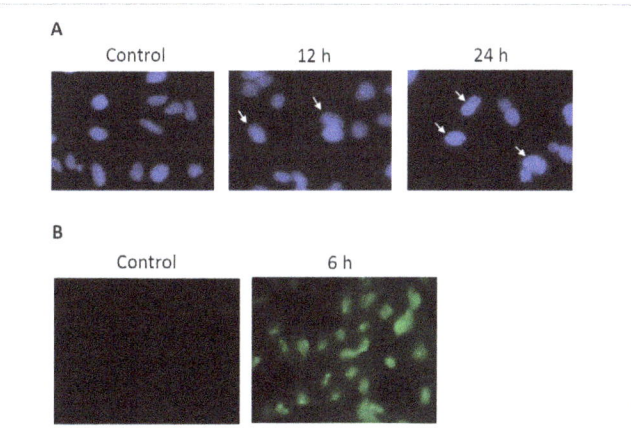

Figure 4: Apoptotic effects of Cordycepin-CMHW in A549 cells: (A) DNA condensation (arrow) in A549 cells can be observed after the treatment of Cordycepin-CMHW (40 μg/mL) for 12 and 24 hrs by inverted phase contrast microscope observations. Magnifications were 200X. (B) TUNEL staining of nuclear mediated apoptotic effect in A549 cells after the treatment with Cordycepin-CMHW (40 μg/mL) for 6 hrs. Magnifications were 200X.

and up-regulating at cleavage of PARP in A549 culture (Figure 5B). These results suggested that cordycepin-CMHW induced apoptosis by activation of caspase signaling pathway in A549 lung carcinoma.

Discussions

Non-small cell lung cancer continues to pose a major health problem to already overstretch; with approximately 221,000 new cases reported in 2015 and ~158,000 deaths (American Cancer Society, http://www.cancer.org/cancer/lungcancer-non-smallcell/). Chemotherapy is a common treatment for non-small cell lung cancer; however, results of a recent trial suggested there is no significant improvement in patients who survive a first encounter with this disease [11].

The medicinal fungus *C. militaris* is a potential harbor of several bio-metabolites for natural drugs to revitalize the various physiological processes, which let it, be marketable in the western world as an alternative medicine [24]. Cordycepin (3'-deoxyadenosine) is a major bioactive component found in *C. militaris* [25]. Although cordycepin administration has shown to inhibit cell proliferations in human non-small cell lung carcinoma [21], the molecular pathways of its anti-cancer effect in such cancer type are not well understood. In the current study, we demonstrated the anti-cancer activity of *C. militaris* hot water extract that harbors cordycepin (cordycepin-CMHW). Our results showed that cordycepin-CMHW can inhibit cell proliferation in human A549 non-small cell lung carcinoma cells *via* the signaling pathway triggered A_3AR stimulation. Further study showed this inhibition was caused by apoptosis. A_3AR is related to cell survival and cell death [22]. As demonstrated by Madi et al., A_3AR was highly expressed in numerous tumors [3]; constitutive activation of this receptor impairs survival of tumor cells [26]. Since the A_3AR signaling

is directed by Akt [5], a serine/threonine protein kinase encharging of cell proliferation and cell death effects, the A_3AR likely function to regulate specific survival activities in tumor cells. Our results showed that cordycepin-CMHW inhibits the phosphorylation of Akt (pAkt), and promoted the activation of WNT/GSK-3β signaling pathway. This is further connected with suppression of proto-oncogene, *c-MYC*. The activation of A_3AR signaling therefore sensitizes cordycepin-CMHW induced tumor growth inhibition in A549 cells. In addition to pAkt, we also found the level of total Akt was inhibited by treating the A549 cells with cordycepin-CMHW. Since up-regulation of Akt was correlated to cancer progression in lung tissue [27]. It is possible that cordycepin-CMHW down-regulated total Akt levels to exert their anti-cancer activity in A549 cells. However, the exact mechanism need to be further examined.

Apoptosis, an additional mechanism of anti-cancer activity triggers by A_3AR [8]. Indeed, A_3AR agonists have been reported to inhibit cell growth and/or induce apoptosis in various tumors [28]. Upon treatment with the cordycepin-CMHW, the A549 cells showed typical apoptotic morphology in culture. Furthermore, the nuclear mediated apoptosis effects (degradation of nuclear DNA into nucleosomal units) can be examined using TUNEL assay. This indicated that cordycepin-CMHW induced apoptosis in A549 cells. Caspases are a family of protease enzymes, which playing essential roles in enhancing apoptotic effects of A_3AR [9,10]. Caspases involved in apoptosis have been sub-classified by their mechanism of action. Specifically, the initiator caspases (caspase-8 and -9) motivate the executioner caspases (caspase-3, -6 and -7), by cleavages for activation, which contributing to the proteolytic of poly ADP ribose polymerase (PARP) and promoting apoptosis by preventing DNA repair-induced survival [29]. In the present work, it was observed that treatment of A549 cells with cordycepin-CMHW leads to induced caspase-9 and caspase-3 activation, and up-regulating at cleavage of PARP in A549 cells. Thus, cordycepin-CMHW is able to induce cell apoptosis by activation of caspase signaling pathway in A549 lung carcinoma. In conclusion, the present study showed that cordycein-CMHW induced tumor growth inhibition in non-small cell lung carcinoma A549 cells involves Akt inactivation and suppressed WNT/GSK-3β pathway. Results also suggested that cordycein-CMHW caused the A549 cell apoptosis by mediating caspase pathway. Taken together, cordycein-CMHW inhibits the growth of A549 cells by suppressing cell proliferation and inducing apoptosis, and may be a potential therapeutic agent for further development for the treatment of non-small cell lung cancer.

Acknowledgments

This work was supported by Ministry of Science and Technology in Taiwan (NSC 101-2324-B-197-002).

Competing Interest

The authors have no competing financial interests to declare.

Authors' Contributions

F.S.H.H. and Y.H.Y. have contributed equally to this work. F.S.H.H. and Y.H.Y. conducted experiments, analyzed data and wrote the manuscript. P.S., W.S.P. and A. D. analyzed and interpreted data, reviewed and edited the manuscript. C.H.H. conducted experiments and analyzed data. Y.L.C. and Y.H.C. designed the experiments, interpreted data, wrote the manuscript and approved the final manuscript.

References

1. Jacobson KA, Gao ZG (2006) Adenosine receptors as therapeutic targets. Nat Rev Drug Discov 5: 247-264.

2. Gao ZG, Jacobson KA (2007) Emerging adenosine receptor agonists. Expert Opin Emerg Drugs 12: 479-492.

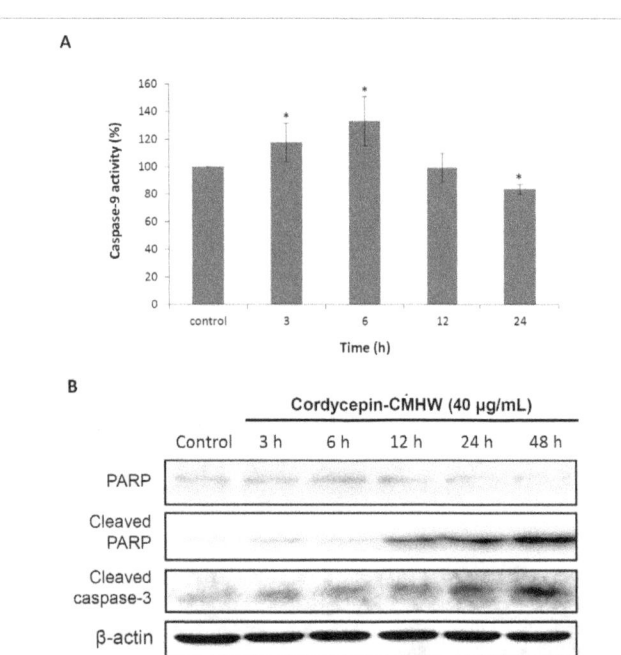

Figure 5: Cordycepin-CMHW mediate caspase and PARP activities in A549 cells: (A) the time-course effects of Cordycepin-CMHW on caspase-9 activity in A549 cells. Controls were set to 100%. The asterisks represent the statistically significant difference in the expression percentage of caspase-9 in A549 cell treated with Cordycepin-CMHW compared with that of the non-treated control ($p<0.05$). (B) A549 cells were treated with cordycepin-CMHW (40 μg/mL) for 0 to 48 hrs and the proteins levels of PARP, cleaved PARP and cleaved caspase-3 were determined by Western blotting. β-actin was used as loading control.

3. Madi L, Ochaion A, Rath-Wolfson L, Bar-Yehuda S, Erlanger A, et al. (2004) The A3 adenosine receptor is highly expressed in tumor versus normal cells: potential target for tumor growth inhibition. Clin Cancer Res 10: 4472-4479.

4. Kamiya H, Kanno T, Fujita Y, Gotoh A, Nakano T, et al. (2012) Apoptosis-related gene transcription in human A549 lung cancer cells via A(3) adenosine receptor. Cell Physiol Biochem 29: 687-696.

5. Merighi S, Benini A, Mirandola P, Gessi S, Varani K, et al. (2005) A3 adenosine receptor activation inhibits cell proliferation via phosphatidylinositol 3-kinase/Akt-dependent inhibition of the extracellular signal-regulated kinase 1/2 phosphorylation in A375 human melanoma cells. J Biol Chem 280: 19516-19526.

6. Fishman P, Bar-Yehuda S, Madi L, Cohn I (2002) A3 adenosine receptor as a target for cancer therapy. Anticancer Drugs 13: 437-443.

7. Chen S, Guttridge DC, You Z, Zhang Z, Fribley A, et al. (2001) Wnt-1 signaling inhibits apoptosis by activating beta-catenin/T cell factor-mediated transcription. J Cell Biol 152: 87-96.

8. Parcellier A, Tintignac LA, Zhuravleva E, Hemmings BA (2008) PKB and the mitochondria: AKTing on apoptosis. Cell Signal 20: 21-30.

9. Antonsson A, Persson JL (2009) Induction of apoptosis by staurosporine involves the inhibition of expression of the major cell cycle proteins at the G(2)/m checkpoint accompanied by alterations in Erk and Akt kinase activities. Anticancer Res 29: 2893-2898.

10. Kim SJ, Min HY, Chung HJ, Park EJ, Hong JY, et al. (2008) Inhibition of cell proliferation through cell cycle arrest and apoptosis by thio-Cl-IB-MECA, a novel A3 adenosine receptor agonist, in human lung cancer cells. Cancer Lett 264: 309-315.

11. Dela Cruz CS, Tanoue LT, Matthay RA (2011) Lung cancer: epidemiology, etiology, and prevention. Clin Chest Med 32: 605-644.

12. Chen Z, Fillmore CM, Hammerman PS, Kim CF, Wong KK, et al. (2014) Non-small-cell lung cancers: a heterogeneous set of diseases. Nat Rev Cancer 14: 535-546.

13. Gridelli C, Massarelli E, Maione P, Rossi A, Herbst RS, et al. (2004) Potential role of molecularly targeted therapy in the management of advanced nonsmall cell lung carcinoma in the elderly. Cancer 101: 1733-1744.

14. Sechler M, Cizmic AD, Avasarala S, Van Scoyk M, Brzezinski C, et al. (2013) Non-small-cell lung cancer: molecular targeted therapy and personalized medicine - drug resistance, mechanisms, and strategies. Pharmgenomics Pers Med 6: 25-36.

15. Cunningham KG, Manson W, Spring FS, Hutchinson SA (1950) Cordycepin, a metabolic product isolated from cultures of Cordyceps militaris (Linn.) Link. Nature 166: 949.

16. Patel S, Goyal A (2012) Recent developments in mushrooms as anti-cancer therapeutics: a review. Biotech 2: 1-15.

17. Yue K, Ye M, Zhou Z, Sun W, Lin X, et al. (2013) The genus Cordyceps: a chemical and pharmacological review. J Pharm Pharmacol 65: 474-493.

18. Zhou X, Luo L, Dressel W, Shadier G, Krumbiegel D, et al. (2008) Cordycepin is an immunoregulatory active ingredient of Cordyceps sinensis. Am J Chin Med 36: 967-980.

19. Cheng YH, Wen CM, Dybus A, Proskura WS (2016) Fermentation products of Cordyceps militaris enhance performance and modulate immune response of weaned piglets. South African Society for Animal Science 46: 121-128.

20. Liu TA, Jan YJ, Ko BS, Chen SC, Liang SM, et al. (2011) Increased expression of 14-3-3beta promotes tumor progression and predicts extrahepatic metastasis and worse survival in hepatocellular carcinoma. Am J Pathol 179: 2698-2708.

21. Tian X, Li Y, Shen Y, Li Q, Wang Q, et al. (2015) Apoptosis and inhibition of proliferation of cancer cells induced by cordycepin. Oncol Lett 10: 595-599.

22. Borea PA, Varani K, Vincenzi F, Baraldi PG, Tabrizi MA, et al. (2015) The A3 adenosine receptor: history and perspectives. Pharmacol Rev 67: 74-102.

23. Wang D, Zhang Y, Lu J, Wang Y, Wang J, et al. (2016) Cordycepin, a Natural Antineoplastic Agent, Induces Apoptosis of Breast Cancer Cells via Caspase-dependent Pathways. Nat Prod Commun 11: 63-68.

24. Das SK, Masuda M, Sakurai A, Sakakibara M (2010) Medicinal uses of the mushroom Cordyceps militaris: current state and prospects. Fitoterapia 81: 961-968.

25. Park BT, Na KH, Jung EC, Park JW, Kim HH, et al. (2009) Antifungal and anticancer activities of a protein from the mushroom Cordyceps militaris. Korean J Physiol Pharmacol 13: 49-54.

26. Bar-Yehuda S, Stemmer SM, Madi L, Castel D, Ochaion A, et al. (2008) The A3 adenosine receptor agonist CF102 induces apoptosis of hepatocellular carcinoma via de-regulation of the Wnt and NF-kappaB signal transduction pathways. Int J Oncol 33: 287-295.

27. Zinda MJ (2001) AKT-1, -2, and -3 are expressed in both normal and tumor tissues of the lung, breast, prostate, and colon. Clin Cancer Res 7: 2475-2479.

28. Gessi S, Merighi S, Sacchetto V, Simioni C, Borea PA, et al. (2011) Adenosine receptors and cancer. Biochim Biophys Acta 1808: 1400-1412.

29. McIlwain DR, Berger T, Mak TW (2013) Caspase functions in cell death and disease. Cold Spring Harb Perspect Biol 5.

42

Different Techniques of Acupuncture – Part of the Traditional Chinese Medicine and "Evidence Based Medicine"

Szilard Hamvas, Monika Havasi, Henrik Szőke, Petrovics Gabor and Gabriella Hegyi*

Faculty of Health Sciences, University of Pecs, Hungary

Abstract

Introduction: Dry needling: e.t. Acupuncture: is one of the most accepted CAM therapies, most well: known branch of the Traditional Chinese Medicine, which flows intensive research a few decades in the US, Europe, even in China. Is backed by proving research results of Evidence Based Medicine for properly as well.

Objective: To summarize the newer understanding of the mechanism of action and indications with regard to harmonization and closer to the TCM/TCM tenets of contemporary classical Chinese medical applying for.

Method: An international literature review, which called CAMbrella, the Pan: European Union project work package based on its research, which took part in the work of the Department of Complementary Medicine in, Health Science Faculty of Pecs University, as well.

Results: Acupuncture and TCM, are one of the most researched area of non–conventional, complementary therapies. We have already demonstrated convincingly established by the management of the majority of acupuncture point physiological responses. The mediator neurohormonal transmitters are already known about now. 40 have been identified which are involved in induced "dry needling" effect.

Discussion: The "Bridge" between the Eastern and Western medicine is the appropriate knowledge transfer, research and application. The performance of in: service training is a university competence. Evidence Based Medicine has an efficient and effective use based on the quality of training in: service training, which is conducted in some Universities for more decades. Further development of this training, quality education can only be realistic to achieve the goals (which effectively give rise to a dedicated TCM Confucius Institute Pecs University).

Keywords: Acupuncture; Dry needling; Traditional Chinese Medicine (TCM); Neurohumoral mechanism

Abbreviations: CAM: Complementary and Alternative Medicine; TCM: Traditional Chinese Medicine (HKO); EBM: Evidence Based Medicine; SZOTE: University of Szeged: Faculty of Medicine; HIETE: Haynal Imre University of Health Science; PTE ETK: University of Pecs, Faculty of Health Sciences; GYEMSZTI: National Institute for Quality and Organizational Development in Healthcare and Medicines; ÁNTSZ: The National Public Health and Medical Officer Service (NPHMOS); Yin: Yang: from the Philosophical Aspect is a Synonym of Matter and Motion, at the Same Time One Refers to the So Called jin Organs (splanchnic), and the Other So Called Transmitting Jang Organs (hollow); AA: Acupuncture Analgesia; KM: Complementery Medicine

Introduction and Definition

Basic questions are arrived in this topic

Speaking about Acupuncture they are a few questions.

A few questions-already answered and still unanswered-are waiting to be clarified:

Do "acupuncture points" really exist? What does it mean a "meridian" and how can it be explained in the classic synonym system?

What is the essence of mechanical peripheral stimulus, the nervous and neurohumoral mechanism mediating acupuncture (e.g., pain-killing)?

Is there an acceptable and relevant professional literature proving the efficiency of clinical acupuncture?

Acupuncture ('dry needling')[1] is one of the basic aspects of Traditional Chinese Medicine (TCM). Its classical base is presented by the "principle of energy flow system", the recognition of the channels (in other words: meridians) and the points of mechanical stimulus, namely the puncture points–acupuncture points-on which the former is based. The application of this principle can be carried out by mechanical stimulus: needle puncture, massage, temperature stimulus, vacuum based suction, as well as by ultrasound, laser, etc. In China it has been known for centuries about different herbs on which meridian they are effective and whether they belong to the type of yin or yang. So the knowledge of channels and points was also taken into consideration in Chinese phytotherapy.[2] In the diagnostic process the examination of the pulse plays an important role: by touching the arteria radialis on the wrist with three fingers both on the surface and deeply, valuable information is received on the organs representing the twelve main meridians. We can say, that we are talking about a diagnostic and therapeutic whole body complex system[3] based on a unitary theoretic foundation which is consistent in itself. Traditional Chinese Medicine has already put down all these in writing in its 2600-year-old basic literature known as 'The Yellow Emperor's Classic of Internal Medicine', which is the most important professional literature even today and was extended later. It is also important to

[2] Materia Medica Institute, Peking (with WHO support).
[3] 'Whole body complex system"-WHO terminology.

[1] It includes Chinese Phytotherapy, Cupping, Tuina massage, nutriceuticals which constitute together TCM.

*Corresponding author: Hegyi Gabriella, Doctorate School, Faculty of Health Sciences, University of Pecs, Hungary, E-mail: drhegyi@hu.inter.net

mention the point system[4] of the ear–as microsystem–acupuncture, which was only discovered a few decades ago, since '…meridians meet on the external ear'–as the above mentioned basic literature says. A newer recognition is the study and application of the Yamamato[4] scalp system. Throughout the acupuncture process extremely tiny filiform needles[5] are put into certain so called 'acupuncture points' under the surface of the skin. The anatomical situation of a point is an entity which is based on classical descriptions, empirical, today's biophysical measurements and new knowledge.

Do "acupuncture point and meridian" really exist?

Is it more efficient to treat an acupuncture point already known than to place the needle into a sham acupuncture point? By examining the efficiency of acupunctural pain-killing [1][6] came to the conclusion that pains induced in acute, laboratory conditions both in humans and animals could only be efficiently alleviated by stimulating acupuncture points, while in the case of treating non-acupuncture points there was no really measurable pain-killing effect observed. This is in accordance with the fact that even so-called placebo pills without active substance were only successful in killing pain in 30% of the cases. At the same time, in the cases of chronic pain this difference is not so obvious. A great number of cases are needed to achieve the statistical significance (a minimum of 122 experimental persons per examination); furthermore this issue has not been closed up to now. Also in Eory's experiments when applying the needle to points considered to have low resistance (acupuncture points are also described as having low resistance and higher impedance, see later) they were able to induce local warming on certain plants (monitored by using infra camera), while in the case of treating points without low electric resistance the plants did not react with an intense growth [2-4].

Do acupuncture points have a specific anatomic structure?

According to the finding of a number of microscopic and electro-microscopic examinations there is no separate structure apart from our skin sense organ representative of special acupuncture points, but a bigger number of sensory nerve endings can be recognized at the indicated points, e.g., GAP junction[9].

Physiological and biophysical description of acupuncture points

In Europe it was the French Niboyet who first described that the areas of the skin surface with low electrical resistance can be identified with acupuncture points.[7] The electrical resistance of human skin as well as its reciproc, namely conductivity varies within wide limits but compared with adjacent skin areas a significant difference can be measured regarding acupuncture points. Simultaneous factors influencing skin resistance must also be taken into consideration since a measurement can be hindered by several influential factors (temperature, surface humidity, calibration of the measuring device). During the measurement we apply a very weak measuring current. In our days 'point detecting' devices are already widespread based on the electrical resistance of the skin and, in case of an alternate current measurement principle, on the measurement of impedance? The German Voll-type point based method of electric diagnostics and

the Japanese so called Ryodoraku ("good conducting connections") method are also based on skin resistance, but with a relatively strong measuring current we can only receive reference values, which means, that these measurements are not suitable for traditional clinical diagnostics, however they give information on the operation of the so called 'control circles' in TCM.

The surface of the skin shows 30-100 mV potential difference in its areas, where it is the surface to be considered more negative compared to the deeper layers [5-7]. When measuring skin potential values acupuncture points are also measurable and bigger differences can be measured in these areas.[8] In case of damage a so called 'damage current' is created depending on the potential difference mentioned above. This partially gives an explanation on the chemical and physical processes induced by the needle applied. The adverb 'partially' needs to be explained here. During acupuncture it is not only the damage potential that induces current, but also the needle itself functions as a thermo element, since when applying the needle there is a temperature difference of more than 10°C.[9]

The electric measurements are reproducible, although the measured resistance decrease can only partially be explained by the thinning of the stratum corneum of the skin, the denser of 'Gap junction' and the higher density of nerves and sensation. In the 70s the so far best indicator of the increased metabolism in points was found by the application of the supersensitive CO_2 respirometer-FREWIL-developed by professor of physiology Frenyó-Eőry.[10] The electrical resistance and the temperature of the skin when at work were measured simultaneously by examining the respiration of the skin. Its result is the following: there is a 52% interconnection between the respiration of the skin and the CO_2 content of the blood running in the capillaries. The physiological role of the significant amount of CO_2 emitted above an acupuncture point might be that it hinders the escape of thermo-energy by enforcing the micro greenhouse effect at the points (by which the relative 'low-thermal' acupuncture point picture on infracamera images can be explained). Bergman (1980) showed that 'acupuncture points' even have infrared emission [8-10].

What is the concept of a "Meridian"? According to our latest knowledge it is a virtual network system which refers to the succesive sequences of the recognized bioactive acupuncture points, so it is not a separately and touchable anatomic structure. This notion is also supported by the newer approach that assigns the points of "meridian" to the embryo structures of spinal cord segmentation in de facto application as well. What is interesting about the concept is that we could get familiar with the zones of head at the end of the 19th century (in addition, in the same area they were also found by Zaricott and McKenzie), furthermore we can meet its empirical experience and recognition in the situation of the sequential points on the "meridian" and its centuries old de facto application as well!

What is the Nervous and Neurohumoral Mechanism Mediating Acupuncture (e.g., Acupunctural Pain-killing)?

The very first clear answer to the nervous mediation of low–frequency Electroacupuncture (EA) applied via inserted needles was given by Chiang [11], whose research is still going on. He stated that the stimuli of type 2 and 3 fibres leading to the muscle induce the so called "spreading" needle sensation that is in connection with the effect that

[4] YNSA: Yamamoto New Scalp Acupuncture, Bristol, 1986, microsystem discovered and published by Toshikatsu Yamamoto, a Japanese professor.
[5] Earlier the needles were made of gold or silver, but recently out of steel with a thicknesses of 0, 30-0, 40 gauge, lenght 1-5 cun (2-10 cm).
[6] Bruce Pomeranz, who was a professor of Department of Physiology at the University of Toronto, has received a Chinese award for his researh in TCM in 1990.
[7] Point detecting devices developed from devices for the measurment of electrical resistance of the skin are based on this finding.

[8] Areas from few square mm to five square cm.
[9] With Shang's words (2001) the acupuncture points are the converging points of surface current.
[10] Frenyo- Eőry, 1984.

gets disturbed by the strong muscle contractions created by stimulation. This explains why an electric stimulation with low frequency and higher current stability is important.[11] The other significant finding is that the induced anesthetic effect is not organ-specific. This is in accord with the following nervous mechanism in case of applying a low frequency and high intensity electro-acupuncture (EA).[11]

An impulse is generated by the activated sensor receptor when a needle is being applied which first runs to the spinal cord then it advances upward through the ascending tracts then through the nuclei of thalamus to the cortex. The fibres responsible for the impulse transmission are myelinated type 2 and 3 afferents with a small diameter. They are responsible for the numbness and the feeling of fullness induced by the spreading needle sensation (but the pain is mediated by the bare type 4 fibres). In case of an activation of skin nerves the A-delta fibres play a role.[12] In the spinal cord the activated nerve cell has a short segmental branch that is endorfinerg. This pre-sinaptically inhibits either through encephalin or dynorphin mediation but not through ß-endorfin one, which means it blocks the transmission of the pain stimuli. Consequently, the encephalins and the dynorphin may block the pain already at the level of the spinal cord. Next the needle stimuli advance through the ascending tracts to the thalamus in the spinal cord. In the peri-aquaeductal grey matter (PAG) of the midbrain it activates the raphe nucleus in the caudal part of the medulla oblongata through encephalin mediation. It sends back descending impulses in the dorsolateral part of the spinal cord (DLT) through monoamine (serotonin and norepinephrine) mediation to the cells of the spinal cord. Both monoamine mechanisms might take part in pain-killing. The originally activated ascending tract in spinal cord also activates the nucleus arcuatus in the hypothalamus-hypophysis complex, while other parts of the hypothalamus receive ß-endorphin from the hypothalamus itself. It effects through the blood current only to a small extent, it rather gets to the cell on a direct retrograde way without getting through the blood-brain barrier (Figures 1 and 2). Anyhow, the destruction of hypophysis in experimental animals inhibits the creation of an acupunctural effect. The hypophysis also releases ACTH in an equimolar amount with ß-endorphin (since their precursor is common).

Adrenocorticotropic Hormone (ACTH) stimulates the adrenal gland to release cortisol, which explains the anti-inflammatory effect of acupuncture in conditions such as asthma, arthritis, etc. At the same time this little amount of cortisol does not have harmful side effects neither does it cause a positive feed-back.

The recent excellent radiological diagnostic techniques (PET, fMRI) prove that acupuncture can activate further parts of central nervous system parts such as nucleus accumbens, amygdala, habenula, thalamic nuclei, etc.[13]

Perhaps the most exciting period of research of analgesic effect of acupuncture was, when it became evident that naloxone-which is an endorphin antagonist-can also inhibit the analgesic effect of acupuncture. In a study of volunteer participants with artificially induced toothache were treated by manual stimulation of Large Intestine 4 (LI4) on hand acupuncture point[14] to relieve pain. One group received intravenous saline; the other group received intravenous naloxone. None of the participants knew which group they were in. (This is a typical example of double blind clinical research.) In the first group

the pain was eliminated in 30 min and the effect persisted longer than one hour. The pain did not subside in naloxone group in spite of dry needling. At the same time the participants of placebo group received placebo injection with the instruction that it was a strong pain-killer medicine. These participants did not experience any alleviation of their pain at all.[15] A subsequent study conducted by Cheng and Pomeraz [6] shows, that an increasing dosage of naloxone causes increasing blocking of acupuncture analgesia (AA). Shortly after the publication, that the dosage of naloxone needed to block AA depended on applied frequency of electro-acupuncture. It is less in case of 2 Hz than in case of 15 Hz and comparatively lot more naloxone was necessary to inhibit pain relief induced by 100 Hz EA. Based on cross-tolerance studies it has become certain that there are different endogenous opiate mediations depending on the frequency of needle stimulation, and all this takes place via different receptors.[16] In 1985 an anti-opioid peptide was first isolated from bovine brain, which was chemically equivalent to angiotensin II. Based on this knowledge the explanation of the antihypertensive effect of acupuncture compared with angiotensin-converting-enzyme inhibitor (ACE inhibitors) is thought provoking. The antihypertensive effect of opioids was already known. Using the opioids as medicine is proved to be difficult because their elimination in the body is too fast. On the other hand if we inhibit the final synthesis of angiotensin II-ACE inhibitors are examples of this-it loses its anti-opioid effect; hence we can lower blood pressure, however it eventually happens due to opioid peptides of the body. Lowering blood pressure in the so called neurogenic stage of hypertension could be achieved more directly through opioids facilitated by acupuncture.[17]

There are some known explanations of the effect of acupuncture

1. **Augmentation theory:** Acupuncture raises the level of triglycerides, certain hormons, prostaglandins, leukocytes, gamma globulins, opsonins, and antibodies (immunstimulatory effect).

2. **Endorphin theory:** Acupuncture stimulates the production of endorphins (especially the enkephalins, and dynorphins) (analgesia).

3. **Neurotransmitter theory:** Acupuncture can influence on the production and secretion of several neurotransmitters (serotonine, noradrenaline) (depression and emotional diseases, the decreased level of serotonin may lead to weight loss).

4. **Circulatory/vasomotoric theory:** Acupuncture liberating vasodilatant substances (especially histamin), (oedemas, neuropathy and post traumatic regenerative conditions).

5. **Gate control theory:** On the level of interneurons of the spine acupuncture stimulated somatosensoric A:delta fibres block the thinner viscerosensor C fibers transmitting the incomming pain information, by which they prevent its spreading into higher level center and prevent the perceiving of pain (anaestesy, analgesy, Diffuse Noxious Inhibiting Control: postulated by le Bars, 2003).

Breakdown of Today's More Acknowledged and thorough Theories

1. Local segmental effect: axon reflex, vasoactive neuropeptides: mostly calcitonin gene related peptid (CGRP), substance P (SP): (Lundeberg, Kashiba, Schaffer, Calsson, 1991, 1992, 1998), endorphin: antiinflammatory effect (Stein, Yassouridis, 1988).

---

[11] Pomeranz, 2001.
[12] The gate control theory of Melzack and Wall.
[13] Yamamoto, T: YNSA publications (1998, 2004, 2010).
[14] The space between I and II metacarpus is the one of the most notable point to pain relief ("Hegu" vagy "Hoku").

[15] Reminder: placebo is only effective in maximum 3% of the cases in acute pain.
[16] Han, 2008. Peking, TCM Academy.
[17] Naturally it may be asked whether effect of acupuncture lowering blood pressure?

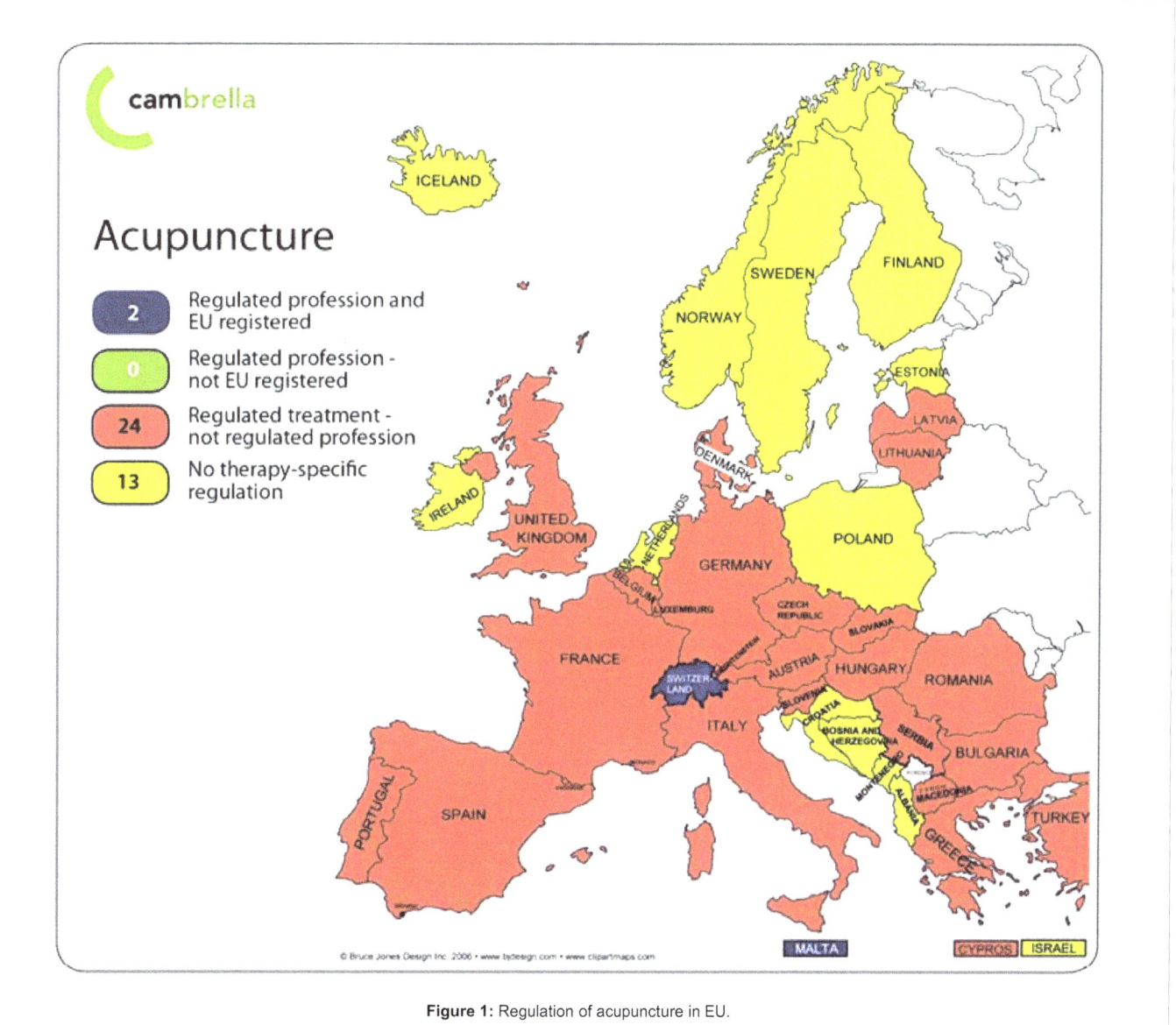

Figure 1: Regulation of acupuncture in EU.

2. Trigger points (70% of them are acupuncture points) treatment ability of myofascial pain syndroms (Irnich, Bayer, Charitee Uni, 2002), myofascial trigger points identical with 70% of acupunctural points (Birch 2003), local trigger points: Aschi points, detoning effect to trigger points (Hong, 1994).

3. Regional perfusion changes: acupuncture/electroacupuncture (Lundeberg, Karolinksa Institute, 1999), periferal vasodilatation (Janson 1989), M: Raynaud electro: stimulation, "segment: reflectoric effect (Sato, 1995, Smidt, 1973), local tissue mediators role (CGRP[18], etc.).

4. Nociceptive afferental inhibition: intensive painful stimulus, A:delta fibres (Sandkuhler, 2001) pain release as observed on animals (Anderson/Lundeberg, 1995), the result is a long lasting blockage of disturbance on A:delta afferent fibres (Liu Chen, Sankuhles, 2000) (Toda/Ichioka, Liu, 1983).

5. Melczak: Wall "gate control" theory: this time has been added and adapted neuromatrix theory. "Gate control" theory has

been added by "neuramatrix" theory, 1999. Differencess between extitatons of A: delta fibres and A: beta fibres, conduction velocity, inhibition of heterosegmental nociceptive stimulus (Sandkuhler, 1996) they are the part of supraspinal descendal inhibiting mechanism.

6. Segmental reflectoric effect: Somatovisceral reflective circle, converging of nociceptive neuron population in spinal cord– Shu points (Janik/Habler, 2002), viscerocutan: visceromotoric reflex: Heasd zones (Head, Zaricott, McKenzie, 1987), connective tissue tone alteration in organ's projection zones (Zimmermann, 2004).

7. Systematic effects: Activating of supraspinal descending braking system (Cao, 2002, Tagechige, 1992), psychic/psychical effect, effect on stress pain (B. Pomeranz, 1996), stress analgesia: through stress: induced reduction of pain sensitivity (Fancelov, 1999), short time activation of endorphin system (but in such an extent explanation of the long term effect is not enough).

[18] Calcitonin gene-related peptide (CGRP) is a member of the calcitonin family of peptides.

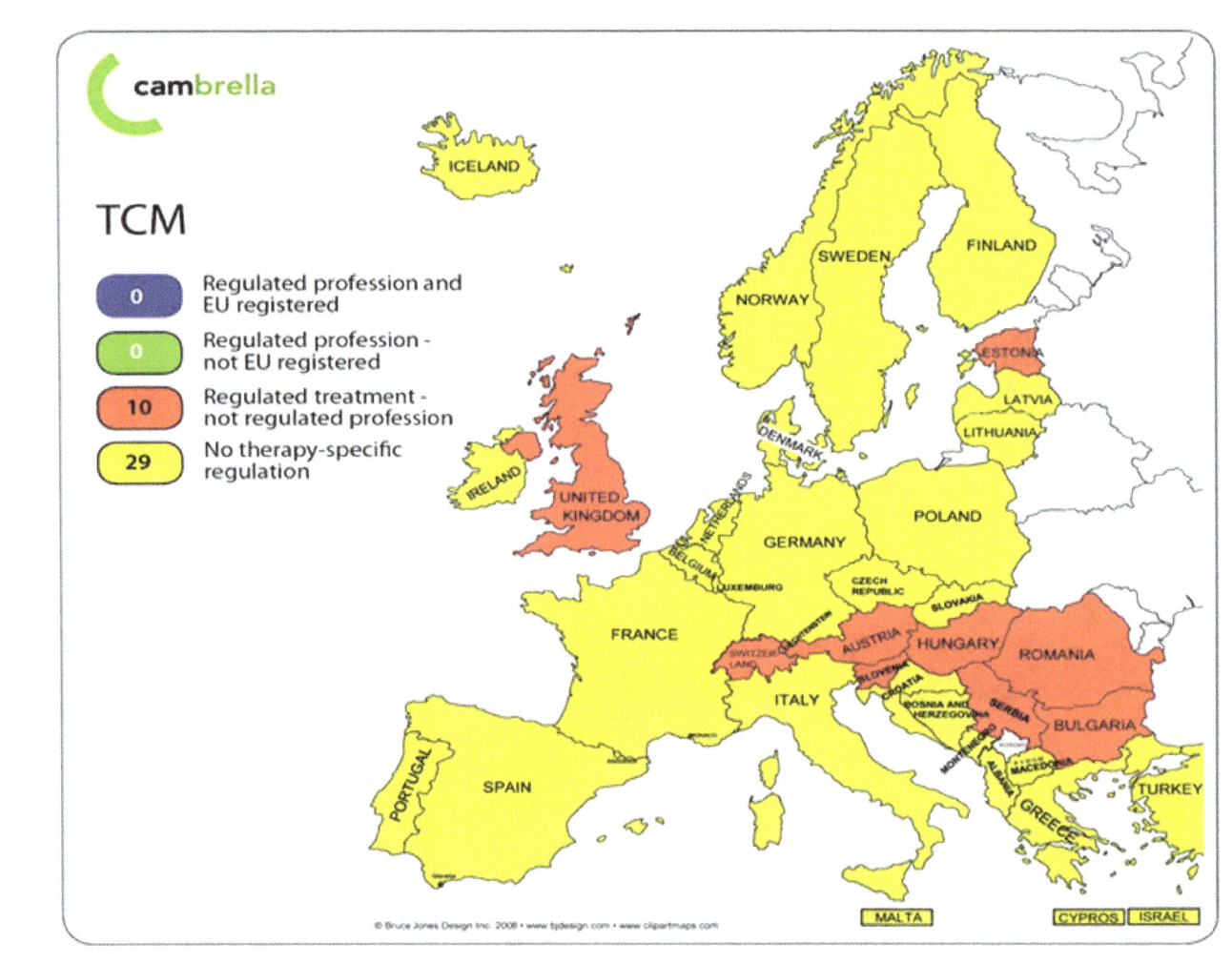

Figure 2: Complex traditional Chinese medicine (Acupunctere, Herbal medicine, Tuina massage, Moxibustion, Cupping) regulation in EU.

8. Diffuse Noxious Inhibiting Control (DNIC): "pain prevents pain" (La Bars, 2002), Villanueva, La Bars, 1995: acupuncture painful stimulation prevents more pain...

9. Endorphin system: endorphinerg system activating (Han, Xie, 1984, Peking), (Tageshire, Pomeranz, 2002, Han Terenius, 1982: the most accepted explanation until this time, decrease of endorphin system regulation, chronic pain syndroms disreglative changes (especially lumboischalgc pain, haedache, fibromylagia).

10. Cerebral effects: fMRI, PET, limbic system activate (Hui, 2000, Hui 2005, Hsieh et al., 2001), hypothalamus, periaquaductal grey matter, gyrus cinguli, cerebellum, semsomororical cortex (Gareus et al., 2002, Biella et al., 2001, Niemtchow, 2007), neural signal modulation in cerebrovascular excitement–migraine effective (Becker, 2004).

11. Autonom vegetative neural effects: under acupuncture done sympatycotomy, followed by strenghtened parasympaticotonus (Ernst, Lee, 1986) causes "poststimulative sympaticolysis" (Anderson, Lundeberg, 1996).

12. Endocrine effects: Hypothalamus activation (Hsieh et al., 2001), the role of hypothalamus: hypophysis axis, explanation

of humoral endocrine changes, increased level of oxytocin after electro:acupuncture, cervical release during childbirth, menses settlement, premenstrual syndrome treatment (Uvnas, Moberg, 1963).

Do we have Acceptable Data about the Clinical Effectiveness of Acupuncture?

Clinical effect of acupuncture can be assessed only based on human individuals, thoroughly prepared by observation. Later we follow basic rules of evidence-based medicine and then verified and confirmed clinical impact studies.

Regular overview summarizing on the evidence based medicine

Overall requirement for effectiveness confirmation is a sufficient amount of performed and well: prepared, random and controlled experiments. Until the 90's experiments of this kind done on individual diseases and its regular evaluation were called metaanalysis.

Today, there is a specific statistical method, where individual examinations are an examined entity. Balanced usage of all the until now gained knowledge about medicine based on facts (evidence based knowledge) is conscientious and open to patient and based on current proven facts decides on the best possible treatment for patients [11,12]. It is expected from the medical doctor that he has possibly the best clinical experiences in given specialization and is educated by the best research results. In system included publications, whatever the results were, have to match certain specification requirements. Only then are we able to guarantee objective and unbiased assessments, thanks to which we are able to prevent pointless repetition of experiments, when the result of the repeated experiment isn't better, therefore it doesn't provide us with newer information from the previous. New outcomes of working hypothesis formulation are important for future research.

In order to eliminate possible bias we use so: called sensitivity analysis. There we compare and examine better and worse results of individual experiments and those are then compared only with results and outcomes of the better experiments. When the outcomes from the previous one are "more optimistic" we are most likely dealing with bias. We are also calling it biased when the outcomes–whether intentionally or not–are evaluating the one and the same experiment numerous times (for example: when the experiment was published more times but under different names).

CAMbrella–the Pan: European Union research project[19] included one worksheet, which was discussing this topic in the recent past, when they analyzed approximately 17.000 articles.

The proven clinical efficacy of the acupuncture

The acupuncture treatment means a diagnosis of the patient as an individual and a planned treatment according to the given clinical pattern [13]. This also means that according to the unique, extremely detailed Chinese pulse and tongue examination there are no two patients totally alike. In this regard, it is a great task to contract the results of certain experiments but the randomization itself is also difficult. While certain problems are always treated on the same point (for instance nausea and vomiting are treated on Pericardium: 6 acupoint[20]), in case of a chronic pain syndrome different treatment protocols must be followed depending on the accompanying symptoms. In order to apply the right acupuncture treatment the criteria are not only the selection of the right puncture points but also the consideration of further factors: Linde et al. [14] examined 5 circumstances: 1) The selected points; 2) The total number of treatments; 3) The number of weekly treatments; 4) The duration of one single treatment; 5) The inducement of needle sensation (in Chinese: De Qi sensation). The adequacy of acupuncture can also be estimated by the minimum number of acceptable treatments. According to the criteria of Molsberger and Bowing [15] it means at least 10 sessions of treatments in which each single treatment session is a minimum of 15 min long and the record of the used acupuncture points. Only 16 out of the 88 clinical studies referring to locomotors and/or neurological diseases examined by them met the criteria above, furthermore only 2 of them fulfilled the criteria of a controlled experiment. Patel et al. suggest that for testing the adequacy of acupuncture the criteria should be the ones predominating in the case of experiments with more positive reactions. Although this approach in itself does not give an answer whether the applied acupuncture has been effective enough against the actual disease, it can be observed that experimental group members preferred treatments tailored individually to selection of points according to the standard formula. But how to integrate individual treatments into controlled experimental methods? "It feels like giving medicine to patients in individual doses instead of the prescription." This contradiction can be dissolved by dividing the

treated group into sub: groups. The certain sub: group members will be treated on the points according to the formula. Following the latter approach it is known that there is no connection between the number of treated points and the successfulness of a treatment, however scientists found a statistically significant relation regarding the number of treatments and the successfulness of the cure. Getting less than 6 treatments was never efficient enough, but those patients who undergone 10 treatments recovered more successfully.

Accepted treatability of certain clinical diseases through acupuncture

Summarizing the results of meta: analyses carried out so far, we can say that, although to a limited extent we can accept it as a fact ("limited evidence") that acupuncture is more effective than pure placebo, sham acupuncture or traditional 'western' medicine in chronic or acute pain syndrome, Pendrick, Harvard Medical School, 2013). According to the efficacy examination of acupuncture treatments for lumbal pain acupuncture is a suitable method but only recommended as a complementary treatment. It was found after the statistical evaluation of 7 studies on fibromyalgia that acupuncture is much more effective than [8] sham acupuncture, but there was not a long: term follow up carried out in the examined studies. Ernst et al., [11] also found using acupuncture is effective to treat acute toothache in a systematic review of 16, than 20 articles. In a systematic review of 22 experiments Melchart et al. [15], found the use of acupuncture was superior in treating headache compared to "sham" acupuncture. They came to the conclusion that, although there is not sufficient data to prove that acupuncture is better than treating with medicine [16] patients with recurrent headache can be encouraged to try acupuncture (1999). Its application is even more recommended to treat tension headaches (Han, Cheung, 2013). In a systematic review of 33 studies suggested that in case of nausea and vomiting the stimulation of Pericardium: 6 acupoint (through massage, needle, etc.) itself is enough to achieve significant effect [17]. The result contributed a lot to the fact that after Nixon's visit to China in 1998 the American National Institute of Health (NIH) came to an agreement to recognize acupuncture as a legal treatment (the establishment of NICAM[21]). It is interesting that in the 4 experiments when patients were stimulated on this point while being anesthetized, nausea was not reducible. Perhaps on this point there is a considerable psychological effect manifested as well, that supposes the conscious mental state [15].

Based on 4 controlled clinical experiments we can state that if we include acupuncture in the common stroke rehabilitation treatments, the chance of a successful rehabilitation significantly increases, in addition the cost of post treatments can also be reasonably decreased (Birch, 2001, Hegyi 2015).

By the examination of patients in controlled clinical experiments we can conclude that: there is sufficient data provided to state that acupuncture and in particular the formularized form of ear acupuncture treatments are suitable to cease alcohol addiction[22], furthermore addicts can be more motivated to go on with other therapies. On the other hand, according to Birch the role of acupuncture is promising but contradictory regarding patients with cocaine and opiate addiction. Further research is required in this field. It is worldwide applied as a complementary treatment for reducing withdrawal symptoms.[23]

According to 4 controlled, randomized clinical experiments it can be said that acupuncture as a complementary treatment can be recommended in treating angina pectoris. The study recommends acupressure as well, which can be carried out as a self-treatment too.

---

[19] CAMbrella, Pan-European Project on CAM in 29 EU-countries, 2010-2012, www.cambrella.eu.
[20] "Nei Guan": It is located on the anterior forearm, two cun–2 finger-above to the wrist crease in the middle

[21] National Institute of Complementary and Alternative Medicine, www.nicam.com.
[22] Actually it only lowers the withdrawal symptoms.
[23] Lincoln Hospital, NY-City, Bronx, Dr. introduced by Dr. Smith: NADA program.

In case of frequent urination, incontinence, recurring lower urinary tract infection and kidney stone acupuncture can be recommended due to having significantly less side effects than common pharmacotherapies.

The relevant literature is about the positively influential intervention to ease delivery and cervical dilatation in case of breech birth and transverse lie (only in case of multipara pregnancy). Birch evaluates 3 studies in his work already mentioned. Based on his studies it can be said that acupuncture is useful for painful period (dysmenorrhea), sterility (due to amenorrhea and luteal insufficiency) and for reduction of hot flushes during menopause, although there is a so far insufficient controlled study provided for a systemic review. Despite this fact its application is successful with a lot of patients.

Allen et al., then others also (Jalinitzhev, 2012) proved that acupuncture is significantly positive for women with depression. Its application in drug addiction already discussed also belongs to the issue of psychiatry and addictology [18,19], as it decreases vegetative symptoms during treatment. [24]

Based on Case Reports and Randomized Controlled Trials Acupuncture Treatment is Applicable in the Following Diseases

- Allergic rhinitis, biliary colic, dysentery [20-26].

- Cramps caused by acut bacterial enteric infection.

- Depression like mood disorders, sleep disorders.

- Depression related to chronic disorders and/or conditions (e.g., post stroke).

- Dysmenorrhoea, menstrual cramps.

- Epigastric pain, (peptic ulcer, acute and chronic gastritis).

- Facial pain (with different etiology), prosopalgia, craniomandibular dysfunctions, temporomandibular joint disorders, neuralgia [10,11,14,15].

- Headaches (especially tension:type headache).

- High blood pressure (essential hypertenison).

- Support and induction of labor: facilitation of dilatation stage, correction of fetal position.

- Knee pain, low back pain (discus hernia, discopathia, postoperative pain).

- Shoulder and neck complaints (neck:shoulder girdle syndrome).

- Leukopenia [16,17].

- Vomiting and nausea [18,26].

- Renal colic.

- Postoperative pain syndromes, postoperative nausea.

- Temporomadibular joint complaints, pain relief before and after dental treatment [11].

- Soft: tissue rheumatic conditions, tennis:elbow, lumbago [27-29].

- Stroke, improving the residual symptoms of transient ischaemic attack, rehabilitation [30-36].

- Habilitation, mental and movement development of disabled children.

- Lability of autonomic nervous system, increased sympathicotonia.

We know different types of acupuncture used all over the world

- Simple dry needling: performed with filiformis thin needles (steel).

- Permanent acupuncture: performed by special constructed needle with lumen, where the absorbable monofilament is placed into the top of lumen and leaded into the skin. This form has a permanent and longer effect of biostimulation on points and deeper neuroanatomical structures. It is used for children and older patients who does not like to frequent treatment by acupuncture. Special effect has to rehabilitation of handicapped children and residual symptoms of post: stroke rehabilitation.

- Acupressure: mechanic stimulation of points with fingertips.

- Laser acupuncture: special light therapy of monochromatic beam, which was introduced by *prof. Mester Endre* (Hungary) and worldwide frequently used. The red beam is used for the laser: acupuncture (680 nm) penetrating 0.8 cm, for trigger point stimulation: The infra: red beam is penetrated deeper (1.2 cm) and used for musculoskeletal stiffness and pain syndromes.

- Ultravoice: acupuncture: not frequently used

- Intradermal permanent needle acupuncture: small steel needle for 2:3 days biostimulation of points

- Epidermal needles for ear acupuncture (ASP needles) only for ear acupuncture for 2:4 days avoiding cartilage damage.

- Electroacupuncture (EA): used as an extension technique of acupuncture based on traditional acupuncture combined with modern electrotherapy, is commonly used for stroke in clinical treatment and researches. However, there is still a lack of enough evidence to recommend the routine use of EA for stroke.

- Massage technique with electrical instruments applied to acupoints.

Outlook

Today's "modern" acupuncture methods combine classical, which methods are evolved based on the empirical, and modern, which are evolving on the modern technical methods. This method is also e.g., Soft Laser Biostimulation, Laser Acupuncture, which especially with children and elderly replaces induced stimulation. These patients tolerate the laser application better. In case of electro: acupuncture we use electric current pulses to induce stimulation. Very often, we use the device also to find the acupuncture points. The effect of magnetic field on acupuncture points is also observed.

Of course, neighboring countries to China (mainly Japan, Korea, and Vietnam) also took on acupuncture. In these three countries they developed and extended different techniques, depending on their specific needs. For example Japanese use very thin needles, so called filiform needles, which are injected through a skin with a tube?

In Vietnam they use also very long needles, 20-30 cm long (for example from both sides of spine longitudinally). This technique is local and Chinese only adopted it and by this they both are influencing

[24] NADA: National Antinicotine and Drog Acupuncture treatment (introduce by Smith, Bronx, NY City, Lincoln Hospital, start of the international program).

its development. In so: called "Embedding acupuncture" absorbable monofilament sewing sutures are used, which are applied on individual points, and for approximately 3 weeks are being resorbed, and this is causing a stimulating effect. By this it is possible to prevent frequent needle application, especially with children and elderly.

TCM as a part of medicine is accepted and applied in 122 countries of the world, and its popularity is increasing, thanks to the strategy of the current Chinese government [25,28].

Apart from that, after finishing a two years course MD`s receive a diploma, which authorizes them to request an authorization to practice in an independent practice. Acupuncture section of TCM in Europe: *Hungary, Germany,* is approved and financially covered by the state insurance as part of the rheumatology and physiotherapy field, but only in state health facilities. Some of the health insurance companies refund these treatments, but only with the additional private health insurance.

Based on these facts, education is part of the university education, which guarantees the necessary level of knowledge. Therefore in the future it will be important to keep it at this level, reasonable to keep it at the level of Bachelor and Master of Science. We also need to emphasize that our goal is not to educate "complementary doctors, workers (professional staff)". Person, who chooses to study medicine, should first get to know the Western medicine. After gaining sufficient amount of knowledge and experience, one can then focus on individual fields of Complementary medicine, and use them later on. We find useful the sharing and passing on of experience from the authentic source to the specialists with EU diplomat, who are interested in broadening their portfolio of healing abilities which are beneficial and safe for the patient. It is also important–mostly per request of the university scholars: that at the universities' students are getting information from authentic sources about given topic, not only partial, often very distorted information.

From this process it is clear, that it is necessary to keep increasing public awareness about topics of healthy life style, keep developing system of education and build a strong and stable position of complementary healing. Prerequisite for adequate education is responsible, specialized and ethically accurate medical professional behavior, which guarantees integrated use of both approaches in use. The term complementary medicine needs to be officially added as the additional option to the standard healthcare. It does have an important spot in the areas of healthy lifestyle counseling, in improving of health culture of public, in prevention of common chronic diseases, in curing early symptoms, but it also has its place in rehabilitation and in curing chronic degenerative problems of geriatric patients. Mostly in cases where due to chronic degenerative diseases of musculoskeletal system there is a high usage of medication and interaction among the medications occurs.

Also from the historical medical point of view it is important to provide complete point of view on individual philosophical aspects of healing methods and its forms (Ayurveda, Tibetan, Chinese, folk eastern kinetic and massage healing techniques) but also about those techniques–even with critical standpoints–which theoretical explanation isn't until today unified. Conditions of research CAM can therefore be supported and executed only in the area of academic institutions–universities. There are accessible sufficient scientific and practical resources, which allow the research also in these areas, on the home university field (similar American organization NICAM has current yearly budget of 122 mil. dollars)

College of complementary medicine takes part mostly in development of curriculum, in pregradual studies, which provides education of students in given topics, continues in educating of doctors for the future. Currently, at the only one workplace in the country, which also works like a "Methodological Center" they also build the post gradual studying plan, necessary minimal requirements for given rules. Since 2004, college regularly maintains and deepens international relations (mostly with Chinese HUU-Hebei United University of Science and Technology: College of Clinical Medicine, Tangshan, Hebei Province, Charitee University of Munich, University of Bristol, Exeter CAM Institute, Chung Gun Memorial University, Taipei University of Taiwan, The Institute of Complementary Medicine (IKOM) University of Bern, South: West University in London) and e.t.

Summary

Acupuncture in a wider meaning like TCM is one of the not so conventional healing methods, which is currently scientifically the best: analyzed field. In European Union it is officially accepted and its usage is in a different extent regulated. It is officially used in 122 world countries (picture 1:2). Basic researches already today provide convincing data about the existence of acupunctural points.

To some extent functions of neurotransmitters are clarified, currently approximately 40 of those that play a role in by acupuncture caused effect are identified. For years it's been known that stimulation of individual peripheral acupunctural points causes activation and deactivation of specific parts of brain. Despite that, there are still a lot of unknown questions regarding clinical effects of acupuncture. It is caused by a small amount of well: controlled, randomized, double blind experiments in this field, but conceptual barriers are appearing. Acupuncture is hard to formulate, individual healing form, which is hard to apply on chosen groups of uniformed healing processes. Still, it is internationally known and people are in an increased amount demanding its application. Health care providers in the EU are also showing interest in this topic. It is the time to consider the possibility of incorporating a patient empowerment model which considers the patient as the most important member of the health team and care managers as key health care collaborators able to enhance and support services to patients provided by physicians in the primary health care system.

We have to mention that in the past some ancient civilization had and has still used food as *medicine*. Traditional Chinese Medicine has also a significant important part of dietary component, which are according to sentences of Greek Hyppocrates: you became what you eat, your food is your health....", but in recent topic we do not deal the complex TCM system, only acupuncture. Nowadays the nutriceuticals industry has grown alongside the expansion and exploration of modern technology and trend, increasingly influenced with some side effects, but it is another story.

Basic prerequisite for accurate usage and its effective application are rooted in regularity, education and more education on an accurate level, which for tens of years have been done by universities. Only continuing support for such education and continuing increase of the quality is the right path in accomplishing of quality education (for this purpose a good quality basis is given by the foundation of Confucius Institute University of Pecs, Faculty of Health Science).

References

1. Pomeranz B, Stux G, Hammerschlag R (2001) Clinical Acupuncture, Scientific Basis. Springer.

2. Eory A, Kuzmann E, Ádám Gy (1970) Exact Mapping of Electrical Skin Resistance Taking into Account the Influential Factors Simultaneously. Magyar Pszichológiai Szemle 4: 514-529.

3. Eory A, Fischer J, Mesko A, McKenna B (1996). Factorial Designs in the Acupuncture Research: Special Features (Advantages and Limitations) Lecture Held at "What To Do If a Randomized Trial Is Not Possible?" International Symposium, Project Münchener Modell, Munich, Germany

4. Eöry A (1984) *In-vivo* skin respiration (CO_2) measurements in the acupuncture loci. Acupunct Electrother Res 9: 217-223.

5. Niboyet JEH (1963) La moindre résistance a l'electricité des surfaces punctiformes et des trajects cutanés concordants avec les points et méridiens basés de l'acupuncture. Imp. Luis-Jean, Lyon

6. Cheng RS, Pomeranz BH (1980) Electroacupuncture analgesia is mediated by stereospecific opiate receptors and is reversed by antagonists of type I receptors. Life Sci 26: 631-638.

7. Allen JJB, Schnyer RN, Hitt SK (1998) The Efficacy of Acupuncture in the Treatment of Major Depression in Women. Psychological Science 9: 397-401.

8. Berman B, Ezzo J, Hadhazy V, Swyers J (1999) Is Acupuncture an Effective Treatment for Fibromyalgia? A Clinical Review Journal of Family Practice 48: 213-218.

9. Clinical Acupuncture, Scientific Basis. Springer.

10. Bullock ML, Culliton PD, Olander RT (1989) Controlled trial of acupuncture for severe recidivist alcoholism. Lancet 1: 1435-1439.

11. Chiang CY, Chang CT (1973) Peripheral Afferent Pathway for Acupuncture Analgesia. Scientia Sinica 16: 210-217.

12. Ernst E, Pittler MH (1998) The effectiveness of acupuncture in treating acute dental pain: a systematic review. Br Dent J 184: 443-447.

13. Ezzo J (2001) Gabriel-Hammerschlag Richard (eds.) Clinical Acupuncture, Scientific Basis. Springer.

14. Linde K, Worku F, Stor W (1996). Randomized Clinical Trials of Acupuncture for Asthma - A Systematic Review. Forschende Komplementärmedizin 3: 148-155.

15. Melchart D, Linde K, Fischer P, White A, Allais G, et al. (1999) Acupuncture for recurrent headaches: a systematic review of randomized controlled trials. Cephalalgia 19: 779-86.

16. NIH Consensus Conference on Acupuncture (1998) JAMA 280: 1518-1524.

17. Shang C (2001) Clinical Acupuncture. In: Stux Gabriel, Hammerschlag Richard (eds), Scientific Basis, Springer.

18. Andrew JV (1996) Can Acupuncture Have Specific Effects on Health? A Systematic Review of Acupuncture Antiemesis Trials. J R Soc Med 89: 303-311.

19. Ezzo JM, Richardson MA, Vickers A, Allen C, Dibble SL, et al. (2006) Acupuncture-point stimulation for chemotherapy-induced nausea or vomiting. Cochrane Database Syst Rev 19: CD002285.

20. Trinh KV, Phillips SD, Ho E, Damsma K (2004) Acupuncture for the alleviation of lateral epicondyle pain: a systematic review. Rheumatol 43: 1085-1090.

21. Linde K, Allais G, Brinkhaus B, Manheimer E, Vickers A, et al. (2009) Acupuncture for tension-type headache. Cochrane Database Syst Rev 21: CD007587.

22. Trinh KV, Graham N, Gross AR, Goldsmith CH, Wang E, et al. (2006) Cervical Overview Group. Acupuncture for neck disorders. Cochrane Database Syst Rev 19: CD004870.

23. White A, Foster NE, Cummings M, Barlas P (2007) Acupuncture treatment for chronic knee pain, a systematic Review Rheumatology 46: 384-390.

24. http://www.samueliinstitute.org/research-areas/military-medical-research

25. www.cambrella.eu

26. Wiesener S, Falkenberg T, Hegyi G, Sarsina P, F.nneb. V (2013) Legal status and regulation of CAM in Europe: Part III - CAM regulations in EU/EFTA/EEA. 1-41. A pan-European research network for Complementary and Alternative Medicine (CAM), Final report of CAMbrella Work Package 2.

27. Hegyi G, Szasz O, Szasz A (2012) Synergy of Oncothermia and Traditional Chinese Medicine. Oncothermia J 7: 373.

28. Hegyi G, Li Jian (2013) Low Back Pain-Complex Approach of Treatment by Different CAM Modalities (Acupuncture and Other Types of Dry Needling, "Targeted RF Noninvasive Physiotherapy" for Low Back Pain) Conf Papers Med Paper.

29. Hegyi G, Fonnebo V, Johanna Hok and Wiesner S (2013) A komplementer medicina jogállása és szabályozasa Europában. Lege Artis Medicinae 23: 350-363.

30. Hegyi G, Máté Á (2013) Back pain and electrostimulation by targeted RF (Boostering), Acupuncture & Electro-Therapeutics Research 38: 39-44

31. Lee MS, Choi TY, Kim J, Kim L, Ernst E (2011) Acupuncture for treating attention deficit hyperactivity disorder: a systematic review and meta-analysis. Chin J Integr Med 17: 257-260.

32. Cho SH1, Whang WW (2009) Acupuncture for alcohol dependence: a systematic review. See comment in PubMed Commons below Alcohol Clin Exp Res 33: 1305-1313.

33. Chen N, Zhou M, He L, Zhou D, Li N (2010).Acupuncture for Bell's palsy. "Cochrane Database of Systematic Reviews". The Cochrane database of systematic reviews 8: CD002914.

34. Sim H, Shin BC, Lee MS, Jung A, Lee H, et al. (2011) Acupuncture for carpal tunnel syndrome: a systematic review of randomized controlled trials. J Pain 12: 307-314.

35. Linde K, Allais G, Brinkhaus B, Manheimer E, Vickers A, et al. (2009) "Acupuncture for migraine prophylaxis". In Linde, Klaus. Cochrane Database Syst Rev 1: CD001218.

36. Ciccone MM, Aquilino A, Cortese F, Scicchitano P, Sassara M, et al. (2010) Feasibility and effectiveness of a disease and care management model in the primary health care system for patients with heart failure and diabetes (Project Leonardo). Vasc Health Risk Manag 6: 297-305.

43

Evaluation of Patients Receiving Jeeva® at an Integrative Pulmonary Care Center

Narinder Singh Parhar[1]*, Gloria St John[1], Ajaipal Singh Gill[1], Frank Son[1] and Sachin A Shah[1,2]

[1]*Parhar Health Systems, Roseville, California, USA*
[2]*Pharmacy Practice, Thomas J long School of Pharmacy and Health Sciences, University of the Pacific, Stockton, California, USA*

Abstract

Introduction: Asthma and COPD contribute significantly to morbidity, mortality, and social-economic burden. Integrative Pulmonary Care center (IPCC) is a specialized program that has an integrative approach to respiratory care. Notably, eligible patients may receive a novel plant based therapeutic option (Jeeva®) in addition to standard of care. Jeeva® integrates several nutraceuticals known to have immune-modulatory, anti-inflammatory and antioxidant properties.

Methods: An evaluation of patient records was performed for all asthma/COPD patients enrolled in the IPCC program who had consented to consume Jeeva®. Demographic data, past medical history, and spirometry data (FEV1, FVC, FEV1/FVC, FEV1% predicted, FVC% predicted, FEV1/FVC% predicted) were collected along with a survey-based assessment of quality-of-life. The primary endpoint was the maximum change in FEV1 and FVC pre-bronchodilator after Jeeva® initiation. A paired students' t-test was utilized to compare the maximum change post- Jeeva® from baseline. Intent-to-treat analysis was performed using the last-observation carried forward methodology.

Results: A total of 26 patients were included for analyses. Median duration of Jeeva® consumption was approximately 6 months (range 1–12 months). There was a statistically significant change in FEV1 and FVC from baseline [1.64 ± 0.72 L to 1.80 ± 0.72 L; (p=0.019) and 2.26 ± 0.80L to 2.50 ± 0.74 L (p=0.004) respectively]. Quality-of-life improved statistically significantly and there was a notable decrease in medication burden.

Conclusion: Patients receiving Jeeva® as part of the IPCC significantly improved pre-bronchodilator FEV1 and FVC from baseline. A small improvement in quality-of-life and medication burden was evident. Further studies looking at Jeeva® in a randomized, placebo-controlled, clinical-trial is warranted.

Keywords: COPD; Asthma; Nutraceuticals

Introduction

Asthma and Chronic Obstructive Pulmonary Disease (COPD) are major causes of morbidity and mortality globally with COPD being the third leading cause of death [1]. More recently, asthma and COPD are being recognized as overlapping conditions aptly termed "asthma–COPD overlap syndrome" (ACOS) [2]. Pharmacologic options for their management often include short and long acting β2-agonists, anticholinergics, inhaled glucocorticoids and Leukotriene modifiers. However, none of the existing medications or regimens has been conclusively shown to modify the long-term decline in lung function [3].

Every year, approximately $30 Billion is spent out-of-pocket by Americans on complementary health approaches. The Integrative Pulmonary Care Center (IPCC) is a private physician's office program that specializes in the care of patients with respiratory conditions using traditional and integrative approaches to care. In addition to standard-of-care, patients can be initiated on a supplement called Jeeva˙ [4]. Patients are also introduced to yoga based breathing exercises, and given the opportunity to work with an exercise physiologist to help correct any defects in posture that limit breathing.

Jeeva˙ is a novel plant based therapeutic option that integrates several nutraceuticals known to have immune-modulatory, anti-inflammatory, and antioxidant properties [5-21]. It includes Arabinogalactan, Acai berry, concentrated Aloe polysaccharides, Bilberry, Gum Acacia, Star Anise, and Turmeric Root in varying doses and is available in a capsule form [16]. To assess the degree of clinical benefit and impact on quality-of-life, we evaluated patients enrolled in the IPCC program being treated with Jeeva˙.

Methods

Upon approval from the Institutional Review Board we performed a review of patients enrolled at an IPCC (http://integrativepulmonarycarecenter.com/) at a private physician's office in Roseville, California [16]. The primary practitioner specializes in internal medicine and holds board certification with the American board of Alternative and Integrative Medicine. All patients voluntarily signed an informed consent document before participating in the program.

Patients were selected for analysis if they had a diagnosis of COPD and/or asthma, and consumed Jeeva˙ (1 capsule twice daily) till at least the next follow-up visit (approximately 2-3 months after enrolment). Those under 18 years of age or pregnant were excluded. Patients were only included if they had a baseline and at least 1 follow up visit with spirometry data (FEV1 and FVC measurements). Forced expiratory volume in one second (FEV1), defines the volume of air that can be forced out in one second after taking a deep breath and forced vital capacity (FVC) measures the volume of air forcibly exhaled from the

*Corresponding author: Narinder Singh Parhar, Sutter Independent Physician 584 N, Sunrise Avenue, #100, Roseville, California
E-mail: Parharmd@gmail.com

point of maximal inspiration both of which are accepted objective markers of pulmonary function.

A comprehensive chart review was conducted to collect age, race, gender, height, weight, smoking status, comorbidities, medication list, spirometry data and adverse effects. Pulmonary function test parameters (FEV1, FVC, FEV1/FVC, FEV1% predicted, FVC% predicted, and FEV1/FVC% predicted) were extracted at baseline and for each subsequent visit with available spirometry data.

Quality-of-life data was collected using the SF-8 survey. Each question was converted to a numerical score with the lowest possible score being 8 and the highest score being 42. It is important to note that a lower score denotes an improvement in quality-of-life.

The primary endpoint was the maximum change in FEV1 and FVC pre-bronchodilator from baseline. Secondary endpoints included the largest change from baseline in FEV1 post bronchodilator, FEV1% predicted pre-bronchodilator, FEV1% predicted post-bronchodilator, FVC post-bronchodilator, FVC% predicted pre-bronchodilator, FVC% predicted post-bronchodilator, FEV1/FVC pre-bronchodilator, FEV1/FVC post-bronchodilator, FEV1/FVC% predicted pre-bronchodilator, FEV1/FVC% predicted post-bronchodilator and SF-8 survey.

A paired students't-test was utilized to compare all endpoints pre- and post- Jeeva® with a p<0.05 considered significant. For patients with missing data, an intent-to-treat (ITT) analysis was performed using the last-observation carried forward methodology.

Results

A total of 26 patients were included for analyses. Sixteen patients were male (62%) and 10 (38%) were Female. The average age and weight were 76 ± 10 years and 179 ± 40 pounds, respectively. Twenty had asthma and 18 had COPD with over 50% having a diagnosis of both. Fourteen (71%) were former smokers and two (4%) were current smokers. Seventeen patients (65%) had hypertension, nine (35%) had diabetes. Relevant comorbid past medical history included allergic rhinitis (38%), anxiety (31%), and chronic bronchitis (8%).

Thirteen patients were on short acting β-2 agonists (50%), four on long acting β-2 agonists (15%), fourteen on inhaled corticosteroids (54%), five on anticholinergics (19%), and one on a leukotriene modifier (4%). Seven were on a long acting β-2 agonist/corticosteroid combination (27%) and four (15%) on a β-2 agonist/anticholinergic combination.

Median duration of Jeeva' consumption was 175 days (range 28–371 days).

FEV1 pre-bronchodilator (Figure 1) improved significantly from baseline (1.64 ± 0.72 L to 1.80 ± 0.72 L; p<0.019). FEV1 post-bronchodilator improved significantly from 1.77 ± 0.68 L to 1.88 ± 0.72 L (p=0.035). FEV1% predicted pre- and post-bronchodilator also improved significantly (Table 1).

FVC pre-bronchodilator (Figure 1) improved significantly from baseline (2.26 ± 0.80 L to 2.50 ± 0.74 L; p=0.004). FVC post-bronchodilator improved from 2.45 ± 0.74 L to 2.57 ± 0.76 L (p=0.054). FVC% predicted pre and post-bronchodilator also improved significantly (Table 1).

FEV1/FVC pre-bronchodilator (Table 1) improved non-significantly from baseline (71.7 ± 14.3 to 74.3 ± 14.2; p=0.221). A trend towards significant improvement was seen with the change in FEV1/FVC post-bronchodilator from 71.9 ± 14.6 to 75.1 ± 14.9 (p<0.056).

Endpoint	Baseline	Maximum change from baseline	p-value
FEV₁ (Liters)	1.64 ± 0.72	1.80 ± 0.72	p=0.019
FEV₁ (Liters) [post- bronchodilator]	1.77 ± 0.68	1.88 ± 0.72	p=0.035
FEV₁% predicted	60.92 ± 22.64	67.08 ± 22.23	p=0.018
FEV₁% predicted [post-bronchodilator]	64.83 ± 21.41	69.04 ± 23.03	p=0.052
FVC (Liters)	2.26 ± 0.80	2.50 ± 0.74	p=0.004
FVC (Liters) [post- bronchodilator]	2.45 ± 0.74	2.57 ± 0.76	p=0.054
FVC% predicted	61.72 ± 18.77	69.40 ± 16.03	p=0.002
FVC% predicted [post- bronchodilator]	66.13 ± 15.77	70.04 ± 15.37	p=0.045
FEV₁/FVC	71.73 ± 14.28	74.29 ± 14.19	p=0.221
FEV₁/FVC [post-bronchodilator]	71.85 ± 14.59	75.05 ± 14.92	p=0.056
FEV₁/FVC% predicted	101.32 ± 20.18	103.64 ± 20.23	p=0.363
FEV₁/FVC% predicted [post-bronchodilator]	101.25 ± 20.55	105.54 ± 21.33	p=0.081

Table 1: Change in Pulmonary Function Endpoints

FEV1/FVC% predicted pre-bronchodilator improved non-significantly from baseline (p=0.363). FEV1/FVC% predicted post-bronchodilator showed a trend towards significant improvement (p=0.081).

Quality of life score improved significantly from 27.4 ± 6.49 to 26.4 ± 6.19 (p<0.017). Nine (35%) of the patients had a reduction or elimination of their pulmonary medication (rescue or maintenance). One (4%) had a reduction in their oxygen use. None of the patients had a respiratory related emergency room visit or hospitalization while in the IPCC program.

Discussion

Asthma and COPD result in a significant social and economic burden [22]. According to the CDC, asthma accounts for one-quarter of all emergency room visits in the U.S. each year and over 3,000 deaths each year [23]. The estimated total cost for the two conditions was approximately $68 billion in 2008 [24]. Recently, the Centers for Medicare and Medicaid Services (CMS) expanded the Hospital Readmission Reduction Program (HRRP) to include COPD. The burden of illness of these patients is such that the CMS will now penalize hospitals for what they deem as unplanned readmission for COPD [25]. This is driven by the fact that 23% of COPD hospitalizations are subsequently readmitted within 30 days post discharge [26].

Our findings indicated a significant benefit in pulmonary function markers in patients enrolled in the IPCC program. Benefits in spirometry endpoints were in line with data from previous analyses where Jeeva® improved pre-bronchodilator FEV1 and FVC by 264 mL and 314 mL from baseline, respectively [4]. This current analysis builds on previous work as it also shows a small improvement in quality-of-life. There was also a reduction in medication use in 38% of the patients. This is important as frequency of rescue inhaler use is a surrogate marker of exacerbation of disease [27].

The respiratory system undergoes various physiological, immunological, and anatomical changes with age [28]. The estimated rate of decline in FEV1 is 25-30 mL/yr starting at age of 35-40 years and can double to 60 mL/yr after the age of 70 years. FVC generally declines at approximately 22 mL/yr in healthy subjects (20 to 60 years) [29]. Figure 2 depicts the hypothetical decline in FEV1 over time [2]. It is

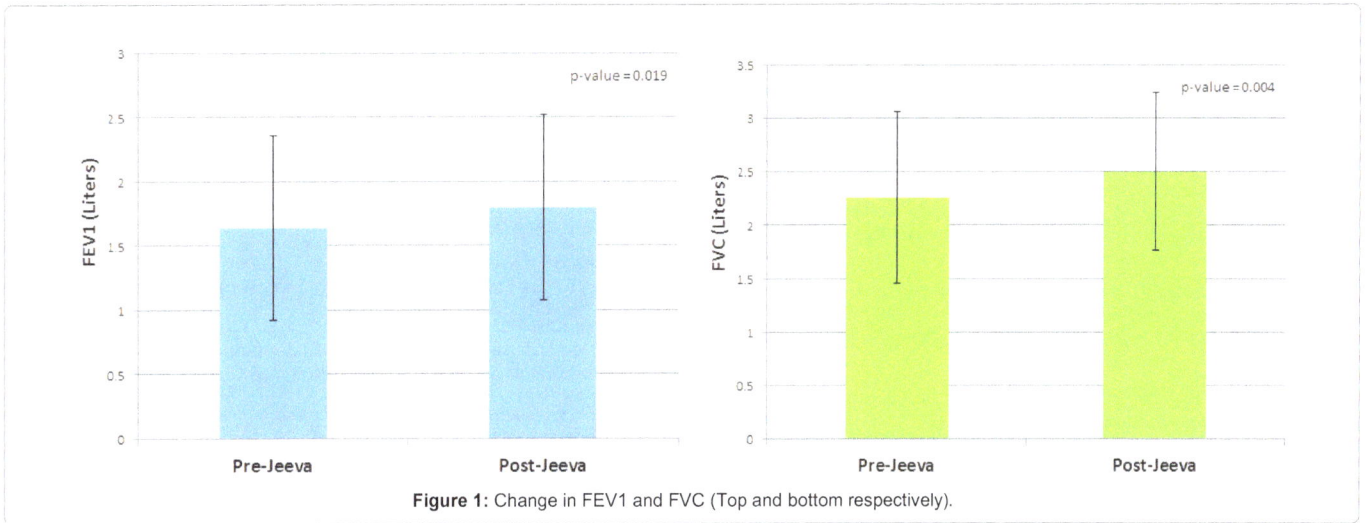

Figure 1: Change in FEV1 and FVC (Top and bottom respectively).

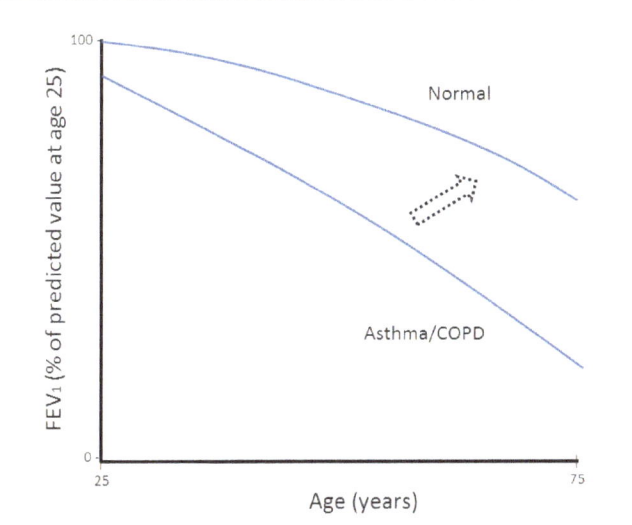

Figure 2: Hypothetical schematic of lung function in Asthma and Chronic Obstructive Pulmonary Disease (COPD), Legend. Change in FEV1 over time in asthma/COPD patients compared to normal decline.

possible that the incorporation of Jeeva˙ to standard-of-care in patients with asthma or COPD can direct them away from the typical decline in FEV1 (depicted by the dotted line arrow) but this needs further evaluation.

The findings from this report and our previous work together support conducting randomized, double-blinded, placebo-controlled trials with Jeeva˙. Other novel, albeit expensive, approaches to optimizing pharmacotherapy include nanoparticle-based drug delivery and innovative inhalers [30,31]. In the future, it would be important to perform cost-effectiveness analyses to assess the ideal integrative approach to minimize the disease burden and optimize quality of life in patients with asthma and COPD.

There are several limitations of note. Primarily, there are innate limitations of a retrospective analysis such as this and it does not infer causality. A lack of placebo arm rules in the possibility of patients simply benefiting from the improved attention received when enrolled in a specialized center such as IPCC. There is compelling data suggesting that a specialized care management model can have a positive outcome on patient health [32]. The compliance rate of yoga breathing was low which could diminish the magnitude of efficacy seen from the IPCC program. However, it strengthens our case for supporting the benefits being primarily driven by Jeeva˙. Hospital admissions were not assessed from a review of medical records but from patient recall which is not always accurate. A lack of a control arm and a small sample size pose inherent limitations in data extrapolation and wide applicability.

Conclusion

Patients receiving Jeeva˙ as part of the IPCC significantly improved pre-bronchodilator FEV1 and FVC from baseline. A small improvement in quality-of-life and medication burden was evident. Further studies looking at Jeeva˙ in a randomized, placebo-controlled, clinical-trial are warranted.

Acknowledgement

The authors would like to thank Athena Xides, Pharm.D. and Kunal Shah, Pharm.D. Candidate for their assistance.

References

1. http://www.who.int/mediacentre/factsheets/fs310/en/

2. Postma DS, Rabe KF (2015) The Asthma-COPD Overlap Syndrome. N Engl J Med 373: 1241-9.

3. Anthonisen NR, Connett JE, Kiley JP, Altose MD, Bailey WC (1994) Effects of smoking intervention and the use of an inhaled anticholinergic bronchodilator on the rate of decline of FEV1. The Lung Health Study. JAMA 272: 1497-505.

4. Shah SA, Lee JJ, Son F, St John G, Parhar NS (2016) Impact of a Novel Plant-based Treatment Option in Improving Pulmonary Function Markers in Patients with Chronic Obstructive Pulmonary Disease and Asthma. Altern Integr Med 2: 215.

5. http://integrativepulmonarycarecenter.com/

6. Kelley GS (1999) Larch Arabinogalactan: clinical relevance of a Novel Immune-Enhancing Polysaccharide. Altern Med Rev 4: 96-103.

7. Chatterjee UR, Ray S, Micard V, Ghosh D, Ghosh K, et al. (2014) Interaction with bovine serum albumin of an anti-oxidative pecticarabinogalactan from Andrographis paniculata. Carbohydr Polym 101: 342-348.

8. Domej W, Oettl K, Renner W(2014) Oxidative stress and free radicals in COPD – implications and relevance for treatment. Int J Chron Obstruct Pulmon Dis 9: 1207-1224.

9. Skyberg JA, Rollins MF, Holderness JS (2012) Nasal Acai Polysaccharides Potentiate Innate Immunity to Protect against Pulmonary Francisella tularensis and Burkholderia pseudomallei Infections. PLoS Pathogens 8: e1002587.

10. Manvitha K, Bidya B (2014) *Aloe vera*: a wonder plant its history, cultivation and medicinal uses. J Pharmacogn Phytochem 2: 85-88.

11. Zhong JS, Huang YY, Zhang TH (2015) Natural phosphodiesterase-4 inhibitors from the leaf skin of aloe barbadensis Miller. Fitoterapia 100: 68-74.

12. Habeeb F, Shakir E, Bradbury F (2007) Screening methods used to determine the anti-microbial properties of Aloe vera inner gel. Methods 42: 315-20.

13. Hohtola A (2010) Bioactive compounds from northern plants. Adv Exp Med Biol 698: 99-109.

14. Burdulis D, Sarkinas A, Jasutiene I (2009) Comparative study of anthocyanin composition, antimicrobial and antioxidant activity in bilberry (Vaccinium myrtillus L.) and blueberry (Vaccinium corymbosum L.) fruits. Acta Pol Pharm 66: 399-408.

15. Braga PC, Antonacci, R, Wang YY, Lattuada N, Dal Sasso M, et al. (2013) Comparative antioxidant activity of cultivated and wild Vaccinium species investigated by EPR, human neutrophil burst and COMET assay. Eur Rev Med Pharmacol Sci 17: 1987-1999.

16. Ali BH, Ziada A, Blunden G (2009) Biological effects of gum Arabic: A review of some recent research. Food Chem Toxicol 48 :1-8.

17. Benmalek Y, Yahia OA, Belkebir A, et al. (2013) Anti-microbial and anti-oxidant activities ofIllicium verum, Crataegus oxyacantha sspmonogyna and Allium cepa red and white varieties. Bioengineered 4: 244-48.

18. De M, De AK, Sen P (2002) Antimicrobial properties of star anise (Illicium verum Hook f). Phytother Res 16: 94-5.

19. Kang P, Kim KY, Lee HS, Min SS, Seol GH, et al. (2013) Anti-inflammatory effects of anethole in lipopolysaccharide-induced acute lung injury in mice. Life Sci 93: 955-961.

20. Shishodia S, Sethi G, Aggarwal BB (2015) Curcumin: getting back to the roots. Ann N Y Acad Sci 1056: 206-17.

21. Bengmark S, Mesa MD, Gil A (2009) Plant-derived health: the effects of turmeric and curcuminoids. Nutr Hosp 24: 273-81.

22. http://www.who.int/healthinfo/global_burden_disease/GBD_report_2004update_full.pdf

23. Bousquet J, Bousquet P, Godard P, Daures JP (2005) The public health implications of asthma. Public Health Reviews. Bull World Health Organ 83: 548-554.

24. http://www.nhlbi.nih.gov/files/docs/research/2012_ChartBook.pdf

25. Braman SS (2015) Hospital readmissions for COPD: We can meet the challenge. J COPD F2: 4-7.

26. Jencks SF, Williams MV, Coleman EA (2009) Rehospitalizations among Patients in the Medicare Fee-for-Service Program. NEJM 360: 1418-28.

27. Jenkins CR, Postma DS, Anzueto AR, Make BJ, Peterson S, et al. (2015) Reliever salbutamol use as a measure of exacerbation risk in chronic obstructive pulmonary disease. BMC Pulm Med 15: 97.

28. Sharma G, Goodwin J (2006) Effect of aging on respiratory system physiology and immunology. Clin Interv Aging 1: 253-260.

29. Swanney MP, Stanton JD, O'Reilly-Nugent A (2014) Natural decline in FEV1 and FVC: Self versus reference equations. ERJ 42:1787.

30. Yhee JY, Im J, Nho RS (2016) Advanced Therapeutic Strategies for Chronic Lung Disease Using Nanoparticle-Based Drug Delivery. J Clin Med 20: 5.

31. Virchow JC, Akdis CA, Darba J, Dekhuijzen R, Hartl S, et al. (2015) A review of the value of innovation in inhalers for COPD and asthma J Mark Access Health Policy 3: 28760.

32. Ciccone MM, Aquilino A, Cortese F, Scicchitano P, Sassara M, et al. (2010) Feasibility and effectiveness of a disease and care management model in the primary health care system for patients with heart failure and diabetes (Project Leonardo). Vasc Health Risk Manag 6: 297-305.

44

Rehabilitation in Secondary Progressive Multiple Sclerosis in Patients: Early Outcomes

Mandolesi S[1], d'Alessandro A[4], Niglio T[3], Gallucci S[2], Cialfi A[2], Mandolesi D[5], Di Donato R[2], Stammegna I[5] and d'Alessandro A[6]*

[1]Department Cardio-vascular and Respiratory Science, "Sapienza" University, Rome, Italy
[2]Department of Rehabilitation, "Villa Dorotea", L'Aquila, Italy
[3]Istituto Superiore di Sanità, Rome, Italy
[4]Faculty of Medicine, University of Foggia, 71122 Foggia FG, Italy
[5]U.R. Occupational Medicine, Sapienza University of Rome, 00185 Rome, Italy
[6]School of Medicine and Health Sciences, "G. d'Annunzio" University, Chieti, Italy

Abstract

Introduction: Multiple Sclerosis (MS) affects approximately 110,000 people in Italy and MS is a leading cause of disability in young adults. Rehabilitation interventions are frequently used as clinical strategies for improving or maintaining functional state.

Methods: We assessed 9 patients with secondary progressive multiple sclerosis (SP-MS): Four female and five male with a mean age of 47.3 years. The mean score EDSS was 7 (values from 3.5 to 8.5). All patients were hospitalized from eight to ten weeks; MSIS-29, EBN, Hamilton, FIM, Barthel, Tinetti and FSS tests were administered. All patients received one weekly spine manipulation in accordance with Palmer, Sutherland, Makenzie procedures both in supine and upright position. Three times a week the patients received also a draining massage of head and lower limbs by Muscular Acoustic Modulator (MAM) device. Eighty minutes a day, for 6 days a week, all patients had neuro-motor rehabilitation.

Results: Only some data from clinical tests showed statistically significant differences, before and after treatments. These data are: FSS scale: $p < 0.01$ (H Kruskal-Wallis=6.7996 with degree of freedom=1); Memory test with deferred Prose: $p < 0.05$ (H Kruskal-Wallis=4.7193 with degree of freedom=1); Memory test with immediate Prose: $p = 0.0920$ Trend (H Kruskal-Wallis=2.8382 with degree of freedom=1).

Conclusion: In our study FIM, Bartel, Tinetti tests showed reductions in clinical disability without statistical significance. We had statistically significant differences, after 6 weeks by this innovative rehabilitation treatment both on the chronic fatigue on the cognitive status in inpatients with SP-MS. These preliminary positive results encourage us to continue research on a larger sample of patients.

Keywords: Rehabilitation; Multiple sclerosis; Venous compression syndrome; Sound vibration

Introduction

Multiple Sclerosis (MS) affects approximately 110,000 people in Italy and is a leading cause of disability in young adults. Rehabilitation interventions are frequently used clinical strategies for improving or maintaining functional status. To date the pharmacological therapeutic approaches are based on the need to put a stop to an immune system that attacks the myelin sheath, which covers the neuronal axons, creating lesions that, with the passage of time, can create irreversible damage.

In MS patients the brain and spinal cord eliminate drain deoxygenated blood and toxins with great difficulty [1]. This failure is due to reduced drain for narrowing of the cerebral veins and blocks that are found in the venous segments located outside the skull, especially in the neck, chest and abdomen. The reduced venous drainage has direct effects on the drainage of Cerebrospinal Fluid (CSF) surrounding the brain and spinal cord whose action is to protect them from trauma, feed them and drain toxic substances.

This cerebral spinal venous insufficiency can be diagnosed through a specific procedure EchoColorDoppler (ECD); which enables the identification of two types of venous blocks: The one inside the vein for valvular anomalies and the external one for compression of the veins caused by the surrounding tissue. The first one may benefit from endovascular treatment (angioplasty), the second by a rehabilitative physical therapy [2].

The anatomy and physiology until now denied the presence of brains, bone marrow, ear and eye, lymphatic drainage system which, therefore, would seem to be isolated organs from this point of view from the rest of the body. We hypothesize that sight, hearing and smell nerves are like compensatory expansion chambers in case of increased intracranial pressure. Russian studies Speransky and more recent Koh et al. instead reported experiments showing drainage from the CSF and brain interstitial system in both cervical and peripheral lymphatic system [3,4]. Our work 2001 showed the presence of an eye lymphatic drainage system. Recent publications of cochlea RM assessment have objectively shown the presence of a hydrops into the cochlea in Meniere's disease patients. The most current research has shown that not only the brain is equipped with its own lymphatic system, but also that such a system consists of two anatomically and functionally distinct parts [5]. A part of this system is a classic lymphatic system composed of true lymphatic vessels. The other, called gliolymphatic system is mainly built by astrocytes. These two brain draining systems

*Corresponding author: d'Alessandro A, School of Medicine and Health Sciences, "G. d'Annunzio" University, Chieti, Italy
E-mail: dalessandraldo@gmail.com

recently discovered, likely to play a substantial role in the pathogenesis of many neuro-immune diseases and neurodegenerative disorders such as multiple sclerosis, Parkinson's disease, and Alzheimer's disease Simka [6].

In 2011 we find the compression syndromes of the jugular and the vertebral veins and are given the indication for specific cervical adjustments of the first vertebrae with positive clinical results [7]. The aim of this procedures was to improve the venous brain drainage and consequently of the CSF. In 2013 starting from the rational that the CSF was correlated with lymphatic system, we treated by sound vibration tissue draining therapy (Dreno-MAM) with positive clinical effects, both MS patients with venous compression syndromes or intravenous blocks [8].

The aim of this pilot study was to evaluate the efficacy of physical rehabilitation treatments on inpatients with Secondary Progressive Multiple Sclerosis (SP-MS).

Methods

Sample

We assessed 9 patients with (SP-MS): four female and five male with a mean age of 47.3 years. The mean score EDSS was 7 (values from 3.5 to 8.5). All patients were hospitalized from eight to ten weeks. The ongoing pharmacological treatments were continued. Each patient provided a signed informed consent to participate to this study.

Measures

Multiple Sclerosis (MS) is a chronic and progressive disabling disease with multiple potential clinical intervention points during its course. It is therefore appropriate to have quality measures specific for this condition that span the course of the disease. International Organization of Multiple Sclerosis Rehabilitation Therapists (IOMSRT) says Evidence Based Medicine (EBM) is: "The conscientious, explicit, and judicious use of current best evidence in making decisions about the care of an individual patient."

Improving the quality of health care is essential in the practice of medicine. Fundamental to these efforts to improve quality is the ability to measure care because we cannot improve what we do not measure. These measures are intended to be used by stakeholders to quantify the quality of care provided to patients with MS. Disease-specific quality measures in physiatry provide a framework that can assist clinicians in practice measurement and modification; these have the potential to benefit both subspecialist and generalist alike. The World Health Organization's International Classification of Impairments, Disabilities and Handicap [9] were used as the conceptual basis for the choice of the best outcomes to be measured. Assessment of neurological status (impairment) was determined by Kurtzke's Functional System Scale (FSS) and Expanded Disability Status Scale (EDSS). This scale is composed of eight subscales, each measuring a specific function within the central nervous system. EDSS score lower than 4 addresses impairment, while grades 4 to 10 are strongly dependent on disability and particularly locomotion. Although some criticisms have been expressed on psychometric properties of this scale not be sufficiently sensitive, it has been used in most clinical trials [10].

Disability was assessed by the motor and the cognitive domains of the Functional Independence Measure (FIM). The underlying rationale for classifying an activity as "independent" or "dependent" is whether another person (a helper) is required and to what extent. There is a good evidence to support the reliability and validity of the FIM to assess disability. Scores were obtained from patient interview by a FIM trained physiatrist. In accordance with the guidelines, scores were consistently determined by actual performance of tasks on a daily basis, rather than each individual optimum performance.

In our study we assessed quality of life by the Multiple Sclerosis Impact Scale (MSIS-29) questionnaire [11]; depression by Hamilton Rating Scale for Depression (HRSD) [12]; cognitive status by Brief Neuropsychological Examination (ENB) questionnaire [13]; chronic fatigue by Fatigue Severity Scale (FSS) questionnaire [14], disability by Functional Independence Measure (FIM) scale [15], activities for daily living (ADLs) by Barthel Index [16] ; gait balance by Tinetti scale [17].

Before and after recovery period MSIS-29, ENB and Hamilton psychological tests, FIM, Barthel, Tinetti and FSS physiatric assessment tests were administered in all patients.

Rehabilitation Program

All patients received one weekly spine manipulation in accordance with Palmer, Sutherland and Makenzie procedures in four steps. In supine position: first step for the opening of foramen magnum; second step for the realignment of C1; third step for realignment of C2. In upright position: fourth step for realignment of other cervical vertebrae and cranial chiropractic adjustment. After manipulation procedure the patients received one acoustic vibration treatment by Muscular Acoustic Modulator (MAM) device on treated areas [18]. The patients received also a draining massage of head and lower limbs, three times a week, by MAM device. Eighty minutes a day, for 6 days a week the patients had individual neuro-motor rehabilitation. The individual neuro-motor rehabilitation consists in passive and active aided mobilizations, stretching of the four limbs and spine, reinforcement and strengthening muscles, motion coordination exercises, functional rehabilitation of gait and proprioceptive exercises.

Statistical Analysis

We used the parametric equivalent of the Kruskal-Wallis test to perform one-way Analysis of Variance (ANOVA) and for testing whether data before and after treatments originate from the same distribution. Kruskal-Wallis test indicates that at least one sample stochastically dominates one other sample. The test does not identify where this stochastic dominance occurs. Anyway, in our pilot study with a very little sample, the Kruskal-Wallis test is enough potent to reject the null hypothesis that the medians of all groups are equal; and the alternative hypothesis is that at least one median of one group is different from the median of the other group.

Results

Only some data from clinical tests showed statistically significant differences, before and after treatments. These data are: FSS scale: $p<0.01$ (H Kruskal-Wallis=6.7996 with degree of freedom=1) (Table 1); Memory test with deferred Prose: $p<0.05$ (H Kruskal-Wallis=4.7193 with degree of freedom=1) (Table 2); Memory test with immediate Prose: $p=0.0920$ Trend (H Kruskal-Wallis=2.8382 with degree of freedom=1) (Table 3). FIM, Bartel and Tinetti tests show the reduction of some aspect of clinical disability but the total scores not were statistically significant.

Discussion

Historically, MS care focused on rehabilitation and symptomatic management; however, this focus broadened with the development of Disease-modifying Therapies (DMTs), resulting in pharmacologic

Fatigue Severity Scale (FSS)
p<0.01 (H di Kruskal-Wallis=6,7996 with degree of freedom=1)

Visit	pt.	Σ	Mean	Variance	Std. Dev.
1	9	499,0000	55,4444	44,5278	6,6729
2	9	375,0000	41,6667	117,5000	10,8397

Visit	Minimum	25%	Median	75%	Maximum	Mode
1	45,0000	50,0000	54,0000	62,000	63,0000	50,0000
2	27,0000	32,0000	41,0000	49,0000	58,0000	27,0000

Table 1: Results of Fatigue Severity Scale (FSS).

Deferred prose memory test (MPD)
p<0.05 (H di Kruskal-Wallis=4,7193 with degree of freedom=1)

Visit	pt.	Σ	Mean	Variance	Std. Dev.
1	9	15,60,000	1,73,333	123,0000	47,958
2	9	19,70,000	2,18,889	I 9,1111	3,0185

Visit	Minimum	25%	Median	75%	Maximum	Mode
1	9,0000	14,0000	18,0000	20,0000	23,0000	18,0000
2	15,0000	21,0000	22,0000	24,0000	25,0000	22,0000

Table 2: Results of Brief Neuropsychological Examination (ENB).

Immediate prose memory test (MPI)
p=0.0920 TREND (H di Kruskal-Wallis=2,8382 with degree of freedom=1)

Visit	pt.	Σ	Mean	Variance	Std. Dev.
1	9	12,40,000	1,37,778	17,9444	4,2361
2	9	16,50,000	18,3333	25,5000 0498	5,0498

Visit	Minimum	25%	Median	75%	Maximum	Mode
1	7,0000	11,0000	14,0000	16,0000	21,0000	16,0000
2	10,0000	15,0000	19,0000	21,0000	25,0000	25,0000

Table 3: Results of immediate prose memory test (ENB).

treatments that effectively reduce relapses and potentially slow the progression of disability. Consequently, DMTs often dominate many discussions regarding MS care, regardless of the fact that they do not reverse disability or restore function, arguably the primary goal of those with MS. Comprehensive, multidisciplinary care goes beyond the management of DMTs in MS treatment plans and strives to improve patient outcomes, functionality, and quality of life, goals that will likely prove to hold considerable importance as health care reimbursement transitions from a fee-for-service to a value-based paradigm. It is therefore likely that achieving improvement in some of the outcomes delineated in the American Academy of Neurology's (AAN) quality measures for MS will necessitate involvement of rehabilitation specialists.

In 2015 the systematic review of the literature (1970–2013) and classified articles using American Academy of Neurology criteria highlights the paucity of well-designed studies, which are needed to evaluate the available MS rehabilitative therapies. Inpatient exercises (3 weeks) followed by home exercises (15 weeks) possibly is effective for improving disability. In the 2015 the Simka review summarises current knowledge on the lymphatic system of the brain. It has long been believed that the central nervous system is characterised by the lack of a lymphatic system and that the role of the lymphatic system is played by Cerebro-spinal Fluid (CSF). Recently, research has shown that not only is the brain equipped with its own unique lymphatic system, but also that this system consists of two anatomically and functionally distinct parts. One part of this system is a classic lymphatic system, i.e., the structure composed of genuine lymphatic vessels. The other, so-called glymphatic system is primarily built by astrocytes. The newly discovered lymphatic system of the brain is likely to play a substantial role in the pathogenesis of many neuro-immune and

neurodegenerative disorders, such as: multiple sclerosis, Parkinson's disease, and Alzheimer's disease [6]. On the basis of this rational and of our previous experience, we used specific vertebral manipulations and applications total body tissue drainage by MAM device.

In 2016, Sandroff says in his Systematic, Evidence-Based Review of Exercise, Physical Activity, and Physical Fitness Effects on Cognition in Persons with Multiple Sclerosis: "Collectively, there is insufficient well-designed research to definitively conclude that exercise, physical activity, and physical fitness are effective for improving cognition in MS" [19].

The AAN systematic review could have, to a greater extent, highlighted the problems created by these methodologic issues and barriers to higher-level research in rehabilitation and argued for solutions that may ultimately influence funding agencies. The question is how to fulfill this need for well-designed trials in rehabilitation. Organizations such as the AAN, CMSC, and IOMSRT have a role in developing and disseminating clearly defined interventions, appropriate endpoints, and effective outcome measures. Collaboration with organizations specific to neurologic rehabilitation, such as the American Physical Therapy Association's Neurology Section, the American Occupational Therapy Association, and the American Speech-Language-Hearing Association, may help enhance and expand MS-specific rehabilitation research currently being performed by rehabilitation scientists and exercise physiologists. Standardized protocols and validated endpoints are needed for all larger studies, especially ones involving multiple centers. It is essential to formulate well-designed trials of rehabilitation therapies and techniques, and to overcome the major challenges of having a placebo group and blinding participants in rehabilitation studies. The need for well-designed research trials of rehabilitation in MS remains ongoing and imperative [20]. The last cited reviews prompted us to use, in our study, the most used questionnaires and physiatric tests. These tools have allowed us, even if in a small sample of patients, to detect positive results both on a cognitive that chronic fatigue impairments.

Conclusion

In our study FIM, Bartel, Tinetti tests showed reductions in clinical disability without statistical significance. We had statistically significant differences, after 6 weeks by this innovative rehabilitation treatment both on the chronic fatigue on the cognitive status in inpatients with SP-MS. These preliminary positive results encourage us to continue research on a larger sample of patients.

Disclosure

Non-financial relationship exists.

References

1. Mancini M, Lanzillo R, Liuzzi R (2014) Internal jugular vein blood flow in multiple sclera patients and matched controls. PLoS ONE 9: e92730.

2. Mandolesi S, Niglio T, Orsini A, De Sio S, d'Alessandro A, et al. (2000) Venous compression syndrome of internal jugular veins prevalence in patients with multiple sclerosis and chronic cerebro-spinal venous insufficiency. Ann Ital Chir 87: 406-410.

3. Speransky AD (1934) A basis for the theory of medicine. New York: International Publisher.

4. Koh L, Zakharov A, Johnston M (2005) Integration of the subarachnoid space and lymphatics: is it time to embrace a new concept of cerebrospinal fluid absorption? Cerebrospinal Fluid Res 2: 6.

5. Wu Q, Dai C, Zhao M (2016) The correlation between symptoms of definite Meniere's disease and endolymphatic hydrops visualized by magnetic resonance imaging. Laryngoscope 126: 974-979.

6. Simka M (2015) Recent advances in understanding the lymphatic and glymphatic systems of the brain Phlebol Rev 3: 69-71

7. Mandolesi S, Ciciarello F, Marceca G (2011) Data analysis of the chronic cerebro-spinal venous insufficiency in patients with multiple sclerosis: new disease classification.

8. d'Alessandro A, Niglio T, Desogus A (2015) New acoustic wave therapy improves quality of life in patients with multiple sclerosis and chronic cerebrospinal venous insufficiency. Ann Ital Chir 86: 336-339.

9. Rae-Grant A, Bennett A, Sanders AE, Phipps M, Cheng E, et al. (2015) Quality improvement in neurology: Multiple sclerosis quality measures: Executive summary. Neurology 85: 1905-1908.

10. Haselkorn JK, Hughes C, Rae-Grant A, Henson LJ, Bever CT, et al. (2015) Summary of comprehensive systematic review: rehabilitation in multiple sclerosis: report of the guideline development, dissemination, and implementation subcommittee of the American Academy of Neurology. Neurology 85: 1896-1903.

11. Hobart J, Lamping D, Fitzpatrick R, Riazi A, Thompson A, et al. (2001) The Multiple Sclerosis Impact Scale (MSIS-29): a new patient-based outcome measure. Brain 124: 962-973.

12. Wiglusz MS, Landowski J, Michalak L (2016) Validation of the polish version of the hamilton rating scale for depression in patients with epilepsy. Epilepsy Behav 62: 81-84.

13. Hämäläinen P, Rosti-Otajärvi E (2016) Cognitive impairment in MS: rehabilitation approaches. Acta Neurol Scand 134: 8-13.

14. Heine M, van den Akker LE, Blikman L, Hoekstra T, van Munster E, et al. (2016) Real-time assessment of fatigue in patients with multiple sclerosis: how does it relate to commonly used self-report fatigue questionnaires? Arch Phys Med Rehabil 97: 1887-1894.

15. Dallmeijer AJ, Dekker J, Roorda LD, Knol DL, van Baalen B, et al. (2005) Differential item functioning of the Functional Independence Measure in higher performing neurological patients. J Rehabil Med 37: 346-352.

16. Mahoney FI, Barthel DW (1965) Functional Evaluation: the Barthel Index. Md State Med J 14: 61-65.

17. Tinetti ME, Williams TF, Mayewski R (1986) "Fall risk index for elderly patients based on number of chronic disabilities". Am J Med 80: 429-434.

18. Saggini (2016) Mechanical vibration in rehabilitation: State of the art. J Nov Physiother.

19. Sandroff BM, Motl RW, Scudder MR, DeLuca J (2016) Systematic, evidence-based review of exercise, physical activity, and physical fitness effects on cognition in persons with multiple sclerosis. Neuropsychol Rev 26: 271-294.

20. Sutliff MH, Bennett SE, Bobryk P, Halper J, Saslow LA, et al. (2016) Rehabilitation in multiple sclerosis: Commentary on the recent AAN systematic review. Neurol Clin Pract 6: 475-479.

Permissions

List of Contributors

Varsha J Galani
Department of Pharmacology, A.R. College of Pharmacy, Vallabh Vidyanagar-388120, Gujarat, India

Sunita S Goswami and Mamta B Shah
Department of Pharmacology, L.M. College of Pharmacy, Navrangpura, Ahmedabad-380009, India

Liudmila B. Boldyreva
The State University of Management, Moscow, Russia

Elena M. Boldyreva
Peoples' Friendship University, Moscow, Russia; Weston Learning Center, Ontario, Canada

Thirunavukkarasu MS and Kapoorchand H
Government Ayurveda Medical College and Hospital, Kottar, Nagercoil, Tamilnadu, India

Ching-Hung Chen
Department of Anesthesiology, Show Chwan Memorial Hospital, Changhua, Taiwan

Chan-Yen Kuo
Graduate Institute of Systems Biology and Bioinformatics, National Central University, Chung-li, Taiwan

Subhas Chandra Datta
Eco-club Research Unit, Kanchannagar D.N.Das High School, Kanchannagar, Burdwan-713102, West Bengal, India

Rupa Datta
Life Science Unit, Burdwan Model School, Dewandighi, Burdwan-713101, West Bengal, India

Shiefa Pinto
Department of Biochemistry, Fr. Muller Medical College, Mangalore, Karnataka, India

Ashalatha V Rao
Department of Biochemistry, K. S. Hegde Medical Academy, Deralakatte Mangalore, Karnataka, India

Anjali Rao
Department of Biochemistry, Kasturba Medical College, Manipal, India

Siddaram Arawatti, Pandey BB and Shringi MK
Department of Shalya tantra, National Institute of Ayurveda, Jaipur, India

Seema Murthy
NKJ Ayurvedic Medical College, Bidar, Karnataka, India

Utubaku AB
Department of Medical Biochemistry, Cross River University of Technology, Calabar, Nigeria

Yakubu OE and Okwara DU
Department of Biochemistry, Federal University Wukari, Nigeria

Rahul Manmode
Department of Chemistry, University of Massachusetts, Lowell-01854, USA

Jagdish Manwar, Satish Padgilwar and Nitin Bhajipale
Department of Quality Assurance, Institute of Pharmacy, Akola-444 004, India

Mustafa Vohra
Department of Alcohol Technology, Vasantdada Sugar Institute, Pune-412 307, India

Bethsaida Yanain Rojas
College of Medicine, Hanyang University, Seoul, South Korea

Eric Richardson
Graduate School of Biomedical Science & Engineering, College of Medicine, Hanyang University, Seoul, South Korea

Dong-Hyun Ahn
Department of Neuropsychiatry, Institute of Mental Health, Hanyang Center for Behavioral Development, Hanyang University, Seongdong-gu, Seoul, South Korea

Rajiv Rastogi
Central Council for Research in Yoga & Naturopathy (CCRYN) 61-65, Institutional Area, Janakpuri, New Delhi-110058, India

Madhumitha Mazumdar
Head, Dept of Oral Medicine, Diagnosis & Radiology, Dr R. Ahmed Dental College& Hospital, Kolkota-14

Aritra Chatterjee
PG Scholar,Dept of Oral Medicine, Diagnosis & Radiology, Dr R. Ahmed Dental College& Hospital, Kolkota-14

Swapan Mazumdar
Consultant Orthodontist, Southern Dental Clinic, Kolkota

Chandrika Mahendra
Formulation Development, The Himalaya Drug Company, Makali, Bangalore

Prahlad S Patki
Head- Medical services & Clinical trials, R&D Center, The Himalaya Drug Company, Makali, Bangalore

Akunna GG, Nwafor J, Egwu OA, Ezemagu UK, Obaje G and Adepoju LH
Department of Anatomy, Federal University Ndufu-Alike Ikwo (FUNAI), Ebonyi State, Nigeria

Akingbade AM
Department of Anatomy, Afe Babalola University, Ado Ekiti, Nigeria

Jahangir A. Satti
Department of Radiation Oncology, Albany Medical College, 43 New Scotland Ave, MC 95, Albany, NY 12208-3478, USA

Ashok Kumar Panda and Saroj Kumar Debnath
Department of Ayurveda Research, Ayurveda Regional Research Institute - A unit of CCRAS, Department of AYUSH, Government of India, Gangtok, Sikkim, India

Gláucia Tamburu Braghetto, Jéssica Oliveira Pigari and Maria José Bistafa Pereira
Ribeirão Preto College of Nursing (EERP/USP), University of São Paulo, Ribeirão Preto, Brazil

Leandra Andréia de Sousa
Ribeirão Preto College of Nursing (EERP/USP), University of São Paulo, Ribeirão Preto, Brazil
Avenida dos Bandeirantes, Campus Universitário, Monte Alegre, Ribeirão Preto, SP, Brazil

Anup Sharma
Indian Institute of Technology, Kharagpur, India

Bulbul Purkait
Department of Biochemistry, Midnapur Medical College and Hospital, Midnapore, India

Hijikata Y
Toyodo Hijikata Clinic, 567-0031 Kasuga 3-11-29 Ibaraki, Osaka, Japan

Varsha J. Galani and Rital R. Panchal
M.Pharm (Pharmacology), A. R. College of Pharmacy & G. H. Patel Institute of Pharmacy, Gujarat, India

Jamal Akhtar
Lecturer, Department of Kulliyat, Hakeem Abdul Hameed Unani Medical College, Eidgah road, Dewas (MP), India

Abid Ali Ansari
Professor & Head Department of Kulliyat, HMS, Unani medical College, Sadashivnagar, Tumkur, Karnataka, India

Nazema Farhin
Department of Kulliyat, Govt. Nizamia Tibbi College, Hyderabad-(AP), India

Rasheed HMA
Professor & Head Department of Kulliyat, Govt. Nizamia Tibbi College, Hyderabad (AP), India

Mandana Bagherian, Adis Keraskian Mojembari and Mohammad Hakami
Department of Psychology, Karaj Branch, Islamic Azad University, Karaj, Iran

Jayagowri Sastry
Head, Department of Clinical Research & Development, Shrimati Kashibai Navale Medical College and General Hospital (SKNMC-GH), Pune, India

Vineeta Deshmukh
Bharatiya Sanskriti Darshan Trust's Ayurved Hospital and Research Center, Pune, India

Vijay Dhoiphode
Tilak Ayurved Mahavidyalaya, Pune, India

Asmita Wele
Bharati Vidyapeeth College of Ayurved, Pune, India

Manisha Solanki
Dhondumama Sathe Homeopathic Medical College, Pune, India

Farha Rizwan
ZVM Unani Medical College, Azam Campus, Pune, India

Amita Gupta
Johns Hopkins School of Medicine, USA

Anita Shankar
Johns Hopkins School of Public Health, USA

Rachuonyo HO
Department of Microbiology, Kenyatta University, Kenya

Ogola PE, Arika WM and Nyamai DW
Department of Biochemistry and Biotechnology, Kenyatta University, Kenya

Wambani JR
Department of Medical Laboratory Sciences, Kenyatta University, Kenya

Perera BPR
Gampaha Wickramarachchi Ayurveda Institute, University of Kelaniya, Sri Lanka

Kumaradharmasena LSP and Kamal S
Department of Shalya Shalakya, Institute of Indigenous Medicine, University of Colombo, Rajagiriya, Sri Lanka

Fernando PIPK and Arawwawala LDAM
Industrial Technology Institute, Bauddhaloka Mawatha, Colombo 07, Sri Lanka

Peiris KPP
Gampaha Wickramarachchi Ayurveda Institute, University of Kelaniya, Sri Lanka

Abe N'doumy Noël
Anthropologist, Research-Teacher, Université Alassane Ouattara, Côte d'Ivoire

Shettar RV
Assistant Professor, P. G. Department of Kayachikitsa, D. G. M. A. M. C. & H, Gadag, India

Bhavya BK
P. G. Scholar, II year Kayachikitsa, D. G. M. A. M. C. & H, Gadag, India

Malik Itrat and Saba Khan
Department of Preventive and Social Medicine, National Institute of Unani Medicine, Bangalore, Karnataka, India

Karthikeyan M
Research Scholar, Department of Pharmacy and Medical Sciences, Singhania University, Rajsathan, India

Balasubramanian T
Associate Professor, Department of Pharmacology, Alshifa College of Pharmacy, Kerala, India

Avinash Shankar
National Institute of Health & Research, Bihar, India

Amresh Shankar and Anuradha Shankar
Centre for Indigenous Medicine & Research, Bihar, India

Zhu P, Zhang M, Yang M, Ying Guo and Sun Y
The 2nd affiliated hospital of Heilongjiang TCM University, China

Puji D
TCM hospital of Daqing City, China

Ao P
The expriment center test cabinet of heilongjiang TCM University, China

Ipseeta Ray Mohanty
Department of Pharmacology, MGM Medical College, Navi Mumbai, India

Suresh Kumar Gupta
Department of Clinical Research and Pharmacology, Delhi Institute of Pharmaceutical Sciences & Research, New Delhi, India

Nimain Mohanty and Yeshwant Deshmukh
Department of Pediatrics, MGM Medical College, Navi Mumbai, India

Dharmavir Singh Arya
Department of Pharmacology, AIIMS, New Delhi, India

Jupitara Deka and J C Kalita
Department of Zoology, Gauhati University, Guwahati-781014, Assam, India

Priya R, ArunaV, Amruthavalli GV and Gayathri R
Dr.JRK's Siddha Research and Pharmaceuticals PVT Ltd, 18, 19, Perumal koil Street, Kundrathur, Chennai-600069, India

Peiyi Chen
Professor, College of Nursing, Guangzhou University of Traditional Chinese Medicine, Guangzhou, China

Yan He
Lecture, Guangzhou Medical University, Guangzhou, China

Ziyu Zhao, Jiapeng Zhang and Jingyun Ye
Master student, College of Nursing, Guangzhou University of Traditional Chinese Medicine, Guangzhou, China

Bedaso Kebede
Veterinary Drug and Animal Feed Administration and Control Authority, Ministry of Livestock and Fisheries, Addis Ababa, Ethiopia

Tsegaye Negese
Hirna Regional Veterinary Laboratory Center, Hirna, Oromia region, Ethiopia

Praveen Hoogar and Ashwini Pujar
Department of Studies in Anthropology, Karnatak University Dharwad, Karnataka State, India

Basavanagouda TT
Karnataka State Tribal Research Institute, Mysore, Karnataka State, India

Abdelmalek SMA, Alkhawaja B and Darwish DA
Department of Pharmacology and Biomedical Sciences, University of Petra, Amman, Jordan

Umakanta Prusty
Regional Research Institute (H), Guwahati, Assam, India

Balkrishna A and Misra LN
Patanjali Research Foundation, Haridwar-249405, Uttarakhand, India

Felix Shih-Hsiang Hsiao
Department of Animal Science and Biotechnology, Tunghai University, Taichung 40704, Taiwan

Yu-Hsiang Yu, Ching-Han Huang, Yi-Lin Chen and Yeong-Hsiang Cheng
Department of Biotechnology and Animal Science, National I-Lan University, Yilan City, Yilan County, Taiwan

Pramod Shah
Department of Biomedical Science and Engineering, National Central University, Taoyuan City 32001, Taiwan

Witold Stanisław Proskura and Andrzej Dybus
Laboratory of Molecular Cytogenetics, West Pomeranian University of Technology, 71-466 Szcz-ecin, Poland

Szilard Hamvas, Monika Havasi, Henrik Szőke, Petrovics Gabor and Gabriella Hegyi
Faculty of Health Sciences, University of Pecs, Hungary

Narinder Singh Parhar, Gloria St John, Ajaipal Singh Gill and Frank Son
Parhar Health Systems, Roseville, California, USA

Sachin A Shah
Parhar Health Systems, Roseville, California, USA
Pharmacy Practice, Thomas J long School of Pharmacy and Health Sciences, University of the Pacific, Stock-ton, California, USA

Mandolesi S
Department Cardio-vascular and Respiratory Science, "Sapienza" University, Rome, Italy

Gallucci S, Cialfi A and Di Donato R
Department of Rehabilitation, "Villa Dorotea", L'Aquila, Italy

Niglio T
Istituto Superiore di Sanità, Rome, Italy

d'Alessandro A
Faculty of Medicine, University of Foggia, 71122 Foggia FG, Italy

Mandolesi D and Stammegna I
U.R. Occupational Medicine, Sapienza University of Rome, 00185 Rome, Italy

d'Alessandro A
School of Medicine and Health Sciences, "G. d'Annunzio" University, Chieti, Italy

Index

www.ingramcontent.com/pod-product-compliance
Lightning Source LLC
Chambersburg PA
CBHW080412190526
45161CB00003B/211